INFECTIOUS DISEASES
EMERGENCY DEPARTMENT
DIAGNOSIS AND MANAGEMENT
First Edition

INFECTIOUS DISEASES
EMERGENCY DEPARTMENT
DIAGNOSIS AND
MANAGEMENT

First Edition

Editors

Ellen M. Slaven, MD
Assistant Professor of Clinical Medicine
Section of Emergency Medicine
Louisiana State University Health Sciences Center
New Orleans, Louisiana

Susan C. Stone, MD, MPH
Assistant Professor of Emergency Medicine
Keck School of Medicine of the University of Southern California
Los Angeles, California

Fred A. Lopez, MD, FACP
Associate Professor and Vice Chair
Department of Medicine
Louisiana State University Health Sciences Center
Assistant Dean for Student Affairs
Louisiana State University School of Medicine
New Orleans, Louisiana

McGraw-Hill
Medical Publishing Division

New York   Chicago   San Francisco   Lisbon
London   Madrid   Mexico City   Milan
New Delhi   San Juan   Seoul
Singapore   Sydney   Toronto

Infectious Diseases: Emergency Department Diagnosis and Management, First Edition

1234567890 DOC/DOC 09876

ISBN 13: 978-0-07-143416-4
ISBN 10: 0-07-143416-X

This book was set in Times Roman by TechBooks.
The editors were Martin J. Wonsiewicz, Christie Naglieri and Penny Linskey
The production supervisor was Sherri Souffrance.
The cover designer was Aimee Nordin.
The index was prepared by Ron Prottsman.
RR Donnelley was printer and binder.

INTERNATIONAL EDITION ISBN 13: 978-0-07-110480-7; ISBN 10: 0-07-110480-1
Copyright 2007 Exclusive rights by the McGraw-Hill Companies, Inc. for manufacture and export. This book cannot be re-exported from the county to which it is consigned by McGraw-Hill. The International Edition is not available in North America.

CIP Data is on file with the Library of Congress

We dedicate this book to the victims of Hurricane Katrina

Ellen M. Slaven, MD
Susan C. Stone, MD, MPH
Fred A. Lopez, MD, FACP

'*In memory of Miles D. McCarthy, PhD and Neil J. Slaven, Jr. And to Margaret T. Slaven and Peter M. DeBlieux, M.D.*'

Ellen M. Slaven, MD

To Val for your love and support.
To Fern for supporting my dreams.
To my father Robert and mother Beverly-you are missed daily.

Susan C. Stone, MD, MPH

To my patients (including those on our LSU Medicine service at Charity Hospital during Hurricane Katrina), the Guida family (who generously hosted my family during and after the hurricane), my parents, my grandmother, Emma, Andrew, and especially my wife, Nora, who allows me to indulge my passion for Medicine.

Fred A. Lopez, MD, FACP

Contents

AUTHORS

Juzar Ali, MD, FRCP(C), FCCP   Professor of Clinical Medicine, Louisiana State University Health Sciences Center, New Orleans, Louisiana
Chapter 11: Tuberculosis

Claudia Barthold, MD   Chief Resident, Section of Emergency Medicine, Louisiana State University Health Science Center, New Orleans, Louisiana
Chapter 10: Community-Acquired Pneumonia and Bronchitis

Diane M. Birnbaumer, MD, FACEP   Professor of Medicine, David Geffen School of Medicine at the University of California, Los Angeles; Associate Program Director, Department of Emergency Medicine, Harbor-University of California-Los Angeles Medical Center, Los Angeles, California
Chapter 39: Fever in the Returning Traveler

Liliana Candia, MDc   Research Fellow in Rheumatology, Section of Rheumatology, Department of Internal Medicine, Louisiana State University Health Sciences Center at New Orleans
Chapter 28: Septic Arthritis

Wallace A. Carter, MD   MD Director, Emergency Medicine Residency, New York Presbyterian, New York, New York; Associate Professor of Emergency Medicine in Medicine, Weill Medical College of Cornell University, New York, New York; Associate Professor of Clinical Medicine, College of Physicians & Surgeons of Columbia University, New York, New York
Chapter 32: Animal Bites and Rabies

Peter DeBlieux, MD   Clinical Professor of Medicine, Department of Medicine, Louisiana State University Health Science Center, New Orleans, Louisiana; Clinical Professor of Surgery, Tulane University, Department of Surgery, Charity Hospital Medical Center of Louisiana at New Orleans
Chapter 10: Community–Acquired Pneumonia and Bronchitis

Bennett P. deBoisblanc, MD, FACP, FCCP, FCCM   Professor of Medicine and Physiology, Department of Medicine, Section of Pulmonary/Critical Care Medicine, Louisiana State University Health Sciences Center, New Orleans, Louisiana
Chapter 9: Influenza
Chapter 12: Anaerobic Lung Abscess

Luis R. Espinoza, MD   Professor and Chief, Section of Rheumatology, Department of Internal Medicine, Louisiana State University Health Sciences Center at New Orleans
Chapter 28: Septic Arthritis

Pieter V. Esterhay, MD   Chief Resident, Emergency Medicine Residency, Tufts University Baystate Medical Center, Springfield, Massachusetts

Jorge A. Fernandez, MD   Clinical Instructor, Keck School of Medicine of the University of Southern California, Los Angeles; Attending Staff, Department of Emergency Medicine, Los Angeles County-University of Southern California Medical Center, Los Angeles, California
Chapter 13: Infective Endocarditis

Julio E. Figueroa, II, MD   Associate Professor, Department of Medicine, Section of Infectious Diseases, Louisiana State University Health Sciences Center, New Orleans, Louisiana

Jordan C. Foster, MD, MSc, FACEP   Assistant Clinical Professor of Medicine, College of Physicians and Surgeons, Columbia University, New York, New York; Site Director, Adult Emergency Department, New York-Presbyterian Hospital/Columbia University Medical Center, New York, New York
Chapter 20: Urinary Tract Infections

Jeffrey E. Frederic, MD   Department of Dermatology, Louisiana State University, Health Science Center, New Orleans, Louisiana
Chapter 23: Adverse Cutaneous Drug Eruptions

Fiona E. Gallahue, MD   Associate Residency Director, New York Methodist Hospital, Brooklyn, New York Chapter 31: Paronychias, Felons, and Tenosynovitis

John R. Godke, MD   Fellow Pulmonary/Critical Care Medicine, Department of Medicine, Section of Pulmonary/Critical Care Medicine, Louisiana State University Health Sciences Center, New Orleans, Louisiana
Chapter 9: Influenza
Chapter 12: Anaerobic Lung Abscess

Robert A. Green, MD   Assistant Professor of Clinical Medicine, College of Physicians & Surgeons, Columbia University, New York, New York; Associate Director, Emergency Medicine, New York-Presbyterian Hospital/Columbia University Medical Center, New York, New York
Chapter 32: Animal Bites and Rabies

Michelle M. Guidry, MD   Clinical Instructor of Medicine, Department of Medicine, Tulane University Health Sciences Center, New Orleans, Louisiana
Chapter 2: Pharyngitis

Michael E. Hagensee, MD, PhD   Associate Professor, Department of Medicine, Section of Infectious Diseases, Louisiana State University Health Sciences Center, New Orleans, Louisiana
Chapter 40: Immunizations

Rodrigo Hasbun, MD   Associate Professor of Medicine, Section of Infectious Diseases, Tulane University School of Medicine, New Orleans, Louisiana
Chapter 5: Meningitis

Sean Henderson, MD   Associate Professor of Emergency Medicine and Clinical Preventive Medicine, Vice-Chair - Department of Emergency Medicine, Keck School of Medicine of the University of Southern California, Los Angeles, California
Chapter 33: Tetanus

Roma Hernandez, MD   Department of Emergency Medicine, Los Angeles County and the University of Southern California Medical Center, Los Angeles, California
Chapter 33: Tetanus

Mark Holodniy, MD, FACP   Division of Infectious Diseases and Geographic Medicine, Stanford University, Stanford, California; AIDS Research Center, VA Palo Alto Health Care System, Palo Alto, California,
Chapter 8: HIV-Associated Central Nervous System Infections
Chapter 19: HIV-Associated Gastrointestinal Infections

Kathleen C. Hubbell, MD, FACEP   Director, Accident Room, Charity Hospital, New Orleans, Louisiana; Clinical Associate Professor of Medicine, Section of Emergency Medicine, Louisiana State University Health Sciences Center in New Orleans
Chapter 29: Plantar Puncture Wounds

Tonya Jagneaux, MD   Fellow, Section of Pulmonary and Critical Care Medicine, Department of Medicine, Louisiana State University Health Sciences Center, New Orleans, Louisiana
Chapter 22: Sepsis

Stephen P. Kantrow, MD Associate Professor, Section of Pulmonary and Critical Care Medicine, Department of Medicine, Louisiana State University Health Sciences Center, New Orleans, Louisiana; Section of Pulmonary and Critical Care Medicine, Department of Medicine, Ochsner Clinic Foundation, New Orleans, Louisiana
Chapter 22: Sepsis

Kerry King MD FACEP Department of Emergency Medicine, Los Angeles County and University of Southern California Medical Center, Los Angeles, California
Chapter 34: Bioterrorism: Anthrax, Smallpox, Plague, and Tularemia

Peter C. Krause, MD Clinical Assistant Professor, Department of Orthopaedic Surgery, Louisiana State University Health Sciences Center, New Orleans, Louisiana
Chapter 27: Osteomyelitis/Infected Prosthetic Devices

Fred A. Lopez, MD, FACP Associate Professor and Vice Chair, Department of Medicine, Louisiana State University Health Sciences Center; Assistant Dean for Student Affairs, Louisiana State University School of Medicine, New Orleans, Louisiana
Chapter 24: Primary Skin Infections: Impetigo, Erysipelas, Cellulitis, Necrotizing Fascititis
Chapter 25: Pyogenic Skin & Soft Tissue Infections

Elizabeth Lynch, MD, FACEP Department of Emergency Medicine, Loma Linda University, Loma Linda, California
Chapter 18: Infectious Diarrhea

Joanne T. Maffei, MD Associate Professor, Department of Medicine, Section of Infectious Diseases/HIV, Louisiana State University Health Sciences Center, New Orleans, Louisiana
Chapter 35: Occupational Exposure in Healthcare Personnel

Javier Marquez, MD Research Fellow in Rheumatology, Section of Rheumatology, Department of Internal Medicine, Louisiana State University Health Sciences Center at New Orleans
Chapter 28: Septic Arthritis

David H. Martin, MD Harry E. Dascomb Professor of Medicine and Microbiology; Chief, Section of Infectious Diseases and Director, Gulf South Sexual Transmitted Infections Tropical Microbicide Cooperative Research Center, Louisiana State University Health Sciences Center, New Orleans, Louisiana
Chapter 36: Sexually Transmitted Diseases

Jorge A. Martinez, MD, JD Clinical Professor of Medicine, Pediatrics, and Public Health, Section of Emergency Medicine, Louisiana State University; Co-Director Louisiana State University Combined Emergency Medicine/Internal Medicine Residency Program, Louisiana State University Health Sciences Center, New Orleans, Louisiana
Chapter 14: Myocarditis and Pericarditis

Maureen McCollough, MD, MPH, FACEP, FAAEM Associate Professor of Clinical Emergency Medicine and Pediatrics, University of Southern California School of Medicine; Director, Pediatric Emergency Department, Los Angeles County, University of Southern California Medical Center, Los Angeles, California
Chapter 21: Febrile Child

Lynne McCullough, MD Assistant Professor of Medicine/Emergency Medicine & Associate Residency Director, University of California, Los Angeles/Olive View-UCLA Emergency Medicine Residency Program, Los Angeles, California
Chapter 17: Peritonitis: Primary SBP & Secondary Peritonitis

Melissa A. McKay, MD Resident, Combined Emergency Medicine/Internal Medicine Residency Program, Louisiana State University Health Sciences Center, New Orleans, Louisiana
Chapter 14: Myocarditis and Pericarditis

Lisa D. Mills, MD   Assistant Professor, Section of Emergency Medicine, Louisiana State University Health Sciences Center, New Orleans, Louisiana; Director, Emergency Medicine Ultrasound, Louisiana State University Emergency Medicine Residency Program; Assistant Professor, Department of Surgery, Tulane School of Medicine New Orleans, Louisiana
Chapter 7: Epidural Abscess and Brain Abscess

Trevor J. Mills, MD, MPH   Associate Professor, Department of Medicine, Section of Emergency Medicine, Louisiana State University Health Sciences Center, New Orleans; Program Director Louisiana State University Emergency Medicine Residency Program, New Orleans, Louisiana; Associate Professor, Louisiana State University School of Public Health, New Orleans, Louisiana
Chapter 6: Acute Encephalitis

Granville Morse, MD   Resident, Louisiana State University Health Sciences Center Emergency Medicine Residency Program, New Orleans, Louisiana

Heather Murphy-Lavoie, MD   Clinical Professor of Medicine, Co-Assistant Director, Hyperbaric Medicine Fellowship, Louisiana State University Health Sciences Center, New Orleans, Louisiana
Chapter 30: Diabetic Foot Ulcers

Lee T. Nesbitt, Jr., M.D.   Henry Jolly Professor and Head of Dermatology, Department of Dermatology, Louisiana State University Health Sciences Center, New Orleans, Louisiana
Chapter 23: Adverse Cutaneous Drug Eruptions

Andrew Nevins, MD   Division of Infectious Diseases and GeographicMedicine, Stanford University, Stanford, California; AIDS Research Center, VA Palo Alto Health Care System, Palo Alto, California
Chapter 8: HIV-Associated Central Nervous SystemInfections
Chapter 19: HIV-Associated GastrointestinalInfections

Robert J. Paquette, MD   Assistant Residency Director, Department of Emergency Medicine, Keck School of Medicine, University of Southern California, Pasadena, California
Chapter 4: Odontogenic Infections, Conjunctivitis, Rhinitis, and Rhinocerebral Mucormycosis

Stephen J. Playe, MD, FACEP   Emergency Medicine Residency Program Director, Tufts University Baystate Medical Center, Springfield, Massachusetts
Chapter 37: Emerging Infections

Jeffrey C. Poole, MD   Clinical Assistant Professor of Dermatology, Louisiana State University Health Science Center, Metairie, Louisiana
Chapter 26: Viral Associated Exanthems

Keith Posley, MD   Clinical Assistant Professor of Medicine, Stanford University Hospital, Palo Alto, California
Chapter 1: Acute Rhinosinusitis

Jason M. Redd, MD   Chief Resident, Department of Emergency Medicine, University of California, Davis Medical Center, Sacramento, California
Chapter 3: Otitis

Charles V. Sanders, MD   Edgar Hull Professor & Chairman, Department of Medicine, Louisiana State University School of Medicine, New Orleans, Louisiana
Chapter 24: Primary Skin Infections: Impetigo,Erysipelas, Cellulitis, Necrotizing Fascititis

Osman R. Sayan, MD, FACEP   Assistant Clinical Professor of Medicine, College of Physicians & Surgeons, Columbia University, New York, New York; Assistant Residency Director, Emergency Medicine, New York-Presbyterian Hospital, New York, New York
Chapter 20: Urinary Tract Infections

Jan M. Shoenberger, MD   Assistant Residency Program Director, Department of Emergency Medicine, Los Angeles County-University of Southern California Medical Center; Assistant Professor, Department of Emergency Medicine, Keck School of Medicine of the University of Southern California, Los Angeles, California
Chapter 15: Hepatitis

Sunil Shroff, MD   Junior Resident, Emergency Medicine Residency, University of California, Los Angeles-Olive View Emergency Medicine, Los Angeles, California
Chapter 17: Peritonitis: Primary SBP & Secondary Peritonitis

Ellen M. Slaven, MD   Assistant Professor of Clinical Medicine, Section of Emergency Medicine, Louisiana State University Health Sciences Center, New Orleans, Louisiana
Chapter 24: Primary Skin Infections: Impetigo, Erysipelas, Cellulitis, Necrotizing Fascititis
Chapter 25: Pyogenic Skin & Soft Tissue Infections

Peter E. Sokolove, MD   Vice Chair of Education, Residency Program Director, and Associate Professor, Department of Emergency Medicine, University of California, Davis Health System, Sacramento, California
Chapter 3: Otitis

Susan C. Stone, MD, MPH   Assistant Professor of Emergency Medicine, Keck School of Medicine of the University of Southern California, Los Angeles, California

Stuart P. Swadron, MD, FRCP(C), FACEP, FAAEM   Residency Program Director, Department of Emergency Medicine, Los Angeles County-University of Southern California Medical Center, Los Angeles, California; Assistant Professor, Department of Emergency Medicine, Keck School of Medicine of the University of Southern California, Los Angeles, California
Chapter 13: Infective Endocarditis

David Talan, MD, FACEP, FIDSA   Professor of Medicine, University of California, Los Angeles, School of Medicine, Los Angeles, California; Chairman, Department of Emergency Medicine, Faculty, Division of Infectious Diseases, Olive View–University of California—Los Angeles Medical Center, Los Angeles, California
Chapter 21: Febrile Child

Cedric J. Tankson, MD   Chief Resident, Department of Orthopaedic Surgery, Louisiana State University Health Sciences Center, New Orleans, Louisiana
Chapter 27: Osteomyelitis/Infected Prosthetic Devices

David E. Taylor, MD   Section of Pulmonary and Critical Care Medicine, Department of Medicine, Louisiana State University Health Sciences Center, New Orleans, Louisiana; Section of Pulmonary and Critical Care Medicine, Department of Medicine, Ochsner Clinic Foundation, New Orleans, Louisiana
Chapter 22: Sepsis
Chapter 36: Sexually Transmitted Diseases

Stephanie N. Taylor, MD   Associate Professor of Internal Medicine and Microbiology, Section of Infectious Diseases, Louisiana State University Health Sciences Center, New Orleans, Louisiana; Medical Director, Delgado Sexual Transmitted Disease Clinic and Training Center, New Orleans, Louisiana

Tamara L. Thomas, MD, FACEP   Associate Professor, Department of Emergency Medicine, Loma Linda University, Loma Linda, California
Chapter 18: Infectious Diarrhea

Rafael E. Torres, MD   Chief Resident, Department of Emergency Medicine, New York Methodist Hospital, Brooklyn, New York
Chapter 31: Paronychias, Felons, and Tenosynovitis

Robert L. Trowbridge, MD   Department of Medicine, Maine Hospitalist Service, Maine Medical Center, Portland Maine; Assistant Professor of Medicine, University of Vermont College of Medicine, Burlington, Vermont
Chapter 16: Hepatobiliary Infections

Keith Van Meter, MD   Clinical Professor of Medicine, Department of Medicine, Louisiana State University Health Sciences Center, New Orleans, Louisiana; Chief, Section of Emergency Medicine Medical Center of Louisiana, New Orleans, Louisiana
Chapter 30: Diabetic Foot Ulcers

Jeff Wiese, MD   Associate Professor of Medicine, Department of Medicine, Tulane University Health Sciences Center, New Orleans, Louisiana
Chapter 2: Pharyngitis

Ronald D. Wilcox, MD   Assistant Professor of Internal Medicine and Pediatrics, Section of Infectious Diseases, Louisiana State University Health Sciences Center, New Orleans, Louisiana; Medical Director, Delta Region AIDS Education & Training Center, New Orleans, Louisiana
Chapter 41: HIV in the Emergency Department

PREFACE

THE FIELD of infectious disease is vast, complex and rapidly expanding. New advances in diagnostic testing (eg. polymerase chain reaction (PCR) technology), the development of new antimicrobial therapies (eg. antiretroviral medications), and even the emergence of novel infectious diseases (eg. severe acute respiratory syndrome (SARS)) requires diligent study by medical practitioners to remain current. This requires great effort for the practitioner of emergency medicine who must maintain up to date medical knowledge in many fields simultaneously.

The editors feel there is a need for a reliable and practical text for those who treat patients with infectious disease in the emergency department: A text that contains comprehensive reviews of common infectious diseases, in addition to practical guidelines on how to treat them. This text is intended to do just that.

Although there are texts available with guidelines for the treatment of infectious diseases "Infectious Diseases: Emergency Department Diagnosis and Management" will provide the emergency medicine physician with a practical and easy to use reference that can be utilized "on the job."

Prominent features of this text include demonstrative case presentations for each chapter. Each chapter also outlines "High Yield Facts" for quick and efficient reference. The chapters are current, brief, and easy to read. Numerous clearly written tables are included throughout the text. Precise recommendations are provided with antimicrobial dosing for both adults and pediatric patients. All of the chapters/recommendations are "evidence based" whenever possible, and when evidence is sparse, or lacking altogether, it is clearly stated. Infectious disease emergencies, such as bacterial meningitis, spinal epidural abscesses, and necrotizing soft tissue infections are included, with emphasis on the need for both medical and surgical intervention.

The intended audience of this text includes house staff and medical students who will find concise plans to aid in recognition, diagnosis and management of the most commonly encountered infectious diseases presenting to emergency departments in North America. Emergency physicians, and other health care practioners, will find this text useful as a quick reference guide as well as a source for more in depth review of many infectious diseases.

Ellen M. Slaven, MD
Susan C. Stone, MD
Fred A. Lopez, MD

1

Acute Rhinosinusitis

Keith Posley

HIGH YIELD FACTS

1. The vast majority of cases of acute infectious rhinosinusitis are nonbacterial and antibiotics do not affect their clinical course.

2. There are no clinical signs or symptoms, physical exam findings, laboratory markers, or radiographic signs that reliably distinguish bacterial from other causes of acute rhinosinusitis.

3. Most cases of acute rhinosinusitis, whether of bacterial or other causes, resolve on their own without specific therapy. Patients with bacterial sinusitis and mild symptoms usually improve without antibiotics.

4. Antibiotics shorten the duration of illness in patients with acute bacterial rhinosinusitis. Patients with symptoms of acute rhinosinusitis are most likely to benefit from antibiotics if their illness has persisted greater than 7 days.

5. If the decision is made to treat acute infectious rhinosinusitis with antibiotics, evidence shows that narrow spectrum antibiotics (i.e., amoxicillin, trimethoprim/sulfamethoxazole) are as effective as broad-spectrum agents for most patients.

CASE PRESENTATION

A 35-year-old woman presents with 3 days of bifrontal headache, myalgias, sore throat, and nasal discharge. Over the past 24 hours the color of the discharge has changed from clear to yellow. She has no major medical problems, but does report seasonal allergies. Her only medication is occasional over the counter loratidine. She does not smoke or drink, and is married with a 1-year-old child who is in day care and just getting over a cold.

On exam she appears well but tired. She is afebrile, speaks with a "nasal" voice, is tender over the right maxillary sinus, and purulent yellow discharge is visible in the right nares. Oropharyngeal exam is notable for some mild cobblestoning of the posterior pharynx. There is no cervical lymphadenopathy detected.

INTRODUCTION

Nonspecific upper respiratory infection, including acute sinusitis, is the third most common diagnosis in adult ambulatory care. Sinusitis itself is among the 10 most common ambulatory diagnoses. In 2001, as many as 28 million office visits resulted in the primary diagnosis of acute sinusitis (1), and in 1996 an estimated 1.7 million patients were treated in emergency rooms for this common condition (2). Overall, sinusitis is the fifth most common diagnosis for which antibiotics are prescribed; in 1992 this resulted in over $200 million being spent on prescriptions for acute rhinosinusitis. Another $2 billion is spent annually on nonprescription remedies (3). Nonspecific acute upper respiratory tract infections, including sinusitis, are the most commonly reported illnesses resulting in missed days of work. The direct medical costs of treating sinusitis, along with the indirect costs of lost productivity, make the overall cost of care for sinusitis staggering. The high prevalence of sinusitis and its associated cost underscores the need for optimizing effective therapy.

DEFINITION, PATHOPHYSIOLOGY, AND MICROBIOLOGY

Most clinicians consider acute sinusitis a bacterial infection. In a prospective observational study, 98% of 176 consecutive ambulatory patients given the diagnosis of sinusitis received antibiotics (4). In the United States, over half of the patients given antibiotics for acute sinusitis are prescribed broad-spectrum agents (5). Over the past decade, however, it has become increasingly apparent that a number of nonbacterial processes, both infectious and noninfectious, can cause symptoms and radiographic changes that previously were considered diagnostic for bacterial sinusitis. For example, 87% of patients with experimentally induced rhinovirus infection had evidence of sinus involvement on computed tomography (6), and 57% of patients with naturally occurring common colds had abnormal sinus radiographs (7). Patients with allergic rhinitis frequently have abnormalities on sinus radiography, and finally patients without symptoms may have abnormal sinus x-rays (8).

In their 1997 position paper, the American Academy of Otolaryngology-Head and Neck Surgery, recognizing that sinusitis is often preceded by rhinitis and rarely occurs without concurrent rhinitis, recast sinusitis as *rhinosinusitis* (9). The group further characterized rhinosinusitis into subgroups based on duration of symptoms. Acute

Table 1–1. Causes of Rhinosinusitis

Host factors
    Allergic rhinitis
    Anatomic abnormalities
    Immunocompromised state
    Neoplasm/mass lesion
    Genetic/congenital
        Cystic fibrosis
        Immotile cilia syndrome
External factors
    Infectious
        Viral
    Bacterial
    Fungal
Toxins
    Tobacco smoke
    Occupational/environmental exposure

rhinosinusitis is defined as having sudden onset and to be of less than 4 weeks duration, while chronic rhinosinusitis by definition lasts greater than 12 weeks. As discussed later, given the myriad conditions that may cause rhinosinusitis, consensus opinion is that the duration of illness should form the basis of most clinical decision making for patients with the various forms of rhinosinusitis.

Pathologically, rhinosinusitis is best described as an inflammatory process that may involve the mucous membranes of the nasal cavity and paranasal sinuses, fluid within these cavities, and possibly the underlying bone (10). A broad range of conditions, ranging from environmental exposures to host factors to infection, can give rise to these changes (Table 1–1). While there may be histological differences among these various causes, the clinical presentation of these disparate conditions may be indistinguishable. Often, more than one process is involved in the patient presenting with acute symptoms.

Typically, acute *bacterial* rhinosinusitis is a secondary infection resulting from sinus ostia obstruction or impairment of mucus clearance mechanisms caused by an acute viral upper respiratory tract infection (11). Allergic rhinitis, nasal polyposis, and anatomic abnormalities (i.e., deviated septum) are other common predisposing conditions.

The microbiology of bacterial rhinosinusitis is complex and depends to a large extent on the chronicity of symptoms. Gwaltney et al. (12) reported the results of maxillary sinusitis aspiration from 383 patients with acute community acquired sinusitis over a 15-year period. Bacteria were recovered from 59% of these aspirates; the most common pathogens were S*treptococcus pneumoniae* (41%) and *Haemophilus influenzae* (35%). Anaerobic pathogens were isolated from 7% of aspirates, usually in association with dental abscesses. Other less common pathogens included *Moraxella catarrhalis*, *Staphylococcus aureus*, and various streptococcal species. Patients with symptoms of longer duration (greater than 12 weeks) are more likely to have mixed infections that may include gram-negative organisms. Of note, much of the data on the bacteriology of acute sinusitis precede the introduction of the conjugated *H. influenza* serotype b (*Hib*) vaccine; currently and in the future, *H. influenzae* may play a less important role in acute bacterial sinusitis.

Less commonly, fungal pathogens may cause rhinosinusitis. Fungi may be present as benign colonizers, may cause a noninvasive hypersensitivity reaction resulting in chronic rhinosinusitis, or in immunocompromised hosts (i.e., organ transplantation, hematalogic malignancies, neutropenia, advanced HIV disease, and diabetes) may present as invasive fungal sinusitis. From the perspective of the Emergency Medicine physician, it is important to maintain a high suspicion for invasive fungal infection in high-risk immunocompromised patients with sinus symptoms, as these conditions can progress rapidly and cause significant local and even fatal complications.

CLINICAL PRESENTATION

The symptoms of acute rhinosinusitis are familiar to the Emergency Medicine physician. They may include (but not be limited to) facial pressure/pain, nasal obstruction, hyposmia, nasal discharge, postnasal drip, sneezing, headache, sinus tenderness, maxillary toothache, and fever. By definition, these symptoms should have been of relatively sudden onset and of less than 4 weeks duration to be considered acute.

Complications of acute bacterial sinusitis, while less common in the antibiotic era, may be severe and should be recognizable to the Emergency Medicine physician. Orbital infection, most commonly associated with ethmoid sinusitis, results from direct extension of infection through the *lamina papyracea* ("paper thin bone"), which forms both the lateral margin of the ethmoid sinus and the medial border of the orbit. Orbital cellulitis typically presents as erythema and edema of the eyelids; the patient is usually febrile and acutely ill. Rapidly progressive ptosis, proptosis, and diminished extraocular movements herald the progression to subperiosteal or orbital abscess, which generally require surgical intervention.

Retrograde extension via venous channels from the sinuses or the orbit may lead to cavernous sinus or cortical vein septic thrombophlebitis. Patients with cavernous sinus thrombosis typically are febrile and toxic-appearing. These patients can be distinguished from uncomplicated orbital cellulitis by the presence of 3rd, 4th, and 6th cranial nerve palsies, fixed and dilated pupils, papilledema on funduscopic exam, obtundation, and diminished vision. Involvement of the optic nerve may lead to permanent vision loss. Further extension of the infection can lead to a variety of intracranial complications ranging from meningitis to subdural empyema to brain abscess. Frontal sinusitis can lead to osteomyelitis of the frontal bones. These patients present with headache, fever, and doughy edema over the involved bone, referred to as "Pott's puffy tumor."

DIAGNOSIS

While a small minority of patients presenting with acute rhinosinusitis have severe, potentially life-threatening symptoms, the primary question for clinicians caring for patients with acute sinus symptoms is: *Might this patient benefit from antibiotics?* This decision depends on the answer to two other questions:

1. *Does this patient have acute rhinosinusitis?*

2. *If so, is it a bacterial process?*

Since only patients with acute *bacterial* rhinosinusitis stand to benefit from antibiotic therapy, the challenge for clinicians is to accurately identify those patients with acute bacterial infection among the larger group of patients whose acute symptoms are due to either viral or noninfectious causes (Fig. 1–1).

The literature on the utility of the various signs, symptoms, and diagnostic tests for establishing the presence of acute bacterial sinusitis is severely limited by the lack of consistent application of a valid reference standard. There is universal agreement that the "gold standard" for diagnosing bacterial sinusitis is sinus puncture, aspiration, and culture of the aspirated fluid (9). Unfortunately, this procedure is technically difficult, potentially uncomfortable for the patient, and expensive. As a result, much of the research in this area has utilized surrogate reference stan-

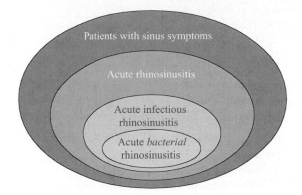

Fig. 1–1. The large majority of patients with sinus symptoms have noninfectious rhinosinusitis.

dards, which make the results of these studies difficult to interpret.

Clinical Exam

Williams et al. (13) prospectively evaluated 247 adult men presenting to a general medical clinic with symptoms of sinusitis or self-suspected sinusitis. They recorded the presence or absence of 16 historical items and 5 physical exam items on a standardized form, and compared these to the results of four-view sinus radiography, which served as the reference standard for this study. Five factors proved to be independent predictors of positive radiographs (Table 1–2). None of these factors, when taken alone, had adequate discriminatory ability; each factor was either not sensitive enough to rule out sinusitis or not specific enough to rule it in. When taken together, however, these individual factors were far more predictive; if none, three, or all five of the factors were present, 9%, 63%, and 92%, respectively, of patients had positive sinus radiographs (Table 1–3). Of note, the clinician's overall "gestalt" (low, intermediate, or high probability of sinus disease) was of similar accuracy as the formal prediction score. The limitation of these data, as stated earlier, is the application of a reference standard that may grossly overestimate the prevalence of bacterial sinusitis (misclassification bias).

No study has prospectively compared symptoms and signs in patients presenting with nasal symptoms to the true gold standard of sinus aspiration and culture, but a study by Hansen and colleagues does merit special attention (14). These investigators studied 174 consecutive

Table 1–2. Physical Exam for Acute Rhinosinusitis

Predictive Characteristic	LR (+)	LR (−)	Sensitivity (%)	Specificity (%)
Maxillary toothache	2.5	0.9	18	93
No improvement with decongestants	2.1	0.7	80	28
History of colored nasal discharge	1.5	0.5	75	52
Abnormal transillumination	1.6	0.05	73	54
Purulent secretion on examination	2.1	0.7	51	76

LR + = likelihood ratio for a positive result.
LR − = likelihood ratio for a negative result.
Source: Modified with permission from (13).

adults suspected of having acute maxillary sinusitis. After a standardized clinical evaluation, each patient had a sinus CT scan, and if any radiographic sign of sinus disease was present the patient underwent sinus puncture and aspiration. The patient was given the diagnosis of acute bacterial sinusitis if the sinus aspirate contained purulent or mucopurulent material. 70% of the patients eventually underwent sinus aspiration, and 53% of the total cohort was given the diagnosis of acute maxillary sinusitis. None of the clinical signs or features collected at presentation independently predicted the presence or absence of purulent sinus aspirate, leading the authors to conclude that, for the diagnosis of acute bacterial maxillary sinusitis, "the clinical exam is more or less worthless."

Taken together, the above two studies are tremendously helpful in understanding the usefulness of the clinical

Table 1–3. Predicted Probability of Radiographic Sinusitis

Number of Predictors	Probability of Radiographic Sinusitis (%)
0	9
1	21
2	40
3	63
4	81
5	92

Predictors of sinusitis are maxillary toothache, history of colored nasal discharge, poor response to nasal decongestants, abnormal transillumination, and purulent secretions on examination.
Source: Modified with permission from (13).

exam. Williams clearly showed that the clinical exam does, in some cases, "rule in" or "rule out" acute rhinosinusitis. Hansen's study shows that, unfortunately, it is not possible to determine if patients with acute rhinosinusitis have bacterial infections. Therefore, based on clinical exam alone, one cannot reliably determine if the patient stands to benefit from antibiotics.

Diagnostic Imaging

Several investigators have studied the value of sinus radiography in evaluating patients for acute bacterial sinusitis, and two recent meta-analyses have been published on this topic (15, 16). In their meta-analysis, Engels et al. (16) demonstrated that the performance of sinus radiography depended in large part on the definition of a positive study. Combining the results from six studies that used sinus puncture as the gold standard, the estimated sensitivity and specificity of radiography using the presence of "opacity or fluid" as the definition of positive were 73% and 80%, respectively. Defining a positive radiograph as "sinus fluid or opacity or mucous membrane thickening" changed the estimate of sensitivity to 90%, but decreased the specificity to 61%. If positive radiographs were defined simply as "opacity," the specificity was high at 85%, but the sensitivity dropped to 41%.

No study to date has compared the performance of cross-sectional imaging, such as computed tomography or MRI, to the gold standard of sinus puncture for the diagnosis of acute bacterial rhinosinusitis. Burke et al. (17) compared sinus radiography to sinus computed tomography in patients with acute sinus symptoms and found that CT is more sensitive for the presence of sinus disease than is radiography. The increased sensitivity came at the cost of lower specificity than plain radiography, thus limiting the ability of CT alone to rule in acute bacterial sinusitis.

Summary

When applied appropriately, clinical evaluation and radiographic studies are sensitive for the presence of sinus disease, but their low specificity limits their ability to distinguish bacterial from nonbacterial processes. A strategy of treating every patient with a clinical or radiographic diagnosis of acute sinusitis with antibiotics results in few missed cases of bacterial sinusitis, but will clearly result in a prescription for antibiotics for a large number of patients with nonbacterial illnesses who will not benefit.

MANAGEMENT

Treatment options for patients with acute rhinosinusitis include antibiotics, topical and systemic decongestants, nasal corticosteroids, and analgesics such as nonsteroidal anti-inflammatory drugs or acetaminophen. To help guide clinical decision making, one must keep in mind that the prognosis for patients with acute rhinosinusitis is quite good regardless of treatment. In a systematic review for the Agency for Health Care Policy and Research, de Ferranti et al. (18) pooled the results of every placebo-controlled trial of antibiotics for acute sinusitis and found that two-thirds of the patients in the placebo groups were cured or improving at the conclusion of the trials. Entry into all of these trials was based on clinical or radiographic criteria; thus it can be assumed that many of these patients had nonbacterial rhinosinusitis. It can be concluded that a large proportion of patients with the clinical diagnosis of acute rhinosinusitis will improve regardless of how they are treated.

Symptom Management

The symptoms of acute rhinosinusitis may cause significant discomfort for the patient and cost to society in the form of missed days of work. Regardless of the decision to prescribe antibiotics, patients should be offered symptomatic treatment. These treatments should be directed at drainage of the nasal passages and sinuses and the relief of sneezing, coughing, and systemic complaints (10).

As a rule, oral decongestants are preferred over nasal preparations to avoid the risk of rebound vasodilatation and pharyngeal irritation that may accompany nasal decongestants (10). There is evidence that clemastine, a first generation antihistamine, reduces sneezing and rhinorrhea in patients with acute rhinosinusitis, albeit with a significant incidence of sedation (19). Loratadine produced a similar benefit without significant sedation (20).

Anti-inflammatory therapy may also be helpful. In patients with experimental acute rhinovirus infections, naproxen was shown to reduce headache, malaise, myalgia, and cough (21). Similarly, intranasal fluticasone reduced the severity and duration of acute sinus symptoms in patients who were also treated with cefuroxime for presumed bacterial sinusitis (22).

Antibiotics

Many randomized studies have been published looking at the effectiveness of antibiotics for acute rhinosinusitis. These studies vary significantly in a variety of key methodological features, including study site (primary care vs. ENT clinics), inclusion and exclusion criteria, method of outcomes assessment, and treatment algorithms. Fortunately, two large meta-analyses have provided a quantitative summary of these data. The study by de Ferranti included 2717 patients from 27 randomized-controlled studies of antibiotics for acute rhinosinusitis (18). A more recent meta-analysis from the Cochrane Collaboration utilized more liberal inclusion criteria and included 13,660 patients from 49 trials (23). Both of these studies yielded similar results.

As mentioned earlier, the patients in the placebo arms of these trials actually fared quite well; two-thirds of them were cured or improved at the conclusion of the study. In addition, there were no documented complications of bacterial sinusitis (orbital cellulitis, brain abscess, etc.) in any of the included clinical trials, underscoring the fact that these complications are rare. In comparison to placebo, treatment with antibiotics further reduced the rate of treatment failures by almost half: 31% in the placebo group failed to improve with treatment as compared to 18% in the treatment group. This corresponded to a significant risk reduction of 46%. In terms of absolute benefit, these data show that eight patients with acute rhinosinusitis need to receive antibiotics to prevent a single treatment failure. As expected, trials that included patients simply on the basis of sinusitis-like symptoms without further diagnostic inclusion had the highest rates of cure or improvement in the placebo group and tended to show a smaller effect of antibiotics. Conversely, studies with more tightly defined patient populations had lower spontaneous resolution rates and showed a clearer benefit from antibiotics.

Given the proven efficacy of antibiotics for acute rhinosinusitis, the next question is: *Which antibiotic to prescribe?* Currently the trend is to prescribe newer, broad-spectrum antibiotics for acute rhinosinusitis (5), but the existing evidence does not support this practice. Many randomized studies directly compared older antimicrobials to newer, broader spectrum agents. In both meta-analyses there was no difference in efficacy (clinical outcomes) in comparing either amoxicillin or folate inhibitors (such as trimethoprim-sulfamethoxazole) to newer, broader spectrum antibiotics. Among the newer antibiotics studied were azithromycin, clarithromycin, cefaclor, cefixime, and cefuroxime. Amoxicillin-clavulanate and the extended-spectrum fluoroquinolones, while popular for the treatment of acute rhinosinusitis, have never been directly compared to the older agents in a clinical trial. Of note is the fact that most of these studies were published in the 1980s and 1990s, at a time when the rates of antimicrobial resistance of *H. influenzae* and *S. pneumoniae* were much lower, and there were fewer immunocompromised patients in the general population. A more recent study retrospectively analyzed the outcomes of a cohort of 17,329 patients prescribed antibiotics for acute sinusitis between July 1, 1996 and June 30, 1997. This study, while methodologically limited, again concluded that prescribing newer, broader spectrum antibiotics did not improve outcomes over amoxicillin, trimethoprim-sulfamethoxazole, or erythromycin.

The benefit from treating acute rhinosinusitis must be weighed against the potential risks. While not rare, direct adverse events from antibiotics tend to be mild and non-life threatening. More importantly, the direct cost of antibiotics must be considered, as well as the potential contribution to the emergence of antimicrobial resistance in a community increasingly exposed to antimicrobial agents.

To summarize the above discussion:

1. Most patients with the clinical diagnosis of acute rhinosinusitis will improve without specific therapy, and therefore do not require antibiotics.
2. Antibiotics result in a higher overall rate of improvement or cure.
3. Available clinical evidence shows that narrow spectrum agents are as effective as newer, broader spectrum antibiotics.
4. The risks of indiscriminant antibiotic use are the direct medical costs and the increased risk of antibiotic resistance in the community.

RECOMMENDATIONS

The American College of Physicians guidelines for the management of acute rhinosinusitis have been endorsed by the Centers for Disease Control and Prevention, the American Academy of Family Physicians, and the Infectious Disease Society of America (Fig. 1–2) (24). Their primary recommendations, as supported by the above evidence, are as follows:

1. *Sinus imaging (radiography or CT) is not recommended for the diagnosis of uncomplicated acute rhinosinusitis.* It is yet to be shown that sinus imaging is superior to clinical assessment for detecting bacterial sinusitis. In the absence of any reliable clinical signs or diagnostic tests, *duration of illness is considered a useful clinical criterion, because acute bacterial sinusitis is not common in patients with less than 7 days of symptoms.*

2. *Acute bacterial rhinosinusitis does not require antibiotic treatment, especially if the symptoms are mild or moderate.* This approach capitalizes on the fact that most patients improve without antibiotics, and minimizes the real and potential risks of overuse of antibiotics. All patients should be offered symptomatic relief.

3. *Patients with severe symptoms at presentation or persistent moderate symptoms (longer than 7 days) and specific findings of acute bacterial rhinosinusitis should be treated with antibiotics.* The specific findings are discussed above, including maxillary pain or tenderness in the face or teeth or persistent purulent sinus drainage.

4. *When an antibiotic is prescribed, it should be the most narrow-spectrum agent with activity against the most likely pathogens, S. pneumoniae and H. influenzae.* Amoxicillin, trimethoprim-sulfamethoxazole, and doxycycline are considered first line agents (Table 1–4).

An important caveat to this last recommendation is that special populations generally are not considered in clinical trials. Clinicians must be aware of factors that predispose patients to antibiotic-resistant pathogens, such as contact with children in daycare centers, recent antibiotic use or hospitalization, or certain chronic medical conditions (e.g., renal dialysis). For these patients, it may be preferable to choose an antimicrobial agent with a broader spectrum of coverage. In addition, knowledge of local antimicrobial

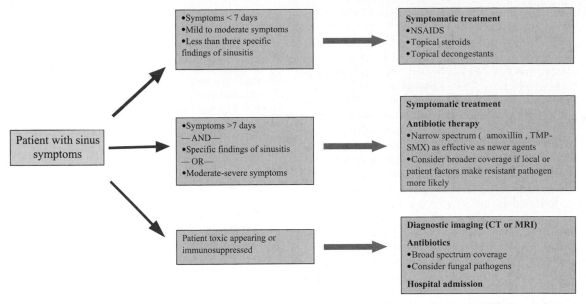

Fig. 1–2. Diagnostic and treatment algorithm for patients presenting with acute (less than 4 weeks duration) sinus symptoms.

susceptibility should contribute to the choice of antibiotic.

DISPOSITION

The vast majority of patients with acute rhinosinusitis are young and otherwise healthy and may be managed as outpatients with either symptomatic relief or antibiotics if deemed appropriate. These patients can be managed expectantly; there is no need for them to be seen in follow-up unless they are not improving after 7 days. Patients who are older with medical co-morbidities are also usually appropriate for outpatient management; for these patients it is important to link their care back to their primary care physician so that they may get ready follow-up if they do not improve. Again, a discrete appointment is not always necessary, but a phone call, fax, or e-mail to the primary care physician will be of tremendous help to the patient should they fail to improve and need to be seen again. While emergent complications may arise, it is generally a costly and inconvenient process for the patient to return

Table 1–4. Commonly Prescribed Antibiotics for Acute Rhinosinusitis[a]

Preferred Agents	Optional Agents[b]
Amoxicillin 500 mg TID	Amoxicillin/Clavulanic acid 500 mg TID or 750 mg BID
Trimethoprim (160 mg)-Sulfamethaxozole (800 mg) one tablet BID	Levofloxacin 250–500 mg q day
Doxycycline 100 mg BID	Azithromycin 500 mg loading dose then 250 mg q day (5-day course)

Consider other agents for patients who are immunosuppressed, severely ill, or have already been treated with antibiotics.

[a]Duration of treatment generally 7–10 days with exception of azithromycin.

[b]There are many other options available; these are listed as examples.

to the emergency department for follow-up of refractory sinus symptoms.

Patients who are immunosuppressed should receive special attention. As alluded to earlier, these patients may present with a paucity of symptoms and still have severe invasive infections. The emergency medicine physician should maintain a low threshold for administering parenteral antibiotics, imaging with CT, and referring to ENT.

Patients with signs of orbital cellulitis, cranial nerve palsies, altered mental status, or other signs of complications of acute sinusitis should be managed as medical emergencies. These patients need parenteral antibiotics and emergent computed tomography of the sinuses and the head, and should see an ENT specialist before leaving the emergency department. For the most part, these cases are managed as inpatients until clear clinical improvement is evident.

CASE OUTCOME

Given the short duration of symptoms, lack of medical co-morbidities, and nontoxic appearance the patient was treated conservatively with over the counter ibuprofen and instructions to use her loratadine daily. She was given a prescription for nasal fluticasone and told to fill it if her symptoms did not improve in 24–48 hours. She missed the next day of work but improved during the day and returned to work the next day. She did not need to fill the prescription for fluticasone as her symptoms steadily improved.

REFERENCES

1. Cherry DKBC, Woodwell DA: Ambulatory Medical Care Survey: 2001 Summary. Advance data from vital and health statistics; no 337. Hyattsvlle, MD, National Center for Health Statistics. 2003.
2. McCaig LFBC: National Hospital Ambulatory Medical Care Survey: 2001 emergency department summary. Advance data from vital and health statistics; no. 335. Hyattsville, MD, National Center for Health Statistics, 2003.
3. Lau J ZD, Engels EA, Balk E, et al.: Diagnosis and treatment of acute bacterial rhinosinusitis. Evidence Report/ Technology Assessment No. 9. Rockville, MD, Agency for Health Care Policy and Research, 1999.
4. Dosh SAHJ, Arch GM, et al.: Predictors of antibiotic prescribing for nonspecific upper respiratory infections, acute bronchitis, and acute sinusitis. J Fam Pract 49(5):407–414, 2000.
5. Steinman MA, Gonzales R, Linder JA, Landefeld CS: Changing use of antibiotics in community-based outpatient practice, 1991–1999. Ann Intern Med 138(7):525–533, 2003.
6. Gwaltney JM, Phillips CD, Miller RD, Riker DK: Computed tomographic study of the common cold. N Engl J Med 330(1):25–30, 1994.
7. Puhakka T, Makela MJ, Alanen A, et al.: Sinusitis in the common cold. J Allergy Clin Immunol 102(3):403–408, 1998.
8. Patel K, Chavda SV, Violaris N, Pahor AL.: Incidental paranasal sinus inflammatory changes in a British population. J Laryngol Otol 110(7):649–651, 1996.
9. Lanza DC, Kennedy DW: Adult rhinosinusitis defined. Otolaryngol Head Neck Surg 117(3 Pt 2):S1–S7, 1997.
10. Gwaltney JM, Jr.: Acute community-acquired sinusitis. Clin Infect Dis 23(6):1209–1223; quiz 1224–1225, 1996.
11. Hickner JM, Bartlett JG, Besser RE, Gonzales R, Hoffman JR, Sande MA: Principles of appropriate antibiotic use for acute rhinosinusitis in adults: background. Ann Intern Med 134(6):498–505, 2001.
12. Gwaltney JM, Jr., Scheld WM, Sande MA, Sydnor A: The microbial etiology and antimicrobial therapy of adults with acute community-acquired sinusitis: A fifteen-year experience at the University of Virginia and review of other selected studies. J Allergy Clin Immunol. 90(3 Pt 2):457–461, 1992; discussion 462.
13. Williams JW, Jr., Simel DL, Roberts L, Samsa GP: Clinical evaluation for sinusitis. Making the diagnosis by history and physical examination. Ann Intern Med 117(9):705–710, 1992.
14. Hansen JG, Schmidt H, Rosborg J, Lund E: Predicting acute maxillary sinusitis in a general practice population. BMJ 311(6999):233–236, 1995.
15. Varonen H, Makela M, Savolainen S, Laara E, Hilden J: Comparison of ultrasound, radiography, and clinical examination in the diagnosis of acute maxillary sinusitis: A systematic review. J Clin Epidemiol 53(9):940–948, 2000.
16. Engels EA, Terrin N, Barza M, Lau J: Meta-analysis of diagnostic tests for acute sinusitis. J Clin Epidemiol 53(8):852–862, 2000.
17. Burke TF, Guertler AT, Timmons JH: Comparison of sinus x-rays with computed tomography scans in acute sinusitis. Acad Emerg Med 1(3):235–239, 1994.
18. de Ferranti SD, Ioannidis JP, Lau J, Anninger WV, Barza M: Are amoxycillin and folate inhibitors as effective as other antibiotics for acute sinusitis? A meta-analysis. BMJ 317(7159):632–637, 1998.
19. Turner RB, Sperber SJ, Sorrentino JV, et al.: Effectiveness of clemastine fumarate for treatment of rhinorrhea and sneezing associated with the common cold. Clin Infect Dis 25(4):824–830, 1997.
20. Braun JJ, Alabert JP, Michel FB, et al.: Adjunct effect of loratadine in the treatment of acute sinusitis in patients with allergic rhinitis. Allergy 52(6):650–655, 1997.
21. Sperber SJ, Hendley JO, Hayden FG, Riker DK, Sorrentino JV, Gwaltney JM, Jr.: Effects of naproxen on experimental rhinovirus colds. A randomized, double-blind, controlled trial. Ann Intern Med 117(1):37–41, 1992.
22. Dolor RJ, Witsell DL, Hellkamp AS, Williams JW, Jr., Califf

RM, Simel DL: Comparison of cefuroxime with or without intranasal fluticasone for the treatment of rhinosinusitis. The CAFFS Trial: A randomized controlled trial. *JAMA* 286(24):3097–3105, 2001.

23. Williams JW, Jr., Aguilar C, Cornell J, et al.: Antibiotics for acute maxillary sinusitis. *Cochrane Database Syst Rev* (2): CD000243, 2003.

24. Snow V, Mottur-Pilson C, Hickner JM: Principles of appropriate antibiotic use for acute sinusitis in adults. *Ann Intern Med* 134(6):495–497, 2001.

2

Pharyngitis

Jeff Wiese
Michelle Guidry

HIGH YIELD FACTS

1. Patients with one or zero Centor criteria (Table 2–1) should neither be tested nor treated.

2. Patients with two Centor criteria should be tested with a rapid streptococcal throat swab test.

3. Patients who meet three or more of the Centor criteria should be treated empirically for group A beta-hemolytic streptococcus without testing.

4. Penicillin V is the recommended treatment for those suspected of having group A beta-hemolytic streptococcal pharyngitis.

5. The primary intention for administration of antibiotics is to prevent rheumatic heart disease; antibiotics reduce length of symptoms by 2 days.

6. Almost all patients with infectious mononucleosis present with a skin rash if administered amoxicillin.

CASE PRESENTATION

A 21-year-old man presents with a sore throat. He reports subjective fevers and swelling of the anterior cervical lymph nodes. He has no cough or sinus congestion. He has no significant past medical history. He takes no medications and has no medication allergies.

His blood pressure is 130/70, his pulse is 100, his respiratory rate is 16, and his temperature is 101° F. Further physical examination reveals an erythematous pharynx with enlarged tonsils covered with white exudates. His anterior cervical lymph nodes are enlarged; there is no additional lymphadenopathy or skin rash. The liver and

Table 2–1. The Centor Criteria for GABHS Strep Throat

1. Fever (subjective or measured)
2. Anterior cervical lymphadenopathy
3. Enlarged tonsils with white exudates
4. Absence of cough

spleen are not enlarged. The pulmonary and cardiac examinations are normal.

INTRODUCTION/EPIDEMIOLOGY

Pharyngitis accounts for 10% of ambulatory care visits and 50% of all outpatient antibiotics (1). Most pharyngitis is due to viral infections, for which supportive care is the indicated treatment (2). Preventing complications (i.e., rheumatic heart disease) from group A beta-hemolytic streptococcal infection (GABHS: Strep throat) is what drives antibiotic use in the management of pharyngitis (3). When antibiotics should be used is controversial: most patients do not require antibiotics, and the primary rationale for antibiotic use is not only to reduce duration of symptoms, but also to prevent secondary complications including rheumatic heart disease and peritonsilar abscesses (4, 5).

There are three goals in evaluating pharyngitis:

1. Decide who should receive antibiotics for suspected GABHS,

2. Ensure other rarer diseases (fungal, diphtheria, gonorrhea) are not present, and

3. Ensure complications of bacterial infection (peritonsilar abscess) are not present.

Historically, throat cultures and the rapid strep assay (latex agglutination antigen tests or ELISA tests) have been used to decide which patients should receive antibiotic therapy. Recent evidence suggests, however, that examination and historical data may be useful in determining which patients should receive testing and which patients may warrant antibiotic therapy without testing (i.e., Centor criteria) (6).

PATHOPHYSIOLOGY/MICROBIOLOGY

Most pharyngitis is due to viral infection from rhinovirus, coronavirus, or adenovirus (3). These viruses favor the back of the throat because it is cool and has less IgA relative to the remainder of the oropharynx. Other important viral infections include Epstein-Barr (EBV) and cytomegalovirus (CMV) mononucleosis, and acute seroconversion to HIV.

Bacterial pharyngitis is primarily due to GABHS, but more rarely is due to *Corynebacterium diphtheriae (diphtheria)*, *Corynebacterium haemolyticum*, *Mycoplasma pneumoniae*, anaerobic streptococci, and *Neisseria gonorrhea* (4).

Fungal pharyngitis is rare and due primarily to oral candidiasis whose presence will be observed in the remainder of the oropharynx.

Noninfectious causes of pharyngitis include postnasal drip, gastric reflux, chronic cough, thyroiditis, and bulimia.

CLINICAL PRESENTATION

Viral Pharyngitis

Historical information is important in identifying viral infections. The presence of rhinorrhea, sinus congestion, conjunctivitis, diarrhea, and cough suggests a rhinovirus or adenovirus infection. Fever is common, and pharyngeal vesicles, tonsilar enlargement with exudates, and lymphadenopathy may also be present. There is no clinically useful diagnostic test; the diagnosis is confirmed by excluding other causes of pharyngitis. The presence of symptoms of other upper respiratory infection(s) is the most diagnostic, as this usually excludes bacterial pharyngitis (5).

Patients with CMV and EBV mononucleosis present with fever, significant malaise and weakness, and an erythematous pharynx with white to purple exudates extending into the nasopharynx. The age of the patient (usually young adults) and the presence of systemic lymphadenopathy (especially postcervical lymphadenopathy) and hepatosplenomegaly are suggestive. A macular skin rash may also be present; the rash will be significantly enhanced if the patient is started on ampicillin (3). Importantly, one-third of patients with mononucleosis present with a secondary bacterial pharyngitis. The lack of ulcers on the pharynx and mouth and the presence of splenomegaly help to distinguish mononucleosis from acute HIV seroconversion.

Eighty-five percent of patients with acute HIV-seroconversion will present with ulcerations in the mouth and pharynx. Fever, lymphadenopathy, and a macular skin rash may also be present, but tonsilar enlargement and exudates are rare. The pharyngitis is less severe than other viral or bacterial causes of pharyngitis. A history of HIV-associated risk factors (i.e., intravenous drug use, unprotected sex, or blood transfusions) is important in deciding who should be tested for HIV.

Bacterial Pharyngitis

Bacterial pharyngitis usually occurs during the winter and early spring months when a GABHS infection following a viral pharyngitis is common (2).

The sudden onset of throat pain, fever, and anterior cervical lymphadenopathy without upper respiratory infection symptoms (cough, rhinorrhea, or nasal congestion) is suggestive of a bacterial infection. The pharynx usually, but not always, demonstrates enlarged tonsils with white exudates. Petechial hemorrhages are occasionally observed on the soft palate. The Centor criteria for bacterial infection includes: (1) fever, (2) anterior cervical lymphadenopathy, (3) enlarged tonsils with white exudates, and (4) absence of cough (7). If three or more criteria are present, the diagnosis is presumed without cultures or rapid strep testing, and empiric therapy should be administered (5, 8).

Gonorrhea pharyngitis has a similar presentation to GABHS pharyngitis, and is suggested by a history of unprotected oral sex and a non-winter-time bacterial pharyngitis (i.e., when bacterial infection secondary to a viral pharyngitis is less common). Urethritis, urethral discharge, or joint pain and swelling are also suggestive. Lymphadenopathy is less common, though pharyngeal exudates are more pronounced.

Diphtheria is rare in an immunized population, though it is observed with greater frequency in alcoholics. A history of nonimmunization or incomplete childhood immunization (e.g., immigrant populations) and a gray pseudomembrane extending over the pharynx, nasal passages, or the tracheo-broncial tree suggest this diagnosis. It is also associated with difficulty in swallowing and shortness of breath (9).

LABORATORY/DIAGNOSTIC TESTING

Diagnostic testing is primarily reserved for excluding GABHS, as therapy for nonbacterial etiologies is supportive care only. The most effective and least expensive strategy is to culture all patients and reserve treatment only for those with a positive culture (8). Practically, however, this strategy is useful only when patient follow-up is assured (5). For this reason a current standard of care is to use the Centor criteria to decide who should receive testing (Table 2–2). An alternative strategy for testing is to test no one, treating only those patients who satisfy three or more of the Centor criteria (4, 8).

Although the rapid-strep throat swab test is more expensive than a throat culture, it is more expeditious and thus more practical in the urgent care setting (8). It is not necessary to obtain throat cultures to document bacterial sensitivities for fear of a treatment failure. Bacteria that fail to respond to antibiotics are usually tolerant to the initial regimen; a second course of the same antibiotic

Table 2–2. Diagnostic Strategy for GABHS Strep Using the Centor Criteria

Number of Criteria Present	Testing	Treatment
None	None	Do not treat
One	None	Do not treat
Two	Test	Treat if test positive
Three	Test	Treat empirically
Four	None	Treat empirically

usually results in success. The exception is in the patient suspected of having gonococcal pharyngitis, for whom a throat and urethral culture should be obtained. A positive result will change therapy (see below) and is important in notifying other patients with a potential exposure. A throat culture for corynebactorium diphtheriae should be reserved only for those patients who are not immunized or are incompletely immunized and a clinical presentation consistent with the diagnosis (see above) (9).

There is no utility in testing for viral pharyngitis, with the exception of testing for mononucleosis. The Monospot test for heterophile antibodies is helpful for diagnosis of mononucleosis due to EBV, but may miss CMV-induced mononucleosis. The primary reason for testing is to document the disease to prevent spread and to investigate an epidemiologic outbreak (i.e., a school cafeteria not sanitizing its glasses), and to avoid giving penicillin antibiotics (as might be done if streptococcal pharyngitis is suspected).

An HIV ELISA test should be ordered only if the patient has appropriate historical risk factors and a clinical presentation suggestive of HIV seroconversion.

MANAGEMENT

Viral Pharyngitis

Treatment for viral pharyngitis includes supportive care: warm liquids (soups, teas), salt-water gargling, and non-steroidal analgesics. Antibiotics are of no use and may introduce additional complications (allergic reactions, diarrhea, candidal infections). Zinc lozenges may reduce the duration of symptoms by 1 day if initiated on the first day of symptoms (10).

Treatment for mononucleosis is also supportive with special instructions to avoid saliva contact with any person for at least 10 weeks (no kissing, shared glasses, etc.). Patients should be advised to avoid any activity that may increase risk for splenic rupture.

If the diagnosis of HIV infection is confirmed by Western-blot, a viral load and CD4 count should be obtained in order to determine the need for antiretroviral therapy. This enables later evaluation of therapeutic efficacy when repeat viral load and CD4 counts are obtained.

BACTERIAL PHARYNGITIS

Penicillin is the mainstay of therapy for bacterial infection (Table 2–3). A 5-day regimen is as successful (94%) as a 10-day course. Oral therapy is as successful as intravenous or intramuscular therapy. Amoxicillin should be avoided since mononucleosis patients misdiagnosed with bacterial infection will demonstrate a significant rash in response to this therapy (4, 11).

If compliance is of concern, a single dose of intramuscular benzathine penicillin G can be instituted. A 3-day course of azithromycin (500 mg once daily) may also be used, though the cost is considerably more.

Second-generation cephalosporins (cefuroxime, 250 mg BID for 5 days) may result in greater bacteriologic eradication, but there is no evidence to suggest that it is more efficacious than penicillin in resolving symptoms or preventing complications.

Azithromycin (500 mg po on day 1, followed by 250 mg daily for 4 days) appears to be the best therapy for penicillin-allergic patients unless cost is of concern. Erythromycin (500 mg four times a day for 10 days) is a cheaper alternative, although resistance may be as great as 25% in some communities. Some second generation cephalosporins such as cefuroxime may also be used; cross-reactivity to a penicillin-allergy occurs in 8% of patients.

Failure to respond to antimicrobial therapy is usually due to inadequate duration of treatment, and not due to

Table 2–3. Antibiotics: Outpatient Treatment of Pharyngitis

Nonpenicillin allergic patient *with* good assurance of compliance:
  Penicillin V, 500 mg po BID × 5–10 days
Nonpenicillin allergic patient *without* good assurance of compliance:
  Benzathine Penicillin G, 1.2 million units IM × 1
Penicillin-allergic patient:
  Erythromycin, 500 mg po QID for 10 days
  Azithromycin, 500 mg po 1st day then 250 mg po q day × 4 days

bacterial resistance. Patients with recurrence or failure of initial therapy usually respond to continuation or re-initiation of the initial therapy (2).

Patients with confirmed gonococcal pharyngitis should receive one dose of 125 mg of intramuscular ceftriaxone and 100 mg of doxycycline twice a day for 7 days. A one-time, 1 g oral dose of azithromycin can be substituted for doxycycline if compliance is of concern. All sexual partners should also be notified and treated.

Patients with confirmed diphtheria are admitted to the hospital for observation for potential surgical removal of the pseudomembrane should respiratory function be compromised. Therapy includes diphtheria antitoxin and preferably penicillin or erythromycin.

A one-time dose of dexamethasone (10 mg IM or po) has been shown to reduce pain in patients with bacterial pharyngitis (12). Steroids should not be used unless antibiotics are also administered and should probably be reserved for those patients who have odynophagia due to tonsilar enlargement sufficient enough to limit adequate oral intake. Patients who cannot maintain oral intake may need to be hospitalized for intravenous fluid support.

Special Circumstances

Peritonsilar cellulitis and abscess

Though rare, bacterial pharyngitis may extend into the surrounding soft tissues of the pharynx, resulting in a peritonsilar cellulitis or abscess(es). This constitutes a medical emergency, as extension into the retropharyngeal space containing the internal carotid artery may result in death.

Patients with a peritonsilar abscess typically present with extended symptoms of a bacterial pharyngitis and complain of a "muffled" voice. The abscess is rarely bilateral; uvula deviation to the opposite side and of the soft palate medially are the keys to diagnosis. This finding should prompt immediate ENT consultation for needle aspiration of the abscess for confirmation, followed by OR drainage.

In the absence of ENT support, the abscess may be drained with a 21-gauge needle inserted into the peritonsilar fold, just superior and medial to the upper pole of the tonsil. Extreme caution must be exercised in aspirating from the abscess, as the carotid artery lies directly behind the abscess. The needle must not be inserted greater than 1 cm to avoid puncturing the internal carotid artery. To prevent this complication, one should remove the plastic cap of a 19-gauge needle and cut off the distal 0.5 cm of the cap and reapply the clipped cap to the needle. The plastic cap will prevent the needle from extending more than 0.5 cm into the peritonsilar fold. One should aspirate as the needle is inserted into the peritonsilar fold. Pre- and postoperative antibiotics should be administered (see above).

Lemierre Syndrome

Lemierre syndrome (i.e., jugular vein septic thrombosis or phlebitis) is extension of a preceding *Fusobacterium necrophorum* pharyngitis into the internal jugular vein, with potential for pulmonary and systemic septic emboli. Rarely, this may also include extension to the carotid artery or the retropharyngeal space with direct extension inferiorly into the mediastinum. A history of prolonged bacterial pharyngitis, neck pain and tenderness, and co-existent pneumonia or chest pain should prompt consideration of the diagnosis. Treatment includes intravenous antibiotics (see above) targeting *F. necrophorum*. Typically, this includes high doses of intravenous penicillin or clindamycin. Surgical drainage of infected areas may also be required.

DISPOSITION

The vast majority of patients with pharyngitis may be treated as outpatients. Admission should be reserved for patients who are unable to maintain oral intake due to tonsilar enlargement, or those with complications such as peritonsilar abscesses or the Lemierre syndrome.

Patients should be told to expect persistence of symptoms for up to 10 days. The mean duration of symptoms in untreated patients with GABHS is 10 days. In those given antibiotics within the first 2 days of symptoms, the mean duration of symptoms is 8 days. Patients who fail to show improvement within 1 week or those who experience signs and symptoms of peritonsilar abscess or the Lemierre syndrome (see above) should be instructed to present to their physician immediately.

CASE OUTCOME

The patient satisfied all four of the Centor criteria. No laboratory testing was performed. He was empirically treated with penicillin. His symptoms resolved 7 days after administration of therapy.

REFERENCES

1. Armstrong GLPR Outpatient visits for infectious diseases in the United States, 1980 through 1996. *Arch Intern Med* 159: 2531–2536, 1999.
2. Bisno A, Gerber M, et al. Practice guidelines of the diagnosis and management of group A streptococcal pharyngitis. *Clin Infect Dis* 35:113–125, 2002.

3. Bisno A: Acute pharyngitis. *New Engl J Med* 344:205–211, 2001.

4. Cooper R, et al.: Principles of appropriate antibiotic use for acute pharyngitis in adults: Background. *Ann Int Med* 2001:509–517, 2001.

5. McIssac W, Kellner J, et al.: Empirical validation of guidelines for the management of pharyngitis in children and adults. *JAMA* 291:1587–1595, 2004.

6. Ebell M, Smith M, et al.: Does this patient have strep throat. *JAMA* 284:2912–2918, 2000.

7. Centor R, Witherspoon J, et al.: The diagnosis of strep throat in adults in the emergency room. *Med Decis Making* 1:239–246, 1981.

8. Neuner J, Hamel M, et al.: Diagnoses and management of adults with pharyngitis. *Ann Int Med* 139:113–122, 2003.

9. Bisgard K, Hardy I, Popovic T, et al.: Respiratory diphtheria in the United States, 1980 through 1995. *Am J Public Health* 88:787–791, 1998.

10. Marshall S: Zinc gluconate and the common cold. Review of randomized controlled trials. *Can Fam Physician* 44:1037–1042, 1998.

11. Hirshmannn J: Antibiotics for common resporatory tract infections in adults. *Arch Int Med* 162:256–264, 2002.

12. Wei J, Kasperbauer J, et al.: Efficacy of single-dose dexamethasone as adjuvant therapy for acute pharyngitis. *Laryngoscope* 112:87–93, 2002.

3

Otitis

Jason M. Redd
Peter E. Sokolove

HIGH YIELD FACTS

1. Diagnosis of acute otitis media requires a history of acute onset of signs and symptoms, the presence of middle ear effusion, and signs and symptoms of middle ear inflammation.
2. A cloudy, opacified, bulging or immobile tympanic membrane is most suggestive of acute otitis media.
3. 48–72 h of observation and symptomatic treatment without antibiotics can be considered in select patients.
4. Amoxicillin (80–90 mg/kg per day) is first line therapy for most patients with acute otitis media.

CASE PRESENTATION

A 3-year-old girl presents with left ear pain and fever for 2 days. Her father reports that she had cold symptoms about a week ago. She denies ear drainage or recent ear infection. Her ear pain has not interfered with her daily activity or sleep. She has no significant past medical history. She takes no medications and has no medication allergies.

She is well-developed, interactive, and does not appear to be in significant pain. Her vital signs are all normal, except for a temperature of 38.5°C. Her physical examination is remarkable for a bulging, immobile, erythematous left tympanic membrane. The ear canal is normal and without discharge. There is no swelling or tenderness over the mastoid region. Other than mild nasal congestion, the remainder of her physical examination is normal.

OTITIS MEDIA

Introduction/Epidemiology

Otitis media causes more physician visits than any other childhood illness and is the most common reason children are prescribed antibiotics (1). In the United States, an estimated $5 billion per year is spent on the more than 5 million annual diagnoses of otitis (2).

Acute otitis media is a middle ear effusion associated with the rapid onset of one or more signs or symptoms of inflammation of the middle ear, such as otalgia, otorrhea, fever, or irritability. Otitis media with effusion is a middle ear effusion without manifestations of an acute infection, and may occur as a result of, or in the absence of, acute otitis media (3). Hearing loss may be present in both conditions.

By the age of 3 years, most children will have had at least one episode of acute otitis media, with a peak incidence between ages 6 and 11 months. Recurrent otitis is common, with up to 20% of children experiencing three or more episodes in their first year (4). Risk factors for acute otitis media include male gender, day care attendance, parental smoking, a family history of middle ear disease, craniofacial abnormalities (e.g., cleft palate or Down syndrome), use of a pacifier, and immunosuppression (5, 6). Breast feeding decreases the incidence of acute otitis media (7).

Pathophysiology/Microbiology

While the pathogenesis of otitis media is multifactorial, dysfunction of the eustachian tube is a critical element in the disease process. In the healthy ear, the eustachian tube effectively performs three physiologic functions: pressure regulation between the middle ear and atmospheric pressure (ventilation); protection of the middle ear from nasopharyngeal pressure variations and ascending secretions or pathogens; and clearance of secretions from the middle ear into the nasopharynx (8). In most children, the inciting event leading to otitis media is a viral upper respiratory tract infection or allergy, which results in mucosal congestion and inflammation of the nose, nasopharynx, and eustachian tube. Obstruction of the eustachian tube may result, leading to negative pressures in the middle ear. Mucociliary clearance is also compromised by the inflammation, and an accumulation of fluid develops in the middle ear. Viruses and bacteria in the upper respiratory tract can be aspirated or insufflated into the middle ear, stimulating a host inflammatory response. Infants and children are at increased risk for otitis media due to their short, horizontal, floppy, narrow eustachian tubes that function relatively poorly.

While eustachian tube dysfunction is a core factor in the development of otitis media, host immune response and microbial load are also important elements. The impaired immune system is a function of age, genetic predisposition, and atopy. The relative microbial load is altered by environmental factors such as day care attendance, season of the year, and contact with siblings (9).

The most common bacterial isolates of middle ear aspirates are *Streptococcus pneumoniae*, nontypable *Haemophilus influenzae*, and *Moraxella catarrhalis*. Approximately 25% of pneumococci in the United States are penicillin resistant as a result of alterations in their penicillin binding proteins, while 20–50% of *H. influenzae* and virtually all strains of *M. catarrhalis* are beta-lactamase-positive (10). Risk factors for disease due to resistant organisms include prior exposure to antibiotics, young age, day care attendance, and prior hospitalization.

Viruses are also frequently associated with otitis media (11, 12). They may occur singly or as a coinfectant with bacteria. The most common viruses involved are respiratory syncytial virus, rhinoviruses, influenza viruses, and adenoviruses (11, 13).

Clinical Presentation

Most of the symptoms commonly associated with otitis media are nonspecific, such as fever, irritability, vomiting, diarrhea, anorexia, cough, and pulling or rubbing of the ears (14). This is especially true of children less than 2 years old, in whom it is difficult to assess ear pain. Older children may be able to report more specific symptoms such as ear pain or hearing loss. While otalgia is a positive predictor of acute otitis media, it is not universally present. Fever, however, is a poor predictor, and occurs in less than half of children with acute otitis media in most studies (14–16). Upper respiratory symptoms such as cough and rhinorrhea are present in most children with acute otitis media, as upper respiratory infection predisposes to middle ear infection.

The diagnosis of acute otitis media rests on the demonstration of a middle ear effusion in association with local or systemic signs of inflammation. Otoscopic visualization of the tympanic membrane is facilitated by pulling up and back on the ear to straighten the canal. A cloudy, opacified, bulging, or immobile tympanic membrane as found on pneumatic otoscopy is most suggestive of acute otitis media (17). Otorrhea may be seen in cases of tympanic membrane perforation. Other signs of a middle ear effusion include loss of tympanic membrane landmarks, and the presence of air-fluid levels or bubbles behind the tympanic membrane. A markedly red tympanic membrane is also suggestive of acute otitis media, while normal color is a negative predictor (17). Prominent blood vessels around the circumference or overlying landmarks of the tympanic membrane may be confused with erythema, but do not support the diagnosis of acute otitis media. Erythema, tenderness, or swelling around the ear is not expected with uncomplicated acute otitis media and is suggestive of mastoiditis.

While not available in most emergency departments, tympanometry and acoustic reflectometry are two other modalities for detecting middle ear effusion. Tympanometry measures the mobility of the tympanic membrane while exposed to a continuous sound frequency. It requires a tight seal in the ear canal and a cooperative patient. Acoustic reflectometry measures sound reflectivity from the tympanic membrane and rates the probability of middle ear effusion. It does not require a tight seal but is dependent on user technique. Both devices are available in hand-held models.

Laboratory/Diagnostic Testing

Most patients with otitis media will require no laboratory or diagnostic testing. However, cranial imaging or aspiration of middle ear fluid may be necessary in complicated cases. Indications for tympanocentesis may include patients with otitis media who are toxic or seriously ill, are unresponsive to antibiotic therapy, are neonates, are immunocompromised, are already receiving antibiotics, or have a suppurative complication (18). Patients with signs or symptoms suggestive of meningitis require cerebrospinal fluid analysis. CT scanning or MRI may be necessary to diagnose or fully define abscesses, lateral or cavernous sinus thrombosis, carotid artery thrombosis, and mastoiditis (19).

Management

Rational management of acute otitis media begins with an understanding of the natural course of untreated disease. Meta-analyses of randomized, placebo controlled trials have shown that approximately 80% of children have resolution of acute otitis media by 1 week without antibiotic treatment (20–24). There are less data on children younger than 2 years, but studies suggest a lower rate of spontaneous resolution of about 30% after several days (25, 26). The benefit of antibiotic therapy is one additional cure for every 7–8 patients treated (20). The effect of antibiotics on pain control is not evident within the first 24 h of therapy, as children managed either with or without antibiotics have about a 60% rate of symptomatic relief (27). Between 2 and 7 days, there is only a modest benefit of antibiotics compared with observation alone. Antibiotics result in one additional patient without pain for about every 15 patients treated (24). These benefits in clinical cure rate and symptomatic improvement must be weighed against the risks of antibiotics, which include allergic reactions,

Table 3–1. Recommended Criteria for Initial Antibacterial-Agent Treatment or Observation in Children with Acute Otitis Media

Age	Certain Diagnosis	Uncertain Diagnosis
<6 months	Antibacterial treatment	Antibacterial treatment
6 months–2 years	Antibacterial treatment	Antibacterial treatment if severe illness; observation option if nonsevere illness[a]
≥2 years	Antibacterial treatment if severe illness; observation option if nonsevere illness[a]	Observation option[a]

Reproduced with permission from *Pediatrics* 113: 1451–65, 2004.

[a]Observation is an appropriate option only when follow-up can be ensured and antibacterial agents started if symptoms persist or worsen. Nonsevere illness is mild otalgia and fever <39°C in the past 24 h. Severe illness is moderate to severe otalgia or fever ≥39°C. A certain diagnosis of acute otitis media meets all three criteria: (1) rapid onset, (2) signs of middle ear effusion, and (3) signs and symptoms of middle-ear inflammation.

vomiting, diarrhea, accelerated bacterial resistance, and undesirable changes in nasopharyngeal flora (9).

The American Academy of Pediatrics (AAP) and American Academy of Family Physicians (AAFP) recently developed practice guidelines for acute otitis media in otherwise healthy children 2 months through 12 years of age, based on a comprehensive review of the literature (28). Children excluded from these guidelines are those with signs or symptoms of systemic illness unrelated to the middle ear, acute otitis media within the previous 30 days, acute otitis media with underlying chronic otitis media with effusion, and those with cleft palate, craniofacial abnormalities, genetic conditions such as Down syndrome, immunodeficiencies or cochlear implants. Given the findings that most children do well without antibiotics, they recommend an "observation option" with only symptomatic treatment for selected children (Table 3–1). Antibiotics may be delayed for 48–72 h in children 6 months to 2 years of age with nonsevere illness and an uncertain diagnosis, and in children 2 years of age and older without severe symptoms, whether the diagnosis is certain or uncertain. There must be an adult able to observe the child, recognize signs of serious illness, and provide access to medical care if necessary. If there is worsening of illness or no improvement in 48–72 h, antibiotics may be started or the child may be reevaluated by a physician. A safety-net antibiotic prescription may be given at the initial visit to be filled if there is no improvement after the 48–72 h observation period (29–31) With close follow-up, there are few episodes of mastoiditis or other suppurative complications when antibiotics are initially withheld (22, 23). This strategy of watchful waiting is similar to the long-time practice in some European countries, such as the Netherlands (32).

When antibiotics are to be initiated, amoxicillin should be prescribed for most children due to its clinical effectiveness, safety, palatability, and low cost (20, 22, 28, 33). The recommended dose for all children is 80–90 mg/kg per day (28). Although lower doses of amoxicillin are effective in most cases, the higher dose yields middle ear concentrations which exceed the minimum inhibitory concentration of all intermediate resistance and many highly resistant *S. pneumoniae* strains (34–36).

While patients with acute otitis media are traditionally treated with antibiotics for 7–10 days, the optimal duration of treatment is controversial. Patients with acute otitis media often improve clinically without antibiotics, contributing to the "Pollyanna phenomenon," where patients improve regardless of the selected antibiotic or duration of treatment (37). A number of studies, mostly involving patients at least 2 years of age, have shown no difference between short course (3–5 days) and traditional course (7–10 days) treatment regimens (38). In two studies of children under age 2 years, comparing 5-day versus 10-day treatment regimens, a benefit was found for traditional duration therapy at 12–14 days after treatment, but the benefit did not persist at 4–6 weeks (38, 39). The AAP/AAFP clinical practice guideline recommends treatment for 10 days for children less than age 2 years or for older children with severe disease (28, 34). Other antibiotics used to treat acute otitis media include amoxicillin/clavulanate, cefdinir, cefpodoxime, cefuroxime, clarithromycin, erythromycin-sulfisoxazole, and sulfamethoxazole-trimethoprim. Single-dose ceftriaxone has a clinical effect comparable to that of a 7–10 day course of oral amoxicillin (22). However, ceftriaxone is more expensive and requires parenteral administration.

Whether the patient was initially managed with observation or initial antibiotics, a reevaluation must be made in 48–72 h if there is no improvement. Table 3–2 lists the AAP/AAFP recommended antibiotic regimens for initial

Table 3–2. Recommended Antibacterial Agents for Patients who Are being Treated Initially with Antibacterial Agents or Have Failed 48–72 h of Observation or Initial Management with Antibacterial Agents

Temperature ≥39°C and/or Severe Otalgia	At Diagnosis for Patients being Treated Initially with Antibacterial Agents		Clinically Defined Treatment Failure at 48–72 h After Initial Management with Observation Option		Clinically Defined Treatment Failure at 48–72 h After Initial Management with Antibacterial Agents	
	Recommended	Alternative for Penicillin Allergy	Recommended	Alternative for Penicillin Allergy	Recommended	Alternative for Penicillin Allergy
No	Amoxicillin 80–90 mg/kg per day	Nontype I: cefdinir, cefuroxime, cefpodoxime; type I; azithromycin, clarithromycin	Amoxicillin 80–90 mg/kg per day	Nontype I: cefdinir, cefuroxime, cefpodoxime; type I; azithromycin, clarithromycin	Amoxicillin-clavulanate (90 mg/kg per day of amoxicillin with 6.4 mg/kg per day of clavulanate)	Nontype I: ceftriaxone, 3 days; type I: clindamycin
Yes	Amoxicillin-clavulanate (90 mg/kg per day of amoxicillin with 6.4 mg/kg per day of clavulanate)	Ceftriaxone, 1 or 3 days	Amoxicillin-clavulanate (90 mg/kg per day of amoxicillin with 6.4 mg/kg per day of clavulanate)	Ceftriaxone, 1 or 3 days	Ceftriaxone, 3 days	Tympanocentesis, clindamycin

This table is reproduced with permission from *Am Acad Pediatr* 113:1451–65, 2004.

use, observation failure, and initial treatment failure. Children initially observed who have not improved should be started on high dose amoxicillin (80–90 mg/kg per day) if other causes of illness are excluded. For unimproved patients with either severe illness or who had initially been treated with amoxicillin, high dose amoxicillin/clavulanate (90 mg/kg per day of amoxicillin component, with 6.4 mg/kg per day of clavulanate in two divided doses) should be started (28).

All patients with pain should be treated with full-dose acetaminophen or ibuprofen irrespective of whether they receive antibiotics initially. This is most important in the first 24 h after diagnosis and especially before bedtime. Narcotic analgesics may be required for severe pain. Antihistamines and decongestants have not been found to be of benefit in acute otitis media (40), and antihistamines may prolong the duration of middle ear effusion (41). Topical anesthetic (benzocaine) or naturopathic agents may provide transient additional symptom relief for patients over the age of 5–6 years with intact tympanic membranes (42, 43).

Special circumstances

Acute myringitis is an inflammation of the layers of the tympanic membrane that may occur in association with acute otitis media. The two forms of myringitis, bullous and hemorrhagic, are caused by similar bacteria and viruses as acute otitis media, with *S. pneumoniae* being the major pathogen and relatively more common than in otitis (44–46). Bullous myringitis is associated with more severe symptoms and may require aggressive pain management (47, 48). A significant number of patients treated for acute otitis media will have otitis media with effusion which persists after treatment. Chronic middle ear effusion can interfere with hearing and lead to speech and language delay. However, the rates of spontaneous resolution are favorable, with the majority of cases resolving by 3 months after an episode of untreated acute otitis media (23, 49, 50). Thus, a watchful waiting period of several months has been suggested before intervention is considered (23, 50).

Intratemporal Complications

Most patients with otitis media will have hearing loss as long as there is a middle ear effusion. The hearing loss is usually conductive and temporary. In addition, disturbances in vestibular, balance, and motor functions can be seen during the acute episode and possibly as a sequela of resolved otitis media and middle ear effusion (51).

The second most common complication of acute otitis media is perforation of the tympanic membrane. Perforations usually quickly heal spontaneously but may persist with or without chronic suppurative otitis media. Topical antibiotic preparations may be beneficial in both acute and chronic otitis with associated tympanic membrane perforation or while a tympanostomy tube is in place (52). When possible, fluoroquinolone drops (e.g., ofloxacin) are recommended rather than potentially ototoxic aminoglycoside-containing preparations (53–56).

Due to the connection of the middle ear and mastoid air cells, most episodes of acute otitis media are associated with some degree of mastoid inflammation. Most commonly the mastoid periosteum is uninvolved, signs and symptoms of mastoid infection are absent, and the inflammation resolves without further complication. Progression to periosteitis or osteitis (acute coalescent mastoiditis), with or without a subperiosteal abscess, occurs rarely and does not appear to be prevented by prior antibiotic treatment (57, 58). In addition to the usual pathogens cultured in acute otitis media, *Streptococcus pyogenes*, *Streptococcus aureus*, and *Pseudomonas aeruginosa* are found relatively more often in mastoiditis (57–61). While some cases require surgical intervention, many can be managed conservatively with parenteral antibiotics (60–63). Some studies suggest the incidence of mastoiditis may be increasing (60, 64, 65).

Other intratemporal complications of acute otitis media include facial nerve paralysis, labrynthitis, petrositis, and external otitis (infectious eczematoid external otitis) (59). With the exception of external otitis, treatment includes parenteral antibiotics, surgical drainage, or myringotomy. Cholesteatoma can also be a sequela of otitis media and is usually treated surgically. This most often results from tympanic membrane retraction, leading to a pocket that protrudes into the middle ear. Dead skin cells accumulate within this pocket to form a cholesteatoma, which can erode into adjacent bone.

Intracranial Complications

Intracranial complications of acute otitis media include meningitis, epidural abscess, brain abscess, subdural empyema, lateral venous sinus thrombosis, cavernous sinus thrombosis and carotid artery thrombosis. In developed countries these complications are relatively rare and are usually associated with chronic ear disease. Meningitis is the most common of these complications and more often results from hematogenous spread rather than direct extension. Treatment for these conditions includes surgical drainage and parenteral antibiotics. In the case of meningitis, surgery is generally deferred except in cases with mastoid osteitis or with worsening of the clinical condition despite 48 h of antibiotic therapy (66). Common pathogens include *S. pneumoniae*, *S. pyogenes*, *S. aureus*, and *P. aeruginosa* (57, 67, 68). Warning signs of an intracranial complication include fever, headache, vestibular symptoms, meningeal signs, seizures and altered mental status (52, 68, 69). Early recognition is critical to reduce morbidity and mortality (70).

Disposition

Children younger than 2 years of age are generally seen in 10–14 days for follow-up. However, older children with resolution of symptoms and no risk factors for recurrent otitis media may not need follow-up after an acute episode (71). All patients with complications needing parenteral antibiotics or surgical intervention require otolaryngology consultation and admission. Other complications such as a perforated tympanic membrane or external otitis can be managed as an outpatient with otolaryngology referral. Febrile neonates should be evaluated with blood, urine, and cerebrospinal fluid cultures and hospitalized for parenteral antibiotics. Adults with persistent otitis media with effusion of unclear etiology should be referred to rule out nasopharyngeal carcinoma (72, 73).

Case Outcome

The patient was administered a 15 mg/kg dose of acetaminophen in the emergency department, and her father was instructed to administer this dose every 4–6 h as needed for discomfort. After discussing the benefits and adverse effects of antibiotics with the patient's father, it was decided to withhold antibiotics for a 72-h "watchful waiting" period. The patient was scheduled for telephone follow-up with her pediatrician in 72 h for reassessment of her clinical condition. The father was also given a 5-day prescription for amoxicillin (80 mg/kg/day) to be filled only if the patient had worsening pain, was not improving at 72 h, or would be unavailable for follow-up. When telephoned by her pediatrician's office 3 days later, the patient was afebrile, clinically improving, and had not needed to fill her "safety net" antibiotic prescription.

OTITIS EXTERNA

Introduction/Epidemiology

Otitis externa is an infection or inflammation of the external auditory canal. Also known as "swimmer's ear," it affects individuals of all ages, with a peak in 7–12-year olds and a decline in those over 50 years of age (74). Otitis externa occurs most often in the summer and is common in the tropics. Risk factors include trauma to the external auditory canal (e.g., cotton swabs or hearing aids), high humidity, warmer temperatures, and maceration of the skin from prolonged moisture exposure.

Pathophysiology/Microbiology

The external auditory canal is lined with squamous epithelial cells and cerumen glands. Gland secretions and desquamated cells form an acidic, lysozyme-containing lipid layer, which protects the canal skin and inhibits bacterial growth. Disruption of this barrier by excessive moisture or local trauma allows maceration of the skin and elevation of the local pH, with subsequent bacterial or fungal overgrowth. Consideration should also be given to a retained foreign body within the canal.

A recent multicenter study in the United States found the most common pathogens in otitis externa to be *P. aeruginosa* (38%), *Staphylococcus epidermidis* (9%), *S. aureus* (7.5%), and Microbacterium species (9.3%). Aspergillus and Candida, the only fungi and yeast recovered, accounted for 1.7% of the total isolates (74), although some studies have reported up to 10% of cases due to fungi.

Clinical Presentation

Otalgia and otorrhea are the most common presenting symptoms of otitis externa. Ear discomfort can progress from pruritus to severe pain that is exacerbated by any movement of the ear, including chewing. Canal occlusion from intense swelling and edema of the skin can result in conductive hearing loss. Signs include erythema and edema of the external canal with pain on movement of the tragus or auricle. Otorrhea and debris can obscure the canal, making it difficult to distinguish otitis externa from acute otitis media with tympanic membrane rupture. Infection may spread to the periauricular soft tissues and lymph nodes. Fungal infections often present with prominent pruritus rather than pain and may have a black, gray, or fluffy white discharge.

Other conditions of the external auditory canal may appear similar to otitis externa. Furunculosis is a small localized, erythematous swelling which usually occurs in the hair-bearing part of the canal and most often is due to *S. aureus*. Herpes zoster oticus (Ramsey Hunt syndrome) causes swelling and vesicles of the canal with facial nerve paralysis.

Laboratory/Diagnostic Testing

While usually unnecessary, laboratory and diagnostic testing can be helpful in some cases. Adults with unexplained external otitis should be screened with a blood glucose and/or urine dipstick to rule out occult diabetes mellitus. Gram stain and culture of canal discharge can be performed in cases of treatment failure, suspected fungal infections, or severe disease. Febrile or toxic patients should have a standard laboratory assessment. A markedly elevated ESR may be seen in cases of necrotizing otitis externa (75). CT or MRI scanning can confirm soft tissue and bone involvement.

Management

Management of otitis externa involves analgesia, external auditory canal cleansing, and topical medications. Cleansing can be accomplished with gentle suctioning and irrigation, using water, saline, 2% acetic acid, Burow solution, or hydrogen peroxide. Irrigation should be avoided or performed very cautiously if the tympanic membrane cannot be visualized or if perforation is suspected, to avoid ossicle disruption and cochlearvestibular damage (76). When irrigation is performed, particular care must be taken to remove as much moisture from the canal as possible after the procedure. At times cleansing will be difficult or impossible due to pain or canal edema. A wick of cotton, gauze, or hydroxycellulose placed into the canal can facilitate drainage and medication delivery. The wick is left in place for 2–3 days, and topical drops are applied to the exposed end.

While older acidifying agents such as acetic acid are still used for prevention or treatment of mild otitis externa, most physicians use a topical antibiotic. The combination agent containing hydrocortisone, neomycin, and polymyxin B has been used effectively for many years and is still commonly used today. However, because of a relatively high incidence of contact hypersensitivity reactions and the potential risk of ototoxicity with a nonintact tympanic membrane, some authors prefer to prescribe the newer fluoroquinolone agents (56, 77, 78). In addition to having few adverse effects, fluoroquinolone dosing frequency is twice a day. Ofloxacin, is currently the only FDA approved agent for use in patients with perforated tympanic membranes. Fluoroquinolones are more expensive, however, and broader use may lead to the development of fluoroquinolone resistance. Oral antibiotics may be necessary in cases with fever, associated otitis media, or skin and periauricular extension, but they should otherwise not be used in uncomplicated cases of otitis externa.

Most cases of otitis externa resolve after 5–7 days with treatment and strict avoidance of moisture in the ear canal. Topical medications should be discontinued at this time, as overuse can lead to dermatitis or fungal colonization, due to alterations in the normal flora of the ear. Fungal infections can often be managed with canal suctioning and acidifying drops, although topical antifungals, such as clotrimazole 1% solution, may be necessary (76). Resistant *Aspergillus* infections may require oral itraconazole.

Special circumstances

Necrotizing Otitis Externa

Further extension of infection into surrounding cartilage, periosteum, and bone can result in necrotizing otitis externa (malignant otitis externa) and skull base osteomyelitis. Signs and symptoms include pain, tenderness, and swelling around the periauricular area, headache, otorrhea, granulation tissue in the floor of the external canal, facial paralysis, and other cranial nerve deficits. Necrotizing otitis externa occurs primarily in elderly diabetics but can be seen in immunocompromised children and AIDS patients as well (75). *P. aeruginosa* is the predominant pathogen, but *S. aureus*, *Proteus mirabilis*, *Klebsiella*, *S. epidermidis*, and *Aspergillus* have also been reported (75). A high index of suspicion must be maintained in at-risk patients who have symptoms disproportionate to exam findings. Particular consideration should be given to systemic therapy, even in cases of suspected early necrotizing otitis externa and in immunocompromised patients. Ciprofloxacin has become the drug of choice for soft tissue and bone complications of otitis externa, although combination therapy with an aminoglycoside and an antipseudomonal beta-lactam antibiotic can also be used (75). With the exception of diagnostic biopsies, surgical management is often unnecessary.

Disposition

All patients with external otitis should be instructed on prevention and avoidance of precipitants of infection, including thorough canal drying and the use of acidifying or astringent drops after swimming or bathing. Patients with worsening symptoms or no response to treatment in 5–7 days must be followed up with their primary care physician or an otolaryngologist for evaluation of possible necrotizing otitis externa. Consultation with an otolaryngologist is mandatory in suspected cases of necrotizing otitis externa, and confirmed cases require parenteral antibiotics and hospital admission.

REFERENCES

1. Freid VM, Makuc DM, Rooks RN: Ambulatory health care visits by children: Principal diagnosis and place of visit. *Vital Health Stat* 13(137):1–23, 1998.

2. Bondy J, Berman S, Glazner J, Lezotte D: Direct expenditures related to otitis media diagnoses: Extrapolations from a pediatric medicaid cohort. *Pediatrics* 105(6):E72, 2000.

3. Bluestone CD: Definitions, terminology, and classification, in Rosenfeld RM, Bluestone CD (eds.): *Evidence-Based Otitis Media. 2nd ed.* Hamilton (Ont.), London, B.C. Decker, 2003; pp 120–135.

4. Teele DW, Klein JO, Rosner B. Epidemiology of otitis media during the first seven years of life in children in greater Boston: A prospective, cohort study. *J Infect Dis* 160(1): 83–94, 1989.

5. Uhari M, Mantysaari K, Niemela M: A meta-analytic review of the risk factors for acute otitis media. *Clin Infect Dis* 22(6):1079–1083, 1996.

6. Casselbrant ML, Mandel EM: Epidemiology, in Rosenfeld RM, Bluestone CD (eds.), *Evidence-Based Otitis Media, 2d ed.* Hamilton (Ont.), London, B.C. Decker, 2003; pp 147–162.

7. Paradise JL, Elster BA, Tan L: Evidence in infants with cleft palate that breast milk protects against otitis media. *Pediatrics* 94(6 Pt 1):853–860, 1994.

8. Bluestone CD: Eustachian tube function and dysfunction, in Rosenfeld RM, Bluestone CD (eds.), *Evidence-Based Otitis Media, 2d ed.* Hamilton (Ont.), London, B.C. Decker, 2003; pp 163–179.

9. Rovers MM, Schilder AG, Zielhuis GA, Rosenfeld RM: Otitis media. *Lancet* 363(9407):465–473, 2004.

10. Klein JO: Bacterial resistance and antimicrobial drug selection, in Rosenfeld RM, Bluestone CD (eds.), *Evidence-Based Otitis Media, 2d ed.* Hamilton (Ont.), London, B.C. Decker, 2003; pp 429–437.

11. Heikkinen T, Thint M, Chonmaitree T: Prevalence of various respiratory viruses in the middle ear during acute otitis media. *N Engl J Med* 340(4):260–264, 1999.

12. Nokso-Koivisto J, Raty R, Blomqvist S, et al.: Presence of specific viruses in the middle ear fluids and respiratory secretions of young children with acute otitis media. *J Med Virol* 72(2):241–248, 2004.

13. Ruuskanen O, Heikkinen T: Otitis media: Etiology and diagnosis. *Pediatr Infect Dis J* 13(1 Suppl 1):S23–6, 1994; discussion S50-4.

14. Niemela M, Uhari M, Jounio-Ervasti K, Luotonen J, Alho OP, Vierimaa E: Lack of specific symptomatology in children with acute otitis media. *Pediatr Infect Dis J* 13(9):765–768, 1994.

15. Howie VM, Schwartz RH: Acute otitis media. One year in general pediatric practice. *Am J Dis Child* 137(2):155–158, 1983.

16. Palmu AA, Herva E, Savolainen H, Karma P, Makela PH, Kilpi TM: Association of clinical signs and symptoms with bacterial findings in acute otitis media. *Clin Infect Dis* 38(2): 234–242, 2004.

17. Rothman R, Owens T, Simel DL: Does this child have acute otitis media? *JAMA* 290(12):1633–1640, 2003.

18. Rosenfeld RM, Bluestone CD: Clinical efficacy of surgical therapy, in Rosenfeld RM, Bluestone CD (eds.), *Evidence-*

Based Otitis Media, 2d ed. Hamilton (Ont.), London, B.C. Decker, 2003; pp 227–240.

19. Vazquez E, Castellote A, Piqueras J, et al.: Imaging of complications of acute mastoiditis in children. *Radiographics* 23(2):359–372, 2003.

20. Rosenfeld RM, Vertrees JE, Carr J, et al.: Clinical efficacy of antimicrobial drugs for acute otitis media: Metaanalysis of 5400 children from thirty-three randomized trials. *J Pediatr* 124(3): 355–367, 1994.

21. Del Mar C, Glasziou P, Hayem M: Are antibiotics indicated as initial treatment for children with acute otitis media? A meta-analysis. *BMJ* 314(7093):1526–1529, 1997.

22. Marcy M, Takata G, Chan LS, et al.: *Management of Acute Otitis Media.* Rockville, MD, U.S. Dept. of Health and Human Services, Public Health Service, Agency for Healthcare Research and Quality, 2001.

23. Rosenfeld RM, Kay D: Natural history of untreated otitis media, in Rosenfeld RM, Bluestone CD (eds.), *Evidence-Based Otitis Media, 2d ed.* Hamilton (Ont.), London, B.C. Decker, 2003; pp 180–198.

24. Glasziou PP, Del Mar CB, Sanders SL, Hayem M: Antibiotics for acute otitis media in children. *Cochrane Database Syst Rev* (1):CD000219, 2004.

25. Damoiseaux RA, van Balen FA, Hoes AW, de Melker RA: Antibiotic treatment of acute otitis media in children under two years of age: Evidence based? *Br J Gen Pract* 48(437):1861–1864, 1998.

26. Damoiseaux RA, van Balen FA, Hoes AW, Verheij TJ, de Melker RA: Primary care based randomised, double blind trial of amoxicillin versus placebo for acute otitis media in children aged under 2 years. *BMJ* 320(7231):350–354, 2000.

27. Rosenfeld RM: Clinical efficacy of medical therapy, in Rosenfeld RM, Bluestone CD (eds.), *Evidence-Based Otitis Media, 2d ed.* Hamilton (Ont.), Saint Louis, B.C. Decker 2003; pp 199–226.

28. American Academy of Pediatrics and American Academy of Family Physicians: Diagnosis and management of acute otitis media. *Pediatrics* 113(5):1451–1465, 2004.

29. Cates C: An evidence based approach to reducing antibiotic use in children with acute otitis media: Controlled before and after study. *BMJ* 318(7185):715–716, 1999.

30. Little P, Gould C, Williamson I, Moore M, Warner G, Dunleavey J: Pragmatic randomised controlled trial of two prescribing strategies for childhood acute otitis media. *BMJ* 322(7282):336–342, 2001.

31. Siegel RM, Kiely M, Bien JP, et al.: Treatment of otitis media with observation and a safety-net antibiotic prescription. *Pediatrics* 112(3 Pt 1):527–531, 2003.

32. Damoiseaux RA, de Melker RA, Ausems MJ, van Balen FA: Reasons for non-guideline-based antibiotic prescriptions for acute otitis media in The Netherlands. *Fam Pract* 16(1): 50–53, 1999.

33. McCracken GH, Jr.: Prescribing antimicrobial agents for treatment of acute otitis media. *Pediatr Infect Dis J* 18(12): 1141–1146, 1999.

34. Dowell SF, Butler JC, Giebink GS, et al.: Acute otitis media: Management and surveillance in an era of pneumococcal resistance—a report from the drug-resistant *Streptococcus pneumoniae* Therapeutic Working Group. *Pediatr Infect Dis J* 18(1):1–9, 1999.

35. Dagan R, Hoberman A, Johnson C, et al.: Bacteriologic and clinical efficacy of high dose amoxicillin/clavulanate in children with acute otitis media. *Pediatr Infect Dis J* 20(9): 829–837, 2001.

36. Piglansky L, Leibovitz E, Raiz S, et al.: Bacteriologic and clinical efficacy of high dose amoxicillin for therapy of acute otitis media in children. *Pediatr Infect Dis J* 22(5):405–413, 2003.

37. Marchant CD, Carlin SA, Johnson CE, Shurin PA: Measuring the comparative efficacy of antibacterial agents for acute otitis media: The "Pollyanna phenomenon." *J Pediatr* 120(1):72–77, 1992.

38. Cohen R, Levy C, Boucherat M, Langue J, de La Rocque F: A multicenter, randomized, double-blind trial of 5 versus 10 days of antibiotic therapy for acute otitis media in young children. *J Pediatr* 133(5):634–639, 1998.

39. Cohen R, Levy C, Boucherat M, et al.: Five vs. ten days of antibiotic therapy for acute otitis media in young children. *Pediatr Infect Dis J* 19(5):458–463, 2000.

40. Flynn CA, Griffin G, Tudiver F: Decongestants and antihistamines for acute otitis media in children. *Cochrane Database Syst Rev* (1):CD001727, 2002.

41. Chonmaitree T, Saeed K, Uchida T, et al.: A randomized, placebo-controlled trial of the effect of antihistamine or corticosteroid treatment in acute otitis media. *J Pediatr* 143(3): 377–385, 2003.

42. Hoberman A, Paradise JL, Reynolds EA, Urkin J: Efficacy of Auralgan for treating ear pain in children with acute otitis media. *Arch Pediatr Adolesc Med* 151(7):675–678, 1997.

43. Sarrell EM, Cohen HA, Kahan E. Naturopathic treatment for ear pain in children. *Pediatrics* 111(5 Pt 1):e574–e579, 2003.

44. Palmu AA, Kotikoski MJ, Kaijalainen TH, Puhakka HJ: Bacterial etiology of acute myringitis in children less than two years of age. *Pediatr Infect Dis J* 20(6):607–611, 2001.

45. Kotikoski MJ, Palmu AA, Nokso-Koivisto J, Kleemola M: Evaluation of the role of respiratory viruses in acute myringitis in children less than two years of age. *Pediatr Infect Dis J* 21(7):636–641, 2002.

46. Kotikoski MJ, Kleemola M, Palmu AA: No evidence of *Mycoplasma pneumoniae* in acute myringitis. *Pediatr Infect Dis J* 23(5):465–466, 2004.

47. McCormick DP, Saeed KA, Pittman C, et al.: Bullous myringitis: A case-control study. *Pediatrics* 112(4):982–986, 2003.

48. Kotikoski MJ, Palmu AA, Puhakka HJ: The symptoms and clinical course of acute bullous myringitis in children less than two years of age. *Int J Pediatr Otorhinolaryngol* 67(2): 165–172, 2003.

49. Takata G, Chan LS, Mangione-Smith RM, United States. Agency for Healthcare Research and Quality, Southern California Evidence-Based Practice Center/RAND: *Diagnosis, Natural History, and Late Effects of Otitis Media with Effusion.* Rockville, MD, U.S. Dept. of Health and Human Services, Public Health Service, Agency for Healthcare Research and Quality; 2003.

50. Rosenfeld RM, Culpepper L, Doyle KJ, et al.: Clinical practice guideline: Otitis media with effusion. *Otolaryngol Head Neck Surg* 130(5 Suppl):S95–S118, 2004.

51. Casselbrant ML, Furman JM, Mandel EM, Fall PA, Kurs-Lasky M, Rockette HE: Past history of otitis media and balance in four-year-old children. *Laryngoscope* 110(5 Pt 1): 773–778, 2000.

52. Bluestone CD: Suppurative complications, in Rosenfeld RM, Bluestone CD (eds.), *Evidence-Based Otitis Media, 2d ed.* Hamilton (Ont.), London: B.C. Decker;482–504, 2003.

53. Bath AP, Walsh RM, Bance ML, Rutka JA: Ototoxicity of topical gentamicin preparations. *Laryngoscope* 109(7 Pt 1): 1088–1093, 1999.

54. Gates GA: Safety of ofloxacin otic and other ototopical treatments in animal models and in humans. *Pediatr Infect Dis J* 20(1):104–107, 2001; discussion 20-2.

55. Perry BP, Smith DW: Effect of cortisporin otic suspension on cochlear function and efferent activity in the guinea pig. *Laryngoscope* 106(12 Pt 1):1557–1561, 1996.

56. Roland PS, Stewart MG, Hannley M, et al.: Consensus panel on role of potentially ototoxic antibiotics for topical middle ear use: Introduction, methodology, and recommendations. *Otolaryngol Head Neck Surg* 130(3 Suppl):S51–S56, 2004.

57. Leskinen K, Jero J: Complications of acute otitis media in children in southern Finland. *Int J Pediatr Otorhinolaryngol* 68(3):317–324, 2004.

58. Luntz M, Brodsky A, Nusem S, et al.: Acute mastoiditis—the antibiotic era: A multicenter study. *Int J Pediatr Otorhinolaryngol* 57(1):1–9, 2001.

59. Bluestone CD: Clinical course, complications and sequelae of acute otitis media. *Pediatr Infect Dis J* 19(5 Suppl): S37–S46, 2000.

60. Katz A, Leibovitz E, Greenberg D, et al.: Acute mastoiditis in Southern Israel: A twelve year retrospective study (1990 through 2001). *Pediatr Infect Dis J* 22(10):878–882, 2003.

61. Butbul-Aviel Y, Miron D, Halevy R, Koren A, Sakran W: Acute mastoiditis in children: *Pseudomonas aeruginosa* as a leading pathogen. *Int J Pediatr Otorhinolaryngol* 67(3):277–281, 2003.

62. Goldstein NA, Casselbrant ML, Bluestone CD, Kurs-Lasky M: Intratemporal complications of acute otitis media in infants and children. *Otolaryngol Head Neck Surg* 119(5): 444–454, 1998.

63. Tarantino V, D'Agostino R, Taborelli G, Melagrana A, Porcu A, Stura M: Acute mastoiditis: A 10 year retrospective study. *Int J Pediatr Otorhinolaryngol* 66(2):143–148, 2002.

64. Spratley J, Silveira H, Alvarez I, Pais-Clemente M: Acute mastoiditis in children: Review of the current status. *Int J Pediatr Otorhinolaryngol* 56(1):33–40, 2000.

65. Zapalac JS, Billings KR, Schwade ND, Roland PS: Suppurative complications of acute otitis media in the era of antibiotic resistance. *Arch Otolaryngol Head Neck Surg* 128(6): 660–663, 2002.

66. Barry B, Delattre J, Vie F, Bedos JP, Gehanno P: Otogenic intracranial infections in adults. *Laryngoscope* 109(3):483–487, 1999.

67. Dhooge IJ, Albers FW, Van Cauwenberge PB: Intratemporal and intracranial complications of acute suppurative otitis media in children: Renewed interest. *Int J Pediatr Otorhinolaryngol* 49(Suppl 1):S109–S114, 1999.

68. Kangsanarak J, Fooanant S, Ruckphaopunt K, Navacharoen N, Teotrakul S: Extracranial and intracranial complications of suppurative otitis media. Report of 102 cases. *J Laryngol Otol* 107(11):999–1004, 1993.

69. Kraus M, Tovi F. Central nervous system complications secondary to oto-rhinologic infections. An analysis of 39 pediatric cases. *Int J Pediatr Otorhinolaryngol* 24(3):217–226, 1992.

70. Albers FW: Complications of otitis media: The importance of early recognition. *Am J Otol* 20(1):9–12, 1999.

71. Hathaway TJ, Katz HP, Dershewitz RA, Marx TJ: Acute otitis media: Who needs posttreatment follow-up? *Pediatrics* 94(2 Pt 1):143–147, 1994.

72. Sham JS, Wei WI, Lau SK, Yau CC, Choy D: Serous otitis media. An opportunity for early recognition of nasopharyngeal carcinoma. *Arch Otolaryngol Head Neck Surg* 118(8): 794–797, 1992.

73. Woollons AC, Morton RP: When does middle ear effusion signify nasopharyngeal cancer? *NZ Med J* 107(991): 507–509, 1994.

74. Roland PS, Stroman DW: Microbiology of acute otitis externa. *Laryngoscope* 112(7 Pt 1):1166–1177, 2002.

75. Rubin Grandis J, Branstetter BFt, Yu VL: The changing face of malignant (necrotising) external otitis: Clinical, radiological, and anatomic correlations. *Lancet Infect Dis* 4(1):34–39, 2004.

76. Sander R: Otitis externa: A practical guide to treatment and prevention. *Am Fam Physician* 63(5):927–936, 41–42, 2001.

77. Dohar JE: Evolution of management approaches for otitis externa. *Pediatr Infect Dis J* 22(4):299–305, 2003.

78. Beers SL, Abramo TJ: Otitis externa review. *Pediatr Emerg Care* 20(4):250–256, 2004.

4

Odontogenic Infections, Conjunctivitis, Rhinitis, and Rhinocerebral Mucormycosis

Robert J. Paquette

HIGH YIELD FACTS

1. Odontogenic infections are usually polymicrobial (predominantly Gram positives and anaerobes).
2. Remember to evaluate diabetic ketoacidosis patients for mucormycosis infections.
3. Severe odontogenic infections can lead to airway compromise. Practice early and aggressive airway management in these patients.
4. Gonococcal conjunctivitis is an aggressive disease entity that requires parenteral antibiotics and emergent ophthalmologic consultation.

ODONTOGENIC INFECTIONS

Case Presentation

A 42-year-old homeless man presents with a chief complaint of fever and sore throat for 5 days. He tells you he was having a great deal of pain secondary to an "infected tooth" prior to the onset of the sore throat. He denies any significant past medical history, medications, or allergies. He is sitting upright holding his head in the "sniffing position" and refuses to lie down. His voice is very muffled and he appears frightened. His vital signs are a pulse of 137, blood pressure of 160/95, respiratory rate of 24, and temperature of 104°F. His exam is significant for severe trismus, extensive firm erythematous swelling of his anterior–superior neck, and notable elevation of his tongue.

Introduction/Epidemiology

There are a great variety of odontogenic infections that can involve the deep tissue planes of the head and neck. Over the last 50 years, there has been a dramatic drop in the

morbidity and mortality of odontogenic infections (1). The reasons for these findings are multiple. Most important is the discovery of antibiotics. Additionally, advances in airway management and surgical techniques have helped to improve outcomes. The responsibility of the emergency physician today is to make a rapid diagnosis and quickly institute appropriate therapies, especially airway management and early surgical consultation.

Pathophysiology/Microbiology

The microbiology of odontogenic infections is almost always polymicrobial in nature. Specific organisms frequently cited include *Staphylococcus aureus*, *Streptococcus species*, and an array of anaerobic organisms such as *Prevotella*, *Porphyromonas*, and *Fusobacterium species* (2).

Most odontogenic infections follow a common pattern. First, a tooth's pulp becomes infected (pulpitis) from either a primary infectious/corrosive source (e.g., dental carries) or an oral surgical procedure (e.g., root canal). This pulpitis progresses to abscess formation. Eventually, the abscess tracts through the bones of the jaw rupturing into a facial compartment (3). The clinical presentation, specific diagnosis, and resulting therapy will be determined by which facial compartment(s) is (are) involved.

Submandibular Infections

Odontogenic infections that cause submandibular edema result from infections of either the submandibular space, the sublingual space, or the submental space (Figure 4–1). With the exception of primary submental infections that arise from mandibular incisors, submandibular swelling is usually due to an infected mandibular molar. However, it should be noted that there are communications between these compartments. A unilateral submandibular space infection can spread across the entire submandibular region to become the life threatening disease process of Ludwig angina. In the Ludwig angina, a predominately cellulitic process engulfs both submandibular spaces and the sublingual space resulting in a massive soft tissue swelling that pushes the tongue upward and posterior. Such severe swelling ultimately results in loss of the airway and asphyxiation (4).

Buccal Space Infections

The buccal space lies between the buccinator muscle and the skin of the lateral cheek. Infected molars of either the maxilla or mandible that rupture superior to, or inferior to,

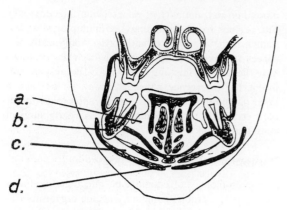

Fig. 4–1. Submandibular anatomy (obtained with permission from Hohl TH, Whitacre RJ, Hooley JR, et al: (28), p 69).
a. Sublingual space
b. Body of mandible
c. Submandibular space
d. Submental space

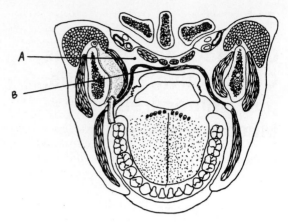

Fig. 4–2. Pharyngeal space anatomy (obtained with permission from Hohl TH, Whitacre RJ, Hooley JR, et al: (28), p 85).
A. Parapharyngeal space
B. Retropharyngeal space

the attachments of the buccinator will result in a buccal space infection. This space communicates with the infraorbital and the superficial temporal spaces.

Infraorbital Space Infections

The infraorbital space (or canine space) lies between the deep lavator anguli oris muscle and the superficial levator superioris muscle. Infected maxillary canine or incisor teeth are the cause of this infection. Because of the loose connective tissue in the region, these infections can spread rapidly into the inferior eyelid and the superficial temporal space. Given this infection's proximity to central facial veins, a feared though rare complication is cavernous sinus thrombosis.

Pharyngeal Space Infections

The pharyngeal space is subdivided into two smaller spaces, the parapharyngeal and the retropharyngeal spaces (Figure 4–2). As the name implies, the parapharyngeal spaces are just lateral to the pharynx and the retropharyngeal space is just posterior. The parapharyngeal space encloses the carotid sheath, the cervical sympathetic chain, and cranial nerves IX, X, XI, and XII.

Odontogenic involvement of the parapharyngeal space can result from extension of third molar abscesses, pericoronitis, or from extension of other evolving deep space infections (e.g., the Ludwig angina) (5). There are two

dreaded complications of parapharyngeal abscesses. The first complication is abscess extension into the retropharyngeal space which then can migrate into the chest resulting in mediastinitis. The second complication is Lemierre syndrome or septic thrombophlebitis of the internal jugular vein. The Lemierre syndrome results most commonly from a dental or pharyngeal *Fusobacterium necrophorum* infection that spreads into the parapharyngeal space (6). Local spread into the internal jugular vein results in a septic thrombophlebitis that frequently leads to showers of septic pulmonary emboli. With modern supportive therapies the mortality has dropped significantly but the morbidity of this disease remains very high.

Clinical Presentation

As a general rule, all the above mentioned infections will have nonspecific clinical markers of systemic illness such as fever, chills, and malaise. More specific clinical identifiers are listed below.

Unilateral submandibular space and submental space infections will present with localized swelling, erythema, and tenderness. Patients may have mild trismus and mild dysphagia. Sublingual space involvement additionally has an associated elevation of the floor of the mouth and tongue. Frequently the patient will keep their mouth open at rest, drool, and have noticeable difficulty speaking and breathing. The Ludwig angina, which involves bilateral submandibular spaces and the sublingual space, results in profound brawny edema of the entire superior-anterior neck, dysphagia, and tongue retropulsion and elevation (7). These patients are toxic-appearing and frequently insist on a "tripod" sitting position to help better stent open their narrowing upper airway.

Buccal space and canine space infections result in an erythematous swelling of the lateral cheek that may extend to the lower lid of the eye and the lateral edge of the lip. Differentiation of these entities can be made based on the degree of cheek swelling, presence of a nasolabial fold, and the involved teeth. Buccal space infection usually has more of a "bulging" swelling laterally, and retention of the ipsilateral nasolabial fold.

Pharyngeal space infections can be challenging to clinically diagnose. Symptoms include neck pain, toxicity, dysphagia, and possibly dyspnea. Parapharyngeal infections may demonstrate torticollis, trismus, or swelling of the anterolateral neck and posteriolateral oropharynx. There may be evidence of cranial nerve abnormalities or Horner syndrome if the infection irritates local cranial nerves (8). Lemierre syndrome patients are universally toxic. They can have the signs and symptoms listed above as well as septic arthritis and evidence of septic emboli to the lungs (6, 8).

Retropharyngeal infections also present similarly to parapharyngeal infections. Frequently there is no external neck swelling, but posterior pharyngeal bulging and nuchal rigidity may be found (5).

Laboratory/Diagnostic Testing

Odontogenic infections are primarily clinical diagnoses. With the exception of imaging studies such as contrast facial or neck CT scanning, laboratory studies add little to the diagnosis. Patients benefiting most from imaging are those in whom the diagnosis is not clear (e.g., retropharyngeal abscess), or those who have extensive infections. (9, 5). For example, a nontoxic patient with a minor canine space infection can be treated without radiographic studies.

Blood chemistries can be useful in identifying sequellae such as electrolyte abnormalities (e.g., DKA) or glucose out of control.

Management

The management principles for deep space odontogenic infections are essentially the same regardless of the exact diagnosis. Three things must be addressed with every patient: airway, antibiotics, and early surgical consultation. As mentioned above, many of these infections can result in loss of upper airway patency. The emergency physician's most important decision with these cases is to determine the need for early intubation. Severe swelling, stridor, tachypnea, air hunger, and tripoding are all extremely worrisome signs of impending airway collapse. Once the decision to intubate has been made, the preferred technique is awake fiberoptic nasotracheal intubation (1). This technique permits the patient to retain vital airway reflexes that help stent open swollen supraglottic regions until the airway has been secured. Standard rapid sequence intubation can result in precipitous airway collapse that may not be amenable to bag-valve mask ventilation.

Antibiotic therapy is directed at the two main classes of bacteria that comprise these predominantly polymicrobial "oral flora" infections: Gram positives and anaerobes. Most sources state that the exact choice of antibiotic will depend on the severity of infection. For most mild odontogenic infections, penicillin or cephalexin is effective (Table 4–1) (3). Because of increasing penicillin resistance, moderate to severe infections should be started on clindamycin, ampicillin-sulbactam, or a combination of penicillin G and metronidazole (10, 11). Given the rise of particularly resistant pathogens such as methicillin-resistant *S. aureus*, any life-threatening odontogenic infection should also be started on vancomycin (12).

Lastly, the ultimate management of most odontogenic infections is surgical. The primary problem is trapped purulent material. For many mild to moderate odontogenic infections, simple tooth extraction or minor intraoral incision and drainage is curative. For others such as the

Table 4–1. Antibiotic Therapy for Odontogenic Infections

Minor infections/nontoxic patient[a]
  Penicillin VK 500 mg po qid × 7–10 days (first choice)
  Cephalexin 500 mg po qid × 7–10 days
  Clindamycin 300 mg po qid × 7–10 days
Moderate to severe infections (hospitalized patients)[b]
  Clindamycin 900 mg IV tid × 10 days
  Ampicillin/sulbactum 3 g IV qid × 10 days
  Penicillin G and metronidazole 500 mg IV qid ×
    10 days
  Cefuroxime 1g IV tid × 10 days

[a]Oral flora have high rates of resistance to macrolides making them a poor choice.
[b]Consider adding vancomycin to regimen if patient is toxic.

Ludwig angina and Lemierre syndrome, particularly invasive deep space exploration may be necessary. Get an oral maxillofacial (OMF) surgeon involved early.

Disposition

Disposition decisions for odontogenic infections are the same as with other infectious etiologies. The decision to admit will depend on the patient's clinical appearance, the presence of comorbidities, and the patient's ability to tolerate oral intake. Clearly, nontoxic patients with no impending airway issues can be started on antibiotics and referred to OMF as an outpatient.

Case Outcome

The patient was immediately started on high flow oxygen, had intravenous access placed, and was brought to the operating room for awake intubation over a fiberoptic scope. Following intubation, ampicillin-sulbactam and vancomycin were initiated. The patient underwent surgical debridement and was admitted to the surgical ICU. The patient remained hospitalized for 3 weeks with steady improvement and was eventually discharged.

INFECTIOUS CONJUNCTIVITIS

Case Presentation

A 31-year-old male presents to the emergency room complaining of 8 h of swelling, redness, and copious purulent discharge from the right eye. On further questioning, he also reports dysuria and penile discharge for the last 3 days. On exam, he has unremarkable vital signs and large amounts of pus in the right eye. His visual acuity is normal on the left and 20/80 on the right. With fluorescein staining, a small corneal ulcer is seen.

Introduction/Epidemiology

Infectious conjunctivitis is a common entity seen in the emergency department. Although the majority of cases are benign and resolve uneventfully, there are a few important variants that the emergency physician must be vigilant for.

Pathophysiology/Microbiology

The common final pathway of all infectious conjunctivitis is the inflammation of the conjunctiva. Viruses are the most common pathogens followed by bacteria. Adenoviruses specifically are the most common viral culprits

(13). Much less common, yet still important to keep in the differential, are the herpes simplex viruses. Among bacteria, *S. aureus* is the most common organism (13). Contact lens use should increase your suspicion for *Pseudomonas*. Other important bacteria include *Haemophilus influenza*, *Streptococcus* spp., *Chlamydia trachomatis*, and *Neisseria gonorrhea* (13, 14).

Clinical Presentation

Differentiation of viral and bacterial conjunctivitis has traditionally been based on clinical features. Most viral infections present with conjunctival injection, mild chemosis, thin watery discharge, and complaints of eye burning or foreign body sensation. Herpetic infections may have the addition of vesicular lesions on the eyelids or conjunctiva. Herpes simplex infections also have the potential to spread to the cornea resulting in dendritic ulcerations of the cornea.

Bacterial infections will present with many of the same findings as viruses. In fact, some studies suggest that trying to differentiate viral and bacterial causes based on clinical findings is fraught with error (15). Traditional signs that help identify bacterial infections include mucopurulent discharge and mild eyelid swelling. Special note should be given to *N. gonorrhea* infections and neonatal conjunctivitis. *Neisseria* should be suspected in copiously purulent, aggressive cases of conjunctivitis in sexually active patients. It progresses rapidly and can quickly result in corneal ulceration and perforation if not treated properly (14).

Neonatal conjunctivitis (ophthalmia neaonatorum) is conjunctival infection acquired when the infant passes through the birth canal or is otherwise contaminated in the neonatal period. Important etiologies include *N. gonorrhea*, *C. trachomatis*, and herpes simplex viruses (16). The presentation is as described above. Diagnosis is important as this entity requires systemic as well as topical therapy.

Laboratory/Diagnostic Testing

For most cases of conjunctivitis, all that is needed is a thorough history and physical. A slit lamp exam, including fluorescein staining, should be performed to rule out other important causes of red eye, as well as to rule out sequellae of external eye infections such as corneal ulcerations. Routine culturing is generally only performed in cases of neonatal conjunctivitis and suspected cases of gonococcal conjunctivitis because of their higher rates of morbidity (13). Additionally, all cases of neonatal

Table 4–2. Antibiotic Therapy for Infectious Conjunctivitis

Simple bacterial conjunctivitis
    Polymyxin B-trimethoprim 1–2 gtts q 3–6 h ×
       7–10 days
    Tobramycin 1–2 gtts q 1–4 h × 7–10 days[a]
    Ofloxacin 1–2 gtts q 1–4 h × 7–10 days[a]
Herpes simplex conjunctivitis
    Acyclovir 500 mg po 5 × /day × 10 days
    Valcyclovir 1000 mg po bid × 10 days
Suspected gonococcal conjunctivitis
    Ceftriaxone 1 g IV QD × 5 days
              Plus
    Doxycycline 100 mg po bid × 14 days[b]
              Plus
    Erythromycin ointment $1/2$ inch q 4 h

[a]Optimal choices in contact lens wearing patients (*Pseudomonas*).
[b]Coverage for potential coinfection with *Chlamydia*.

conjunctivitis should undergo a sepsis evaluation to rule out systemic toxicity (16).

Management

Because of the difficulties in differentiating viral from bacterial infections, most routine infectious conjunctivitis is treated in the same manner (17). This includes cool compresses, temporary cessation of contact lens use, and topical antibiotics. Broad spectrum antibiotics such as polymyxin-trimethoprim and tobramycin drops are recommended (Table 4–2) (13). If *Pseudomonas* is suspected, fluoroquinolone or aminoglycoside agents are preferred. Patients with herpetic conjunctivitis should be given oral acyclovir or valcyclovir (18).

Gonococcal conjunctivitis requires both topical and systemic antibiotics as well as frequent irrigation of the infected eye. When treating suspected gonococcus, *Chlamydia* is also empirically treated given the frequent co-infection rate. A combination of intravenous ceftriaxone, oral doxycycline, and topical erythromycin ointment adequately treats most patients (see table) (13, 14). When treating neonatal conjunctivitis, the physician must be sure to provide parenteral coverage of gonococcus, *Chlamydia*, and herpetic etiologies.

Disposition

Given the relatively benign course of most conjunctivitis, the vast majority of emergency department patients will do well with outpatient management and timely follow-up. Exceptions to this rule include those with suspected gonococcal conjunctivitis and neonatal conjunctivitis. These groups generally require admission for intravenous antibiotics, frequent irrigations, and emergent evaluation by an ophthalmologist.

Case Outcome

The diagnoses of gonococcal conjunctivitis, urethritis, and corneal ulcer were made clinically and the patient's eye and urethra were cultured. Immediately afterwards, the patient was started on intravenous ceftriaxone, oral doxycycline, and erythromycin ointment. Ophthalmology was consulted and the patient was admitted to the hospital for continued parenteral antibiotics and frequent eye irrigations. The patient's infections resolved and he was discharged home without sequellae.

INFECTIOUS RHINITIS AND RHINOCEREBRAL MUCORMYCOSIS

Introduction/Epidemiology

Infectious rhinitis is an extremely common affliction, yet it generally has a very low morbidity. With the exception of rare entities such as mucormycosis, most rhinitis will be managed with simple outpatient therapies.

Pathophysiology/Microbiology

By far, the most common pathogens responsible for infectious rhinitis are viruses. Specific agents include rhinoviruses, adenoviruses, influenza, and parainfluenza (19). All of these agents have a strong affinity for attachment points on the nasal epithelium. Spread usually occurs by direct contact with body-fluid-covered fomites or through inhalation of aerosolized fluid droplets. Inflammation spreads along the confluent nasal and sinus epithelium causing swelling, discharge, and irritation.

Bacterial rhinitis is usually secondary to a viral infection and frequently involves organisms that are normally commensal. During times of weakened host defenses, organisms such as *H. influenza*, *Streptococcus pneumoniae*, and *Moraxella* can in turn become pathologic (20, 21).

Mucormycosis is a general term for invasive, frequently fatal, infections with environmentally ubiquitous fungi of the order Mucorales (22). These fungal infections are almost exclusively found in patients with pre-existing, serious immunocompromise. Rhinocerebral mucormycosis has a specific predilection for patients with diabetic ketoacidosis. The fungus travels to the nasal mucosa via fomite or aerosolization and begins to grow. Spread occurs through hyphal invasion of blood vessels that results in an expanding area of thrombosis and tissue necrosis (23). Constant progression ultimately results in cerebral extension and death.

Clinical Presentation

Viral rhinitis will present as the classic upper respiratory infection: nasal congestion, clear nasal discharge, myalgias, and subjective fevers. These symptoms will generally last less than 10 days (24). When nasal symptoms persist longer than 10 days, secretions become increasingly purulent, or facial pain develops, one should suspect possible conversion into bacterial rhinosinusitis (25).

Rhinocerebral mucormycosis symptoms begin surprisingly benign. Nasal or facial pain, possible blood tinged discharge, anterior headache, and fever may be the only complaints. As the necrosis spreads through the facial compartments, facial swelling, diplopia, vision loss, and proptosis may develop (23, 26). When the infection enters the calvarium, findings of cavernous sinus thrombosis, and altered mental status frequently develop. Other important signs of mucormycosis to look for include black necrotic ulcerations on either the nasal septum or the hard palate (26).

Laboratory/Diagnostic Testing

The diagnosis of viral and bacterial rhinitis is clinical. In fact, since viral rhinitis has been shown to cause swelling of the sinus epithelium that can be indistinguishable from bacterial sinusitis on facial CT, CT scanning should be avoided in patients with fewer than 7 days of symptoms (27).

The diagnostic work-up of rhinocerebral mucormycosis is more involved. Since most patients with mucor infections will have severe immunocompromise, basic lab studies such as chemistries, glucose, and CBC are indicated. Additionally, contrast facial CT scans help determine the extent of tissue invasion and help surgeons plan debridement. Ultimately however, diagnosis confirmation requires a tissue biopsy that demonstrates thrombosis and fungal elements (23).

Management

The vast majority of infectious rhinitis cases of less than 10 days duration are viral. As a result, most infectious rhinitis therapy is largely symptomatic. Topical decon

Table 4–3. Antibiotic Therapy for Bacterial Rhinitis

First-line agents[a]
Amoxicillin 875 mg po bid × 14 days
Trimethoprim-sulfamethoxazole 1 DS tab po bid × 14 days
Second-line agents[b]
Amoxicillin-clavulanate 875 mg po bid × 14 days
Cefaclor 500 mg po bid × 14 days
Levofloxacin 500 mg po bid × 14 days

[a]Many communities with significant rates of resistance to these agents.
[b]Best used after treatment failures with first-line agents or in more severe cases.

gestants (e.g., oxymetazoline) and intranasal ipratropium bromide both work to decrease nasal secretions (21, 25). If the patient presents with features of bacterial rhinitis such as duration longer than 10 days, increasingly purulent discharge, or facial pain, antibiotics should be considered. Bacterial rhinitis is treated in the same manner as bacterial sinusitis since the diagnoses are frequently indistinguishable. Antibiotics such as trimethoprim-sulfamethoxazole, ampicillin, quinolones, second generation cephalosporins, and amoxicillin-clavulanate are all acceptable choices (Table 4–3) (21, 25). Therapy is for 10–14 days.

The management of mucormycosis involves correction of underlying metabolic derangements, aggressive surgical debridement, and intravenous amphotericin B (22).

Disposition

Patients with viral and bacterial rhinitis are universally managed as outpatients. Clearly, patients with suspected rhinocerebral mucormycosis will require ICU admission for aggressive medical management and urgent consultation with an ENT surgeon for surgical debridement.

REFERENCES

1. Flynn TR: Odontogenic infections. *Oral Maxillofac Surg Clin North Am* 3(2):311–329, 1991.
2. Brook I: Anaerobic bacteria in upper respiratory tract and other head and neck infections. *Ann Otol Rhinol Laryngol* 111:430–440, 2002.
3. Swift FQ, Gulden WS: Antibiotic therapy—managing odontogenic infections. *Dent Clin N Am* 46:623–633, 2002.
4. Ferrera PC, Busino LJ, Snyder HS: Uncommon complications of odontogenic infections. *Am J Emerg Med* 14(3):317–322, 1996.

5. Pynn BR, Sands T, Pharoah MJ: Odontogenic infections: Anatomy and radiology. *Oral Health* 7–21, 1995.

6. Golpe R, Marin B, Alonso M: Lemierre's syndrome (necrobacilliosis). *Postgrad Med J* 75:141–144, 1999.

7. Spitalnic SJ, Sucov A: Ludwig's angina: Case report and review. *J Emerg Med* 13(4):499–503, 1995.

8. Flynn TR: The swollen face: Severe odontogenic infections. *Emerg Med Clin N Am* 18(3):481–519, 2000.

9. Yonetsu K, Izumi M, Nakamura T: Deep facial infections of odontogenic origin: CT assessment of pathways of space involvement. *Am J Neuroradiol* 19:123– 128, 1998.

10. Baker KA, Fotos PG: The management of odontogenic infections. *Dent Clin N Am* 38(4):689–706, 1994.

11. Sands T, Pynn BR, Katsikeris N: Odontogenic infections: Microbiology, antibiotics and management. *Oral Health* 11–28, 1995.

12. Brook I: Microbiology and management of deep facial infections and Lemierre syndrome. *ORL* 65:117–120, 2003.

13. Syed NA, Hyndiuk RA: Infectious conjunctivitis. *Infect Dis Clin N Am* 6(4): 789–805, 1992.

14. Ullman S, Roussel TJ, Forster RK: Gonococcal keratoconjunctivitis. *Surv Ophtho* 32(3):199–208, 1987.

15. Rietveld RP, van Weert HC, ter Riet G, Bindels PJ: Diagnostic impact of signs and symptoms in acute infectious conjunctivitis: Systematic literature search. *Brit Med J* 327:789, 2003.

16. de Toledo AR, Chandler JW: Conjunctivitis of the newborn. *Infect Dis Clin N Am* 6(4):807–813, 1992.

17. Birinyi F, Mauger TF: Ophtholmologic conditions, in Knoop KJ, Stack LB, Storrow AB (eds.), *Atlas of Emergency Medicine, 1st ed.* New York, McGraw-Hill, 1997; p 30.

18. Kaufman HE: Treatment of viral diseases of the cornea and external eye. *Prog Retin Eye Res* 19(1):69–85, 2000.

19. Fairbanks DNF, Raphael GD: Nonallergic rhinitis and infection, in Cummings CW, Fredrickson JM, Harker LA, et al. (eds.), *Otolaryngology—Head and Neck Surgery, 2d ed.* St. Louis, MosbyYear Book, 1993; p 783.

20. Van Cauwenberge P, Ingels K: Effects of viral and bacterial infection on nasal and sinus mucosa. *Acta Otolaryngol* 116:316–321, 1996.

21. Wilson WR: Nasal and sinus congestion and infection, in Wilson WR, Nadol JB, Randolph GW (eds.), *The Clinical Handbook of Ear, Nose and Throat Disorders, 1st ed.* Boca Raton, Parthenon Publishing Group, 2003; p 185.

22. Peterson LK, Wang M, Canalis RF, et al: Rhinocerebral mucormycosis: Evolution of the disease and treatment options. *Laryngoscope* 107:855–862, 1997.

23. Sugar AM: Mucormycosis. *Clin Infect Dis* 14(Supp1):S126–S129, 1992.

24. Tami TA: Infectious and inflammatory disorders, in Seiden AM, Tami TA, Pensak ML, et al. (eds.), *Otolaryngology—The Essentials, 1st ed.* New York, Thieme, 2002; p 107.

25. Dykewicz MS: Rhinitis and sinusitis. *J Allergy Clin Immunol* 111(2):S520–S529, 2003.

26. Gonzalez CE, Rinaldi MG, Sugar AM: Zygomycosis. *Infect Dis Clin N Am* 16(4):895–914, 2002.

27. Gwaltney JM, Philips CD, Miller RD, Riker DK: Computed tomographic study of the common cold. *N Engl J Med* 330:25–30, 1994.

28. Hohl TH, Whitacre RJ, Hooley JR, et al.: *Diagnosis and Treatment of Odontogenic Infections.* Seattle, Stoma Press, 1983.

5

Meningitis

Rodrigo Hasbun

HIGH YIELD FACTS

- *Streptococcus pneumoniae* is the leading etiologic agent of bacterial meningitis.

- A screening head computed tomography (CT) scan should only be done if the age is greater than 60 years, patient is immunocompromised, has a history of a central nervous system (CNS) lesion or a history of seizure within 1 week of presentation, or has mental status changes or focal neurological findings upon physical examination.

- The meningeal signs are poor screening tools to decide which patients should undergo lumbar puncture to rule out meningitis.

- Adjunctive dexamethasone should be started 15 minutes before the first dose of antibiotic therapy and continued only in patients with pneumococcal meningitis.

- The aseptic meningitis syndrome (meningitis with a negative Gram stain and culture) has a broad differential diagnosis that includes both infectious and noninfectious etiologies, some requiring urgent therapy for cure and survival.

CASE PRESENTATION

A 35-year-old white male with a history of a splenectomy presents to the emergency department with a 24-h history of fever, headache, stiff neck, and photophobia. The physical examination of the patient reveals a temperature of 104°F, blood pressure of 85/50 mm, heart rate of 115, and respiratory rate of 28. He is alert and oriented with a Glasgow coma scale of 15. Fundi show no papilledema. His neck is stiff but the Kernig and Brudzinski signs are negative. His neurological examination is normal. No rash is present.

A head CT scan is not ordered and the patient undergoes a lumbar puncture. The opening pressure is 350 mm H20 and the cerebrospinal fluid (CSF) appears cloudy.

The CSF Gram stain reveals lancet-shaped gram-positive diplococci with numerous leukocytes. The CSF glucose is 30 mg/dL and the protein is 250 mg/dL.

INTRODUCTION

Bacterial meningitis remains a disease with significant morbidity and mortality. Major epidemiological changes, including the decline of *Haemophilus influenzae* meningitis and the emergence of drug-resistant *S. pneumoniae*, have changed the empiric therapy of patients with bacterial meningitis. *S. pneumoniae* is now responsible for almost half of all episodes. This chapter will focus on issues related to the epidemiology of bacterial meningitis, diagnosis (i.e., the need for a screening head CT scan, the diagnostic accuracy of the meningeal signs), and the prognosis (and the impact of timing of the initial dose of antibiotic) and make recommendations for the empirical antibiotic therapy of patients with bacterial meningitis. Also included is a review of the differential diagnosis of patients presenting with the aseptic meningitis syndrome.

EPIDEMIOLOGY/MICROBIOLOGY

There have been two major changes in the epidemiology of meningitis that affect the empirical management of patients presenting with suspected meningitis. First, there is widespread use of the conjugate vaccine against *H. influenzae* type b in infants in the developing countries. Before the advent of the vaccine, *H. influenzae* type b accounted for 70% of cases of bacterial meningitis among children less than 5 years of age. In 1995, the Center for Disease Control (CDC) sponsored multistate surveillance study of bacterial meningitis documented a 94% reduction in the number of cases of *H. influenzae*, making *S. pneumoniae* the most common pathogen identified (1). Because *H. influenzae* was, in the past, responsible for the majority of cases of bacterial meningitis in children less than 5 years of age, the median age of persons with bacterial meningitis has now increased from 15 months to 25 years of age. In the CDC study, the most common etiologic agents of bacterial meningitis were *S. pneumoniae* (47%), followed by *Neisseria meningitidis* (25%) and group B streptococcus (12%). Both *H. influenzae* and *Listeria monocytogenes* accounted for approximately 8% each of the cases of bacterial meningitis. The etiologic agents associated with meningitis varied by age group. Group B streptococcus was the leading pathogen in the neonatal period accounting for approximately 70% of cases; but invasive disease and meningitis have also been described in adults with comorbid conditions (2). Both *S. pneumoniae* (45%) and *N. meningitidis* (31%) were the leading pathogens in infants 1–23 months of age. *N. meningitidis* caused the majority of cases among patients between 2 and 18 years of age. In adults older than 19 years of age, *S. pneumoniae* accounted for 62% of the episodes of bacterial meningitis. As in previous surveillance studies, case fatality rates varied by pathogen. *S. pneumoniae* (21%) and *L. monocytogenes* (15%) had the highest mortality rates, while group B streptococcus (7%), *H. influenzae* (6%), and *N. meningitidis* (3%) were associated with lower mortality.

The second important epidemiologic trend is the emergence of penicillin- and cephalosporin-resistant *S. pneumoniae*. Although the first penicillin-resistant *S. pneumoniae* isolate was described in 1967, it was not until the last decade that worldwide infection with multidrug-resistant *S. pneumoniae* has increased (3). The resistance of *S. pneumoniae* to penicillin and other β-lactams is due to variations in the structure and molecular size of penicillin-binding proteins. In the 1995 multistate surveillance study by the CDC (1), 29/84 (35%) cerebrospinal fluid isolates of *S. pneumoniae* that underwent susceptibility testing were resistant to penicillin (14% highly resistant; mean inhibitory concentration (MIC) $>2\mu$g/m). These changes in the resistance patterns of *S. pneumoniae* mandate susceptibility testing for all isolates and have changed the empiric antibiotic management of patients with bacterial meningitis.

CLINICAL PRESENTATION

Patients with bacterial meningitis present with acute onset of fever, headache, stiff neck, nausea/vomiting, and mental status changes. In a recent large European prospective study of 696 cases of bacterial meningitis, the classic triad of fever, stiff neck, and altered mental status was present in only 44% of patients (4). However, 95% of all patients had at least two of the four symptoms of headache, fever, neck stiffness, and altered mental status. A rash was present in 26% of patients, more commonly seen in those infected with *N. meningitides*, and in 89% of the cases the rash was described a petechial. Only 5% of patients experienced a seizure prior to presentation. Focal neurologic deficits were noted in 33% of patients, and 14% were described as comatose (4).

LABORATORY/DIAGNOSTIC TESTING

Role of Cranial Imaging in Suspected Meningitis

For practicing physicians in emergency departments, it has become routine to obtain a head CT scan before performing a lumbar puncture in adult patients with suspected meningitis. This is done to "rule out" the possibility of an intracranial abnormality associated with increased intracranial pressure that could theoretically place the patient at risk for cerebral herniation after CSF removal. However, considerable controversy in the literature and in clinical practice exists as to whether a screening CT scan should be done routinely or only in selected patients. Besides the cost implication of this practice, there is a potential delay in diagnosis and therapy of patients with suspected meningitis that could compromise clinical outcome. To better define the role of cranial imaging prior to lumbar puncture, a prospective observational study of 301 adult patients with suspected meningitis in the emergency department was done in New Haven, CT (5). Of the 301 patients, 235 (78%) underwent a head CT scan before the lumbar puncture. In 56 of the 235 patients (24%), the results of the CT scan were abnormal; 11 patients (5%) had mass effect. Baseline clinical variables that were associated with an abnormal head CT scan were: age greater than 60 years, immunocompromise, history of a CNS lesion, history of seizure within 1 week of presentation, as well as the following neurological abnormalities: abnormal level of consciousness, an inability to answer two consecutive questions correctly or to follow two consecutive commands, gaze palsy, abnormal visual fields, facial palsy, arm and leg drift, and abnormal language. None of these features were seen in 96 of the 235 patients (41%) who underwent a screening CT scan. The CT scan was normal in 93 of these 96 patients, yielding a 97% negative predictive value. Of the three misclassified patients, only one had a mild mass effect on CT, and all three subsequently underwent lumbar puncture, with no evidence of brain herniation 1 week later. Avoiding cranial imaging in this low risk subgroup would reduce unnecessary costs and delays in the diagnosis and therapy of patients with suspected meningitis.

Diagnostic Accuracy of the Meningeal Signs

For more than a century the Kernig sign (in a sitting position, or when lying supine with the hip flexed, extension of the knee is limited due to pain), Brudzinski sign (flexion

Table 5–1. Typical CSF Finding in Bacterial vs Viral Meningitis

CSF Parameter	Bacterial	Viral
Opening pressure	>180 mm H_2O	<180 mm H_2O
WBC count	$1000–5000/mm^3$	$100–1000/mm^3$
% neutrophils	$\geq 80\%$	Unusual except early
Protein	100–500 mg/dL	50–100 mg/dL
Glucose	≤ 40 mg/dL	Normal
Serum/CSF glucose ratio	<0.6	>0.6
Gram stain	$+60–90\%$	Negative
Culture	$+70–85\%$	Negative
Bacterial antigen	$+50–100\%$	N/A

of the neck resulting in flexion of the hip and knee), and nuchal rigidity have been used in the assessment of patients with suspected meningitis and physicians routinely rely upon them to determine which patients should undergo lumbar puncture. Despite their widespread use, the meningeal signs have never been studied rigorously. A recent prospective cohort study of 297 patients with suspected meningitis was completed in New Haven, CT to investigate the diagnostic accuracy of the three meningeal signs (6). Of the 297 patients, 80 (27%) patients had meningitis (i.e., more than 5 leukocytes/mL of CSF). The sensitivity of all three meningeal signs was low; both Kernig and Brudzinski signs had a sensitivity of 5% and a negative predictive value of 72% and nuchal rigidity had a sensitivity of 30% and a negative predictive value of 73%. Furthermore, the diagnostic accuracy of these meningeal signs did not improve in the subset of patients with more significant inflammation (100 or more leukocytes/mL of CSF) or in the subset of patients with a positive CSF culture. Better clinical diagnostic signs are needed and decisions regarding lumbar puncture should not be solely based on the presence or absence of the meningeal signs.

Laboratory

Confirmation of the diagnosis is made by careful analysis of the CSF and blood cultures. Routine studies of CSF include the Gram stain, culture, cell count with differential, and measurements of glucose and protein. An opening pressure should be obtained and documented in the procedure note. The Gram stain is readily available and is frequently positive. Up to 90% of children with pneumococcal meningitis have a positive Gram stain (7). Gram-negative pathogens are less frequently seen on the Gram stain as are pathogens encountered following neurosurgery (8). Despite identifying bacteria on CSF Gram stain, empiric antibiotic therapy should be modified based

on culture results, not the Gram stain, due to the possibility of error. *L. monocytogenes*, for example, a gram-positive bacillus, is frequently misidentified as a gram-positive cocci (9).

Typical findings of CSF in patients with bacterial and viral meningitis are compared in Table 5–1. In the setting of viral meningitis the opening pressure is usually normal and the white blood cell (WBC) count is $100–500/mm^3$. Neutrophils may predominate early in the course of infection but lymphocytes are the common finding. In bacterial meningitis, the opening pressure is usually elevated and the WBC count is $1000–5000/mm^3$. The sensitivity of the Gram stain is not influenced by prior antibiotic therapy (4). Usually neutrophils predominate but a lymphocytic predominance may be found in neonates and infections with *L. monocytogenes*. Although meningitis is defined as having ≥ 5 WBCs in the CSF, normal CSF was found in 10% of patients with *N. meningitides* meningitis, thus mandating that CSF should always be examined by the Gram stain and culture (10).

Blood cultures should always be obtained, provided acquisition does not delay antibiotic administration. Blood cultures reveal pathogens causing bacterial meningitis in up to 90% of cases caused by *H. influenzae* type b, 85% caused by pneumococcus, and approximately 50% caused by *N. meningitidis* (11). In a recent Dutch study, 404/611 (66%) of the patients with bacterial meningitis had positive blood cultures (4).

Routine blood testing (complete blood count with differential, serum chemistries, BUN, creatinine, and glucose) is not useful for diagnosing meningitis but may provide prognostic information. Peripheral WBC $<500/mm^3$, hemoglobin <11 g/dL, and platelet count $<100,000$ mm^3 are all associated with greater mortality (8). Van de Beek and colleagues (4) found that an elevated erythrocyte sedimentation rate (ESR) and a reduced platelet count were associated with an unfavorable outcome.

The utility of routine use of rapid antigen assays of CSF has been the subject of debate. Latex agglutination tests and countercurrent immunoelectrophoresis detect specific polysaccharide surface antigens from *S. pneumoniae*, *H. influenzae* type b, *N. meningitidis* groups A, B, C, Y, W-135, group B streptococci, and *Escherichia coli* k1. Various studies report wide ranges of sensitivity and specificity (12). These tests have the greatest accuracy in detecting *H. influenzae* type b, but since the dramatic decline in invasive disease due to implementation of the vaccine they may be less useful. Experts suggest they could be used in situations when the Gram stain is negative (12).

Polymerase chain reaction (PCR) is an emerging technology that is based on the ability to detect DNA of pathogens, living or dead, and amplifying it many times over until such a quantity is obtained that can be detected by a species specific DNA primer. The advantages of PCR testing include rapidly available results, often within hours, and the detection of organisms even if they have been killed by prior antimicrobial administration. Primers are available for the most common pathogens. Radstrom et al. utilized PCR primers for *N. meningitidis*, *S. pneumoniae*, *H. influenzae*, group B streptococcus, and *Staphylococcus epidermidis* for simultaneous detection of meningeal pathogens and reported a sensitivity of 94% and specificity of 96% (13). Because this technique amplifies even the smallest amount of DNA of pathogenic organisms it is extremely sensitive, and is most useful on sterile clinical specimens, especially CSF. PCR applied to serum may be too sensitive. Dagan et al. (14) reported a high false positive rate in healthy control subjects while studying pneumococcal infections, including meningitis, and is presumed to be due to nasopharyngeal carriage of pneumococci.

Another advantage of PCR technology is the ability to amplify specific gene sequences. One group of researchers has developed a strategy to amplify the pneumococcal penicillin-binding protein 2B gene to detect the presence of penicillin-susceptible and penicillin-resistant strains in CSF (15). Sensitivity and specificity were 100%, and the testing required only 15 μL of CSF. Presently, information on antibiotic sensitivity depends upon the ability to recover the organism from culture, requiring at least 48 h.

MANAGEMENT

Empirical Antibiotic Therapy

If the lumbar puncture is delayed, or the results of the CSF Gram stain are pending, empirical antibiotic therapy should be promptly instituted. As outlined in Table 5–2,

Table 5–2. Empirical Therapy in Patients with Suspected Bacterial Meningitis Pending Results of Blood and CSF Cultures

Predisposing Factor	Antibiotic of Choice
Age	
<3 months[a]	Ampicillin plus cefotaxime[b]
3 months–50 years	Third-generation cephalosporin plus vancomycin
>50 years	Ampicillin plus third-generation cephalosporin plus vancomycin
Impaired cellular immunity	Ampicillin plus third-generation cephalosporin and vancomycin
Postneurosurgery, head trauma, or with a CSF shunt	Vancomycin plus ceftazidime

[a] Preterm, low-birth-weight neonates are at higher risk for nosocomial meningitis with staphylococci or gram-negative bacilli and should be covered with vancomycin and ceftazidime.
[b] Ceftriaxone is preferred over cefuroxime except in the neonatal period.
Source: Adapted from (7).

the empirical regimens for patients with presumed bacterial meningitis are based on age and underlying comorbidities (16, 17). For children less than 3 months of age, the most likely pathogens are group B streptococcus, *L. monocytogenes* and *E. coli*, and empirical therapy consists of ampicillin and a third-generation cephalosporin (most commonly cefotaxime) and vancomycin. Ceftriaxone is avoided in this age group because it binds albumin and alters bilirubin metabolism. In the 3-month-to-50-year-old age group, the most likely pathogens include *S. pneumoniae* and *N. meningitidis* and empirical therapy should be a third-generation cephalosporin and vancomycin. In those older than 50 years of age, the most commonly implicated agents are *S. pneumoniae, L. monocytogenes*, and gram-negative bacilli, and therapy should include ampicillin and a third-generation cephalosporin plus vancomycin. In patients with CSF shunts or with recent neurosurgical procedures, the likely etiologic agents are staphylococci, diphtheroids, and gram-negative bacilli, including *Pseudomonas aeruginosa*. The combination of vancomycin and ceftazidime would be most appropriate in this setting. In patients with impaired cellular immunity

Table 5–3. Recommended Antibiotic Therapy for Culture-Confirmed Bacterial Meningitis in Adults

Meningeal Pathogen	Antibiotic of Choice
S. pneumoniae	
Penicillin MIC <0.1 μg/mL	Penicillin G 4 million units IV q4 h[a]
Penicillin MIC 0.1–1.0 μg/mL	Ceftriaxone 2 g IV q12 h
Penicillin MIC >2.0 μg/mL	Vancomycin 1 g IV q12 h plus
	Ceftriaxone 2 g IV q12 h[b]
H. influenzae	
β-lactamase negative	Ampicillin 2 g IV q4 h
β-lactamase positive	Ceftriaxone 2 g IV q12 h
N. meningitides	Penicillin G 4 million units IV q4 h
Group B streptococci (*Streptococcus agalactiae*)	
L. monocytogenes	Ampicillin 2 g IV q4 h plus
	Gentamicin 1–1.7 mg/kg q8 h

[a]IV = intravenous and q = every.
[b]Consider the addition of rifampin 600 mg po qd if adjunctive dexamethasone is used and if the isolate is susceptible to rifampin.
Source: Adapted from (7).

(e.g., lymphoreticular tumors, recent chemotherapy and high-dose corticosteroids) of any age group, *L. monocytogenes* should be a consideration and ampicillin should be added to the empirical regimen. As shown in Table 5–3, the antibiotic therapy can be changed once the isolate and the susceptibility of the organism are known.

Timing of the Initial Dose of Antibiotic

A common reason for malpractice litigation is the delayed institution of antibiotic therapy in a patient with bacterial meningitis. Standard textbooks argue that adverse clinical outcome from delayed therapy necessitates prompt administration of empirical antibiotics (18, 19). Such sources assume that a delay of only hours could adversely affect the prognosis of these patients, but published data are inconclusive since clinical outcome is influenced by many other confounding factors (e.g., age, comorbidity, severity of illness, and virulence of the pathogen) (20). A retrospective cohort study of 269 adults with community acquired bacterial meningitis investigated the relationship between the timing of the initial dose of effective antibiotic and the clinical outcome after controlling for recognized confounding factors (21). In this study, three baseline clinical features (hypotension, altered mental status and seizures) were independently associated with adverse clinical outcome (death or neurological morbidity

at discharge) and were used to create a prognostic model. The model stratified patients into three prognostic stages with low risk (9%; stage I), intermediate risk (33%; stage II), and high risk (56%; stage III) of adverse clinical outcome ($P = 0.001$). For the total cohort, the median delay in antibiotic therapy was 4.0 h and was not significantly different in patients with or without an adverse outcome within any prognostic stage. However, analysis of patients whose prognostic stage advanced from arrival in the emergency department until the initial antibiotic dose unveiled a clear association between antibiotic timing and clinical outcome. Patients who arrived in the emergency department in stage I or II but who advanced to stage III at the time of initial antibiotic therapy had significantly more adverse clinical outcomes that those who remained in the original emergency department prognostic stage at the time of antibiotic initiation. The results of this study suggest that the impact of antibiotic timing on clinical outcome varies with the severity of illness at presentation and not with a specific time delay.

Despite the widespread recommendations of initiating antibiotic therapy before the head CT scan or the lumbar puncture, two studies have shown that 41% of 301 patients with suspected meningitis and only 35% of patients with documented bacterial meningitis received empirical antibiotic therapy appropriately (4, 5). The sensitivity of the CSF Gram stain (80%) is not affected by prior antimicrobial therapy and should not be a reason to withhold antibiotic therapy while awaiting results of a head CT scan or the lumbar puncture (4).

Specific Antibiotic Therapy

Streptococcus pneumoniae

The treatment of pneumococcal meningitis has been modified in the last decade because of the emergence of penicillin- and cephalosporin-resistant isolates (17). All CSF *S. pneumoniae* isolates should undergo susceptibility testing and be categorized as susceptible (MIC < 0.1 mg/L), relatively resistant (MIC 0.1–1.0 mg/L) or highly resistant (MIC > 2 mg/L) to penicillin. For susceptible strains of *S. pneumoniae*, penicillin G remains the drug of choice. The antibiotic coverage of pneumococcal meningitis with unknown susceptibilities is problematic. Resistance to other antimicrobials has been described, including cephalosporins, chloramphenicol, trimethoprim-sulfamethoxazole, and erythromycin (3). Resistance to vancomycin has not been reported.

Chloramphenicol, third-generation cephalosporins, vancomycin, imipenem, and meropenem have been used in treating patients with penicillin-resistant *S. pneumoniae* meningitis (17). Chloramphenicol has been associated with poor clinical results; in one study, 20 out of 25 children had serious neurological sequelae and/or mortality. This was most likely due to the high minimum bacterial concentrations (MBCs) that resulted in subtherapeutic bactericidal activity. Third-generation cephalosporins have been effective in treating penicillin-resistant isolates, but clinical failures have occurred in patients with pneumococcal strains with MICs for cefotaxime or ceftriaxone of >2 mg/L. The current 2002 guidelines by the National Committee for Clinical Laboratory Standards state that CSF isolates of *S. pneumoniae* with a MIC of 1 μg/ml should be considered as having intermediate resistance, and isolates with MIC $\geq$ 2 μg/mL should be considered resistant (22). Vancomycin was evaluated in 11 adults with penicillin-resistant *S. pneumoniae* meningitis; four of them had poor outcomes (23). In two of the failures, the CSF vancomycin levels at 48 h were undetectable, and CSF penetration of vancomycin is further decreased by the concomitant use of dexamethasone (24). Meropenem has been evaluated in three randomized clinical trials in children with bacterial meningitis and has shown similar efficacy when compared to cefotaxime and ceftriaxone, but the number of patients with penicillin-resistant pneumococcus in the studies have been low (25–27). Meropenem also has activity against *L. monocytogenes*

in vitro and has received approval by the Food and Drug Administration (FDA) for its use in pediatric bacterial meningitis.

Another group of antimicrobial agents that appear promising are the new fluoroquinolones. They have excellent in vitro activity against the majority of the meningeal pathogens, have reproducible inflammation-independent (i.e., not decreased by the administration of steroids) CSF penetration, and have both in vitro and in vivo activities against penicillin and cephalosporin-resistant pneumococci (28). A randomized clinical trial assessed the efficacy of trovafloxacin with ceftriaxone in pediatric bacterial meningitis (29). Clinical and microbiological outcomes were similar in both groups and the incidence of joint abnormalities was low and not statistically significant between the two (<1% in the trovafloxacin arm and 2% in the comparator arm).

In experimental models of penicillin-resistant pneumococcal meningitis, the combination of vancomycin and ceftriaxone has been synergistic even when the MIC to ceftriaxone was greater than 4 mg/L (30). However, in animals being treated concomitantly with dexamethasone, the effectiveness of vancomycin was reduced. Only those animals being treated with the combination of ceftriaxone and rifampin achieved sterile CSF when dexamethasone was added. Based on these studies and on the limited clinical data, the recommendation is to use a combination of vancomycin and ceftriaxone in patients with suspected pneumococcal meningitis with unknown susceptibilities. If adjunctive dexamethasone is given, I recommend considering the addition of rifampin (see Table 5–3). Meropenem is a FDA approved alternative therapy in meningitis in children above the age of 3 months. The new fluoroquinolones show great promise but the clinical data are currently limited.

Neisseria meningitides

N. meningitides accounts for 25% of all cases of bacterial meningitis and is the leading pathogen in patients between 2 and 18 years of age (2). Penicillin remains the drug of choice for patients with meningococcal meningitis. However, susceptibility patterns are changing and clinical isolates with intermediate resistance to penicillin (MIC of 0.1–1.0 mg/L) have been reported in Spain, South Africa, North Carolina, and most recently from France (31). In this French study, 30% of 2167 clinical isolates from 1999–2002 were resistant to penicillin. The resistance in these isolates is mediated by alterations in the penicillin-binding proteins, but rare isolates of β-lactamase-producing strains with MICs of >250 mg/L have been described. Patients infected with intermediate resistant strains have been effectively managed with penicillin. In meningitis caused by the highly resistant β-lactamase-producing strains, an alternative agent like ceftriaxone should be used.

Listeria monocytogenes

L. monocytogenes should always be considered in patients who have cellular immunodeficiency or are at the extremes of age (age less than 3 months and patients older than 50 years) (2). This is very important because third-generation cephalosporins are inactive against Listeria, and ampicillin at high doses should be added to the empiric regimen if this pathogen is suspected. Listeria can also cause parenchymal brain lesions (e.g., cerebritis, brain abscess) and can cause a meningoencephalitis picture with focal neurological signs, seizures, and altered mental status. Listeria meningitis carries a mortality rate of 15%. Based on in vitro and in animal model data showing synergy, most authorities recommend adding gentamicin to ampicillin in cases of Listeria meningitis (9). Vancomycin and chloramphenicol are not suitable alternatives because of high failure rates. In the penicillin-allergic patient, trimethoprim-sulfamethoxazole should be used because of its bactericidal activity against *L. monocytogenes*, its good CSF penetration, and because it has been used successfully in patients (40).

Role of Adjunctive Steroids

Despite the use of antibiotics the mortality rate of adults with bacterial meningitis is 25% and has not changed significantly in the last three decades (32). Animal models have implicated locally generated cytokines (interleukin-1, interleukin-6 and tumor necrosis factor) within the subarachnoid space as inducers of CSF inflammation (33). This inflammatory process is responsible for much of the neurological sequelae of bacterial meningitis. Several studies of experimental meningitis have shown a reduction of CSF leukocytosis and brain edema in those animals treated with adjunctive dexamethasone (34). A meta-analysis of 11 randomized studies in children with bacterial meningitis demonstrated that the addition of adjunctive dexamethasone reduced CSF inflammation and the incidence of hearing loss (35). In contrast, a recently published study done in Malawi showed no impact of dexamethasone in the outcome of children with bacterial meningitis (36). Despite the clinical data, controversy continues for three reasons. First, the majority of patients enrolled in these studies were children with *H. influen-*

zae meningitis, currently a rare cause. Second, with the emergence of penicillin-resistant *S. pneumoniae*, the CSF penetration of vancomycin could be decreased by the adjunctive use of dexamethasone hampering microbiologic cure. Third, bacterial meningitis is now more frequent in the adult population where less clinical data exist. There exists only one randomized, double-blinded and placebo-controlled study evaluating steroids in adults with bacterial meningitis (37). In this European trial, de Gans and colleagues randomized 301 patients with bacterial meningitis to adjunctive dexamethasone versus placebo in addition to standard antibiotic therapy. Adjunctive dexamethasone was associated with a reduction in mortality (RR, 0.48; 95 CI 0.24–0.96; $P = 0.04$). The benefit of steroids was strongest for the *S. pneumoniae* subgroup where patients randomized to steroids had a mortality rate of 26% compared to 52% in the placebo group (RR, 0.50; 95 CI 0.30–0.83; $P = 0.006$).

Although uncertainties remain, in children more than 2 years old and with bacterial meningitis we recommend the use of adjunctive dexamethasone, particularly those suspected to be infected with *H. influenzae*. Dexamethasone should be given intravenously 15 minutes before or simultaneously with the initial antibiotics at a dose of 0.15 mg per kilogram of body weight every 6 h for 4 days. In adults, dexamethasone 10 mg intravenously should be started empirically 15 minutes before or concomitantly with bactericidal antibiotic therapy in all patients with suspected bacterial meningitis. Dexamethasone therapy should be continued only on those patients with proven pneumococcal meningitis.

SPECIAL CIRCUMSTANCES

Prevention

Vaccination

Secondary cases can be prevented by the administration of the meningococcal vaccine and by antibiotic prophylaxis of contacts of patients with meningococcal disease. Nasopharyngeal colonization with *N. meningitides* occurs in 5–10% of the population in the United States, but invasive disease occurs in only 1–2 per 100,000 population. Increasing reports of outbreaks in college dormitories have prompted the Advisory Committee on Immunization Practices to recommend considering vaccination of incoming college students (38). Invasive meningococcal disease occurs in patients without bactericidal or opsonizing antibodies. Meningococcal polysaccharide vaccines that induce serum bactericidal antibodies have been shown to be efficacious in controlling outbreaks and epidemics. The current available polysaccharide vaccines target the serogroups A, C, Y, and W-135. Unfortunately, these vaccines are less immunogenic in children less than 2 years of age, have a T-cell-independent mechanism without a booster response, and do not create herd immunity by decreasing nasopharyngeal carriage (39). As with *H. influenzae* and *S. pneumoniae*, serogroup A, C, Y, W-135 meningococcal polysaccharides have been chemically conjugated to carrier proteins. These improved vaccines are currently undergoing clinical trials and have shown to induce a T-cell-dependent response that improves immune response in infants and lead to booster response phenomena with subsequent doses. The conjugate vaccines may also provide herd immunity by decreasing nasopharyngeal colonization. Serogroup B accounts for one-third of all cases of meningococcal disease in the United States and almost two-thirds of the cases in France (31, 39). Unfortunately, the immunogenicity of the capsule of the serogroup B meningococcus is poor because the capsule possesses a component (polysialic acid) that is present in fetal neural tissue. Noncapsular antigens (e.g., outer membrane proteins) have been investigated in the prevention of meningococcal disease in outbreak settings. Other targets for vaccination against serogroup B include other outer membrane proteins, pili, exotoxins, Neisserial surface protein A, transferring-binding proteins, and intranasal vaccines.

Chemoprophylaxis

The risk of meningococcal disease is up to 1000 fold higher among close contacts (i.e., household, day care, or nursery school) of an index case than in the general population. Sulfonamides were the first drugs to be used to prevent secondary cases but because of the development of resistance, and the inability to control an epidemic at Fort Ord in 1965, sulfonamides were abandoned and used only if the isolate was known to be susceptible. Rifampin was then used at a dose of 600 mg orally twice a day and became the standard chemoprophylactic regimen in the United States. Rifampin though has some limitations: failure to eradicate the carrier state in up to 10–25% of patients; development of rifampin resistance; contraindication in pregnancy; and the requirement for 2 days of administration. Other alternatives include intramuscular ceftriaxone (250 mg for adults and 125 mg for children) and the fluoroquinolones. Several studies have evaluated the use of fluoroquinolones in the eradication of the carrier state of *N. meningitidis* (28). One single oral dose of ciprofloxacin (250, 500, or 750 mg), or ofloxacin 400 mg,

has eradicated the carrier state with good efficacy and prevented secondary cases of meningococcal meningitis.

THE ASEPTIC MENINGITIS SYNDROME

A 35-year-old female presents to the emergency department on Labor Day with a 3 day history of severe headache, nausea, vomiting, and stiff neck. Her physical and neurological examinations are unremarkable. Her CSF shows 110 WBCs with a 95% lymphocyte count. Her CSF protein is 85 mg/dl and her CSF glucose is 52 mg/dL. The CSF Gram stain shows white cells but no organisms are seen.

Definition

The aseptic meningitis syndrome was originally described by Wallgren in 1925 (41). The criteria for diagnosis included an acute presentation, CSF pleocytosis without bacteria (on Gram stain or culture), the absence of a focal central nervous system lesion or a systemic illness that could present as meningitis, and a benign clinical course. Most likely, Wallgren was referring to viral meningitis in his description of the syndrome. The term "aseptic meningitis syndrome" is now used more broadly and encompasses many treatable and untreatable causes, as well as many infectious and noninfectious etiologies (42).

Etiologic Agents of the Aseptic Meningitis Syndrome

In the 1950s diagnostic virology capabilities flourished and large-scale epidemiological studies of the aseptic meningitis syndrome were performed that identified seasonal patterns and a major role for viral etiologies, especially nonpolio enteroviruses. Over the last 40 years, case reports have documented a wide spectrum of both infectious as well as noninfectious causes of the aseptic meningitis syndrome (see Tables 5–4 and 5–5). This is probably due to an increase in the immunosuppressed population and improvements in the diagnostic microbiology, virology, and neuroradiology fields.

The aseptic meningitis syndrome has a diverse spectrum of etiologies that can be classified into four different categories. (1) Urgent treatable cause: This group includes patients with meningitis that require urgent therapy and admission for cure and survival. Etiologies determined to represent urgent treatable causes include bacterial meningitis; fungal meningitis; *herpes simplex virus, varicella zoster virus,* or *cytomegalovirus*

Table 5–4. Infectious Etiologies of the Aseptic Meningitis Syndrome

Viral etiologies

Enteroviruses[a]	Polioviruses
Human immunodeficiency virus	Varicella-Zoster
Lymphocytic choriomeningitis virus	Cytomegalovirus
Mumps virus	Epstein-Barr virus
Herpes simplex types 1 and 2	Influenza A and B
Arboviruses[b]	Measles
Reovirus tupe 1	Adenoviruses
Parvovirus B-19	Rubella

Bacterial etiologies

Bacterial meningitis	*Chlamydia* sp
Parameningeal focus[c]	*Rickettsia* sp.
Leptospirosis	*Ehrlichia* sp.
Bacterial endocarditis	*Brucella* sp.
Lyme disease	*Bartonella henselae*
Treponema pallidum	Nocardia/actinomycosis
Mycobacterium tuberculosis	Mycoplasma

Fungal | **Parasitic**

Cryptococcus neoformans	Naegleria
Coccidiodes immitis	Acanthamoeba
Histoplasma capsulatum	Taenia solium
Candida species	Schistosomiasis
Aspergillus	Angiostrongylus cantonensis
Paracoccidiodes	Toxoplasma gondii

[a] Most common cause of aseptic meningitis.
[b] In the United States, the more important arboviruses include West Nile, St. Louis, California, Eastern Equine, Western Equine, and Venezuelan encephalitis.
[c] Brain abscess, sinusitis, otitis, mastoiditis, subdural abscess, epidural abscess, venous sinus thrombophlebitis, pituitary abscess, cranial osteomyelitis.
Source: Adapted from (32).

Table 5–5. Noninfectious Etiologies of the Aseptic Meningitis Syndrome

Medications	*Systemic illnesses*
Nonsteroidal antiinflammatory drugs	Connective tissue disorders
Antimicrobial agents	Sarcoidosis
Muromonab-CD3 (OKT3)	Behcet disease
Azathioprine	Vasculitis and Kawasaki disease
Carbamazepine	Vogt-Koyanagi-Harada syndrome
Immune globulin	Serum sickness
Ranitidine	
Phenazopyridine	

Tumors	**Procedure-related**
Intracranial tumors and cysts	Spinal anesthesia
Meningeal carcinomatosis	Postneurosurgery
Lymphoma	Intrathecal injections
Leukemia	Chymopapain injections

Source: Adapted from (32).

meningoencephalitis; rickettsial meningoencephalitis; bacteremia; meningeal carcinomatosis; central nervous system vasculitis; parameningeal mass lesions (e.g., *tumor* or *abscess*); or subarachnoid hemorrhage. (2) Treatable but not urgent cause: This group includes patients with meningitis that require therapy but not urgently. Etiologies determined to represent nonurgent treatable causes of the aseptic meningitis syndrome include Lyme disease, neurosyphilis, and acute primary HIV infection. (3) Untreatable cause: This group includes patients who have an established diagnosis for their meningitis but for which there is currently no therapy available. Etiologies in this group include the enteroviruses, arboviruses (*St. Louis encephalitis* and *West Nile virus*), and Epstein-Barr virus infection. However, diagnosis of these pathogens remains essential in defining the changing epidemiology of the aseptic meningitis syndrome. Also, many of these patients will require supportive care (e.g., *West Nile virus*). (4) Unknown cause: This group represents approximately 70% of all patients who present with aseptic meningitis syndrome and includes patients for whom no etiologic agent was identified (43).

Empirical Management

Management of adults with aseptic meningitis syndrome who present to the emergency department is controversial. Physicians recognize that aseptic meningitis may have etiologies that require urgent therapy, but are uncertain of the probability for an urgent treatable cause in an individual patient. This has fostered costly diagnostic testing, unnecessary hospitalization, and empiric antimicrobial therapy for most patients (43). Investigators have attempted to use either clinical features or technological assays of the initial CSF sample to differentiate between adult patients with bacterial meningitis and "viral meningitis." Spanos and colleagues (44) developed a predictive model to help to distinguish between acute bacterial meningitis and acute viral meningitis in patients greater than 1 month of age. However, several methodologic concerns exist regarding this model. First, the study group was limited to hospitalized, immunocompetent patients at tertiary care centers with a discharge diagnosis of meningitis. This restriction of the cohort raises concerns about the generalizability of the model. The patients who were not hospitalized, immunocompromised and those presenting with aseptic meningitis but who had other urgent treatable causes (e.g., bacteremia, parameningeal focus, fungal, meningeal carcinomatosis, etc.) were excluded. Because the cohort was assembled retrospectively, all the potential clinical variables

that could have been predictive in a model were not assessed in every case.

Other investigators have attempted to use CSF assays to distinguish between viral and bacterial meningitis. Technological assays that have been used include enteroviral RNA PCR, cytokine levels, ferritin, C-reactive protein, histamine, enzymes, metabolites of biogenic amines, and a broad-range bacterial PCR assay(42). The role of many of these tests in the acute care setting remains unclear because the results of most of these tests are not available within the time frame needed to make management decisions and many are not available in all hospital laboratories. A recent unpublished prospective study of 151 patients with aseptic meningitis syndrome presenting to the emergency departments of the Medical Center of Louisiana in New Orleans and at Tulane University Hospital have identified independent baseline clinical factors associated with an urgent treatable etiology (45). The factors are divided into abnormal host variables (age >65 years, HIV/AIDS, intravenous drug use), abnormal examination variables (Glasgow Coma Scale <15, vesicular or petechial rash), and abnormal CSF variables (elevated CSF protein >100 mg/dL and CSF glucose <45 mg/dL).

DISPOSITION AND OUTCOME

In the recent Dutch study, the overall mortality rate of bacterial meningitis was 21%, pneumococcal meningitis had a higher case rate than meningococcal meningitis (30% vs. 7%, $P < 0.001$) (4). Factors associated with death or with severe neurological sequelae were mostly driven by the presence of systemic compromise (positive blood culture, tachycardia, elevated ESR, thrombocytopenia, low CSF WBC, and abnormal mental status) and the presence of pneumococcal meningitis (presence of otitis media or sinusitis, absence of petechial rash, and advanced age).

Given the high mortality and morbidity associated with bacterial meningitis, all patients with suspected bacterial meningitis, based upon clinical and laboratory findings, should be admitted to the hospital with intravenous empiric antibiotics and steroids pending the results of CSF and blood cultures.

In patients presenting with the aseptic meningitis syndrome, the disposition is controversial and should be based on a case-by-case basis. Admission should be warranted if variables associated with an urgent treatable cause are present (immunosuppression (HIV/AIDS), intravenous drug users, age >65, abnormal mental status changes, vesicular or petechial rash, decreased CSF glucose <45 mg/dL, and increased CSF protein >100 mg/dL). If the patient is discharged, close follow-up should be arranged prior to disposition.

CASE OUTCOME

Empirical intravenous vancomycin and ceftriaxone therapy was administered. The patient developed seizures after the initiation of antibiotic therapy and required mechanical ventilation. He died 3 days later.

Key issues are as follows:

- Despite antibiotic therapy pneumococcal meningitis is still associated with a 30% mortality rate.

- Dexamethasone therapy decreases mortality in patients with pneumococcal meningitis and should be started empirically before the first dose of antibiotic therapy.

- Antibiotic therapy should be started before lumbar puncture and should not be delayed because of the head CT scan.

CONCLUSION

Despite the availability of effective antibiotic therapy, the morbidity and mortality of patients with bacterial meningitis remains unacceptably high. Treatment of bacterial meningitis is currently evolving because of major epidemiological shifts. Routine use of the *H. influenzae* conjugate vaccine has markedly reduced the incidence of this pathogen and has made *S. pneumoniae* the predominant organism causing bacterial meningitis in the United States. The emergence of penicillin- and cephalosporin-resistant *S. pneumoniae* has further complicated the therapeutic approach of patients presenting with bacterial meningitis.

The differential diagnosis of the aseptic meningitis syndrome is becoming more complex for the emergency department physician; outcome studies could aid in the future in accurately selecting a subgroup of patients that can be safely managed as outpatients.

In the future, improvement in the outcome of patients with bacterial meningitis will depend on the continued development of new antimicrobial agents, continued global surveillance of antimicrobial resistance, widespread use of effective conjugate vaccines, and better selection of patients for treatment with adjunctive corticosteroids.

REFERENCES

1. Schuchat A, Robinson K, Wenger JD, et al.: Bacterial meningitis in the United States in 1995. *N Engl J Med* 337:970–976, 1997.
2. Dunne D, Quagliarello VJ: Group B streptococcal meningitis in adults. *Medicine* 72:1–10, 1993.
3. Doern G, Heilmann K, Huynh H, Rhomberg P, Coffman S, Brueggemann A: Antimicrobial resistance among clinical isolates of *Streptococcus pneumoniae* in the United States during 1999–2000, including a comparison of resistance rates since 1994–1995. *Antimicrob Agents Chemother* 45(6):1721–1729, 2001.
4. van de Beek D, de Gans J, Spanjaard L, et al.: Clinical features and prognostic factors in adults with bacterial meningitis. *N Engl J Med* 351:1849–1859, 2004.
5. Hasbun R, Abrahams J, Jekel J, Quagliarello VJ: Computed tomography of the head before lumbar puncture in adults with suspected meningitis. *N Engl J Med* 345:1727–1733, 2001.
6. Thomas K, Hasbun R, Jekel J, Quagliarello V: The diagnostic accuracy of Kernig's, Brudzinski's sign, and nuchal rigidity in patients with suspected meningitis. *Clin Inf Dis* 35:46–52, 2002.
7. Arditi M Three-year multicenter surveillance of pneumococcal meningitis in children: Clinical characteristics, and outcome related to penicillin susceptibility and dexamethasone use. *Pediatrics* 102:1987–1997, 1998.
8. Kaplan SL: Clinical presentations, diagnosis and prognostic factors of bacterial meningitis. *Infect Dis Clin N Am* 13:579–594, 1999.
9. Lorber B. Listeriosis. *Clin Infect Dis* 24:1–11, 1997.
10. Coll M, Uriz M, Pineda V, et al.: Meningococcal meningitis with 'normal' cerebrospinal fluid. *J Infect* 29:289–294, 1994.
11. George RH: Timing of lumbar puncture in severe childhood meningitis. *Br Med J* 291:1123–1124, 1985.
12. Finlay FO, Witherow H, Rudd PT: Latex agglutination testing in bacterial meningitis. *Arch Dis Child* 73:160–161, 1995.
13. Radstrom P, Backman A, Qian N, Kragsbjerg P, Pahlson C, Olcen P: Detection of bacterial DNA in cerebrospinal fluid by an assay for simultaneous detection of *Neisseria meningitidis*, *Haemophilus influenzae*, and Streptococci using a seminested PCR strategy. *J Clin Microbiol* 32:2738–2743, 1994.
14. Dagan R, Shriker O, Hazan I, et al.: Prospective study to determine clinical relevance of detection of pneumococcal DNA in sera of children by PCR. *J Clin Microbiol* 36:669–673, 1998.
15. Du Plessis M, Smith AM, Klugman KP: Rapid detection of penicillin-resistant *Streptococcus pneumoniae* in cerebrospinal fluid by a seminested-PCR strategy. *J Clin Microbiol* 36:453–457, 1998.
16. Quagliarello VJ, Scheld WM: Treatment of bacterial meningitis. *N Engl J Med* 708–716, 1997.

17. Hasbun R, Aronin S, Quagliarello V: Treatment of bacterial meningitis. *Comp. Ther.* 25(2):73–81, 1999.

18. Tunkel AR, Scheld WM: Acute meningitis. In Mandell, Douglas (ed.), *Bennett's Principles and Practice of Infectious Diseases, 5th ed.* Churchill Livingston, Philadelphia, PA, 2000; pp 959–997.

19. Roos K, Tyler K: Acute bacterial meningitis. In Braunwald E, Fauci AS, Kasper DL, Hauser SL, Longo DL, Jameson JL (eds.), *Harrison's Principles of Internal Medicine, 15th ed.*, McGraw Hill, 2001; pp 2462–2467.

20. Radetsky M: Duration of symptoms and outcome in bacterial meningitis: An analysis of causation and the implication of a delay in diagnosis. *Pediatr Infect J* 11:694–698, 1992.

21. Aronin S, Peduzzi P, Quagliarello VJ: Community acquired bacterial meningitis: Risk stratification for adverse clinical outcome and impact of antibiotic timing. *Ann Int Med* 29(11):862–869, 1998.

22. Performance standards for Antimicrobial Susceptibility Testing: Twelfth Informational Supplement. NCCLS document M100-S12. Wayne, PA, National Committee for Clinical Laboratory Standards, 2002.

23. Viladrich PF, Gudiol F, Linares J, et al.: Evaluation of vancomycin for therapy of adult pneumococcal meningitis. *Antimicrob Agents Chemother* 35:2467–2472, 1991.

24. Paris MM, Hickey SM, Uscher MI, et al.: Effect of dexamethasone on therapy of experimental penicillin- and cephalosporin-resistant pneumococcal meningitis. *Antimicrob Agents Chemother* 38:1320–1324, 1994.

25. Klugman KP, Dagan R, and the Meropenem Study Group: Randomized comparison of meropenem with cefotaxime for treatment of bacterial meningitis. *Antimicrob Agents Chemother* 39:1140–1146, 1995.

26. Schmutzhard E, Williams KJ, Vukmirovits G, et al.: A randomized comparison of meropenem with cefotaxime or ceftriaxone for the treatment of bacterial meningitis in adults. *J Antimicrob Chemother* 36(Suppl A):85–97, 1995.

27. Odio CM, Puig JR, Feris JM, et al.: Prospective, randomized, investigator-blinded study of the efficacy and safety of meropenem vs. cefotaxime therapy in bacterial meningitis in children. *Pediatr Infect Dis J* 18:581–590, 1999.

28. Hasbun R, Quagliarello VJ: Use of the quinolones in treatment of bacterial meningitis, in Andriole VT (ed.), *The Quinolones, 3d ed.* New York, Academic Press, 2000; pp 325–342.

29. Saez-Llorens X, Mccoig C, Feris J, et al.: Quinolone treatment for pediatric bacterial meningitis: A comparative study of trovafloxacin and ceftriaxone with or without vancomycin. *Pediatric Infect Dis J* 21(1):14–22, 2002.

30. Friedland IR, Paris MM, Ehrett S, Hickey S, Olsen KD, McCracken GH Jr.: Evaluation of antimicrobial regimens for treatment of experimental penicillin- and cephalosporin-resistant pneumococcal meningitis. *Antimicrob Agents Chemother* 37:1630–1636, 1993.

31. Antignac A, Ducos-Galand M, Guiyole A et al.: *Neisseria meningitides* strains isolated from invasive infections in France (1999–2002): Phenotypes and antibiotic susceptibility patterns. *Clin Infect Dis* 37(7):912–920, 2003.

32. Durand ML, Calderwood SB, Weber DJ, et al.: Acute bacterial meningitis in adults: A review of 493 episodes. *N Engl J Med* 328:21–28, 1993.

33. Quagliarello VJ, Scheld WM: Bacterial meningitis: Pathogenesis, pathophysiology and progress. *N Engl J Med* 327: 864–872, 1992.

34. Tauber MG, Khayam-Bashi H, Sande MA: Effects of ampicillin and corticosteroids on brain water content, cerebrospinal fluid pressure, and cerebrospinal fluid lactate levels in experimental pneumococcal meningitis. *J Infect Dis* 151:528–534, 1985.

35. McIntyre PB, Berkey CS, King SM, et al.: Dexamethasone as adjunctive therapy in bacterial meningitis: A meta-analysis of randomized clinical trials since 1988. *JAMA* 278:925–1031, 1997.

36. Molyneaux EM, Walsh AL, Forsyth H, et al.: Dexamethasone treatment in childhood bacterial meningitis in Malawi: A randomized controlled trial. *Lancet* 360:211–218, 2002.

37. Gans J, Diederick V, et al.: Dexamethasone in adults with bacterial meningitis. *N Engl J Med* 347:1549–1556, 2002.

38. Harrison LH: Preventing meningococcal infection in college students. *Clin Infect Dis* 30:648–651, 2000

39. Rosenstein NE, Perkins BA, Stephens DS, Popovic T, Hughes JM: Meningococcal disease. *N Engl J Med* 344: 1378–1388, 2001.

40. Levitz RE, Quintiliani R: Trimethoprim-sulfamethoxazole for bacterial meningitis. *Ann Intern Med* 100:881–890, 1984.

41. Wallgreen A: Une nouvelle maladie infectieuse du system nerveux central? *Acta Padiatr* 4:158–182, 1925.

42. Hasbun R: The aseptic meningitis syndrome in adults. *Curr Inf Dis Rep* 2:345–351, 2000.

43. Elmore JG, Horwitz RI, Quagliarello VJ: Acute meningitis with a negative Gram's stain: Clinical and management outcomes in 171 episodes. *Am J Med* 100:78–84, 1996.

44. Spanos A, Harrell FE, Durack DT: Differential diagnosis of acute meningitis: An analysis of the predictive value of initial observations. *JAMA* 262:2700, 1989.

45. Hadi C, De Salvo K, Hasbun R: Aseptic meningitis syndrome in adults: Predictors for an urgent treatable etiology in three urban hospitals. Abstract #750. Presented at *the 41*st *Annual Meeting of IDSA*, October 9–12, 2003, San Diego.

6

Acute Encephalitis

Trevor J. Mills

HIGH YIELD FACTS

1. In the acute setting, the specific etiology of encephalitis will rarely be determined. Untreated Herpes virus encephalitis has a high mortality, therefore, acyclovir (10 mg/kg IV q 8 h) should be initiated early in all cases of encephalitis.

2. Since encephalitis and meningitis share many presenting symptoms, patients with suspected encephalitis should receive early empiric antibiotic therapy for bacterial meningitis.

3. The evaluation of patients suspected of having encephalitis mandates a detailed geographic and travel history.

CASE PRESENTATION

A 23-year-old woman presents to the emergency department with her family who state that the patient is "not herself." They report that for the last 3 days the patient has been emotionally labile with subjective fever. On presentation she appears agitated. Vital signs are temperature 39.2°C, heart rate 110 beats/minute, blood pressure 105/65, and respiratory rate 18 breaths/minute. Shortly after arrival she has a generalized seizure requiring large doses of benzodiazepines to control. After the seizure she becomes unresponsive and is intubated for airway protection in the setting of a depressed mental status. Computed tomography (CT) of the head is normal. Lumbar puncture yields CSF revealing 500 red blood cells, 80 neutrophils, increased protein, normal glucose, and an increased opening pressure.

INTRODUCTION/EPIDEMIOLOGY

It is postulated that Alexander the Great died of West Nile Encephalitis (WNE) (1). He traveled in areas with endemic disease and died after a 2-week course of escalating fevers, fluctuating energy, delirium, and terminal flaccid paralysis. While the theories of his death may provide hours of heated discussion, the reality is, today, we have only slightly more to offer to victims of encephalitis than we did in 323 BC.

Encephalitis is defined by inflammation of the brain parenchyma. Classically, patients with encephalitis present with fever, altered mental status, and neurological disorders. The clinical presentation of encephalitis is similar to bacterial meningitis in the presence of headache and fever. However, encephalitis differs from bacterial meningitis in that bacterial meningitis often presents with headache, fever, and nuchal rigidity, whereas encephalitis almost always presents with headache, fever, and altered mental status, ranging from mood disorders to focal neurological deficits to coma. There is also a subtle distinction between encephalitis and aseptic meningitis. Aseptic meningitis involves inflammation of the meninges, sparing the brain parenchyma, and like bacterial meningitis, patients often have normal cerebral function. A few viruses can cause both encephalitis and meningitis, for example the enteroviruses, and the two syndromes are sometimes blurred, resulting in patients being given the diagnosis of "meningoencephalitis."

This chapter will focus on infectious causes of encephalitis in the immunocompetent adult host. For a discussion of bacterial and aseptic meningitis refer to Chapter 5. Infectious brain disorders in the setting of HIV are described in Chapter 8, and Chapter 32 includes a discussion of rabies. A discussion of neonatal Herpes encephalitis is presented in Chapter 26.

The Center for Disease Control and Prevention (CDC) estimates that there are approximately 20,000 cases of encephalitis in the United States (US) each year. The epidemiology of encephalitis demonstrates two distinct patterns, endemic causes and epidemic causes (Table 6–1).

Endemic causes of encephalitis include both infectious and postinfectious conditions. Acute infections that may cause encephalitis include the herpes viruses, rabies, the enteroviruses, the paramyxoviruses, the arenaviruses, rubella, and yellow fever. Herpes simplex virus type I (HSV-1) accounts for 10–20% of all such cases of encephalitis and is the most common cause of infectious encephalitis in the US (2). Herpes simplex virus type 2 (HSV-2) occurs in infants as a result of transmission during delivery. Infections with the rabies virus are rare, but result in encephalitis with a mortality rate greater than 95% (3). The enteroviruses are a significant cause of meningoencephalitis in the neonatal period, but infrequently cause encephalitis in older infants, children, or adults.

Rare causes of nonepidemic viral encephalitis include the paramyxoviruses (measles, mumps), the arenaviruses

Table 6–1. Epidemiology of Viral Encephalitis in the United States

Name	Pattern	Age	Frequency	Geography
HSV-1	Endemic	All ages	2–4000 cases/year	Equal in all states/regions
HSV-2	Endemic	Neonates	2–3/10,000 births	Equal in all states/regions
Rabies	Endemic	All ages	1–2 cases/year	All states, rural areas
Enteroviruses	Endemic	Neonates	2–4000 cases/year	All states
CE	Epidemic	Children	70 cases/year	East, Central
EEE	Epidemic	>50 years, <15 years	4 cases/year	Eastern Seaboard, Midwest, Gulf Coast
WEE	Epidemic	Young	16 cases/year	West of the Mississippi, rural areas
SLE	Epidemic	Young, elderly	128 cases/year	Midwest, South
WNE	Epidemic	Young, elderly	2900 cases in 2002	Continental US

(lymphocytic choriomeningitis and Lassa viruses) rubella, and yellow fever. However, in the US, measles, mumps, and rubella infections have been greatly reduced by the widespread availability of vaccines.

Encephalitis can also follow an acute viral infection with many common viruses. Postinfectious causes of encephalitis include upper airway infections, mostly caused by varacella and influenza viruses. Measles is a worldwide cause of postinfectious encephalitis.

In contrast to the endemic causes of encephalitis, epidemic outbreaks of encephalitis are the result of arthropod-borne infections and have distinct geographic and seasonal patterns. All of the arthropod-borne encephalitis viruses occur more frequently in the summer and fall, because they are dependent on seasonal vectors, for example mosquitoes. In the US, the main arthropod-borne causes of encephalitis include five major categories of viruses: California serogroup Encephalitides (CE), Eastern Equine Encephalitis (EEE), Western Equine Encephalitis (WEE), Saint Louis Encephalitis (SLE), and WNE.

California serogroup Encephalitides is one of the most prevalent arthropod-borne viruses in the US and accounted for 752 cases of encephalitis in the 1990s. La Crosse virus is the most common CE subtype and occurs in the Central States, Eastern Seaboard, and Gulf Coast. Serious infections are most commonly seen in the pediatric age groups and it has an estimated 1% mortality (4).

Eastern Equine Encephalitis also occurs along the Eastern seaboard, Midwest, and Gulf coast. There were only four reported cases in humans in 1997, with an average of 4 cases a year and an incidence of 0–14 cases a year. However, it is a highly virulent infection and there is a high mortality rate in individuals who develop the disease (50–70%).

Western Equine Encephalitis is found predominately west of the Mississippi River and occurs most often during the months of June and July. Most illnesses occur in very young children. There are approximately 16 cases a year, with a mortality rate of approximately 2–5% (5).

Saint Louis Encephalitis is the leading cause of epidemic mosquito borne encephalitis in the US, with an average of 128 documented cases a year. SLE is distributed throughout the continental US and has a mortality rate of 5–15% (6). The very young and very old are at greatest risk of permanent neurological deficits and death.

West Nile viral infections have recently risen to prominence in the US, with the first cases reported in New York City in 1999. By 2002 there were 4161 reported cases in 41 states, and a record 8500 cases were reported in 2003 (7). About 30% of cases of West Nile viral infections will progress to WNE.

Besides the five major causes of arthropod-borne encephalitis in the US, there are several less prevalent causes of epidemic outbreaks of viral encephalitis. Powassen Encephalitis (PE) is the only tick-borne cause of encephalitis naturally occurring in the US. Four cases were reported in Maine and Vermont in 2001, the first cases since 1994 (8).

Venezuelan Equine Encephalitis (VEE) occurs in Central and South America, with a disease presentation much like WEE and EEE. Adults often have a nonspecific illness and severe disease is mostly limited to children. The last cluster of cases reported within the US came from Mexico to Texas in 1971.

Along with VEE, there are a number of special considerations for evaluation of travelers and immigrants with suspected encephalitis. Japanese Encephalitis is widespread throughout China, Southeast Asia, and India and it causes the greatest number of arthropod-borne viral encephalitis worldwide, estimated at more than 50,000 cases each year (9). Tick-borne encephalitis (TBE) occurs in Russia and throughout Europe. Depending on the sub-type, TBE may have a mortality rate of 5–25%. Along with the tick vector, TBE can be transmitted to humans by infected cow's and goat's milk. Murray Valley Encephalitis is endemic in New Guinea and Australia and affects mainly children.

PATHOPHYSIOLOGY/MICROBIOLOGY

Encephalitis may arise from hematogenous transmission or neuronal spread. Herpes Viruses and rabies virus both initially arise from a cutaneous exposure and are then transmitted via peripheral neuronal pathways back to the gray matter of the central nervous system (CNS).

In contrast to the neuronal spread of rabies and Herpes virus, the majority of arthropod-borne viruses are transmitted via hematogenous spread from mosquito bites. Birds serve as the amplifying host. After the initial human inoculation, viral replication ensues with seeding of the retiuloendothelial system and then, to CNS involvement. Along with mosquito bites (and rarely, tick bites), there are now reports of arthropod-borne disease transmission from blood transfusions (10), organ transplants (11), and maternal fetal transmission (12).

Regardless of the path of transmission, once the offending virus reaches the CNS, the result is perivascular inflammation, inflammatory response, and frank hemorrhage usually in the gray matter, and/or the gray-white junction.

In comparison to acute viral encephalitis, in post-infectious encephalitis, no pathogens are detected or recovered from the CNS. Perivascular inflammation and demylenation are prominent features. It is postulated that the damage to the CNS is an immune mediated process.

CLINICAL PRESENTATION

Encephalitis is often difficult to diagnose because of its nonspecific clinical presentation. The hallmarks of the disease include fever, neurological abnormalities, and altered mental status. Frequently, there is an initial "flu-like" syndrome early in the disease process. Headache, mood disorders, nausea, vomiting, and neurological symptoms, including parasthesias, paralysis, cranial nerve palsies, generalized weakness, and seizures, are common presenting symptoms. The elderly and very young have the greatest risk of morbidity and mortality. Not all cases will progress to a fulminate disease state, especially in healthy hosts, and many people recover from mild cases without seeking medical attention. Thus, the true prevalence of encephalitis is probably underestimated because of its non-specific symptoms and variable course.

The viruses that cause encephalitis manifest different clinical presentations depending on the CNS structures they infect.

Herpes simplex virus type 1 results in encephalitis with a rapid decline in consciousness within hours following the onset of illness. Fever is seen in up to 90% of patients, and headache, focal or generalized seizures, and partial paralysis may be present. A previous history of HSV is present in up to 30% of patients. However, active herpes labialis is only detected in 10% of cases of HSV-1 encephalitis. Because HSV-1 has a predilection for the medial-temporal and inferior-frontal lobes, mood and behavior disorders, such as hypo-mania and hyper-sexuality, can occur. Likewise, in early HSV-1 encephalitis, dysarthria, gustatory and olfactory hallucinations may also exist. Approximately 5% of HSV encephalitis is a result of HSV type II infection. In contrast to HSV-1, concurrent mucocutaneous lesions are very common in HSV-2 encephalitis. California Encephalitis presents with a flu-like illness, including fever, headache, nausea, vomiting, and lethargy. Serious sequelae include seizures, paralysis, coma, and neurological deficits. EEE presents with fever, general muscle pains, headache, seizures, and coma. Even in recovery from the acute stage, many patients will suffer permanent neurological deficits. WEE infections cause mostly mild viral like syndromes. Patients infected with WEE have headache, fever, nausea, vomiting, and malaise that may progress to altered mental status and gross neurological deficits. Children more frequently develop permanent neurological deficits, found in 5–30% of severe pediatric cases. SLE often presents with a mild viral like syndrome, with severe disease resulting in headache, fever, and meningoencephalitis. The elderly are at greatest risk for encephalitis and death. West Nile Encephalitis can present with a meningoencephalitis, or true encephalitis. Fever is present in more than 90% of cases and is associated with headache, weakness, nausea, and vomiting in 50%. Peripheral neuropathy, focal paralysis, diffuse weakness or a Guillain-Barre-like syndrome may also occur with WNE (13).

LABORATORY/DIAGNOSITIC TESTING

The laboratory investigation of suspected encephalitis should include serum CBC, electrolytes, BUN and creatinine, urinalysis, blood cultures, and urine cultures. While none of the aforementioned tests will specifically diagnose encephalitis, they may be useful in excluding other reasons for fever and altered mental status.

In the emergency department, lumbar puncture (LP) for cerebral spinal fluid (CSF) analysis will provide the largest clues toward diagnosis. However, in the setting of focal neurological deficits, altered mental status, age greater than 60 years, or immunocompromised status, CT of the head should be performed prior to LP, to reduce the possibility of herniation from mass lesion (14).

When performing the LP, the opening pressure of the CSF should be measured during LP, because it may be elevated with encephalitis. Cerebral spinal fluid should be obtained for protein, glucose, Gram-stain, cell count with differential, bacterial cultures, viral cultures, fungal cultures, acid-fast bacillus, India ink stain, and VDRL testing. Cerebral spinal fluid analysis will help rule out acute bacterial and fungal causes of meningitis. In encephalitis, the CSF usually shows a low number of WBCs (10–200), with a predominance of lymphocytes. CSF protein may be slightly elevated, but glucose is usually normal. Additionally, polymerase chain reaction (PCR) testing of the CSF can help detect HSV, the enteroviruses, and WNE. In particular, PCR of the CSF for HSV DNA has an extremely high sensitivity (98%) and specificity (94–100%) (15, 16). Polymerase chain reaction for detection of enteroviruses can yield a diagnosis in up to 75% of patients with culture negative aseptic meningitis. The IgM antibody for West Nile Virus can also be isolated in CSF and serum. Serum ELISA testing for IgM can isolate many of the arthropod-borne viruses. Serum ELISA testing for the arthropod-borne viruses will be available mostly at state-run laboratories.

Imaging studies include CT of the head or magnetic resonance imaging (MRI). Both may help to rule out other disease processes that mimic encephalitis, such as intracranial hemorrhage, brain masses, or meningitis. Early in the course of encephalitis, CT is usually normal, while MRI may be normal or show changes consistent with edema and inflammation of the basal ganglia, cortex, and gray–white matter junction. Magnetic resonance imaging in the setting of HSV encephalitis can show focal edema and hemorrhage in the frontal and temporal lobes. Eastern Equine Encephalitis produces focal abnormalities involving the basal ganglia and thalami.

MANAGEMENT

Emergency department management of the patient with suspected encephalitis involves administration of intravenous acyclovir (10 mg/kg every 8 h), empiric antibiotics for coverage of bacterial meningitis, and supportive care. Since HSV encephalitis is the only treatable cause of viral encephalitis, and acyclovir has a low adverse reaction/complication rate, empiric administration of intravenous acyclovir is indicated in all cases of suspected encephalitis. Acyclovir may be discontinued when HSV infection is eliminated from the differential diagnosis by PCR of the CSF. For specific antibiotics for the empiric treatment of bacterial meningitis see Chapter 5.

Supportive care should include the establishment of intravenous access, fluid resuscitation as needed, and continuous cardiac and blood pressure monitoring. If the patient has a seizure, then anticonvulsant medications and seizure precautions should be implemented. Systemic administration of steroids should be reserved for patients with signs and symptoms of eminent herniation, such as decreased mental status, oculomotor paresis, and hemiparesis or total paralysis.

All cases of confirmed encephalitis should be reported to the local and state health department.

PREVENTION

The primary prevention mechanism of arthropod-borne diseases should include clothing barriers and insect repellants. For those travelers who request additional assistance in the prevention of encephalitis, there are vaccinations for people who may have a high probability of exposure to endemic JE, rabies, and yellow fever.

DISPOSITION

Patients with suspected encephalitis should be admitted to an intensive care unit with input from a combination of critical care, neurologists, and infectious disease specialists.

CASE OUTCOME

The emergency physician immediately recognized the potential for encephalitis and administered intravenous acyclovir and antibiotics and admitted her to the intensive care unit. HSV 1 was detected in the CSF by PCR. After a week of intensive care, she made a full recovery.

REFERENCES

1. Marr JS, Calisher CH: Alexander the Great and West Nile virus encephalitis. *Emerg Infect Dis* 9:12, 1599–1603, 2003.

2. Whitley RJ: Viral encephalitis. *N Engl J Med* 323:242–250, 1990.

3. Centers for Disease Control and Prevention: First human death associated with Raccoon Rabies, Virginia 2003. *MMWR Morb Mortal Wkly Rep* 52:1002–1003, 2003.

4. McJunkin JE, Reyes ED, Irazuztz JE, et al. : La Crosse encephalitis in children. *N Engl J Med* 344:801–807, 2001.

5. Goddard J: Viruses transmitted by mosquitoes: La Crosse encephalitis. *Infect Med* 17:407–410, 2000.

6. Tsai TF: Arboviral infections in the United States. *Infect Dis Clin North Am* 5:89–93, 1991.

7. West Nile virus activity, United States, Nov 13–19, 2003 *MMWR Morb Mortal Wkly Rep* 52:1132, 2003.

8. Outbreak of Powassan encephalitis, Maine and Vermont, 1999–2001. *MMWR Morb Mortal Wkly Rep* 50:761, 2001.

9. Tsai TF: Factors in the changing epidemiology of Japanese encephalitis and West Nile fever, in Saluzzo JF, Dodet B (eds.): *Factors in the Emergence of Arbovirus Diseases.* Paris, Elsevier, 1997; pp 179–189.

10. Pealer LN, Marfin AA, Petersen LR: Transmission of West Nile virus through blood transfusion in the United States in 2002. *N Engl J Med* 349:1236–1245, 2003.

11. Iwamoto M, Jernigan DB, Gausch A, et al.: Transmission of West Nile virus from an organ donor to four transplant recipients. *N Engl J Med* 348:2196–2203, 2003.

12. Intrauterine West Nile virus infection, New York 2002. *MMWR Morb Mortal Wkly Rep* 51:1135, 2002.

13. Sejvar JJ, Haddad MB, Tierney BC, et al.: Neurologic manifestations and outcome of West Nile virus infection. *JAMA* 290:511–515, 2003.

14. Hashburn R, et al.: Computed tomography of the head before lumbar puncture in adults with suspected meningitis. *N Engl J Med* 345:1727–1733, 2001.

15. Lakeman FD, Whitley RJ: Diagnosis of herpes simplex encephalitis: Application of polymerase chain reaction to cerebrospinal fluid from brain-biopsied patients and correlation with disease. *J Infect Dis* 171:857–863, 1995.

16. Aurelius E, Johansson B, Skoldenberg B, et al.: Rapid diagnosis of herpes simplex encephalitis by nested polymerase chain reaction assay of cerebrospinal fluid. *Lancet* 337: 189–192, 1991.

17. Provisional surveillance summary of the West Nile virus epidemic, United States, January–November 2002. *MMWR Morb Mortal Wkly Rep* 51:1129, 2002.

18. Whitley RJ, Kimberlin DW: Viral encephalitis. *Pediatr Rev* 20:192–198, 1999.

19. Chou JT, Rossignol PA, Ayres JW : Evaluation of commercial insect repellents on human skin against Aedes aegypti. *J Med Entomol* 34:624–630, 1997.

20. Johnson R: Acute encephalitis. *Clin Infect Dis* 23:219–224, 1996.

7

Epidural Abscess and Brain Abscess

Lisa D. Mills

HIGH YIELD FACTS

1. Patients with intracranial and spinal epidural abscesses may be afebrile at presentation.

2. The clinical scenario guides the selection of empiric antibiotic choice.

3. Early neurosurgical or spinal orthopedic consultation comprises a mandatory aspect of the management of central nervous system abscess.

4. Magnetic resonance imaging (MRI) is the imaging study of choice for the diagnosis of central nervous system abscesses. Computed tomography (CT) with contrast misses small abscesses and early cerebritis.

CASE PRESENTATION

A 34-year-old man returns to the emergency department for the third visit in 10 days. He reports low back pain that is no longer relieved by acetaminophen with hydrocodone. He states that the pain is now radiating down his right leg. He denies fever, trauma, incontinence, and extremity weakness.

His vital signs reflect an afebrile, normotensive patient without tachycardia or tachypnea. He is agitated and complains of severe pain. Physical examination reveals midline tenderness to palpation midline, along the thoracic vertebral bodies 10–12. The neurologic examination is normal. He has "track marks" along both forearms that are not infected, although the patient adamantly denies intravenous drug use.

INTRODUCTION/EPIDEMIOLOGY

Focal central nervous system infections occur extracranially and intracranially. Extracranial abscesses located between the meninges and the vertebral body are spinal epidural abscesses. Spinal epidural abscesses can occur along any level of the spine; however, the thoracic and lumbar spine are more commonly affected than the cervical spine (1). Intracranial abscesses can be located outside of the dura or within the brain parenchyma. Intracranial abscesses located outside of the meninges are epidural abscesses. Abscesses located within the brain parenchyma are called brain abscesses.

Spinal epidural abscesses occur more frequently than intracranial epidural abscesses at a rate of 9:1 (2). Spinal epidural abscess accounts for 2–28 per 100,000 hospital admissions per year and occurs at a rate of 1 per 1930 epidural catheters (3–5). The incidence of spinal epidural abscess has been increasing since the 1980s (3, 6, 7). The peak incidence is in patients aged 60–70 years (3).

Despite advances in imaging, antimicrobial therapy, and surgical interventions, there remains significant morbidity and mortality associated with spinal epidural abscess (8). Significant morbidity occurs in approximately 33% of patients (7). Mortality ranges from 18 to 23% (9, 10). Risk factors for poor outcomes include the presence of co-morbidities, previous spinal surgery, presence of severe neurologic deficit, and infection with methcillin-resistant *Staphyloccus aureus* (MRCS) (8). Delay of surgery for more than 24 h in patients with neurologic deficit results in less recovery of neurologic function (7). Early diagnosis and intervention are the most effective means to decrease the morbidity and mortality of spinal epidural abscess.

Brain abscesses are responsible for 1 in 10,000 hospital admissions annually (11). Brain abscesses occur predominately in men and the average age is 30–40 years. The exception is infection stemming from a paranasal focus, in which case, the median age is 10–30 years. Endocarditis resulting from intravenous drug use is an important risk factor for the development of brain abscesses. Twenty-five percent of focal intracranial infections occur in children less than 15 years (12, 13). Twenty to forty percent of intravenous drug users with endocarditis develop central nervous system infections. The incidence of intracranial abscess is increasing.

Factors likely contributing to the increased incidence of brain abscess are the growing number of people living with immune compromised conditions and increasing numbers of intracranial surgical procedures (16, 13).

Even with appropriate treatment, brain abscesses are fatal in up to 30% of cases (13). Mortality has decreased dramatically with the advent of CT scanning which allows for more prompt diagnosis (17). Persistent neurologic deficit is seen in 30–50% of cases (11, 18). Morbidity and mortality due to brain abscesses are associated with four factors: fulminant clinical presentation, primary source of infection, multiple abscesses, and neurologic deficits at the time of diagnosis. Patients with a rapid progression of symptoms and decreased level of consciousness are more likely to do poorly. Otorhinoghenic sources are associated with decreased mortality (18). Early diagnosis and treatment are essential in decreasing morbidity and mortality (19).

PATHOPHYSIOLOGY/MICROBIOLOGY

Abscesses are focal collections of purulent fluid and necrotic tissue. The events leading to abscess formation included focal infection, inflammation, liquefactive necrosis, and capsule formation. In the brain, the early inflammatory process manifests as cerebritis. In the spine, the focal area of inflammation may present as diskitis. Abscesses mature when a fibrous capsule forms to isolate the necrotic area.

Spinal epidural abscess can occur in the ventral or dorsal aspects of the spinal canal. In the dorsal aspect of the spine, the dura mater does not adhere to the vertebral body, leaving a true epidural space. Anteriorly, the dura mater adheres to the vertebral bodies to the level of the lumbar spine. Where the dura mater adheres to the vertebral body, the epidural space is only a potential space. At the lumber spine, an epidural space exists in the anterior spinal canal. The epidural space in the spinal canal facilitates vertical extension of an infectious process. At the base of the skull, the epidural space again becomes a potential space. This is due to the adherence of the dura mater to the skull at the foramen magnum. Infectious processes must dissect the dura away from the skull to progress through the space. As a result, intracranial epidural abscesses tend to be restricted to a focal space and advance slowly.

Risk factors for epidural abscess include immunocompromise, overlying suppurating infection, trauma, and invasive procedures of the central nervous system. Diabetes is present in 27% of cases. Surgical procedures to the spine precede 17% of spinal epidural abscess (20). Blunt thoracic trauma precedes spinal epidural abscess in 30% of cases (22). Intravenous drug use is present in 33% of cases of spinal epidural abscess.

Because multiple organisms cause epidural and brain abscesses, the clinical scenario provides important clues to the causative organisms. Soft tissue infections and manipulation of the spinal canal during surgery or percutaneous procedures predispose patients to spinal epidural abscesses. Posterior spinal epidural abscesses are thought to be caused by hematogenous spread from distant foci of infection, such as cardiopulmonary or pelvic infections. Anterior spinal epidural abscesses are associated with

Table 7–1. Pathogens of Spinal Epidural Abscess

S. aureus	63%
M. tuberculosis	25%
Aerobic gram-negative bacilli	16%
Aerobic streptococci	9%
Staphylococcus epidermidis	3%
Anaerobes	2%
Others	1%
Unknown	6%

diskitis and vertebral osteomyelitis (3, 19). The majority of spinal epidural abscesses are caused by *S. aureus*, accounting for 60% of cases (2). *Mycobacterium tuberculosis* causes up to 25% of spinal epidural abscesses. Other common causes of spinal epidural abscess are listed in Table 7–1 (20, 7). No source of infection is identified in one-third of spinal epidural abscesses.

Intracranial epidural abscesses are usually a result of extension of local infection or direct inoculation during surgical procedures. Sinusitis, otitis media, and mastoiditis are common pre-existing conditions in patients with intracranial epidural abscess (21). Aerobic and microaerophillic streptococcus are the most common pathogens. Anaerobes, such as peptostreptococcus, are less commonly involved. Rarely, aerobic gram negative bacilli and fungi cause intracranial epidural abscesses (21). Infections following intracranial surgery are most commonly caused by staphylococci species and gram-negative bacteria.

Brain abscesses primarily arise from contiguous infection or hematogenous spread. The common sources include paranasal, dental, otologic infections, and cardiopulmonary. Otogenic abscesses are usually the result of chronic, not acute otitis (24, 25). Sinus infections spread to the brain in a predictable pattern. Frontal and ethmoid sinus infections lead to infections in the frontal lobes. Infections in the sphenoid sinuses rarely cause intracranial abscesses. Dental infections generally spread to the frontal lobes and cause a single abscess (26). Twenty-five per cent of brain abscess can be traced to a cardiac or pulmonary source, including endocarditis. Cardiopulmonary sources tend to give rise to multiple abscesses located in the distribution of the median cerebral artery at the gray white matter junction (26).

Gram-positive aerobic are the leading pathogens of brain abscess. Seventy per cent of brain abscesses are caused by aerobic and microaerophilic streptococcal species. The human oropharynx, appendix, and genital tract serve as reservoirs for streptococcus species. The

Table 7–2. Common Pathogens of Brain Abscesses

Streptococci species	70%
(aerobic, anaerobic, microaerophilic)	
S. aureus	10–15%
Anaerobes	40–100%
Bacteroides species	
Prevotella melaninogenica	
Enteric gram-negative bacilli	23–33%
Pseudomonas species	
Escherichia coli	
Klebsiella species	
Negative cultures	4%

most common streptococcus found in brain abscess is streptococcus milleri (30). *S. aureus* causes brain abscesses following trauma and neurosurgery (21, 28). When *S. aureus* is present, it is commonly the sole cultured pathogen (17).

Aerobic gram-negative bacilli are found in 23–33% of brain abscesses. They usually are found in mixed culture with Proteus species and *Pseudomonas aeruginosa* in abscesses of otic origin. Gram-negative organisms are more common in patients with immunocompromised conditions (21, 28). Rarely are they found in brain abscesses. Gram-negative bacilli follow neurosurgery or trauma (18, 30).

Both anaerobic and aerobic organisms cause brain abscesses. Anaerobic bacteria may be the primary pathogens or found in a mixed infection. They are present in 40–60% of brain abscesses. The most common anaerobic organisms are anaerobic streptococci and bacteroides species (21, 28). Anaerobic infections most often originate from the oropharynx, although they may hematogenously spread from pelvic or abdominal infections (27).

Organisms commonly associated with meningitis, such as *Streptococcus pneumonia*, *Haemophilus influenzae*, *Neisseria meningitides*, and *Listeria monocytogenes*, cause <1% of brain abscess. Facultative gram-negative organisms, such as *Citrobacter diversus*, *Proteus* species, *Serratia marcescens*, and Enterobacter species, rarely cause meningitis. However, when these organisms infect the meninges, brain abscesses often develop (28). Table 7–2 lists common pathogens of brain abscesses.

CLINICAL PRESENTATION

Epidural and brain abscesses affect the central nervous system in two ways, compression and direct invasion. In the fixed compartment of the skull and the spinal canal, expanding abscesses compress central nervous system tissue, creating pain and neurologic dysfunction. An abscess may also directly invade surrounding structures including blood vessels, spinal cord, and ventricles. This can lead to tissue destruction as the infection progresses. Clinical signs and symptoms of these abscesses depend upon their location, size, and extent of tissue invations and include pain, muscle weakness, seizures, and incontinence.

Patients with brain and epidural abscess commonly present with headache or back pain. These complaints are common among emergency department patients. Initially, patients may not have neurologic deficits to indicate a serious pathologic condition. These infections require a high index of suspicion for a timely diagnosis. Thus, it is not surprising that 30% of brain and epidural abscesses are misdiagnosed on the initial emergency department visit (20, 32, 34).

Spinal epidural abscesses most commonly present with pain. Seventy-four percent of patients complain of back or neck pain, usually focal pain with point tenderness. Three percent of patients complain of headache (33). Patients with acute spinal epidural abscess usually appear ill. Sixty-six percent have fever (20, 33).

Without treatment, symptoms of spinal epidural abscess progress from focal pain to pain radiating along a nerve root distribution. As the abscess increases in size neurologic deficits develop. The most common neurologic deficits are weakness (26%), incontinence (24%), and sensory deficits (13%) (33). Mild neurologic deficits can rapidly progress to paralysis. The severity of neurologic symptoms often does not correlate with the observed degree of cord compression. This may indicate vascular obstruction to the spinal cord (2). If symptoms of spinal cord compression occur, emergent intervention is necessary to prevent permanent paralysis.

Intracranial epidural abscess and brain abscess present with signs and symptoms of intracranial mass effect. Fever is present in only 50% of patients (11). Headache is the most common symptom, occurring in 55–70% of patients with intracranial abscess. The headache tends to be one sided and moderate to severe in intensity (28). Less than 50% of patients have the classic triad of headache, fever, and neurologic deficit (35). As intracranial pressure increases due to the expansion of the abscess, the headache becomes more painful and may be associated with nausea and vomiting. Neck stiffness occurs in 15% of patients with brain abscess. This is more commonly associated with extension of the abscess into the lateral ventricle or abscesses in the occipital lobe (28).

The most common neurologic signs resulting from brain abscess are altered mental status and hemiplegia.

These are present in approximately 50% of cases at the time of diagnosis (36, 37). Often, neurologic deficits manifest according to the location of the abscess. Patients with cerebellar abscess may present with ataxia, nausea, vomiting, and nystagmus. Abscesses located in the brainstem tend to spread along the length of the brain stem, resulting in a complex mix of neurologic deficits (36). Seventy-five percent of patients with an intracranial abscess present to the physician within 2 weeks of the onset of the infection (37). Brain abscess should be included in the differential diagnosis of patients with headache and a suppurating infection or in patients with headache, fever, and signs or symptoms of increased intracranial pressure.

Patients with intracranial epidural abscesses develop signs and symptoms due to increased intracranial pressure. These patients present with headache, nausea, vomiting, neurologic deficits, and altered mental status (2, 32). Gradenigo syndrome is a manifestation of intracranial epidural abscess that consists of unilateral face pain and lateral rectus palsy. It is caused by impingement on cranial nerves 5 and 6 by an abscess in the apex of the temporal space (2). The clinical presentation is similar to brain abscess.

DIAGNOSTIC TESTING/LABORATORY

Radiographic imaging is the gold standard in the diagnosis of central nervous system abscess. Magnetic resonance imaging is the most sensitive study for the detection of central nervous system abscess. Because MRI is not always available on an emergency basis, CT is the alternative. CT is 95–99% sensitive (39). CT with intravenous contrast may identify signs of central nervous system infection such as inflammation and mass effect (38).

The progression of acute brain infection can be followed with CT or MRI. Days 1–3 of the infection are characterized by focal infection and inflammation, known as cerebritis. On CT and MRI this presents as a nonenhancing, low density lesion. Late cerebritis presents on days 4–9. It appears as a ring-enhancing lesion on CT and MRI with contrast. Capsule and frank abscess form on days 10–14. On CT and MRI a thick capsule is seen. MRI is more effective than CT at demonstrating early cerebritis, small lesions, multifocal lesions, and brain edema (39–41, 48).

Spinal epidural abscesses often present with back pain. Plain radiographs of the spine may reveal signs of osteomyelitis if the infectious process has been present for more than 3 weeks (42). CT with intravenous contrast of the spine provides evidence of abscess and infectious processes involving the bones or soft tissues of the spine.

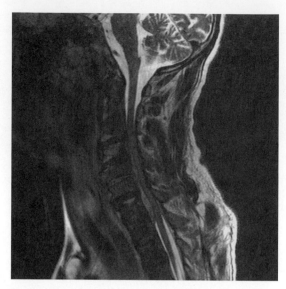

Fig. 7–1. T-2 weighted MRI of an epidural abscess of the cervical spine.

MRI better defines the extent of the abscess and spinal cord involvement. On MRI, the epidural abscess is iso- or hypointense on the T1-weighted images and hyperintense on T2-weighted images. Gadolinium enhancement shows linear enhancement surrounding the non-enhancing purulent collection (43) (Fig. 7–1 and Fig. 7–2).

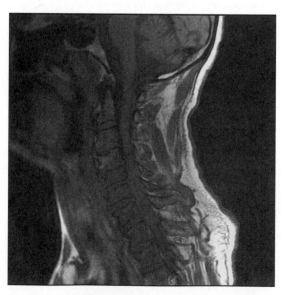

Fig. 7–2. T-1 weighted MRI of an epidural abscess of the cervical spine.

Laboratory testing includes a complete blood cell count with differential and blood cultures. The white blood cell count may be elevated or normal. The erythrocyte sedimentation rate is usually above 30 mm/h, although neither are reliably elevated in the diagnosis of brain abscess (18, 44). Blood cultures are positive in only 10% of patients with brain abscesses (28). However, the organisms cultured from the blood correlate with those isolated from the central nervous system abscesses (20).

Lumbar puncture is contraindicated in all epidural abscess and brain abscess. Twenty per cent of patients with central nervous system abscess who undergo lumbar puncture die or have marked neurologic deterioration after lumbar puncture (13). The focal mass effect is a risk for herniation with lumbar puncture.

MANAGEMENT

Management of patients with central nervous system abscess requires early consultation with a neurosurgeon or orthopedic surgeon and early administration of appropriate antibiotics. The prognosis in spinal epidural abscess is improved when decompression is achieved within 24 h of presentation (34, 45). Empiric antibiotics are indicated as soon as the diagnosis is suspected. The selection of antibiotics is dictated by the clinical circumstances. No single antimicrobial agent is sufficient for empiric therapy in central nervous system abscess. A combination of agents is required (46, 47, 51).

In patients with central nervous system abscesses resulting from trauma or surgery, gram-positive cocci, such as *S. aureus*, and gram-negative bacilli, including Pseudomonas species. Three drug therapy is generally indicated for empiric coverage. Nafcillin provides adequate coverage for gram-positive organisms. Vancomycin is an alternative if the patient is allergic to penicillin or if MRSA is prevalent in the population. Ceftriaxone or cefotaxime provides adequate gram-negative coverage, unless Pseudomonas is suspected. If Pseudomonas species is suspected, ceftazidime or cefepime should be used. Metronidazole provides excellent anaerobic coverage, due to its enhanced central nervous system penetration.

Brain abscesses resulting from sinus, oral, and ear infections involve oropharyngeal flora. Penicillin G is the mainstay of therapy in these cases. Aerobic and anaerobic streptococci will be covered by penicillin G. Penicillin G covers all oral flora, but may not cover all pathogens in the abscess. Metronidazole may be utilized as an alternative, but must be used with an antibiotic that provides aerobic coverage (35). Aminoglycosides, macrolides, tetracyclines, and first-generation cephalosporins do not effectively penetrate the central nervous system. These antibiotics should not be used to treat brain abscesses (50).

Recent experience indicates that certain patients may be candidates for antibiotic treatment without surgical intervention (47). Mature brain and epidural abscesses may lend themselves to CT-guided aspiration (48). These decisions should be made in consultation with a neurosurgeon (31).

Steroids are not a routine part of the management of central nervous system abscess. They are reserved for patients with midline shift or severe brain edema (46). The decision to administer steroids to a patient with a brain abscess should be made in consultation with a neurosurgeon.

SPECIAL CONSIDERATIONS

Immunocompromised Patients

Patients who are immunocompromised are at risk for developing brain abscess from a wider variety of pathogens. Patients with AIDS or those taking immune-modulating doses of glucocorticoids are at risk for infection with *L. monocytogenes*. Ampicillin should be added to the empiric antibiotic regimen for these patients. Antitoxoplasma agents should be empirically given until toxoplasma is definitively ruled out.

Immunocompromised patients are also at risk for fungal infections, including *Aspergillus* species, *Cryptococcus neoformans*, and *Coccidiodides immitis*. These pathogens enter the body through the lungs, seeding the brain hematogenously.

Mucormycosis is a rare fungal infection associated with brain abscess in the setting of coexisting overwhelming infections. Seventy percent of infections occur in diabetics. It usually begins as a sinusitis and progresses to brain abscess. These patients appear acutely ill. The prognosis for brain abscess in immunecompromised patients is poor. Aggressive therapy offers the best prognosis.

Cyanotic Cardiac Lesions

Patients with cyanotic heart lesions are at risk for brain abscess. This is more common in children. Brain abscess should be considered in the differential diagnosis of headache in all patients with cyanotic heart lesions (26).

Worldwide

Parasites are common pathogens of brain abscess in patients living in areas with underdeveloped sewage and sanitation systems. Cysticercosis is the most common brain infection in Mexico. Cysticercosis is treated with mebendazole. Other parasites that cause brain abscess include *Entamoeba histolytica* and *Schistosoma* species. Treatment of these infections requires a multidisciplinary approach including neurosurgeons and infectious disease specialists.

DISPOSITION

If central nervous system abscess is suspected, MRI or CT with contrast is performed. Empiric antibiotics should be started and the patient admitted. Patients with confirmed central nervous system abscess require admission to the hospital for prolonged courses of intravenous antibiotics and repeat imaging to ensure improvement.

CASE OUTCOME

Due to physical exam findings consistent with intravenous drug use and the prolonged course of the back pain, a CT scan of the lumbar spine was ordered. Blood cultures were drawn. The empiric antibiotic regimen included vancomycin, metronidazole, and cefotaxime. The CT images suggested diskitis at the fourth lumbar vertebra with possible epidural abscess. The patient was admitted to the neurosurgery service while arrangements were being made for an emergent MRI.

REFERENCES

1. Koppel BS, Tuchman AJ, Mangiardi JR: Epidural spinal infection in intravenous drug use. *Arch Neurol* 45:1331–1337, 1988.
2. Gellin BG, Weingarten K, Gamache FW, et al.: Epidural abscess, in Scheld WM, Whitley RJ, Durack DT (eds.), *Infections of the Central Nervous System, 2d ed*. New York, Raven Press, 1991.
3. Martin RJ, Yuan HA: Neurosurgical care of spinal epidural, subdural, and intramedullary abscesses and arachnoiditis. *Orthop Clin N Am* 27:125–136, 1996.
4. Lavin ML, Kaminski HJ, Ross JS, Ganz E: Spinal epidural abscess: A 10 year perspective. *Neurosurgery* 27:177–181, 1990.
5. Wang LP, Hauerberg J, Schmidt JF: Incidence of spinal epidural abscess after epidural analgesia. *Anesthesiol* 91(6), 1999.
6. Lindner A, Warmuth-Metz M, Becker G, Toyka VV: Iatrogenic spinal epidural abscess: Early diagnosis essential for good outcome. *Eur J Med Res* 2:201–205, 1997.
7. Rigamonti D, Liem L, Sampath P, et al: Spinal epidural abscess: Contemporary trends in etiology, evaluation, and management. *Surg Neurol* 52:189–197, 1999.
8. Ericsson M, Algers G, Schliamser SE: Spinal epidural abscess in adults: Review and report of 29 cases. *Neurosurgery* 22:249–257, 1990.
9. Curling OD, Gower DJ, McWhorter JM: Changing concepts in spinal epidural abscess: A report of 29 cases. *Neurosurgery* 27:185, 1990.
10. Hlavin ML, et al: Spinal epidural abscess: A ten-year perspective. *Neurosurgery* 27:177, 1990.
11. Wispelwey B, Scheld WM: Brain abscess. *Sem Neurol* 12:273, 1992.
12. Kagawa M, Takeshita M, Yatos, et al.: Brain abscess in congenital cyanotic heart disease. *J Neurosurg* 58:913, 1983.
13. Yen P, Chan S, Huang T: Brain abscess with reference to otolaryngologic sources of infection. *Otolaryngol Head Neck Surg* 113:15, 1995.
14. Tunkel AR, Pradham S: CNS infections in injection drug users. *Infect Dis Clin N Am* 16(3), 2002.
15. Tunkel AR: *Neurol Clin* 11(2):419–440, 1993.
16. Tyler KL, Martin JB, Scheld WM: Focal suppurative infections of the central nervous system, in Tyler KL, Martin JB (eds.), *Infectious Diseases of the Central Nervous System*, Philadelphia, Aduis, 1993.
17. Tunkel AR, Wispelwey B, Scheld WM: in Mendell, Douglas, Benetts (eds.), *Principles and Practice of Infectious Disease, 5th ed*. Philadelphia, Churchill Livingston, 2000.
18. Wispelwey B, Dacey RG, Scheld WM: Brain abscess, in Scheld WM, Whitley RJ, Durack DT (eds.), *Infections of the Central Nervous System 2d ed*. Philadelphia, Lippincott-Raven, 1997.
19. Mackenzie AR, Laing RBS, Smith CG, et al.: Spinal epidural abscess: The importance of early diagnosis and treatment. *J Neurol Neurosurg Psychiatry* 65:209–212, 1998.
20. Nussbaum ES, Rigamonti D, Standiford, et al.: Spinal epidural abscess: A report of 40 cases and review. *Surg Neurol* 38:225–231, 1992.
21. Ariza J, Casanova A, Viladrich Pf, et al.: Etiologic agents and primary source of infection in 42 cases of focal intracranial suppuration. *J Clin Microbiol* 24:899, 1989.
22. Vike BH, Honingford EA: Cervical spine epidural abscess in a patient with no predisposing risk factors. *Ann Emerg Med* 27:777–780,1996.
23. Griffiths DL. Tuberculosis of the spine: A review. *Adv Tuber Res* 20:92, 1980.
24. Mathews T, Marus G: Otogenic intradural complications: A review of 37 patients. *J Laryngol Otol* 102:121, 1988.
25. Heilpern KL, Lorber B: Focal intracranial infections. *Infect Dis Clin N Am* 10(4), 1996.

26. Saez-Lorens X. Brain abscess in children. *Semin Pediatr Infect Dis* 14(2):108–114, 2003.
27. Le Moal G, Landron C, Grollier G, et al.: Characteristics of brain abscess with isolation of anaerobic bacteria. *Scand J Infect Dis* 35:318, 2003.
28. Chun CH, Johnson JD, Hofstetter M: Brain abscess, a study of 45 consecutive cases. *Medicine* 65:415, 1986.
29. Hlavin ML, Kaminski HJ, Fenstermaker RA, et al.: Intracranial suppuration: A modern decade of postoperative subdural empyema and epidural abscess. *Neurosurgery* 34:974–980, 1994.
30. Gossling J: Occurrence and pathogenicity of the strep milleri group. *Rev Infect Dis* 10:257, 1988.
31. Mampalam TJ, Roseblaum ML: Trends in the management of bacterial brain abscess: A review of 102 cases over 17 years. *Neurosurgery* 23:451, 1988.
32. Brock DG, Bleck TP: Extra-axial suppurations of the central nervous system. *Semin Neurol* 12:263, 1992.
33. Reihsaus E, Waldbaur H, Seeling W: Spinal epidural abscess meta-analysis of 915 patients. *Neurosurg Rev* 232:175–204, 2000.
34. Rigamonti D, Liem L, Wolf AL, et al.: Epidural abscess in the cervical spine. *Mt Sinai J Med* 61(4):357–362, 1994.
35. Wispelwey B, Scheld WM: Brain abscess: Etiology, diagnosis, and treatment. *Infect Med* 9:13, 1990.
36. Seydoux C, Francioli P: Bacterial brain abscesses: Factors influencing mortality and sequelae. *Clin Infect Dis* 15:394, 1992.
37. Hogan RE: Sudden "stroke-like" onset of hemiparesis due to bacterial brain abscess. *Neurology* 44:569, 1994.
38. Zimmerman RA, Girard NJ: Imaging of intracranial infection, in Scheld WM, Whitley RJ, Durack DT (eds.), *Infections of the Central Nervous System, 2d ed*. Philadelphia, Lippincott-Raven, 1997, pp 923–944.
39. Bowen BC, Post MJD. Diagnostic imaging of central nervous system infection and inflammation, in Schlossberg D (ed.), *Infections of the Nervous System*. New York, Springer-Verlag, 1990; p 315.
40. Dagirmanjiam A, Schills J, McHenry MC: MR imaging of spinal infection. *MRI Clin N Am* 7(3):525, 1999.
41. Wiengarten K, Zimmerman RD, Becker RC, et al.: Subdural and epidural empyemas: MR imaging. *AM J Neuroradiol* 10:81, 1989.
42. Roca RP, Yoshikawa TT: Infections in heroin users. *Clin Orthoped Res* 144;238–240, 1979.
43. Numaguchi Y, Rigamonti D, Rothman M: Spinal epidural abscess: Evaluation with gadolinium-enhanced MR imaging. *Radiographics* 1993.44. Wispelwey B: Brain abscess, in Mandell GL, Bleck TP (eds.), *Atlas of ID (Central Nervous System and Eye Infections)*, Vol 3. Philadelphia, Churchill Livingston, 1995.
45. Liem LK, Rigamonti D, Wolf AL, et al.: Thoracic epidural abscess. *J Spinal Disord* 7:449, 1994.
46. Sjolin J, Lilja A, Eriksson N, et al.: Treatment of brain abscess with cefotaxime and metronidazole: Prospective study on 15 consecutive patients. *Clin Infect Dis* 17:857, 1993.
47. Carpenter JL: Brainstem abscesses: Cure with medical treatment, case report and review of the literature. *Clin Infect Dis* 18:219, 1994.
48. Case record of the Massachusetts General Hospital (case 430 – 1993). *N Engl J Med* 329:1335, 1993.
50. Yamamoto M, Jimbo M, Ide M, et al.: Penetration of intravenous antibiotics into brain abscesses. Experience with 9 cases. *Minim Invasive Neurosurg* 39:108–112, 1996.
51. Aseni V, Carton JA, Maradona JA, et al: Imipenem therapy of brain abscesses. *Eur J Clin Microbiol Infect Dis* 15:653–657, 1996.

8

HIV-Associated Central Nervous System Infections

Andrew Nevins
Mark Holodniy

HIGH YIELD FACTS

1. Opportunistic infections (i.e., toxoplasmosis) affecting the central nervous system (CNS) are extremely unlikely in patients with CD4 counts $>200/mm^3$. Thus, it is important to know where the patient is on the HIV disease spectrum (i.e., asymptomatic with high CD4 counts versus AIDS) in determining the differential diagnosis of CNS infections.

2. Patients who present with acute febrile illnesses associated with CNS symptoms and are not known to be HIV-infected should undergo a risk assessment for HIV infection. Those patients with significant risk factors (injection or other recreational drug use, hepatitis C virus (HCV) infection, history of (or current) sexually transmitted diseases (STDs)) should be offered rapid HIV testing.

3. Patients with significant cerebrospinal fluid (CSF) findings should be admitted and receive empiric antibacterial agents until bacterial cultures are negative and/or other serologic or culture tests reveal the diagnosis.

4. Noncontrast computed tomography (CT) brain scans have poor sensitivity in revealing significant pathology associated with HIV-associated CNS infections. Contrast-enhanced CT scans or magnetic resonance imaging (MRI) studies are preferred in revealing syndromes such as ventriculitis, basilar meningitis, abscess, or lymphoma.

CASE PRESENTATION

A 47-year-old man presents to the emergency department with a 3-day history of frontal headache, photophobia, anorexia, and low-grade fevers. He has a history of AIDS, and was hospitalized 6 months ago with cryptococcal meningitis. He denies any recent travel or exposure to animals. He cannot remember his most recent CD4 count, but thinks it is "low." He admits to relatively good compli-

ance with his antiretroviral regimen and oral fluconazole preventative therapy.

On exam, he is mildly ill-appearing with a temperature of 101.2°F. His neck is minimally stiff and he has no sinus tenderness. Oral exam reveals mild thrush. Ear exam is normal. There are no rashes on his skin. The rest of his exam, including neurologic exam, is within normal limits. A noncontrast CT scan of his head is obtained while he is being evaluated in the emergency department and is reported as normal. A lumbar puncture is performed which reveals spinal fluid with a glucose of 35 mg/dL, a protein of 220 mg/dL, and a white blood cell (WBC) count of $827/mm^3$, with a differential of 70% lymphocytes, 14% monocytes, 10% neutrophils, and 2% basophils.

INTRODUCTION/EPIDEMIOLOGY

It is estimated that there are over 40 million people worldwide with HIV-1 infection (1). In the United States, an estimated one million people are infected with approximately 40,000 new infections documented per year (2). HIV-1 infection is caused by a lentivirus (retrovirus) and in most patients without HIV-specific treatment results in profound loss of T-cell mediated (primarily CD4 cell loss) immunity over several years with subsequent development of acquired immunodeficiency syndrome (AIDS) resulting in opportunistic infections (OIs), HIV-associated malignancies, or death. AIDS is defined as having HIV-1 infection with a CD4 count of less than $200/mm^3$ or 14%. HIV-1 is transmitted mainly through sexual contact, needle sharing (injection drug use or transfusion), or during pregnancy or subsequent breast feeding.

Treatment for HIV-1 infection with highly active antiretroviral therapy (HAART) has resulted in dramatic reductions in AIDS-associated OIs and death (3). HAART significantly reduces HIV replication, resulting in CD4 T-cell increases and subsequent restoration or partial restoration of immune system function. Over 20 antiretroviral (ARV) medications and additional fixed dose combination products in four classes are currently U.S. FDA approved for use in HIV-1 infection. HAART involves combination treatment with three or more medications given daily. National treatment guidelines have been developed to help guide clinicians in the most appropriate combination regimens to be prescribed for a given patient (3). Although the benefit of HIV treatment is clearly recognized, emerging data indicate that long-term HAART can be associated with significant metabolic disturbances (i.e. lipodystrophy, diabetes), CNS-associated side effects, drug–drug interactions, and drug resistance with subsequent treatment failure.

Despite these recent treatment advances, CNS infections are still seen in patients with HIV-1 infection, although the number of serious OIs has declined significantly over the last 5 years (4). Three major groups of patients presenting with CNS infections are those with documented HIV infection who present with common bacterial or viral pathogens, those with known AIDS who present with opportunistic infections, and those who are not known to be HIV-infected yet present with opportunistic infections.

PATHOPHYSIOLOGY/MICROBIOLOGY

Organisms associated with CNS infection in HIV-infected patients are listed in Table 8–1 and can be classified into those which result in meningitis, encephalitis, focal brain lesions and myelitis (spinal cord infections). Pathogenic processes can be further classified into those

Table 8–1. Common Pathogens Associated with CNS Infections in HIV Patients

Bacteria
  S. pneumoniae
  N. meningitidis
  L. monocytogenes
  H. influenzae
  M. tuberculosis
  M. avium complex (MAC)
  N. asteroides
  T. pallidum (syphilis)
Fungi
  C. neoformans
  H. capsulatum
  C. immitis
  A. fumigatus
  Candida species
Viruses
  Herpes viruses (Herpes Simplex 1 and 2, Varicella Zoster, Cytomegalovirus)
  JC Virus (progressive multifocal leukoencephalopathy)
  Enteroviruses (Coxsackieviruses, Echoviruses)
  Adenovirus
  West Nile virus and other arboviruses
Parasites
  T. gondii

occurring as a result of recent exposure and those infections acquired earlier in life and for which acute disease is the result of reactivation of existing infection due to immunodeficiency. Routine bacterial pathogens (in decreasing order of prevalence) such as *Streptococcus pneumoniae, Neisseria meningitidis, Listeria monocytogenes, Haemophilus influenzae, Nocardia asteroides, Treponema pallidum* (syphilis), *Borrelia burgdorferi* (Lyme disease), and viral infections such as HIV, enteroviruses, or arboviruses (including West Nile virus) are usually the result of more recently acquired infection. Infections with these pathogens can occur at any stage of HIV infection. Bacterial infections in HIV-infected patients are significantly more common than in HIV-uninfected patients (5). Organisms such as *Toxoplasma gondii, Histoplasma capsulatum, Mycobacterium tuberculosis, Cryptococcus neoformans, Coccidiodes immitis, Aspergillus fumigatus*, and herpes viruses such as Cytomegalovirus (CMV), Herpes simplex (HSV) or Varicella zoster (VZV), are either acquired in childhood or after some prior subclinical exposure during adulthood and are subsequently kept in check by an intact immune system. Therefore, these agents usually cause disease as a result of reactivation, rather than new infection, and are more likely to cause disease in patients with profound immune suppression associated with AIDS (CD4 count $<100/mm^3$).

Organisms more likely to result in meningitis include *S. pneumoniae, N. meningitidis, L. monocytogenes, H. influenzae, T. pallidum, M. tuberculosis, C. neoformans,* and *C. immitis.* Viruses including HIV, enteroviruses, and arboviruses may present with an encephalitis- or meningoencephalitis-type picture. Organisms more likely to result in focal brain lesions include *T. gondii,* and less commonly *M. tuberculosis, Cryptococcus, Nocardia,* and *Aspergillus* species. Herpes viruses can result in meningitis, retinitis, meningoencephalitis, or myelopathies. JC virus has been shown to be the causative agent in progressive multifocal leukoencephalopathy (PML).

Other causes of CNS disease that are important to mention as they figure prominently in the differential diagnosis of CNS infections in HIV-infected patients include the AIDS dementia complex (ADC) and primary CNS lymphoma secondary to EBV infection. It is also important to note that several HIV-specific medications can cause CNS-type symptoms and patients may present to the emergency department if they had not been previously counseled on expected side effects. A comprehensive list of side effects is beyond the scope of this chapter. The reader is referred to the U.S. Department of Health and Human Services (HHS) guidelines on antiretroviral therapy for a complete listing (3). However, some ARV medications such as zidovudine (ZDV, AZT, Retrovir®, Combivir®, Trizivir®) can cause significant headache or flu-like symptoms, and efavirenz (Sustiva®) can cause hallucinations and sleep disturbances. Furthermore, a number of medications commonly utilized in the setting of HIV, including isoniazid (INH) and trimethoprim-sulfamethoxazole (TMP-SMX), may cause aseptic meningitis.

Many of these organisms are acquired as a result of inhalation or through contact with contaminated material or soil, or through direct percutaneous or sexual contact. Sinopulmonary bacterial infections and infective endocarditis can result in subsequent blood stream infection with resultant infectious embolic dissemination or direct extension into surrounding meningeal, brain, or spinal cord tissue. In general, organisms cause local meningeal or brain parenchymal inflammation, which results in white blood cell recruitment with subsequent inflammatory cytokine release. Extensive recruitment of white blood cells results in local destruction of brain tissue, which can further result in surrounding edema and neurologic sequelae.

CLINICAL PRESENTATION

CNS infections manifesting as meningitis usually present with constitutional symptoms such as headache, stiff neck (meningismus), photophobia, and fever. In more severe cases, nausea, vomiting, gait disturbances, altered sensorium, and seizures can occur. These latter symptoms are usually associated with increased intracranial pressure. Intracranial abscesses and other focal brain lesions can also result in these symptoms and may present with additional symptoms suggestive of a mass effect (i.e., weakness, plegia, and sensory deficits). CNS infections of the spinal cord or infectious myelopathies usually present with neurologic deficits (sensory or motor) that are localized to the spinal cord level (6). Physical examination to elicit the Kernig sign, Brudzinski sign, and nuchal rigidity has not been found to be predictive of meningitis (7). Rash may be present in certain kinds of infections such as *N. meningitidis* or acute HIV infection (see below).

Patients who are acutely infected with HIV can present with meningoencephalitis (8). The syndrome usually begins within 2 weeks of infection. Patients usually complain of a flu-like illness manifested by fever, cervical lymphadenopathy, a macular truncal rash, aphthous oral ulcers, and meningitis-type symptoms (9). One percent or more of patients presenting with acute meningitis-type symptoms have been reported to be acutely HIV-infected (10). Although many people do not seek medical attention, as the symptoms are relatively mild and nonspecific, some patients will present with this syndrome, which can last from 1 to several weeks. Routine HIV enzyme immunoassay (EIA) and Western Blot assays (including rapid HIV tests) may be negative or indeterminate at this point, however (11). Patients are viremic, and although not approved for HIV diagnosis, plasma HIV-1 viral load (HIV RNA) assays will be positive. However, these test results would not be available in the emergency department due to the prolonged turn-around time (TAT).

Patients who are chronically HIV-infected can suddenly develop meningoencephalitis presumably due to HIV infection itself (12). In addition, patients receiving HAART who suddenly discontinue these medications can also present with an acute retroviral syndrome (resembling acute HIV infection) including meningitis (13, 14). Finally, patients with advanced HIV infection who initiate HAART can develop immune reconstitution inflammatory syndrome (IRIS), which is manifested by clinical deterioration despite improvement in the immune system. Atypical presentation of CNS tuberculosis, cryptococcal meningitis, PML, or cytomegalovirus uveitis as a consequence of IRIS has been described (15).

The presentation of routine bacterial or viral meningitis, and of viral encephalitis or meningoencephalitis, is not inherently different in HIV-infected patients. Symptoms usually develop within 1–3 days. Symptoms associated with focal brain lesions such as from toxoplasmosis, CNS lymphoma, or PML are nonspecific and usually develop over weeks and include altered mental status, hemiparesis, and visual disturbances, among others. Syphilitic CNS infections can also present with a vasculitic syndrome resulting in symptoms resembling stroke. Stroke and seizures are often seen as a consequence of CNS OIs and are more common in HIV-infected young people (aged 25–45 years) compared to age matched uninfected controls (16, 17). Cognitive-behavioral illnesses such as ADC and PML are of insidious onset and include memory and concentration difficulties, depression, personality changes, and possibly gait disturbances (18, 19). Finally, patients may present with visual complaints including visual field deficits, eye pain, floaters, and blurred vision, among others. Fundoscopic examination may reveal retinitis as a result of herpes viruses (primarily CMV), toxoplasmosis, or *Candida*. More extensive CNS involvement may be present as evidenced by additional symptoms described above.

LABORATORY/DIAGNOSTIC TESTING

The workup for CNS infections usually begins with a brain imaging study and lumbar puncture in order to obtain cerebrospinal fluid. Routine CSF tests should always include a WBC count and differential, total protein, and glucose. Additional tests could include syphilis-associated Venereal Disease Research Laboratory (VDRL) test; cryptococcal antigen (CRAG); routine bacterial, fungal and mycobacterial cultures; and polymerase chain reaction (PCR) tests for HSV, CMV, EBV, or JC virus, depending on the differential diagnosis.

In order to interpret CSF findings, one must first understand what abnormalities are present with HIV infection alone. HIV is a neurotropic virus and is found throughout brain tissue and CSF. During acute HIV infection, most patients will have a lymphocytic pleocytosis, normal glucose, and mildly elevated protein levels. During chronic HIV infection (after more than 6 months), and in the absence of other CNS infections, more than a third of patients will have normal CSF findings (20, 21), although over half will have minimally increased lymphocyte counts ($<50/mm^3$), normal glucose, and mildly elevated protein (range 50–70 g/dL) levels. These mild abnormalities persist over time (22, 23).

Other viral or bacterial infections will result in further abnormalities. Numerous studies have concluded that bacterial infections in general have CSF WBC counts $>2000/mm^3$ with a neutrophil predominance ($>1000/mm^3$), CSF glucose is usually decreased (<40 mg/dL), and total protein is usually elevated (>100 mg/dL). In addition, a CSF: serum glucose ratio of <0.3 has been found to be predictive of bacterial meningitis (24, 25). Viral infections manifest with moderately elevated CSF WBC counts ($<1000/mm^3$) with mononuclear cell predominance. CNS involvement with CMV typically produces a mononuclear cell reaction in CSF. However, in CMV-associated myelopathy a neutrophil-predominant reaction has been described (26, 27). The timing of lumbar puncture relative to the onset of symptoms may show fewer cells early in bacterial infection followed by a rapid increase in neutrophils over time (28). Glucose levels are usually normal and protein is normal to minimally elevated. Other tests that have proven useful in predicting CNS bacterial infection include serum and CSF procalcitonin (a prohormone of calcitonin produced by c-cells in the thyroid) and C-reactive protein (CRP) (29–31).

A CSF Gram stain is positive in only 20–50% of bacterial infections. Bacterial cultures for common pathogens are usually positive in 24–72 h. However, bacterial culture results may be difficult to interpret in the face of ongoing OI antimicrobial prophylaxis with a sulfonamide and/or macrolide antibiotic. PCR tests for HSV, CMV, JC virus (for PML), and EBV (for lymphoma) are very useful and have adequate sensitivity and specificity. However, their long turnaround time renders them less helpful in the emergency department in establishing a diagnosis. Viral culture for herpes viruses is of little clinical utility. Diagnosis of tuberculosis meningitis is somewhat more difficult. Tuberculous meningitis-associated CSF findings are nonspecific. Although culture remains the gold standard, it is positive in only a minority of cases and usually takes weeks for results to come back. PCR tests for the diagnosis of tuberculosis are sometimes used but may not be very useful (32). Neurosyphilis is usually a late complication of syphilitic infection. HIV-infected patients who are found to have positive serum rapid plasma reagin (RPR) or syphilis EIA tests should undergo lumbar puncture to rule out neurosyphilis whether they currently have symptoms or not. CSF WBC count of $>20/mm^3$ and positive CSF VDRL reactivity are usually used to define presence of neurosyphilis (33). Serum RPR titer $>1:32$ and a CD4 count $<350/mm^3$ have been found to be highly predictive of neurosyphilis (34). Serum RPR titer is also used to monitor treatment outcome, where a fourfold or greater reduction in titer is usually associated with a positive treatment response. Although most patients will demonstrate a reduction in CSF VDRL titer after treatment, some HIV-infected patients fail to normalize their VDRL titer (33). Evaluation for retreatment in these cases may be necessary.

CNS toxoplasmosis generally results in nonspecific CSF findings. Diagnosis is usually made in those patients with symptoms, brain imaging abnormalities (see below), serum, or CSF toxoplasma antibody specific tests, toxoplasma PCR or brain biopsy. In some patients toxoplasmosis blood tests will be negative despite biopsy proven disease (35). Cryptococcal meningitis results in an elevated opening pressure, markedly elevated CSF protein and decreased glucose. A serum or CSF CRAG titer is invariably positive and reduction in titer can be used to monitor treatment efficacy. CSF culture or India ink prep demonstrating the organism will be positive in a majority of patients.

Brain imaging remains an important component of the workup for HIV-associated CNS infections. Noncontrast CT scans can reveal edema, blood, mass effect, and large intracranial lesions such as abscess or tumor in the cerebrum. CT scans cannot visualize the posterior fossa or brainstem, however, and contrast is required to better define abscesses. MRI scans, on the other hand, are generally more sensitive in defining abscesses, white matter diseases such as PML and ADC, and ventriculitis. MRI scans can also be used to visualize processes in the posterior fossa, brain stem, and spinal cord (36–38).

With regard to specific diseases, toxoplasmosis will usually appear on CT scan as numerous hypodense lesions which ring-enhance with contrast. MRI is usually more sensitive in defining multiple lesions and surrounding edema and is best demonstrated on T2-weighted images. Lesions can be located anywhere in the brain parenchyma, but tend to favor the basal ganglia and corticomedullary junction. Primary CNS lymphoma is more likely to present with a solitary mass lesion located in the periventricular white matter or corpus collosum. CMV infection is often not detected by CT scan, whereas MRI scan may better reveal a periventriculitis (seen best on T2-weighted images as hyperdense lesions) or basilar meningitis. Because of the general lack of inflammatory response, PML appears on CT as hypodense, nonenhancing lesions in the subcortical white matter and on MRI as multiple small T2-weighted hyperdense lesions. ADC usually does not reveal any specific neuroimaging findings on imaging studies except for cortical atrophy in advanced cases. Cryptococcal meningitis also does not reveal any specific imaging abnormalities, unless a cryptococcal abscess (cryptococcoma) is present. Table 8–2 presents laboratory and imaging findings for the major HIV-associated CNS infections. Figure 8–1 details an algorithm for using imaging results to determine a diagnosis.

MANAGEMENT

The initial evaluation of patients who present to the emergency department with CNS-associated symptoms includes a thorough history and physical examination. In patients known to be HIV-infected, one must ascertain the stage of HIV infection and whether the patient is currently receiving HIV treatment or appropriate antimicrobial prophylaxis for OIs. Many patients, although not necessarily receiving HIV specific medications, will know their approximate CD4 count, or it can be obtained from health care personnel caring for the patient. In patients with CD4 counts $>200/mm^3$, it is unlikely that OIs will be the etiology of CNS symptoms, and this would only be likely in those patients who recently initiated HAART and have an IRIS-type syndrome. Patients with CD4 counts $<200/mm^3$ and who are not receiving antimicrobial prophylaxis with trimethoprim-sulfamethoxazole,

dapsone, and/or azithromycin are at high risk for not only *Pneumocystis carinii* pneumonia (PCP), but also toxoplasmosis and disseminated *Mycobacterium avium* complex (DMAC) infection. Most patients do not routinely receive prophylaxis against fungal infections such as cryptococcus or viral infections such as CMV or other herpes viruses, unless they are known to have had prior active infection and are currently receiving secondary preventative treatment. Recent travel or exposure history may also be important in the differential diagnosis for determining the likelihood of exposure and subsequent infection with organisms such as *H. capsulatum* or *C. immitis*.

Although the examination may reveal obvious pathology such as seizures, focal neurologic deficits, and altered sensorium, these are nonspecific findings and are unlikely to yield a specific diagnosis. Imaging and lumbar puncture are the required next procedures. If there is any delay in obtaining these procedures, empiric antibacterial therapy is required.

An algorithm for the workup of HIV-associated CNS infections is presented in Figure 8–1. It is highly recommended that MRI be used as the preferred imaging modality because it is more sensitive in discerning CNS abnormalities than noncontrast CT. Typically, however, a diagnostic workup begins with a noncontrast CT scan. If the CT scan is negative and there is no evidence of increased intracranial pressure (i.e., dilated ventricles, mass effect, etc.), a lumbar puncture to obtain CSF should be performed. If CSF findings are within normal limits, it is unlikely that bacterial or viral meningitis (except possibly HIV meningoencephalitis) is present, and no specific treatment would be required. In patients with a CSF lymphocytosis, mildly elevated protein, and normal glucose, viral meningitis (with enteroviruses or adenovirus) is highly likely. Until more specific tests like CRP or procalcitonin are validated and become readily available, most emergency department staff would initiate antibacterial therapy. If a significantly elevated CSF WBC count (with neutrophil predominance) is present with associated decreased glucose and elevated protein, bacterial or cryptococcal meningitis should be highly suspected. Cryptococcal meningitis is more likely to occur in those patients with known or presumed CD4 counts $<100/mm^3$. Bacterial and fungal cultures and serum and CSF CRAG titers should be obtained. Empiric antibacterial therapy should be initiated as outlined in Table 8–3. Typical empiric regimens might include vancomycin, ceftriaxone, and/or ampicillin, which will cover the majority of community-acquired bacterial pathogens. In those facilities where CRAG results are rapidly obtained and,

Table 8–2. Major CNS Infections in HIV Infected Patients

	Clinical Course	**Typical CD4 Count/mm^3**	**CSF Findings**	**MRI/CT Scan**	**Diagnosis**
AIDS dementia complex	Subacute or chronic	<100	↑ protein, but often normal	Atrophy and ill-defined white matter changes	Neuropsychiatric tests; mental status exam is insensitive
Toxoplasmosis	Acute	<100	↑ protein with monos; normal in ~25%	Single or multiple ring enhancing lesions with mass effect	Typical CT scan with response to empiric therapy; serum IgG+ in 85–95%
CNS Lymphoma	Usually subacute	<100	↑/↑↑ protein; normal in 40%	Solid enhancing lesions, with or without mass effect, often periventricular	Typical scan but no response to empiric toxoplasma therapy; CSF PCR for EBV
Cryptococcal meningitis	Acute, subacute, or chronic	<100	↑ protein with ↓ glucose; ↑↑ monos	Cystic lesions in basal ganglia, or no focal lesions	CSF CRAG, CSF culture, serum CRAG
CMV	Acute or subacute	<50	↑ protein with lymphs; may be normal	Periventricular inflammation/enhance ment	CSF PCR or CMV
PML	Subacute	<50	Normal	Punctuate, nonenhancing multifocal lesions without mass effect in subcortical white matter	Typical clinical course with CT scan; CSF PCR for JC virus
Tuberculosis	Chronic	<350	↑↑ protein, ↓ glucose; ↑↑ monos	Normal or with intracerebral lesions	PPD variable; CXR findings or culture + from any site; CSF culture + in 10–20% CSF PCR
Neurosyphilis	Asymptomatic Subacute mental status changes Meningeal Meningovascular Tabes dorsalis General paresis Ocular	Any	Variable; ↑ protein, ± VDRL in ~60%	Variable, often normal	CSF VDRL almost 100% specific; blood VDRL and FTA-ABS +

PML = progressive multifocal leukoencephalopathy, CSF = cerebrospinal fluid, EBV = Epstein-Barr virus, CMV = cytomegalovirus, CRAG = cryptococcal antigen, monos = monocytes, lymphs = lymphocytes.

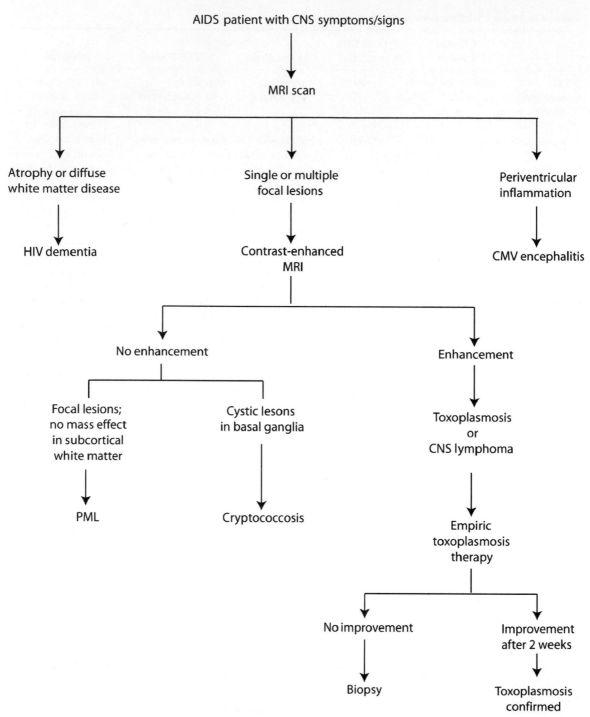

Fig. 8–1. Imaging workup for CNS-associated infections in AIDS patients (reproduced from Johnson R, Griffin JW (eds): *Current Therapy in Neurologic Disease, 4th ed.* St. Louis, Mosby-Year Book, 1993; p 151).

Table 8–3. Empiric Treatment Regimens for HIV-Associated CNS Infections

Organism	Treatment
S. pneumoniae	Ceftriaxone, 2g IV q12h; may add vancomycin IV until sensitivity of organism is known
H. influenzae	Ceftriaxone, 2g IV q12h
N. meningitidis	Ceftriaxone, 2g IV q12h or penicillin G, 2mU IV q4h
L. monocytogenes	Ampicillin, 2g IV q4h
C. neoformans	Fluconazole, 400 mg IV/PO qd or, for more severe disease, amphotericin B, 0.5–0.8 mg/kg IV qd + 5-flucytosine, 50–150 mg/kg/d PO divided qid until response, then change to fluconazole.
T. gondii	Pyrimethamine, 200 mg PO × 1, followed by 75–100 mg PO qd + sulfadiazine, 1–1.5 g PO q6h + folinic acid, 10–15 mg PO qd OR TMP-SMX, 10/50 mg/kg IV/PO qd divided q8h (clindamycin, 600 mg IV/PO q6h for sulfa-allergic patients)
M. tuberculosis	Isoniazid, 300 mg PO qd + rifampin, 600 mg PO qd + ethambutol, 15 mg/kg PO qd + pyrazinamide, 25 mg/kg PO qd (in conjunction with county health department); treatment of known multidrug resistant TB cases should be managed by an infectious diseases specialist.
Cytomegalovirus	Ganciclovir, 5 mg/kg IV q12h
Herpes Simplex Virus	Acyclovir, 10 mg/kg IV q8h
T. pallidum	Penicillin G, 3–4 million units IV q4h (for penicillin-allergic patients, either desensitize to penicillin or consult with an infectious diseases specialist)

found to be positive, treatment should be initiated with intravenous amphotericin B and oral 5-flucytosine (5-FC).

If the CT scan reveals a solitary or multiple focal lesions in a patient with presumed or confirmed AIDS (CD4 count <100/mm^3), cerebral toxoplasmosis or lymphoma should be suspected. In this setting, if a previous toxoplasma serology is known and is positive, or if the serostatus is unknown, then treatment should be initiated with a combination of pyrimethamine, leucovorin, and either sulfadiazine, clindamycin, or atovoquone. If recent toxoplasmosis serology is previously known to be negative, empiric treatment can be withheld pending further workup. Empiric toxoplasmosis therapy should not be withheld even if lymphoma is suspected based on imaging studies, as CSF cytology, EBV PCR, or stereotactic biopsy may be required to confirm this diagnosis and results would not be available for emergency department staff.

In those patients with negative noncontrast CT scan results, and in whom the neurologic exam suggests focal findings, a contrast-enhanced CT scan or MRI scan should be obtained, if available, to visualize the brain stem (basilar meningitis) and posterior fossa or to provide further detail in delineating focal lesions or ventriculitis. In patients in whom CMV retinitis or CNS disease such as meningoencephalitis is demonstrated, intravenous ganciclovir should be initiated. In AIDS patients with imaging findings consistent with PML, no specific acute treatment is required.

DISPOSITION

The vast majority of HIV-infected patients with presumptive CNS infections should be admitted. Admission is required for patients with AIDS who have significant CSF and/or imaging abnormalities, neurologic deficits, and signs of systemic illness.

CASE OUTCOME

A presumptive diagnosis of bacterial meningitis was made and the patient was given intravenous ceftriaxone and ampicillin in the emergency room and admitted to the medicine ward. CSF cryptococcal antigen and toxoplasmosis serology were reported negative later that evening. An MRI scan of the brain with gadolinium contrast performed the next day did not show evidence of abscess, ventriculitis, or meningitis. Routine bacterial cultures of CSF were negative after 3 days. CSF cytology was initially interpreted as being suspicious for cells consistent with CNS lymphoma. A repeat lumbar puncture demonstrated a reduced but significant number of mature lymphocytes with normal morphology as well as normalization of protein and glucose. PCR tests for HSV and EBV were negative. The patient's symptoms improved dramatically over the next few days and he was discharged home with a presumptive diagnosis of viral meningitis, most consistent with an enterovirus infection.

REFERENCES

1. UNAIDS. AIDS Epidemic Update, December 2003.
2. CDC. HIV/AIDS Surveillance Report U.S. HIV and AIDS cases reported through December 2002 End Year Edition Vol. 14, 2002.
3. DHHS Guidelines for the Use of Antiretroviral Agents in HIV-1-Infected Adults and Adolescents. http://www. aidsinfo.nih.gov/guidelines. October 29, 2004.
4. Sacktor N, Lyles RH, Skolasky R, et al.: HIV-associated neurologic disease incidence changes: Multicenter AIDS cohort study, 1990–1998. *Neurology* 56:21–26, 2001.
5. Almirante B, Saballs, M, Ribera E, et al.: Favorable prognosis of purulent meningitis in patients infected with human immunodeficiency virus. *Clin Infect Dis* 27:176–180, 1998.
6. Di Rocco A: Diseases of the spinal cord in human immunodeficiency virus infection. *Semin Neurol* 19:151–155, 1999.
7. Thomas KE, Hasbun R, Jekel J, Quagliarello VJ: The diagnostic accuracy of Kernig's sign, Brudzinski's sign, and nuchal rigidity in adults with suspected meningitis. *Clin Infect Dis* 35:46–52, 2002.
8. Ho DD, Sarngadharan MG, Resnick L, et al.: Primary human T-lymphotropic virus type III infection. *Ann Intern Med* 103:880–883, 1985.
9. Daar ES, Little S, Pitt J, et al.: Diagnosis of primary HIV-1 infection. Los Angeles County Primary HIV Infection Recruitment Network. *Ann Intern Med* 134(1):25–29, 2001.
10. Pincus JM, Crosby SS, Losina E, et al.: Acute human immunodeficiency virus infection in patients presenting to an urban urgent care center. *Clin Infect Dis* 37(12):1699–1704, 2003.
11. Clark SJ, Kelen GD, Henrard DR, et al.: Unsuspected primary human immunodeficiency virus type 1 infection in seronegative emergency department patients. *J Infect Dis* 170(1):194–197, 1994.
12. Wendel KA, McArthur JC: Acute meningoencephalitis in chronic human immunodeficiency virus (HIV) infection: Putative central nervous system escape of HIV replication. *Clin Infect Dis* 37:1107–1111, 2003.
13. Brenton G, Duval X, Gervais A, et al.: Retroviral rebound syndrome with meningoencephalitis after cessation of antiretroviral therapy. *Am J Med* 114:769–770, 2003.
14. Worthington MG, Ross JJ: Aseptic meningitis and acute HIV syndrome after interruption of antiretroviral therapy: Implications for structured treatment interruption. *AIDS* 17:2145–2146, 2003.
15. Shelburne SA III, Hamill RJ: The immune reconstitution inflammatory syndrome. *AIDS Rev* 5:67–79, 2003.
16. Garg RK: HIV infection and seizures. *Postgrad Med J* 75(885):387–390, 1999.
17. Qureshi AI, Janssen RS, Karon JM, et al.: Human immunodeficiency virus infection and stroke in young patients. *Arch Neurol* 54(9):1150–1153, 1997.
18. Koutsilieri E, Scheller C, Sopper S, et al.: Psychiatric complications in human immunodeficiency virus infections. *J Neurovirol* 8 (Suppl 2):129–133, 2002.
19. Dworkin MS: A review of progressive multifocal leukoencephalopathy in persons with and without AIDS. *Curr Clin Top Infect Dis* 22:181–195, 2002.
20. Appleman ME, Marshall DW, Brey RL, et al.: Cerebrospinal fluid abnormalities in patients without AIDS who are seropositive for the human immunodeficiency virus. *J Infect Dis* 158:193–199, 1988.
21. Marshall DW, Brey RL, Cahill WT, et al.: Spectrum of cerebrospinal fluid findings in various stages of human immunodeficiency virus infection. *Arch Neurol* 45:954–958, 1988.
22. Friedmann PD, Samore MH: Diagnostic characteristics of cerebrospinal fluid analysis for secondary meningitis in HIV-infected adults. *J Investig Med* 46:153–160, 1998.
23. Marshall DW, Brey RL, Butzin CA, et al.: CSF changes in a longitudinal study of 124 neurologically normal HIV-infected U.S. Air Force personnel. *JAIDS* 4:777–781, 1991.
24. Phillips EJ, Simor AE: Bacterial meningitis in children and adults. *Postgrad Med* 103:102–117, 1998.
25. Spanos A, Harrell FE Jr., Durack DT: Differential diagnosis of acute meningitis. An analysis of the predictive value of initial observations. *JAMA* 262:2700–2707, 1989.
26. Anders HJ, Goebel FD: Neurological manifestations of cytomegalovirus infection in the acquired immunodeficiency syndrome. *Int J STD AIDS* 10:151–159, 1999.
27. Roullet E: Opportunistic infections of the central nervous system during HIV-1 infection (emphasis on cytomegalovirus disease). *J Neurol* 246:237–243, 1999.
28. Straussberg R, Harel L, Nussinovitch M, Amir J: Absolute neutrophil count in aseptic and bacterial meningitis related to time of lumbar puncture. *Pediatr Neurol* 28:365–369, 2003.
29. Jereb M, Muzlovic I, Hojker S, Strle F: Predictive value of serum and cerebrospinal fluid procalcitonin levels for the diagnosis of bacterial meningitis. *Infection* 29:209–212, 2001.
30. Viallon A, Zeni F, Lambert C, et al.: High sensitivity and specificity of serum procalcitonin levels in adults with bacterial meningitis. *Clin Infect Dis* 28:1313–1316, 1999.
31. Nathan BR, Scheld WM: The potential roles of C-reactive protein and procalcitonin concentrations in serum and cerebrospinal fluid in the diagnosis of bacterial meningitis. *Curr Clin Top Infect Dis* 22:155–165, 2002.
32. Schutte CM: Clinical, cerebrospinal fluid and pathological findings and outcomes in HIV-positive and HIV-negative patients with tuberculous meningitis. *Infection* 29(4):213–217, 2001.
33. Marra CM, Maxwell CL, Tantalo L, et al.: Normalization of cerebrospinal fluid abnormalities after neurosyphilis therapy: Does HIV status matter? *Clin Infect Dis* 38(7):1001–1006, 2004.
34. Marra CM, Maxwell CL, Smith SL, et al.: Cerebrospinal fluid abnormalities in patients with syphilis: Association with clinical and laboratory features. *J Infect Dis* 189(3):369–376, 2004.

35. Garly ML, Petersen E, Pedersen C, Lundgren JD, Gerstoft J: Toxoplasmosis in Danish AIDS patients. *Scand J Infect Dis* 29(6):597–600, 1997.
36. Wilson BG: CT assessment of CNS complications of AIDS. *Radiol Technol* 73:424–437, 2002.
37. Lizerbaum EK, Hesselink JR: Neuroimaging of AIDS. I. Viral infections. *Neuroimag Clin N Am* 7:261–280, 1997.
38. Thurnher MM, Thurnher SA, Schindler E: CNS involvement in AIDS: Spectrum of CT and MR findings. *Eur Radiol* 7:1091–1097, 1997.

9

Influenza

Bennett P. deBoisblanc
John R. Godke

HIGH YIELD FACTS

1. Influenza characteristically presents in well-defined epidemics as an acute respiratory illness associated with high fever, chills, headache, myalgias, and malaise.

2. The keys to diagnosis include knowledge of influenza activity in the community, characteristic signs and symptoms, and a positive rapid diagnostic test.

3. Suspected cases should be placed in respiratory isolation since influenza is highly contagious.

4. Administration of amantadine, ramantidine, zanamivir, or oseltamivir within 48 h of symptom onset can reduce the severity of symptoms, the duration of viral shedding, and perhaps the risk of secondary complications.

5. Routine, system-oriented vaccination of high-risk individuals presenting to the emergency department for unrelated complaints should be employed.

CASE PRESENTATION

A 45-year-old man with a history of moderate persistent asthma presents to the emergency department in January during a period when there is a moderate amount of influenza activity in the community. He gives a history of fever, cough, and myalgias beginning 24 h previously.

On physical exam he is diaphoretic and has labored breathing with use of accessory muscles of respiration. His blood pressure is 145/90, his pulse is 120, his respiratory rate is 32, and his temperature is 39.0°C. His pulsus paradoxus is measured as 24 mm Hg. His oxyhemoglobin saturation by pulse oximetry is 89%. Auscultation of his chest reveals diffuse wheezing but no crackles. His chest x-ray shows hyperinflation of both lungs but there are no parenchymal infiltrates.

INTRODUCTION/EPIDEMIOLOGY

Influenza is usually a self-limited, acute viral respiratory illness that has the potential to cause significant morbidity and mortality of global dimensions. It typically occurs in regional epidemics lasting 8–10 weeks during the winter months. During an average epidemic in the United States, approximately 30,000 deaths occur in excess of what would be normally observed. Put in perspective, influenza kills more Americans every year than any other infectious disease including AIDS. Every decade or so, changes in the virulence and antigenic makeup of influenza viruses permit these viruses to span the globe in a nonseasonal pandemic characterized by a high attack rate and a mortality rate in excess of three times that seen during a typical year. The most dramatic example of a severe pandemic occurred between 1918 and 1919, when the "Spanish flu" killed approximately 700,000 Americans during a 12-week period. This figure is even more dramatic when one considers that in 1918 the U.S. population was only 1/3 of what it is today and that most of the deaths occurred among young adults between the ages of 20 and 45 years. It is estimated that as many as 50 million persons worldwide died during this same period (1).

The social implications of influenza are significant as well. The annual financial burden of influenza in the United States is estimated to be in excess of $12–$14 billion. These costs are partly due to the typical 150–450% rise in acute care visits during influenza outbreaks, but the greatest financial impact of influenza is due to absenteeism from work. Some estimates suggest that 10–12% of all work-associated absenteeism is related to influenza (2–4).

MICROBIOLOGY AND PATHOPHYSIOLOGY

Influenza viruses are enveloped, single-stranded RNA viruses approximately 100 nm in size. These viruses belong to the family *Orthomyxoviridae* and are divided into three genera: A, B, and C. Influenza C rarely causes disease in man. Both A and B viruses are capable of causing severe human disease, but influenza A poses the greatest problem because of its unique ability to stay below the human immunity radar by continually mutating its antigenic proteins.

Transmission of influenza to a susceptible host usually occurs via droplet nuclei and small particle aerosols generated by coughing or sneezing. When inhaled, influenza virions bind to sialic acid residues on respiratory epithelial cells via hemagglutinin (H) spikes that protrude from the viral envelope. Binding, and therefore infection, can be blocked by specific secretory IgA.

The viral envelope itself is composed of a lipid bilayer, the inside layer of the envelope contains matrix (M) proteins that are the target of certain antiviral drugs. If sufficient binding of hemagglutinin spikes to sialic acid residues occurs, the influenza virus gets adsorbed into the host cell cytoplasm. Once inside of an epithelial cell, insertion of viral genes into the host's genome begins the process of viral replication. The infected cell then undergoes lysis releasing up to 1 million viral copies. Neuraminidase (N) spikes on the viral envelope allow the new virions to escape and infect additional cells. This process may be repeated until the entire respiratory mucosa has been infected.

Humoral immunity directed against strain-specific hemagglutinin and neuraminidase is protective but antigenic drift, caused by subtle changes in an influenza virus's hemagglutinin and neuraminidase, allows new strains of influenza A viruses to avoid the herd immunity that has developed to previous strains. Two minor antigenic variant strains of type A influenza, A(H1N1) and A(H3N2), and type B influenza viruses are currently circulating globally.

Antigenic shift, on the other hand, refers to major changes in the hemagglutinin or neuraminidase. Antigenic shift can result in more widespread and lethal pandemic forms of influenza. Passage of influenza A viruses through natural reservoirs, such as foul and swine, may allow for major genetic reassortments and the creation of hybrid viruses. These hybid viruses may harbor a combination of animal and human viral genes. The only way humans can respond to the ever-changing antigenic makeup of influenza viruses is to continually update their humoral immunity. When hybrid viruses contain hemagglutinin or neuraminidase to which humans have not been recently exposed, such as the occurrence in 1997 when an H5N1 avian-human hybrid emerged in Hong Kong, another pandemic is possible. Three times during the present century, an avian influenza virus crossed species to humans and started a pandemic. Similarly, human influenza A(H3N2) has crossed to swine and is now a major cause of zoonosis in North America. Once established, these hybrid viruses can circulate for several decades.

In response to the global threat of another pandemic, the World Health Organization (WHO) has established a worldwide network of National Influenza Centers to track influenza epidemiology for the purposes of updating the influenza vaccines (4–9).

Epithelial cells, monocytes, and macrophages are highly susceptible to an infection with influenza viruses. Within 24–48 h, infected monocytes undergo apoptosis. Prior to apoptosis these monocytes initiate a cell-specific immune response that includes the transcription and subsequent release of pro-inflammatory cytokines such as tumor necrosis factor (TNF), Interleukin-1 (IL-1) IL-6, and type I interferons. Infection of monocytes also induces the selective expression of monocyte-specific chemokines that explains the mononuclear cell infiltration of the respiratory mucosa. In contrast, the release of the neutrophil-specific chemokines, important for host defenses against bacterial infections, is suppressed (10). The resultant suppression of neutrophil chemotaxis and the enhanced adherence of bacteria to the denuded respiratory mucosa may explain the increased risk of secondary pneumonia that occurs 7–14 days after infection.

Interferons are detectable in respiratory secretions beginning 3–6 days after infection and hallmark the end of viral shedding. Strain-specific humoral immunity develops within 5 days in patients previously exposed to related influenza viruses or within 10–14 days in patients not previous exposed, e.g. young children. Subclinical infection occurs frequently among previously immunized close contacts of cases, as evidenced by a four-fold rise in strain-specific antihemagglutinin.

CLINICAL PRESENTATION

The symptoms of acute influenza are distressing to the affected individual even in mild cases and often prompt an acute health care visit. Typically a patient experiences an explosive onset of high fever, rigors, malaise, paroxysmal cough, headache, and myalgias beginning 18–72 h after exposure. Because influenza viruses can infect the respiratory epithelium from the nose and paranasal sinuses all the way to the alveoli, symptoms and signs of rhinitis, pharyngitis, laryngitis, tracheobronchitis, or viral pneumonia may be present. Patients may complain of extreme fatigue, burning watery eyes, profuse clear nasal discharge, earache, sore throat, loss of voice, or burning substernal chest pain during coughing paroxysms. Myalgias can be so generalized and severe that even the extraocular muscles may be affected resulting in a wax figure-like gaze. The headache can be severe and is typically retrobulbar and associated with photophobia, raising the suspicion of bacterial meningitis. Contrary to popular belief, gastrointestinal symptoms are uncommon. Symptoms usually begin to spontaneously wane within 72 h but coughing paroxysms may persist for weeks.

On physical examination, the temperature may exceed 39°C during the first day, especially in children. The face is usually flushed and the skin hot and moist. The conjunctivae, tympanic membranes, and nasal turbinates are often inflamed. "Shotty" cervical lymphadenopathy is common in children. Although minor wheezing and occasional crackles are often observed, excessive tachycardia, tachypnea, and hypoxemia should suggest a complicated course due to a co-morbid condition.

Taken in isolation, influenza symptoms are not specific enough to make a definitive diagnosis. The differential diagnosis of the symptom complex associated with influenza includes other respiratory viruses, especially respiratory syncytial virus (RSV). RSV infection can occur throughout the winter especially in young children. However, in the setting of a local epidemic of influenza, the above symptoms are highly suggestive of influenza. Because attack rates during an epidemic may exceed 50% of individuals in a susceptible population, simultaneous presentation of similar cases is often a clue to the diagnosis. The greatest confusion occurs when RSV and influenza are simultaneously circulating in the community. In one report of routine virological surveillance of flu-like illness occurring during the winters of 1997–1999, approximately 30% of swab specimens yielded influenza viruses and 20% RSV (11). Influenza vaccination within the preceding months does not exclude the possibility that a patient has developed influenza but prior vaccination will often attenuate the severity of the symptoms. The highest infection rates occur in children and young adults because of their lack of immunity from prior exposure to the virus, while morbidity from influenza is usually highest among infants, the elderly, and those with comorbidities.

During pandemics, severe presentations occur more commonly and carry a high mortality rate. Serious morbidity or mortality from influenza may result from direct viral injury of organs such as the lung, from an overzealous host response to infection, from an exacerbation of an underlying condition, or from a secondary bacterial pneumonia.

Occasionally during epidemic influenza outbreaks, a patient will present to the emergency department with primary viral pneumonia manifested by severe hypoxemia and diffuse pulmonary infiltrates characteristic of the acute respiratory distress syndrome (ARDS). The respiratory secretions in patients with viral pneumonia may resemble "port wine" while the Gram stain of these secretions reveals a paucity of bacteria. The development of primary viral pneumonia appears to be more common among pregnant patients and those with preexisting cardiovascular disease. In other cases disseminated intravascular coagulation (DIC), delirium or coma, or rhabdomyolysis may be observed (12–16). A variety of clinical central nervous system manifestations, such as the Reye syndrome, acute necrotizing encephalopathy, and myelitis as well as autoimmune conditions (such as the Guillain-Barre syndrome), may occur during the course of influenza infection (17). Neurological involvement is fortunately rare but is often associated with serious sequelae or death. Some epidemiologic studies have suggested a link between influenza and the subsequent development of schizophrenia (18).

Exacerbation or unmasking of underlying comorbid conditions may also bring patients with influenza to the emergency department. Following infection with influenza virus, the entire respiratory epithelium of the tracheobronchial tree can slough. The denuded airways become extremely inflamed often resulting in airway hyperreactivity. Wheezing and coughing can last weeks to months. During this period, patients with asthma and COPD are susceptible to severe, even life-threatening exacerbations. Because the presentation of severe asthma or COPD may completely obscure concomitant influenza symptoms, a diagnosis of underlying influenza may only become apparent if a rapid influenza test is performed.

Influenza has also been associated with increase in cardiovascular mortality. The peak annual incidence of myocardial infarction and stroke typically occurs during influenza epidemics. Both acute coronary syndromes and ischemic stroke share a common pathogenesis involving atherosclerotic plaque rupture and intravascular thrombosis, processes that could be initiated by a systemic inflammatory response. In one study, 19% of those suffering an acute myocardial infarction recall having had a viral respiratory tract infection in the prior 2 weeks. Furthermore, administration of influenza vaccination has been associated with a 50% reduction in the incidence of sudden cardiac death, acute myocardial infarction, congestive heart failure, and ischemic stroke (19a). As is the case in acute exacerbations of asthma and COPD, in the setting of congestive heart failure, stroke, or acute myocardial infarction the diagnosis of acute influenza must often be pursued utilizing a rapid flu test since typical influenza symptoms may be inapparent.

Approximately three-fourths of all deaths attributable to influenza are due to infectious complications, most commonly bacterial pneumonia. The elderly and patients with chronic cardiopulmonary or metabolic diseases are at greatest risk for this complication. The reappearance of fever, the onset of purulent sputum production, or the development of pleuritic chest pain 7–14 days after the acute presentation should raise suspicion of secondary bacterial pneumonia. The signs, symptoms, and x-ray findings of postinfluenza bacterial pneumonia are indistinguishable from bacterial pneumonia not associated with influenza and are discussed elsewhere (see Chapter 10). It has been suggested that 50% of all bacterial pneumonias occur following influenza. The most common bacterial pathogens isolated are *Streptococcus pneumoniae*, *Haemophilus influenzae*, and *Staphylococcus aureus*. Occasionally bacterial pneumonia will develop within the first week of acute influenza presenting the clinician with a picture of mixed viral and bacterial pneumonia.

LABORATORY/DIAGNOSTIC TESTING

Selection of appropriate laboratory testing should be guided by the presenting signs and symptoms of a patient. A complete blood count, a basic metabolic profile, and blood and sputum bacterial cultures are not necessary in straightforward, uncomplicated cases. However, in complicated cases and in cases where the diagnosis of influenza remains uncertain, additional laboratory testing is appropriate.

A definitive virological diagnosis can be made by viral culture, antigen detection, RNA detection by PCR, and serological analyses. Obtaining acute and convalescent serum samples 2 weeks apart for the identification of hemagglutination-inhibiting antibodies is sensitive and specific for the diagnosis of acute influenza but this approach does not offer information in a time frame that can impact clinical decision making. For this reason, serological testing is used for epidemiologic purposes only. Viral culture of a nasopharyngeal wash or swab takes 5–10 days for confirmation and is most commonly performed by a state-based lab (Table 9–1). Viral culture is most useful to confirm that influenza is present in a community and to identify the particular strain that is circulating. It can also be used to identify other viral infections that cause clinical symptoms similar to the flu. Like serologic confirmation, viral culture is not timely enough to impact patient care.

Rapid flu tests are used to definitively diagnose influenza A and B, and to differentiate influenza from other viral and bacterial infections in a time frame that allows antiviral medications to be used. The newly licensed rapid tests detect viral antigens or viral RNA in respiratory secretions. These tests are now reliable enough to be used in both outpatient and inpatient settings. On average, rapid in-office tests are more than 70% sensitive and 90% specific for influenza (20, 21). Commercially available assays vary in complexity, specificity, sensitivity, time to obtain results, specimen analyzed, and cost (Table 9–1). The results of rapid flu tests are particularly useful in selecting appropriate antiviral therapy, avoiding inappropriate antibiotic therapy, and in promptly initiating measures to decrease the spread of disease.

MANAGEMENT

Otherwise healthy patients with uncomplicated influenza should receive only symptomatic treatment if they present to the emergency department more than 48 h after the onset of symptoms. Common "over-the-counter" flu preparations that contain a combination of antipyretics, analgesics, decongestants, and antitussives are sufficient for the majority of patients. Children should avoid aspirin-containing compounds because of the risk of the Reye syndrome. Patients who are experiencing an exacerbation of a co-morbid condition will often require hospital admission. Co-morbid conditions, such as asthma or congestive heart failure, should be managed in the usual fashion. Patients with influenza who present within 48 h of the onset of symptoms may be candidates for antiviral therapy. Antivirals approved by the FDA for the treatment of prophylaxis of influenza are listed in Table 9–2.

Amantadine hydrochloride and its analog rimantadine (Flumadine™) are orally administered drugs that are active at the M_2 transmembrane protein site. Amantadine, 200 mg/day, administered to adults within 48 h of symptom onset reduces the duration of fever by approximately 1 day. Rimantadine, administered 100 mg twice daily, has comparable effectiveness. Advantages of these agents include low cost and high oral bioavailability, while the disadvantages include efficacy only against influenza A viruses, the relative rapid development of resistance, and the adverse effects. Both amantadine and rimantadine have significant gastrointestinal side effects, while central nervous system side effects are common only with amantadine, especially in the elderly and those with renal dysfunction (22).

Persons who have influenza A infection and who are treated with amantadine can shed sensitive viruses early in the course of treatment and after 5–7 days of therapy shed drug-resistant viruses. Resistant viruses have been identified as causes of influenza outbreaks in nursing homes where amantadine was used for the Parkinson disease. Measures should be taken to reduce contact between persons taking and those not taking amantadine or ramantadine (23).

Table 9–1. Influenza Diagnostic Table

Procedure	Influenza Types Detected	Acceptable Specimens	Time for Results	Rapid Results Available
Viral culture	A and B	NP swab[a], throat swab, nasal wash, bronchial wash, nasal aspirate, sputum	5–10 days[b]	No
Immunofluorescence DFA antibody staining	A and B	NP swab[a], throat swab, nasal wash, bronchial wash, nasal aspirate, sputum	2–4 h	No
RT-PCR[c]	A and B	NP swab[a], throat swab, nasal wash, bronchial wash, nasal aspirate, sputum	1–2 days	No
Serology	A and B	Paired acute and convalescent serum samples[d]	>2 weeks	No
Enzyme immuno assay (EIA)	A and B	NP swab[a], throat swab, nasal wash, bronchial wash	2 h	No
Directigen flu A[e] (Becton-Dickinson)	A	NP swab[a], throat swab, nasal wash, nasal aspirate	<30 minutes	Yes
Directigen flu A+B[e,f] (Becton-Dickinson)	A and B	NP swab[a], throat swab, nasal wash, nasal aspirate	<30 minutes	Yes
FLU OIA[e] (Thermo Electron)	A and B[g]	NP swab[a], throat swab, nasal aspirate, sputum	<30 minutes	Yes
FLU OIA A/B[e,f] (Thermo Electron)	A and B	NP swab[a], throat swab, nasal aspirate, sputum	<30 minutes	Yes
XPECT flu A/B (Remel)	A and B	Nasal wash, NP swab[a], throat swab	<30 minutes	Yes
NOW flu A test[e,f] (Binax)	A	Nasal wash, NP swab[a]	<30 minutes	Yes
NOW flu B test[e,f] (Binax)	B	Nasal wash, NP swab[a]	<30 minutes	Yes
QuickVue influenza test[h] (Quidel)	A and B[g]	NP swab[a], nasal wash, nasal aspirate	<30 minutes	Yes
QuickVue influenza A+B test[h] (Quidel)	A and B[f]	NP swab[a], nasal wash, nasal aspirate	<30 minutes	Yes
ZstatFlu[h] (ZymeTx)	A and B[g]	Throat swab	<30 minutes	Yes

[a]NP = nasopharyngeal.
[b]Shell vial culture, if available, may reduce time for results to 2 days.
[c]RT-PCR = reverse transcriptase polymerase chain reaction.
[d]A fourfold or greater rise in antibody titer from the acute- (collected within the first week of illness) to the convalescent-phase (collected 2–4 weeks after the acute sample) sample is indicative of recent infection.
[e]Moderately complex test—requires specific laboratory certification.
[f]Distinguishes between influenza A and B virus infections.
[g]Does not distinguish between influenza A and B virus infections.
[h]CLIA-waived test. Can be used in any office setting. Requires a certificate of waiver or higher laboratory certification.
Adapted with permission from (19b).
List may not include all test kits approved by the U.S. Food and Drug Administration.
Disclaimer: Use of trade names or commercial sources is for identification only and does not imply endorsement by the Centers for Disease Control and Prevention or the Department of Health and Human Services.

Table 9–2. Antivirals Approved by the FDA for the Prevention or Treatment of Influenza

Drug	Activity	Indication	Dose	Duration
Amantadine	Influenza A	Prophylaxis	Adults: 200 mg p.o. daily Children <9 years: 4.4–8.8 mg/kg/day Adults >65 years, liver or renal disease: 100 mg p.o. daily	Duration of epidemic or up to 2 weeks following vaccination
		Treatment	Same as prophylaxis	Begin within 48 h; continue for 7 days
Rimantadine	Influenza A	Prophylaxis	Adults: 100 mg p.o. BID Children <10 years: 5 mg/kg/day Adults >65 years, liver or renal disease: 100 mg p.o. daily	Duration of epidemic or up to 2–4 weeks following vaccination
		Treatment	Same as prophylaxis	Begin within 48 h; continue for 7 days
Oseltamivir	Influenza A or B	Prophylaxis	Children >13 years and adults: 75 mg p.o. daily	Duration of epidemic or up to 2 weeks following vaccination
		Treatment	Children >13 years and adults: 75 mg BID	Begin within 48 h; continue for 5 days
Zanamivir	Influenza A or B	Treatment	Children > 7 years and adults: Two inhalations (10 mg) BID Not indicated in presence of obstructive lung disease	Begin within 48 h; continue for 5 days

Two neuraminidase inhibitors, zanamivir (Relenza™) and oseltamivir (Tamiflu™), have been FDA-approved for treating both influenza A and B infections in adults and children. These drugs demonstrate potent antiviral activity in vitro against all strains of influenza A and B, including H5N1 and H9N2 avian strains recently implicated in human cases (24). They reduce the duration of illness by about 1.5 days when started within 36–48 h of illness onset (25). Studies to address other groups at increased risk for influenza complications, such as pregnant women and children below 1 year of age, have not been performed (26).

Zanamivir is delivered directly to the primary site of viral replication by inhalation from a dry powder inhaler (10 mg via the Diskhaler twice daily for 5 days). Treatment of influenza within 48 h of the onset of symptoms results in a faster return to normal activities, better sleep, reduced requirement for relief medication, and a reduced incidence of antibiotic use and complications. Compared to placebo, zanamivir reduces the duration of symptoms by 1.5 days in otherwise healthy patients and by 2.5 days in high-risk patients. In patients with asthma or chronic

pulmonary disease, zanamivir reduces the rate of pulmonary complications and does not adversely affect pulmonary function (27–29).

Oseltamivir is an oral drug that lacks the potential for significant drug-drug interactions. Transient gastrointestinal disturbance is the major adverse effect and can be reduced by taking oseltamivir after a light snack (30, 31). Clinical benefits are only seen when oseltamivir is applied within 48 h after onset of symptoms. Oseltamivir, administered 75 mg twice daily for 5 days, reduces the duration of symptoms by up to 1.5 days and the severity of illness by up to 38% compared with placebo when initiated within 36 h of symptom onset in otherwise healthy adults with naturally acquired febrile influenza. The incidence of secondary complications and the use of antibiotics may also be reduced in oseltamivir recipients, but it does not prevent pneumonia or hospitalization secondary to influenza. Earlier treatment results in better treatment effects. Treatment within 12 h after onset of symptoms reduces the duration of illness by approximately 75 h, while delaying treatment until 24 h after the onset of symptoms reduces symptoms by approximately 50 h (32).

Drug resistance to the neuraminidase inhibitors is not a problem at present because, although such mutants occur, they are less virulent and spread less easily (33).

DISPOSITION

Patients with suspected acute influenza should be placed in respiratory isolation. Viral shedding in respiratory secretions begins prior to the onset of the acute illness and persists for approximately 5 days. Because virions may remain viable for several hours at room temperature, transmission via fomites is possible. Strict attention to handwashing is critical following even casual contact, such as a handshake.

Influenza poses special hazards inside health care facilities and can cause explosive outbreaks of illness. During epidemics in the community, testing for influenza should be requested in all patients with compatible symptoms admitted to the hospital, and measures should be introduced for the prevention or early control of an outbreak. Health-care workers are at risk of acquiring influenza and thus serve as an important reservoir for patients under their care. Influenza and other respiratory viruses can cause nonfebrile illness while remaining transmissible (34). Annual influenza immunization of health-care workers is a primary means of preventing nosocomial influenza, although it is substantially underutilized (35). Health-care providers, staff, or visitors who exhibit typical symptoms of influenza should be prevented from visiting the hospital during a known influenza outbreak in the community.

INFLUENZA PROPHYLAXIS DURING UNRELATED EMERGENCY DEPARTMENT VISITS

Physicians should consider offering influenza prophylaxis to high-risk patients presenting to the emergency department for unrelated health-care visits. A missed opportunity for either vaccination or drug prophylaxis might result in serious morbidity or mortality for such patients. Up to 70% of patients who die of influenza-related complications each year had a visit to a health-care provider for an unrelated problem at some time during the vaccination season but were not vaccinated. Examples of missed opportunities include visits for asthma exacerbations, chest pain, or minor injuries in the elderly. A system-oriented approach to vaccination, e.g. an automatic standing order to offer vaccination to all at-risk individuals at the time of emergency department discharge, results in a much higher rate of vaccination than does a reminder to a patient to obtain vaccination.

Risk factors for severe postinfluenza complications include age over 65 years, chronic cardiopulmonary disease, renal disease, diabetes, or residence in a closed community such as a nursing home. Pregnant patients expected to be at term during an influenza period should also be vaccinated, since acute influenza is a common cause of preterm labor and neonatal mortality. When given annually, inactivated trivalent influenza vaccines can reduce severe complications from influenza among the elderly by 30–60%. Among children with asthma, otitis media and asthma exacerbations are reduced by 20–75%. Finally, vaccination of residents and staff of long-term care facilities reduces mortality among residents by over 40% (36).

Two influenza vaccines are available in the United States, an inactivated, trivalent intramuscular formulation and a live, attenuated intranasal trivalent preparation. The intramuscular formulation is approved for use in patients over 6 months of age. Influenza in infants younger than 6 months of age can be prevented by maternal vaccination. The injectable, inactivated trivalent influenza vaccine may be safely given during pregnancy as it does not contain live virus. Family members and other close contacts should be vaccinated with the injectable vaccine to reduce the possibility of transmission to individuals at risk (37, 38). The live intranasal vaccine (FluMist™) is indicated for use only in healthy persons between 5 and 49 years of age. Intranasal administration is generally more acceptable, especially to children, but the shedding of live virus poses a risk to pregnant mothers and to immune compromised contacts (39). The attenuated intranasal vaccine reduces the number of cases of serologically confirmed influenza A by approximately 50% compared to approximately 70% for the intramuscular vaccine.

The intramuscular trivalent vaccine is well tolerated in high-risk patients. Adverse reactions are generally mild and similar to those observed in healthy people (i.e., soreness/redness at site of vaccination, low-grade fever, aches), although the achievable titers of antihemagglutinin antibodies are generally lower (40). Because immunization with inactivated vaccine does not induce significant changes in either viral load or CD4+ cell counts, it can be safely administered to HIV-infected individuals (41).

Because vaccination does not offer protection for several days, asymptomatic individuals exposed to active cases should receive prophylaxis with an antiviral drug. Antiviral prophylaxis should also be considered for unvaccinated or recently vaccinated high-risk individuals during epidemic influenza. The M_2 blockers, amantadine and rimantadine, are licensed for the prophylaxis in diverse high-risk populations, including children. When used prophylactically, amantadine and rimantadine may prevent up to two-thirds of serologically confirmed clinical influenza A cases. Neither drug, however, has achieved widespread acceptance because of the rapid development of viral resistance, lack of activity against influenza B, and concerns about possible adverse events. Complete cross-resistance occurs with these compounds. Resistant strains are transmissible and are fully pathogenic.

The neuraminidase inhibitors, zanamivir and oseltamivir, have been shown to be approximately 75% effective in preventing laboratory-confirmed infection when administered prophylactically during the influenza season. Oral oseltamivir (administered 75 mg once or twice daily for 6 weeks) during a period of local influenza activity significantly prevented the development of naturally acquired influenza by >70% compared with placebo in unvaccinated otherwise healthy adults. The drug also demonstrated exceptional efficacy when used adjunctively in previously vaccinated high-risk elderly patients (42). When used for prophylaxis, inhaled zanamivir, administered 10–20 mg/day for 10 days to 4 weeks, prevented influenza A in two-thirds of recipients in a university community. Both zanamivir and oseltamivir can be used prophylactically to prevent spread of infection within families where 80–90% protection has been documented.

CASE OUTCOME

A rapid flu test performed on a nasal wash specimen was positive for influenza A. The patient was admitted to the intensive care unit for close observation. He was treated for both acute influenza A and for an acute asthma exacerbation. He received oseltamivir 75 mg twice daily for 5 days and systemic corticosteroids and nebulized beta$_2$ agonists. He became afebrile within 72 h. His respiratory distress slowly improved over the next 4 days but he continued to wheeze and his peak expiratory flow rate remained below his baseline for two additional weeks. He was able to be discharged home 1 week after hospital admission with close outpatient follow-up. He was vaccinated with the inactivated, trivalent intramuscular vaccine to protect against reinfection with concomitantly circulating influenza B virus.

REFERENCES

1. Barry JM: *The Great Influenza*. New York, Penquin Group, 2004, p 546.

2. Anonymous: Easing the burden: The challenge of managing influenza. *Am J Manag Care* 6:S276–S281, 2000.

3. O'Reilly FW, Stevens AB: Sickness absence due to influenza. *Occup Med (Oxford)* 52:265–269, 2002.

4. Anonymous: Epidemiology and virology of influenza illness. Based on a presentation by Arnold S. Monto, MD. *Am J Manag Care* 6:S255–S264, 2000.

5. Olsen CW: The emergence of novel swine influenza viruses in North America. *Virus Res* 85:199–210, 2002.

6. De Jong JC, Rimmelzwaan GF, Fouchier RA, et al.: Influenza virus: A master of metamorphosis. *J Infect* 40:218–228, 2000.

7. Hilleman MR: Realities and enigmas of human viral influenza: Pathogenesis, epidemiology and control. *Vaccine* 20:3068–3087, 2002.

8. Nicholson KG, Wood JM, Zambon M: Influenza. *Lancet* 362:1733–1745, 2003.

9. Rao BL: Epidemiology and control of influenza. *Natl Med J India* 16:143–149, 2003.

10. Kaufmann A, Salentin R, Meyer RG, et al.: Defense against influenza A virus infection: Essential role of the chemokine system. *Immunobiology* 204:603–613, 2001.

11. Fleming DM: Influenza diagnosis and treatment: A view from clinical practice. *Phil Trans R Soc* B 356:1933–1943, 2001.

12. Grose C: The puzzling picture of acute necrotizing encephalopathy after influenza A and B virus infection in young children. *Pediatr Infect Dis J* 23:253–254, 2004.

13. Morton SE, Mathai M, Byrd RP, Jr., et al.: Influenza A pneumonia with rhabdomyolysis. *South Med J* 94:67–69, 2001.

14. Newland JG, Romero JR, Varman M, et al.: Encephalitis associated with influenza B virus infection in 2 children and a review of the literature. *Clin Infect Dis* 36:e87–e95, 2003.

15. Oba K, Nishihara A, Okamura K, et al.: Two cases of acute myositis associated with influenza A virus infection in the elderly. *J Nippon Med Sch* 67:126–129, 2000.

16. Mori I, Yokochi T, Kimura Y: Role of influenza A virus hemagglutinin in neurovirulence for mammalians. *Med Microb Immunol* 191:1–4, 2002.

17. Studahl M: Influenza virus and CNS manifestations. *J Clin Virol* 28:225–232, 2003.

18. Munk-Jorgensen P, Ewald H: Epidemiology in neurobiological research: Exemplified by the influenza-schizophrenia theory. *Br J Psychiatry - Supplementum* 40: s30–s32, 2001.

19a. Meyers DG: Myocardial infarction, stroke, and sudden cardiac death may be prevented by influenza vaccination. *Curr Atheroscler Rep* 5:146–149, 2003.

19b. Centers for Disease Control. Prevention and control of influenza: Recommendations of the Advisory Committee on Immunization Practices (ACIP). *Morb Mortal Wkly Rep* 53:1–40, 2004.

20. Demmler GJ: Laboratory diagnosis of influenza: Recent advances. *Sem Pediatr Infect Dis* 13:85–89, 2002.

21. Montalto NJ: An office-based approach to influenza: Clinical diagnosis and laboratory testing. *Am Fam Physician* 67:111–118, 2003.

22. Jefferson TO, Demicheli V, Deeks JJ, et al.: Amantadine and rimantadine for preventing and treating influenza A in adults. (Update of *Cochrane Database Syst Rev* (2):CD001169, 2001; PMID: 11405978). *Cochrane Database Syst Rev* CD001169, 2002.

23. Suzuki H, Saito R, Masuda H, et al.: Emergence of amantadine-resistant influenza A viruses: Epidemiological study. *J Infect Chemother* 9:195–200, 2003.

24. Doucette KE, Aoki FY: Oseltamivir: A clinical and pharmacological perspective. *Expert Opin Pharmacotherapy* 2: 1671–1683, 2001.

25. Khare MD, Sharland M: Influenza. *Expert Opin Pharmacotherapy* 1:367–375, 2000.

26. Ison MG, Hayden FG: Therapeutic options for the management of influenza. *Curr Opin Pharmacol* 1:482–490, 2001.

27. Hoffken G, Gillissen A: Efficacy and safety of zanamivir in patients with influenza—impact of age, severity of infections and specific risk factors. *Med Microbiol Immunol* 191:169–173, 2002.

28. Cheer SM, Wagstaff AJ: Spotlight on zanamivir in influenza. *Am J Respir Med* 1:147–152, 2002.

29. Fleming DM: Managing influenza: Amantadine, rimantadine and beyond. *Int J Clin Pract* 55:189–195, 2001.

30. Dutkowski R, Thakrar B, Froehlich E, et al.: Safety and pharmacology of oseltamivir in clinical use. *Drug Saf* 26: 787–801, 2003.

31. Long JK, Mossad SB, Goldman MP: Antiviral agents for treating influenza. *Cleve Clin J Med* 67:92–95, 2000.

32. Gillissen A, Hoffken G: Early therapy with the neuraminidase inhibitor oseltamivir maximizes its efficacy in influenza treatment. *Med Microbiol Immunol* 191:165–168, 2002.

33. Oxford J, Balasingam S, Lambkin R: A new millennium conundrum: How to use a powerful class of influenza anti-neuraminidase drugs (NAIs) in the community. *J Antimicrob Chemother* 53:133–136, 2004.

34. Salgado CD, Farr BM, Hall KK, et al.: Influenza in the acute hospital setting. (Erratum appears in *Lancet Infect Dis* 2 (6):383, 2002.) *Lancet Infect Dis* 2:145–155, 2002.

35. Maltezou HC, Drancourt M: Nosocomial influenza in children. *J Hosp Infect* 55:83–91, 2003.

36. Hak E, Hoes AW, Verheij TJ: Influenza vaccinations: Who needs them and when? *Drugs* 62:2413–2420, 2002.

37. Munoz FM: The impact of influenza in children. *Sem Pediatr Infect Dis* 13:72–78, 2002.

38. Zangwill KM, Belshe RB: Safety and efficacy of trivalent inactivated influenza vaccine in young children: A summary for the new era of routine vaccination. *Pediatr Infect Dis J* 23:189–197, 2004.

39. Mossad SB: Demystifying FluMist, a new intranasal, live influenza vaccine. *Cleve Clin J Med* 70:801–806, 2003.

40. Brydak LB, Machala M: Humoral immune response to influenza vaccination in patients from high risk groups. *Drugs* 60:35–53, 2000.

41. Zanetti AR, Amendola A, Besana S, et al.: Safety and immunogenicity of influenza vaccination in individuals infected with HIV. *Vaccine* 20:B29–B32, 2002.

42. McClellan K, Perry CM: Oseltamivir: A review of its use in influenza. (Erratum appears in *Drugs* 61(6):775, 2001.) *Drugs* 61:263–283, 2001.

10

Community-Acquired Pneumonia and Bronchitis

Peter DeBlieux
Claudia Barthold

HIGH-YIELD FACTS

1. The diagnosis of pneumonia is made through history, physical examination, laboratory data, and, most importantly, the chest radiograph.

2. Atypical pneumonia can be clinically indistinguishable from other etiologies and antibiotic choices should take this into consideration.

3. Clinical judgment, consideration of psychosocial factors, as well as the pneumonia severity index (PSI), help determine inpatient versus outpatient treatment.

4. Immunocompromised patients with pneumonia require special consideration.

5. Viral pathogens can cause primary pneumonia and may lead to bacterial super-infection, both of which can cause significant morbidity and mortality.

CASE PRESENTATION

A 65-year-old woman presents to the emergency department (ED) with a chief complaint of shortness of breath. She states that she has had shaking chills and fever for 2 days accompanied by mild dyspnea on exertion. She has a cough productive of green sputum and complains of generalized malaise. She has a history of hypertension and diabetes and takes medication for each.

She is thin and appears ill but is alert and oriented. Her blood pressure is 142/90, her pulse is 113, her respiratory rate is 28, her oxygen saturation is 91% on room air, and her temperature is 101.2°F. Further physical examination reveals crackles in the left lower lung with egophony, but without wheezing, dullness to percussion, or tactile fremitus.

INTRODUCTION/EPIDEMIOLOGY

Many patients present to emergency departments with complaints of cough, fever, dyspnea, or sputum produc-

tion. Of those who have an infectious etiology of their symptoms, most will have viral upper respiratory infections that require symptomatic treatment only. It is the role of the emergency physician to identify those with pneumonia, as these patients require antimicrobial treatment and consideration for inpatient admission.

According to the National Center for Health Statistics in the year 2001, pneumonia accounted for over 1.3 million hospitalizations in the United States and, when combined with influenza, was listed as the seventh leading cause of death (1). It is the number one cause of death from infectious disease. The cost of treating community-acquired pneumonia (CAP) in the 1990s was estimated at over $8 billion annually. Inpatient costs were estimated at over $4 billion annually for those over 65 years of age and over $3 billion for those younger than 65 (2).

In order to appropriately maximize inpatient resources and practice prudent antibiotic prescribing in an era of increasing antibiotic resistance in organisms, the decisions regarding diagnosis, disposition, and empiric treatment have become increasingly complex. The ED is often the initial location a patient will seek treatment, and the emergency physician must be well versed in these progressive issues.

PATHOPHYSIOLOGY

Community-acquired pneumonia is an acute infection of the pulmonary parenchyma in a patient not hospitalized or residing in a long-term care facility for greater than 14 days prior to the onset of symptoms (3). Symptoms include cough, fever, myalgias, or dyspnea. Chest radiograph may reveal a pulmonary infiltrate. Physical examination demonstrates findings consistent with pulmonary infection such as egophany, tactile fremitus, or crackles. Infection can occur through hematogenous spread (i.e., septic emboli from right sided endocarditis), inhalation of aerosolized infectious particles (as with *Mycobacterium tuberculosis*, influenza or *Legionella pneumophila*), direct extension from surrounding structures (as with a liver abscess or trauma), or, most commonly, by aspiration of oropharyngeal secretions.

There is a series of defense mechanisms the body uses to prevent inhaled or aspirated particles, and secretions from inducing infection. When one or more of these protective systems fail, pneumonia can develop. For example, patients with preexisting neurological impairment may not be able to prevent aspiration due to diminished cough reflex. Patients with chronic lung disease may not have the ciliary function necessary to propel mucus and

Table 10–1. Commonly Recognized Presentations of Pneumonia

Etiology	Common Symptoms	Common Associations or Findings
S. pneumoniae	Fever, chills, or rigors Productive cough Chest pain	Community-acquired Usually sporadic Large outbreaks possible in those sharing living quarters More common in winter
K. pneumoniae	Current jelly sputum Abrupt onset Severe illness	Alcoholics
H. influenza	Fever Cough	Common in both children and adults COPD patients -Splenectomy patients
S. aureus	Hemoptysis Chest pain	Intravenous drug users Endocarditis Septic thrombophebitis Indwelling catheters After influenza A infection
L. pneumophila	Febrile systemic illness Prodrome of fever, malaise Nonproductive cough	Exposure to aerosolized water droplets containing bacteria Outbreak can occur if many are exposed Can have significant gastrointestinal complaints
M. pneumoniae	Minor respiratory illness with insidious onset	Rash, headache, sore throat, bullous myringitis or other extrapulmonary manifestations Young patients Occurs in any season Outbreaks can occur in those sharing close quarters
C. pneumoniae	Nonproductive cough Fever rare Long incubation period	More common in children and the elderly Rare extrapulmonary infection Sore throat and hoarseness
Influenza	Rapid progression of fever, cough, dyspnea, and cyanosis	Underlying pulmonary or cardiac disorders
Aspiration	Progressive fever Purulent sputum Shortness of breath Coarse rhonchi over dependent lung zones	Patients with impaired swallowing ability as in stroke or multiple sclerosis Patients with altered level of consciousness as in seizure or alcohol intoxication
P. aeruginosa or other gram-negative bacteria	Abrupt onset of symptoms Severe symptoms	COPD patients Cystic fibrosis patients

(Continues)

Table 10–1. (*Continued*) Commonly Recognized Presentations of Pneumonia

Etiology	Common Symptoms	Common Associations or Findings
H. capsulatum	Self-limited illness Fever and chill Fatigue Anterior chest discomfort Nonproductive cough	Most people are asymptomatic Found commonly in the Mississippi and Ohio River valleys Most common endemic mycosis in the United States
P. jiroveci	Insidious onset Hacking nonproductive cough Retrosternal chest tightness Dyspnea	Almost exclusively in immunocompromised hosts Hypoxia can be severe

inhaled particles out of the respiratory tract. Recent viral infections may denude epithelium and decrease protective immunoglobulins, reducing barrier protection that makes a secondary bacterial infection more likely. Finally, patients with impaired immune systems because of malignancy, infection with the human immunodeficiency virus (HIV), or chronic corticosteroid use may have diminished ability to fight infections that have set in once other barriers have been breached.

MICROBIOLOGY

There are many bacteria, viruses, and fungi that can each cause acute lung infection. Co-infection from a virus and bacteria or two bacteria is not uncommon (4–6). Identifying the pathogen responsible for the infection can be difficult. In studies on CAP, it is not uncommon to have 20–30% of patients without a known etiology after standard testing (5–7). Commonly performed sputum and blood cultures have poor yields and are associated with a considerable incidence of false positive rates. Agent-specific serological or urine tests, while available for some pathogens, can be difficult to perform, are costly, and offer variable clinical benefit.

The most commonly isolated etiology of CAP is *Streptococcus pneumoniae*. The percent attributable to this bacterium varies from approximately 15% to 40% (4–7). The "atypical" pathogens, specifically *L. pneumophila, Chlamydia pneumoniae*, and *Mycoplasma pneumoniae* are rather a significant cause of community-acquired pneumonia. While the percentages vary based on groups studied, as much as 30% of all community-acquired pneumonias are attributable to these atypical agents (4, 5, 7). Studies have estimated that viral pneumonia accounts

for about 5–10% of CAP (5–7). Other commonly found causative pathogens are *Haemophilus influenzae, Staphylococcus aureus*, and *Moraxella catarrhalis* (4–7) (see Table 10–1).

CLINICAL PRESENTATIONS

Classic Presentation

The classic presentation of CAP is associated with clinical findings and patient populations that are historically attributable to certain pathogens. As with the classic presentation of appendicitis or myocardial infarction, there are constellations of symptoms and signs with which every clinician should be familiar. It is imperative to understand that the disease rarely presents so clearly or consistently. The most commonly recognized presentation of pneumonia is the one classically attributed to infection with *S. pneumoniae*. Patients complain of a sudden onset of a single bone-shaking chill, followed by fever, cough, purulent sputum production, and dyspnea. There is a leukocytosis, a lobar infiltrate with air bronchograms on chest radiograph, positive blood and sputum cultures and successful treatment with beta-lactam antibiotics. *H. influenzae, S. aureus*, and *Klebsiella pneumoniae* are other pathogens that classically present in this manner.

The term atypical has been used to describe pathogens of CAP that do not follow this "typical" pattern. These pneumonias require macrolides, fluoroquinolones or tetracyclines rather than beta lactams for treatment (8). Discovery of the etiology requires special diagnostic testing because traditional blood cultures and sputum cultures are not as useful. They have nonspecific laboratory and radiographic findings (Fig. 10–1). Pneumonias caused by the atypical agents – *M. pneumoniae, C. pneumoniae*,

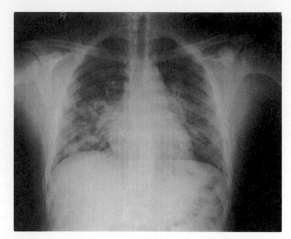

Fig. 10–1. A classic PA and lateral projection in a patient with an atypical pneumonia.

L. pneumophila, or viruses are classically accompanied by numerous extrapulmonary complaints, have a slower onset of respiratory symptoms, and, with the exception of some cases of *L. pneumophila*, are less severe.

While the above presentations and those listed in Table 10–1 are helpful to suggest a diagnosis, there is no rapid and reliable way to differentiate between typical and atypical pneumonia in patients with CAP. No historical or physical examination findings nor radiographic findings can distinguish between typical and atypical causes of CAP (5, 9, 10). Many studies have shown that the presentations are by no means as divergent as the "classic" presentations imply. Some feel that the term atypical is obsolete (8). The variety of typical and atypical causes of pneumonia so often mimic one another that in the ED physicians should consider them almost indistinguishable, never treating one without the other.

Differential Diagnosis of Pneumonia

The gold standard for diagnosing CAP is identification of a pathogen taken directly from infected lung parenchyma by bronchoscopy. This is not feasible in the emergency department. As such, the diagnosis of CAP is achieved by combining a suggestive history, specific abnormalities on physical examination, laboratory results, and findings on chest radiograph. Many of the clinical findings are also common to other diseases and the emergency physician must always consider the differential diagnoses.

Two diseases often incorrectly diagnosed as CAP are pulmonary embolism and exacerbations of congestive heart failure. In any of these three diseases, patients can have leukocytosis, fever, constitutional symptoms,

chest radiograph changes, and/or hypoxia. Additionally, all three can produce adventitial lung sounds on physical examination, a cough, and minor hemoptysis. Acute coronary syndrome can present as a vague history of dyspnea, or chest pain that can be confused with nonspecific respiratory symptoms. Neoplasms can present either as a primary cause of respiratory symptoms, or as the cause of a postobstructive pneumonia. A patient with acute aspiration can have cough, fever, and even an infiltrate on chest radiograph without there being an acute infection. Patients with acute exacerbations of chronic bronchitis will present with productive cough, dyspnea, and hypoxia. Careful examination of all relevant data can help eliminate these and other competing illnesses while securing the diagnosis of CAP.

History

The history of patients with CAP may assist the emergency physician in three ways. Initially, it aids with diagnosis. The patient will likely complain of some combination of lower respiratory tract infection symptoms such as cough, chest discomfort, dyspnea, or sputum production in addition to fever, sweats, and rigors (3). A thorough history can help rule out competing differential diagnoses. Secondly, a full review of systems and inquiry regarding recent travel or sick contacts can be invaluable. For example, a history of chronic alcoholism may raise suspicion for *K. pneumoniae* while recent travel to Toronto or China may raise suspicion for severe acute respiratory syndrome (SARS). Finally, historical factors play a significant role in deciding disposition. Questions regarding past medical history, immunosuppressive conditions or medications, HIV risk factors, and social support allow informed decisions regarding suitability for outpatient treatment. A complete history is fundamentally necessary, but it is important to note that no historical detail can either confirm or refute the diagnosis of CAP without obtaining a chest radiograph (11).

Physical Examination

The emergency physician should complete a thorough physical examination of the patient, paying careful attention to not only the lung examination, but also any clues that could help rule in or out competing diagnoses. Clues may also point out HIV risk factors or conditions common in patients with acquired immunodeficiency syndrome (AIDS) (i.e. "track marks" or thrush) that can significantly change management if CAP is diagnosed. Physical examination findings of mental status, degree of respiratory distress, and vital sign abnormalities play a significant role in disposition and should be specifically noted. Multiple aberrations in vital signs are common in patients with pneumonia but, like other physical examination findings, they are not universally seen. While Gennis et al. (12) did find that CAP was unlikely if there were no vital sign abnormalities, 31% of patients with pneumonia were afebrile, 25% lacked tachypnea, and 50% were not tachycardic. The diagnosis of pneumonia should never be excluded solely on the basis of normal vital signs in light of a suspicious history or physical examination.

The examination of the lungs has four basic components that can all aid in the diagnosis of pneumonia: inspection, palpation, percussion, and auscultation (11). While there are no pathognomonic findings that assure a diagnosis of pneumonia, there are abnormalities that, when weighed with other factors, can strongly support the diagnosis. Careful inspection of the entire thorax should take place in each patient. Deformity of the chest wall can indicate underlying lung disease from chronic obstructive pulmonary disease (COPD), previous trauma, or congenital abnormalities. Retractions or labored breathing indicates respiratory distress. Splinting can occur secondary to the pain of an infiltrate or effusion irritating the adjacent pleura. The emergency physician should palpate the entire chest and ask the patient to repeat the same phrase (e.g., "99"). Assessing for tactile fremitus in this manner allows the emergency physician to compare each hemithorax and may give clues to the location and size of a pleural effusion (decreased or absent fremitus) or infiltrate (increased fremitus). The location and size of an effusion or infiltrate can be assessed by percussion. Dullness to percussion indicates that fluid occupies formerly air filled spaces, or collected within the pleural space.

Finally, the emergency physician should listen closely to the entire chest with the patient inhaling and exhaling. Bronchial breath sounds, which are normally heard over the trachea, may be traced over an area of lung consolidation, as can crackles or rhonchi. Tests for whispered pectroliliquy can be performed by asking the patient to whisper. The spoken words are clearer and louder over areas of consolidation than over unaffected areas of the lung. Asking the patient to say "EEE" and hearing "AYE" is indicative of egophony and is also suggestive of consolidation.

LABORATORY/DIAGNOSTIC STUDIES

Chest Radiograph

There is no combination of physical examination, or historical findings that can confirm or refute the diagnosis

alone (11); thus a chest radiograph, preferably two-views (posterior-anterior and lateral), should be performed on all patients in whom pneumonia is suspected (Fig. 10–2). It is considered critical in the diagnosis of pneumonia (3). Lower respiratory tract infections can present radiologically as diffuse interstitial infiltrate, focal or lobar consolidation, or as multifocal opacities (13). Classic radiological findings are listed in Table 10–2. As with the commonly recognized clinical presentations highlighted in Table 10–1, it is important to note that though potentially helpful, chest radiograph findings alone should not be used to determine a causative pathogen nor to direct therapy. Identifying multilobar disease and/or pleural effusions can help stratify patients into risk groups that aid in admission decisions (14).

Radiographic changes due to CAP may manifest as subtle changes detectable only with close examination of the radiograph. Air filled portions of the bronchial tree that are normally radiologically invisible appear as radiolucent branching structures on a more radioopaque background when surrounded by an area of consolidation. These are known as air bronchograms and are suggestive of a lobar pneumonia. On the lateral chest radiograph, the loss of the progressive lucency typically seen over the lower thoracic vertebral bodies, known as a "spine sign," can suggest a lower lobe pneumonia even if not seen on the posterior-anterior view.

While the absence of an infiltrate can help guide the clinician away from a diagnosis of pneumonia, it does not absolutely refute its presence if history and physical examination strongly suggest it. Infiltrates have been discovered on chest computed tomography (CT) performed after clear chest radiographs were obtained (15). A study involving patients with suspected CAP underwent both chest radiograph and high-resolution chest CT. Eighteen pulmonary infiltrates detected by chest radiograph were also detected by CT, but CT identified eight additional cases of infiltrates not seen on chest radiographs. Bilateral involvement was evident on chest radiograph in less than half of the cases detected by chest CT (15).

Laboratory Studies

Patients suspected of having pneumonia who are being considered for admission should have a complete blood count, basic chemistry, and liver function panel drawn (3, 16, 17). Additionally, other tests needed to fully evaluate competing diagnoses (i.e., D-dimer, brain natriuretic peptide (BNP) and cardiac enzymes) may be indicated. Abnormalities in the blood urea nitrogen, glucose, and sodium levels, and hematocrit, while not useful in making the diagnosis of CAP, are all criteria that may help

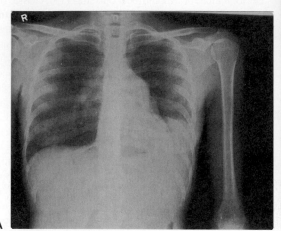
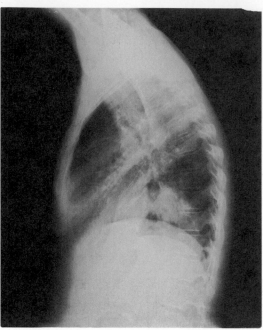

Fig. 10–2. (A and B): While apparent on the PA view, this infiltrate is most clearly defined on the lateral projection.

determine the need for admission. Abnormalities discovered in the liver function panel, or creatinine can indicate underlying chronic or acute liver and renal disease respectively, and factor into disposition decisions as well.

Pulse Oximetry

Hypoxia is related to an increased morbidity and mortality in patients with CAP. A pulse oximetry reading should be documented on all patients suspected of having pneumonia. An arterial blood gas (ABG) analysis should be performed in patients suspected of having pneumonia with significantly abnormal pulse oximetry readings, those with underlying pulmonary diseases, and those who are tachypneic. The PCO_2 measurements can help the physician monitor the patient's ventilatory reserve and elevations can be an indicator of respiratory fatigue in the tachypneic patient.

Diagnosing the Etiology of Pneumonia

It is difficult to determine the microbial etiology of pneumonia based on history or radiographic information alone. Discovering a specific pathogen can prove to be invaluable in the tailoring of antibiotics or the anticipation of complications. The Infectious Disease Society of America (IDSA) notes that microbiological studies can also help

advance epidemiological knowledge, help clinicians implement antimicrobial prophylaxis in cases of tuberculosis, *Neisseria meningitides* or *H. influenzae*, and reduce antibiotic expenses (3). Several tests exist for the clinician to establish the specific etiology of pneumonia, such as sputum and blood cultures, but results are unavailable in the ED. These cultures can be obtained in the ED for the benefit of the admitting physician. Generally, cultures are not appropriate for outpatients, but local practice habit and the preference of the patient's primary care physician should be considered.

Sputum culture

Sputum cultures are recommended by the IDSA in their 2000 guidelines for treating CAP, as well as their 2003 update, for every patient admitted to the hospital with the diagnosis of CAP (3, 17). The American Thoracic Society (ATS), however, recommends sputum Gram stain and culture be done more selectively and only in those in whom a drug-resistant bacterium or an organism not routinely covered by empiric therapy is suspected (e.g., in patients with immunocompromise, those who have failed outpatient therapy, and those with recent hospital admission) (16). If obtained, the sputum Gram stain and

Table 10–2. Classic Radiographic Findings in Community Acquired Pneumonia According to Pathogen

Etiology	Classic Radiographic Findings in Pneumonia
S. pneumoniae	Homogeneous, nonsegmental, parenchymal opacity Can be multilobar Air bronchograms Begins in the periphery of the lobe
K. pneumoniae	Homogeneous, nonsegmental, parenchymal opacity Bulging of interlobar fissures Pleural effusions 60–70%
H. influenzae	Variable but predominantly patchy infiltrates Cavitation in 15% Pleural effusion in 50%
S. aureus	Patchy involvement Lobar enlargement with bulging of interlobar fissures in severe cases Lung abscesses are common Pleural effusions 30–50% Lack of air bronchograms
L. pneumophila	Nonsegmental opacity in peripheral distribution Rapid progression Can have bilateral involvement
M. pneumoniae	Fine reticular pattern followed by patchy, multifocal, ill-defined opacities Pleural effusion in 20% usually small and unilateral
Influenza	Varies from mild interstitial prominence to extensive air-space disease
Anaerobic bacteria	Varies from patchy bilateral infiltrates to confluent unilateral disease Caviation or abscess in 20–60%
P. aeruginosa	All lobes with predominance of lower lobes Multinodular opacities Necrosis and cavitations Unilateral or bilateral pleural effusions
Fungal	Can be normal or have nonspecific changes
P. carinii	Can be normal Granular pattern or hazy, ground-glass opacity in early stages Parenchymal opacity with a granular or reticular-granular pattern in the lung periphery in late stages

Source: Adapted from text in (13).

subsequent culture should be used to broaden antibiotic coverage if an unexpected pathogen is found, not narrow it if a common pathogen is found.

The inherent problem with sputum Gram stain and culture is their lack of specificity and sensitivity. Additionally, a quality specimen can be difficult to obtain. Inferior sputum samples, often resulting from poor collection technique, add little value. If collected, a deep-cough expectorated sputum sample should ideally be obtained before antibiotics are administered and Gram staining and culture should be performed within 2 h of collection (3).

Care should be exercised if induction is needed to obtain a sample. The induction process and procedure should be carried out in a negative pressure flow room to prevent nosocomial spread of highly infective organisms such as *M. tuberculosis* and influenza.

Blood culture

Recent articles and policy decisions highlight the controversy surrounding the decision of whether or not to obtain blood cultures on patients with CAP (18–22). Clinical evidence has suggested that blood cultures in patients with CAP who are ambulatory with mild disease are of little utility (18). There is also growing agreement that patients with severe CAP, who have not responded to treatment as expected, should have blood cultures drawn in hopes of identifying a resistant organism (19).

An article by Metersky et al. (20) found independent predictors of bacteremia to be liver disease, hypotension, hypo- or hyperthermia, tachycardia, uremia, hyponatremia, leukopenia, or leukocytosis. Using these predictors, the authors proposed a decision support tool that, when factoring in recent antibiotic usage, divided patients into categories of low, moderate, and high risk of bacteremia. Obtaining blood cultures from only patients with a moderate or high risk of bacteremia resulted in a significant decrease in the number of blood cultures drawn in a cohort of over 12,000 patients without missing significant numbers of bacteremic patients (20). Conversely, a study of over 14,000 patients with pneumonia found that blood culture collection within 24 h of arrival alone was associated with 10% lower odds of 30-day mortality (21). Hospital policy may preclude emergency physicians from weighing this decision because the Joint Commission on Accreditation of Healthcare Organizations (JCAHO) has made blood culture collection within 24 h one of six core quality measurements for inpatients with CAP (22).

In the latest ATS and IDSA guidelines on CAP, blood cultures are recommended only for hospitalized patients (16, 17). If blood cultures are ordered, two sets of aerobic and anaerobic blood cultures should be drawn from different sites before antibiotics are initiated. Inability to draw blood cultures should *never* delay antibiotics administration.

HIV Test

Community-acquired pneumonia is a common reason for hospital admission for HIV patients. CAP in a patient without risk factors should prompt the clinician to consider an undiagnosed immunocompromised state. With informed consent, patients with pneumonia between the ages of 15 and 54 should undergo HIV testing (3). While HIV does not itself cause pulmonary infiltrates, knowing a patient's HIV status allows the clinician to include or exclude opportunistic infections in the differential diagnosis. Patients with significant risk factors for HIV, those with a chest radiograph consistent with *Pneumocystis jiroveci* (formerly *Pneumocystis carinii*) pneumonia (PCP), or those with the presence of a low absolute lymphocyte count warrant testing for HIV.

Antigen Specific Tests

The pneumococcal urinary antigen assay is noted in the 2003 IDSA update to be an acceptable test when used to augment conventional blood and/or sputum cultures (17). Though not widely used, its rapid result when compared to blood cultures may be helpful to the admitting physician in tailoring antibiotic therapy and anticipating clinical course. A urinary antigen assay as well as a specific respiratory culture exists for *L. pneumophila*. It is generally recommended in patients with an enigmatic pneumonia, during an epidemic of *L. pneumophila* infections, in an immunocompromised host, or if the patient fails to respond to a beta-lactam (17). Use of these tests should be dictated by availability and local practice habit.

Decision of Outpatient versus Inpatient Treatment

The decision to admit or discharge a patient from the ED once the diagnosis of CAP is established is a crucial one. It is intuitive that 21-year-old previously healthy patients with normal vital signs, normal pulse oximetry, an infiltrate on chest radiograph, close primary care provider follow-up, and excellent social support can be treated for their pneumonia as an outpatient. It is also an intuitive clinical choice that a 76-year-old diabetic who is hypotensive and hypoxic with multilobar disease should be treated in the intensive care unit (ICU). Questions regarding admission arise with those patients diagnosed with CAP who do not fall into the extremes of the two scenarios detailed above. Fine et al. (14) have proposed a PSI to aid in measuring a patient's severity of disease and chance of mortality, thus aiding in admission decisions. The PSI stratifies patients with CAP into five risk classes based on a series of historical, physical examination, and laboratory data. The five risk classes are related to the expected 30-day mortality, with risk class I being low risk for mortality and risk class V having the highest risk of mortality. Patients assigned to the lowest risk class, Class I, must be less than 50 years of age without comorbidities and without derangements in their vital signs. The associated mortality of patients assigned to risk class I is 0.1–0.4% and thus suggests these patients be considered candidates for outpatient management (14).

If a patient does not meet the criteria for class I, then risk class is determined using a point system with points being awarded for specific examination, diagnostic test, or historical data. The point system is detailed in Table 10–3. A patient's minimum number of points are determined by age and gender. For example, a 70-year-old

Table 10–3. Pneumonia Severity Index

Characteristic	Points Assigned
Age for men	Age in years
Age for women	Age in years − 10
Nursing-home resident	+10
Neoplastic disease	+30
Liver disease	+20
Congestive heart failure	+10
Cerebrovascular disease	+10
Renal disease	+10
Altered mental status	+20
Respiratory rate at 30/min	+20
Systolic blood pressure < 90 mm Hg	+20
Temperature < 35°C or > or = 40°C	+15
Pulse > or = 125/min	+10
Arterial pH < 7.35	+30
Blood urea nitrogen > or = 30 mg/dL	+20
Sodium < 130 mmol/L	+20
Glucose > or = 250 mg/dL	+10
Hematocrit < 30%	+10
Partial pressure of arterial oxygen < 60 mm Hg	+10
Pleural effusion	+10
Class II: 70, class III: 71–90, class IV: 91–130, class V: > 130	

Source: Adapted from table in (14). Permission from author still pending.

female with CAP will have, at minimum, a PSI of 60 points. Additional points are assigned based on specifics of past medical history, physical examination findings, laboratory data, and radiographic findings. The total number of points awarded determines the patient's class assignment. Class II patients have a mortality risk of 0.6–0.7% and the study authors suggest they be candidates for outpatient management, while class III patients with a mortality of 0.9–2.8% would likely benefit from a brief inpatient stay. Class IV patients are suggested to be placed in inpatient wards and class V patients are suggested to be admitted to the ICU (14).

If a 70-year-old female with CAP has no other points assigned, a score of 60 suggests that outpatient management could be considered on age and gender alone. If, however, she is found to have an altered mental status, breast cancer, glucose of 300 mg/dL, and sodium of 125 mmol/L, her

final score, when calculated by adding the points received for these findings to her initial score of 60, gives her a final PSI of 140. This places her in class V suggesting that she may benefit from management in the ICU.

While the PSI provides a framework for admission criteria in patients with CAP, it does have its limitations. Many psychosocial and historical conditions that make a patient less suitable for outpatient management have no points attributed to them in the calculation of the PSI. For example, no points are awarded for immunocompromised states such as HIV or chronic steroid use. The presence of hypoxia adds only 10 points impacting the patient's risk class minimally, even though it is standard to admit those with acute hypoxia due to pneumonia. Altered mental status is grounds for admission alone and yet is given a weight of only 20 points. The most recent IDSA guidelines (17) addressed the complexity of the decision to admit or discharge patients with CAP by proposing a three-step process to determine the site of treatment. They recommend consideration of (1) the PSI, (2) any factors that could compromise care at home, and, above all else, (3) the clinical judgment of the physician caring for the patient. Factors listed that could compromise care include hypoxemia, either acute or in light of chronic oxygen dependence, hemodynamic instability, and inability to take oral medication (17). Additional factors contributing to a physician's clinical judgment are the presence of unstable living conditions, frail physical condition, history of substance abuse, history of severe psychiatric problems, and homelessness. In addition, the ATS specifically notes that patient preferences should be factored into the final disposition decision (16). These guidelines reinforce the emergency physician's responsibility to use all the available data, their personal experience, and clinical judgment when deciding the ultimate disposition for a patient.

Once the decision to admit a patient with pneumonia has been made the emergency physician, in concert with the admitting physician, must decide if the patient requires admission to an ICU. Patients requiring vasopressors or mechanical ventilation must be treated in an ICU setting. Intensive care should be strongly considered for those patients with multilobar disease, bilateral pleural effusions, hypotension, severe hypoxia, significant tachypnea, or renal failure, especially if more than one of these is present (16) (Fig. 10–3).

Outpatient Treatment

Once the decision is made to send a patient home, the emergency physician must choose an appropriate antibiotic regimen. In Table 10–4 a synthesis of

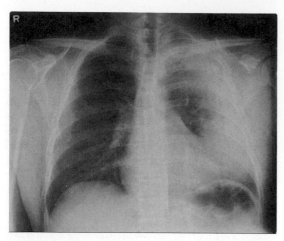

Fig. 10–3. This AP view demonstrates pneumonia involving both the left upper and left lower lungs.

recommendations from the IDSA and ATS is listed. Both agree that azithromycin, clarithromycin, or doxycycline is appropriate outpatient monotherapy for previously healthy patients with CAP. Patients with recent antibiotic usage should be given broader coverage given the risk of a drug-resistant *S. pneumoniae* (DRSP). DRSP should be considered not only in those with recent antibiotic usage but also in patients who have one of the recognized risk factors: age over 65, immunosuppression, multiple comorbidities, or exposure to children in day care (16). Either a respiratory fluoroquinolone (levafloxacin, gatifloxacin, or moxifloxacin) or a beta-lactam (cefdinir, cefpodoxime proxetil, cefprozil, or cefuroxime axetil)

plus an advanced spectrum macrolide (clarithromycin or azithromycin) are recommended for these patients (16).

The respiratory fluoroquinolones are included in the guidelines for outpatient CAP treatment regimens by both the IDSA and the ATS. A recent study demonstrated that a short course of high-dose levofloxacin (750 mg PO Q day × 5 days) was as effective as lower dose-longer course regimens (23). However effective the fluoroquinolones are in treating pneumonia, care must be used to prevent overuse of these agents. Fluoroquinolones are vital in the treatment of pneumonia caused by macrolide and penicillin-resistant organisms. If fluoroquinolones are over-utilized then the incidence of fluoroquinolone-resistant *S. pneumoniae* may increase. Fluoroquinolones should be reserved for those who have macrolide or penicillin allergies, in whom a once-a-day dose is required, or for those the clinician feels other regimens are inappropriate.

A new class of antibiotics, the ketolides, has recently been approved by the United States Food and Drug Administration (FDA) for the treatment of CAP. Telithromycin, a ketolide, has shown promise as a well tolerated first-line therapy for mild to moderate disease (24).

There is no clear length of treatment. Even though short-course regimens are being studied, typical treatment should last a minimum of 7–10 days with repeat evaluation by the patient's primary care physician within that time. Longer courses may be indicated for more severe disease or preexisting illnesses.

Inpatient Treatment

Patients admitted with CAP should receive their first dose of intravenous (IV) antibiotics in the ED. There is a

Table 10–4. Outpatient Treatment

Clinical Case	IDSA 2003	ATS 2001
Previously healthy with no recent antibiotic use	Macrolide OR doxycycline	Advanced generation macrolide OR doxycycline
Comorbidities with recent antibiotic use	A fluoroquinolone alone or an advanced macrolide plus a beta lactam[a]	Beta-lactam plus advanced macrolide or doxycycline OR antipseudomonal fluoroquinolone alone
Comorbidities without recent antibiotic use	An advanced macrolide OR fluoroquinolone	
Influenza with bacterial superinfection	A beta-lactam OR a respiratory fluoroquinolone	

[a]Beta-lactam includes high dose amoxicillin (1 g PO TID), high dose amoxicillin clavulanate (2 g PO BID), cefpodoxime, cefprozil (listed by IDSA only), or cefuroxime.

Source: Adapted from tables and text in (16) and (17). Permission from authors still pending.

decreased mortality, both in-hospital and within 30 days of admission, and decreased length of stay if a patient receives an initial dose of antibiotics within 4 h (25). The timing of administration of the initial dose of antibiotics is already monitored by the JCAHO and the Center for Medicare and Medicaid Services (CMS) and consideration is being given to establishing initial antibiotic administration within 4 h of presentation as a specific quality measure (22). While another study was not able to replicate the benefit of the more rapid administration of antibiotics (26), the emergency physician should give the initial empiric dose of antimicrobial therapy as soon as the diagnosis is made.

The IDSA and ATS also propose specific recommendations for a range of clinical scenarios in patients hospitalized with CAP (see Table 10–5). For admitted patients, azithromycin with a third-generation cephalosporin such as ceftriaxone or cefotaxime is recommended by both organizations. The ATS cites monotherapy with IV azithromycin as an acceptable treatment for previously healthy adults with CAP. Monotherapy with a macrolide

should be avoided in those with risk factors for DRSP (16).

For severely ill patients admitted to the ICU, antibiotic coverage must include activity against *Pseudomonas aeruginosa*. *P. aeruginosa* should also be treated as a possible etiology in CAP in patients with structural lung diseases such as bronchiectasis, chronic corticosteroid therapy, recent broad spectrum antibiotic therapy, and malnutrition (16, 17). This coverage can be achieved by using a combination of antipseudomonal beta-lactams (such as piperacillin-tazobactam, imipenem, meropenem, cefepime), a respiratory fluoroquinolone or an advanced spectrum macrolide, and an aminoglycoside (such as gentamicin). For those with penicillin allergies, aztreonam is an appropriate antipseudomonal penicillin substitute.

Antibiotic coverage may need to be further broadened if methicillin-resistant *S. aureus* (MRSA) is suspected. For example, MRSA coverage should be instituted for patients with CAP who reside in nursing homes known to harbor MRSA, who have an indwelling catheter, who inject illicit drugs, or who have previously diagnosed, or

Table 10–5. Inpatient Treatment

Clinical Case	IDSA 2003	ATS 2001
Inpatient medical ward with no recent antibiotic use	An advanced macrolide plus a beta-lactam[a] OR fluoroquinolone alone	IV azithromycin alone OR doxycycline plus beta-lactam or antipseudomonal fluoroquinolone alone
Inpatient medical ward with recent antibiotic use or comorbidities	An advanced macrolide plus a beta-lactam OR a fluoroquinolone	Beta-lactam plus IV or PO macrolide or doxycycline OR IV antipseudomonal fluoroquinolone alone
ICU with pseudomonas infection not an issue	Beta-lactam plus either an advanced macrolide OR a fluoroquinolone	Beta-lactam plus IV macrolide or fluoroquinolone
ICU with pseudomonas infection not an issue but beta-lactam allergy	A respiratory fluoroquinolone +/− clindamycin	
ICU with pseudomonas infection being an issue	An antipseudomonal agent[b] plus ciprofloxacin OR an antipseudomonal agent plus an aminoglycoside plus a fluoroquinolone or a macrolide	Selected antipseudomonal beta-lactams plus IV antipseudomonal quinolone OR selected antipseudomonal beta-lactam plus IV aminoglycoside plus IV macrolide or IV nonpseudomonal fluoroquinolone
ICU with *Pseudomonas* infection being an issue but beta-lactam allergy	Aztreonam plus levofloxacin OR aztreonam plus moxifloxacin or gatifloxacin +/− an aminnoglycoside	Aztreonam plus IV antipseudomonal fluoroquinolone OR aztreonam plus IV aminoglycoside plus IV macrolide or nonpseudomonal fluoroquinolone

[a]Ceftriaxone, cefotaxime, ampicillin-sulbactam; IDSA includes ertapenem, ATS includes high dose ampicillin.
[b]Piperacillin-tazobactam, imipenem, meropenem, cefepime (piperacillin alone per the IDSA only).
Source: Adapted from tables and text in (16) and (17).

suspected, bacterial endocarditis (16). Treatment must include intravenous vancomycin. If aspiration pneumonia is a consideration, the antibiotic selection must include coverage for anaerobic bacteria. The addition of clindamycin to either a respiratory fluoroquinolone or the combination of cephalosporin/macrolide would be reasonable, or ampicillin/sulbactam, imipenem, or meropenem can be utilized with a macrolide. This can be achieved with the addition of clindamycin, a beta-lactam/beta-lactamase inhibitor such as ampicillin/sulbactam, imipenem or meropenem in addition to a fluoroquinolone or macrolide/cephalosporin combination (3).

OTHER CONSIDERATIONS

Acute Bronchitis

Healthy, young adults with an acute respiratory illness, but who lack chest radiograph abnormalities and signs of pulmonary disease on physical examination are more likely to have acute bronchitis than CAP. Acute bronchitis is a transient (no more than 14 days duration) respiratory illness in patients without chronic lung disease (3). Cough can be accompanied by sputum production, fever, or chest discomfort. The difference between acute bronchitis and pneumonia is the mild nature of the disease, lack of chest radiograph findings, and lack of signs of pulmonary consolidation on physical examination. Greater than 90% of uncomplicated acute bronchitis has a viral etiology (27). Pathogens include both viruses known to cause upper respiratory tract disease, such as adenovirus and rhinoviruses, as well as those known to cause lower respiratory tract disease, such as influenza and respiratory syncytial virus (RSV). Nonviral causes represent 5–10% of all cases of uncomplicated acute bronchitis and include *Bordetella pertussis*, *M. pneumoniae*, and *C. pneumoniae* (27). Differential diagnoses include cough-variant asthma, postnasal drip syndrome, or a simple upper respiratory infection.

Studies examining the utility of antibiotic therapy in acute bronchitis have found no benefit and thus antibiotic therapy is not routinely recommended (28). Treatment for acute bronchitis is primarily symptomatic and supportive. If a patient has suspected pertussis, for example during outbreaks or secondary to known exposures, diagnostic tests should be performed and reported to health agencies if positive. Macrolides are the treatment of choice for pertussis.

For those with depressed immune systems, those who are severely ill, or for those whose symptoms have lasted longer than 2 weeks, a diagnosis of CAP, not acute bronchitis, should be considered. If antibiotic treatment is desired CAP guidelines based on the patient's age and health status should be followed.

Acute Exacerbation of Chronic Obstructive Pulmonary Disease

An acute exacerbation of COPD is defined as illness in a patient with chronic bronchitis or emphysema with at least one of three cardinal symptoms: worsening dyspnea, an increase in sputum purulence, or an increase in sputum production. Exacerbations can be secondary to environmental exposures, concomitant clinical conditions, such as congestive heart failure or pulmonary embolism, and infections including viral or bacterial pathogens. Chest radiographs are recommended in the evaluation of these patients to demonstrate infiltrates or other pathology such as pneumothorax, pulmonary edema, or pleural effusions.

Antibiotic therapy for patient with acute exacerbation of COPD remains controversial. While debate still persists regarding whether or not to give antibiotics to these patients, in the opinion of a consensus group of internists and chest physicians antibiotics are beneficial in treating patients with acute COPD exacerbations (29). The evidence for prescribing antibiotics is strongest for patients with "type-1 exacerbations." These are exacerbations defined by Anthiosen et al. (30) as those with all three cardinal symptoms of COPD exacerbations: worsening dyspnea, an increase in sputum purulence, and an increase in sputum production. The least benefit of antibiotic treatment was found in patients with "type-3 exacerbation"—those with an upper respiratory infection within the past 5 days, fever without other cause, or increased wheezing, cough or heart rate who only had one of the cardinal signs (29). In general, patients hospitalized for COPD exacerbations should receive antibiotics.

There is no standard recommendation for duration of therapy or choice of antibiotics in treating exacerbations of COPD. One study demonstrated that fluoroquinolones, amoxicillin-clavulanate, or advanced macrolides, such as clarithromycin or azithromycin, may be more beneficial than amoxicillin, oral cephalosporins, trimethoprim-sulfamethoxazole, or erythromycin (31). No prospective study has been conducted.

Viral Pneumonia

Viruses can cause significant illness leading to hospitalization and even death (6, 7, 32). RSV, a common disease in childhood, can produce pneumonia in adults. Antigen detection tests are available for RSV, but they are insensitive for detecting disease in adults and are not generally recommended (17). Parainfluenza virus and adenovirus can also cause pneumonia. Unfortunately, no antiviral treatment has been proven effective (17). Suspicion of varicella zoster virus or herpes simplex virus as the cause of pneumonia should occur in patients with immunocompromised states with dermal evidence of varicella or herpes zoster. Prompt treatment with intravenous acyclovir (10 mg/kg IV q 8 h) should be initiated (17).

Influenza can cause both an upper respiratory illness as well as pneumonia. Pneumonia is best differentiated from the more benign upper respiratory illness by the presence of shortness of breath and pulmonary infiltrates on chest radiographs (32). Underlying lung disease appears to be a risk factor. A history of chronic respiratory disease was found more commonly in those with influenza pneumonia than in those with the influenza upper respiratory syndrome (32). Both influenza A and influenza B can cause pneumonia. Influenza B should be treated with oseltamivir and zanamivir while influenza A infections can be treated with amantadine and rimantadine (17). Oseltamivir (75 mg PO BID × 5 days) and zanamivir (10 mg inhaled BID × 5 days) can be used for both, but should be initiated within 2 days of initial influenza symptoms.

Influenza, as well as other viral infections, can predispose a patient to a secondary bacterial infection. If bacterial superinfection is suspected, in those patients previously diagnosed with influenza presenting with significant worsening of their respiratory symptoms, antimicrobial therapy active against *S. pneumoniae*, *S. aureus*, *and H. influenzae* should be initiated. The IDSA recommends amoxicillin-clavulanate or other beta-lactams such as high dose amoxicillin (1 g PO TID), high dose amoxicillin clavulanate (2 g PO BID), cefpodoxime, or cefprozil (17). For penicillin-allergic patients a fluoroquinolone can be used. There are data suggesting that treating upper respiratory infections with antivirals listed above for use in influenza treatment may reduce lower respiratory complications such as bacterial superinfection (33). The best therapeutic intervention for influenza is through vaccination to help prevent the illness altogether.

A newly recognized coronavirus has been identified as the causative agent in SARS, a highly contagious and deadly disease. The illness should be suspected in those who have recently traveled to an area where SARS is present, had contact with someone who has traveled to these areas, or has the disease, and has symptoms of a respiratory illness and fever (17, 34). For suspected cases, local public health agencies should be involved early to aid diagnosis. The patient should be kept in negative pressure respiratory isolation. Treatment is currently aggressive symptomatic and supportive care only as no standard antiviral treatment has been identified.

Pneumonia and HIV-Infected Patients

CAP is the most common reason for hospitalizations in HIV-infected patients (35). There has been a decline in the incidence of PCP, as well as other opportunistic infections, since the introduction of highly active antiretroviral therapy (HAART). However, the incidence of CAP has not decreased as dramatically (36). Low CD4 counts increase the likelihood of pneumonia in the HIV-infected patient, especially if the patient smokes cigarettes or uses intravenous drugs (37). Trimethoprim-sulfamethoxazole prophylaxis is effective in preventing PCP and CAP (37). *Streptococcus pneumonia* is the most commonly isolated bacteria in HIV positive patients with pneumonia (6, 37). *H. influenzae*, *P. aeruginosa*, and *S. aureus* are also common pathogens.

P. jiroveci remains the most common opportunistic infection in patients infected with HIV (35). Symptoms of PCP are more gradual in onset than those with bacterial pneumonia. The classic presentation includes cough with progressive dyspnea associated with ground glass infiltrates on chest radiograph. Chests radiographs are not very sensitive and abnormal findings can be subtle or even absent. The current antibiotic recommendations for immunocompetent patients with CAP do not provide antimicrobial coverage against PCP. The addition of trimethoprim-sulfamethoxazole, dapsone-trimethoprim, or clindamycin-primaquine combinations should be considered in any patient with AIDS and pneumonia if historical details such as progressive dyspnea or chest radiograph findings such as ground glass infiltrates suggest PCP (3). Adjunctive therapy with steroids is indicated in severe disease as demonstrated by hypoxia. If the PaO_2 is below 70 mm Hg prednisone (40 mg PO QDay × 5 days followed by a taper) should be administered. Dexamethasone and methylpresnisolone can also be used. The common bacterial pathogens causing CAP cannot be reasonably excluded in these patients; thus antibiotic therapy should include agents effective against them. Special consideration should be given to the possibility of pulmonary tuberculosis. HIV-infected patients are at increased risk of primary and secondary tuberculosis and may demonstrate very subtle findings on chest radiograph (38). Chest radiography has the greatest variability in those with a CD4 count less than 200 and it occurs in patients with advanced HIV infection, or AIDS, who may have active pulmonary tuberculosis with normal chest radiographs (38).

The emergency physician must always consider early respiratory isolation for any HIV-infected patient with a CD4 count less than 200 and a history consistent with tuberculosis or a new infiltrate on chest radiograph. Patients with advanced HIV infection, or AIDS, and the diagnosis of CAP or those with all, but mild PCP should be admitted. HIV-infected patients with mild PCP and without hypoxia, or significant dyspnea, can be considered for outpatient therapy. Consultation with the patient's physician and consideration of outpatient resources are prudent.

Pneumonia and Immunocompromised Patients without HIV

Patients with neutropenia from cancer or chemotherapy, and organ transplant recipients are at risk for CAP and require special consideration. They may present with very few respiratory symptoms, instead manifesting mental status changes, unexplained tachycardia or fever as signs of their pulmonary infection (39). Historical information regarding chemotherapy, immunosuppressive medications, recent infections, and recent antibiotic usage is critical. For patients with neutropenia and fever, empiric monotherapy with a carbepenem, cefepime, or ceftazidime is warranted (40). Combination therapy, by adding an amioglycoside, may be utilized especially if *P. aeruginosa* is considered a possible pathogen. If MRSA is a concern then vancomycin is an appropriate addition to the antibacterial regimen (40). Antivirals should not be started empirically unless there is evidence of a viral disease. If influenza is identified, treatment with the same antivirals as used for nonimmunocompromised patients should be initiated (40). If herpes simplex or varicella-zoster lesions are found in a patient with pneumonia intravenous acyclovir should be administered (40). Immunocompromised patients with pneumonia require admission. Consultation with the infectious disease specialists and the patient's primary care physician is essential.

Pneumonia and the Elderly or Nursing-Home Patient

Elderly patients with CAP are not as likely to present with classic signs and symptoms, and the emergency physician should include CAP in the differential diagnosis of fever, confusion, lethargy, or anorexia in the elderly (41–43). Nursing home patients develop a median of one episode of pneumonia per 1000 days of resident care (42). Many are initially treated in the nursing home with oral or intramuscular antibiotics and only present to the ED when their condition worsens, or does not improve. Selecting an appropriate empiric antibiotic regimen is made difficult due to the myriad of pathogens encountered in the nursing home environment. In a review of published studies, Muder et al. (42) found that *S. pneumoniae* was the most common etiology of pneumonia in nursing-home patients, with Gram negative bacteria, *H. influenza* and *S. aureus* accounting for many of the remaining cases. Atypical pathogens are found less frequently in nursing home patients than in patients with CAP (4, 7). However, a recent study found a decrease in mortality in elderly patients with pneumonia, including those from long-term care facilities, if they were treated with antibiotics that covered atypical pathogens when compared to a regimen that did not (44). This suggests that there is a role for antibiotic coverage for atypical pathogens when treating pneumonia in the elderly or nursing home patient.

Antibiotic recommendations from the IDSA and ATS are similar for elderly patients with pneumonia regardless of their place of residence (17, 18). However, chronic illness and exposure to antibiotics are common in these patients. A careful history and review of the patient's full medical record may highlight the need for broader antibiotic coverage.

CASE OUTCOME

A chest radiograph was ordered and revealed air bronchograms with a dense opacity in the left lower lobe. There was no effusion present. She had a partial pressure of oxygen of 62 mm Hg on ABG with a pH of 7.40. Her chemistry panel reveals a normal sodium, an increased glucose of 200 mg/dL, a creatinine of 1.9 mg/dL, and a blood urea nitrogen of 35 mg/dL. Her complete blood count reveals a white blood cell count of 15.9 with an 11% bandemia, but a normal hematocrit. Her liver function tests were normal.

She was given supplemental oxygen with an improvement in her oxygen saturation to 96%. In the emergency department she had blood cultures performed and then received an intravenous dose of ceftriaxone and azithromycin. Her PSI was calculated at 85 placing her in class III. She was admitted to an inpatient ward by her primary care physician with a diagnosis of CAP to receive continued antibiotics, antipyretics, hydration, and supplemental oxygen. She continued to improve and was switched to oral antibiotics on day 3 of her hospitalization. She was discharged the following day to follow up with her primary care physician.

REFERENCES

1. National Center for Health Statistics, Division of Data Services. Myattsville, MD; FastStats A to Z, 2001. Available

at http://www.cdc.gov/nchs/faststats.htm. Accessed January 18, 2004.

2. Neiderman MS, McCombs JS, Unger AN, et al.: The cost of treating community-acquired pneumonia. *Clin Ther* 20(4):820–837, 1998.

3. Bartlett JG, Dowell SF, Mandell LA, et al.: Practice guidelines for the management of community-acquired pneumonia in adults. *Clin Infect Dis* 31:347–382, 2000.

4. File TM, Segreti J, Dunbar L, et al.: A multicenter, randomized study comparing the efficacy and safety of intravenous and/or oral levofloxacin versus ceftriaxone and/or cefuroxime axetil in treatment of adults with community-acquired pneumonia. *Antimicrob Agents Chemother* 41(9):1965–1972, 1997.

5. Lieberman D, Ben-Yaakov M, Lazarovich Z, et al.: *Chlamydia pneumoniae* community-acquired pneumonia: A review of 62 hospitalized adult patients. *Infection* 24(2):109–114, 1996.

6. Mundy LM, Auwaerter PG, Oldach D, et al.: Community-acquired pneumonia: Impact of immune status. *Am J Respir Crit Care Med* 152:1309–1315, 1995.

7. Neill AM, Martin JR, Weir R, et al.: Community acquired pneumonia: Aetiology and usefulness of severity criteria on admission. *Thorax* 51:1010–1016, 1995.

8. Gupta SK, Sarosi GA: The role of atypical pathogens in community-acquired pneumonia. *Med Clin N Am* 85(6): 1349–1365, 2001.

9. Farr BM, Kaiser DL, Harrison BDW, et al.: Prediction of microbial aetiology at admission to hospital for pneumonia from the presenting clinical features. *Thorax* 44:1031–1035, 1989.

10. Marrie TJ, Peeling RW, Fine MJ, et al.: Ambulatory patients with community-acquired pneumonia: The frequency of atypical agents and clinical course. *Am J Med* 101:508–515, 1996.

11. Metlay JP: Does this patient have community-acquired pneumonia? Diagnosing pneumonia by history and physical examination. *JAMA* 278(17):1440–1445, 1997.

12. Gennis P, Gallagher J, Falvo C, et al.: Clinical criteria for the detection of pneumonia in adults: Guidelines for ordering chest roentgenograms in the emergency department. *J Emerg Med* 7(3):263–268, 1989.

13. Gharib AM, Stern EJ: Radiology of pneumonia. *Med Clin N Am* 85(6):1461–1491, 2001.

14. Fine MJ, Auble TE, Yealy DM, et al.: A prediction rule to identify low-risk patients with community-acquired pneumonia. *N Engl J Med* 336(4):243–250, 1997.

15. Syrjälä H, Broas M, Suramo I, et al.: High resolution computer tomography for the diagnosis of community-acquired pneumonia. *Clin Infect Dis* 27:358–363, 1998.

16. Neiderman MS, Mandell LA, Anzueto A, et al.: Guidelines for the management of adults with community-acquired pneumonia: Diagnosis, assessment of severity, antimicrobial therapy and prevention. *Am J Respir Crit Care Med* 163:1730–1754, 2001.

17. Mandell LA, Bartlett JG, Dowell SF, et al.: Update of practice guidelines for the management of community-acquired pneumonia in immunocompetent adults. *Clin Infect Dis* 37:1405–1432, 2003.

18. Campbell SG, Marrie TJ, Ackroyd-Stolarz S, et al.: Utility of blood cultures in the management of adults with community acquired pneumonia discharged from the emergency department. *Emerg Med J* 20:521–523, 2003.

19. Luna CM: Blood cultures in community-acquired pneumonia: Are we ready to quit? *Chest* 123(4):997–998, 2003.

20. Metersky ML, Ma A, Bratzler DW, et al.: Predicting bacteremia in patients with community-acquired pneumonia. *Am J Respir Crit Care Med* 169:342–347, 2004.

21. Meehan TP, Fine MJ, Krurnholtz HM, et al.: Quality of care, process and outcomes in elderly patients with pneumonia. *JAMA* 278:2080–2084, 1997.

22. Joint Commission on Accreditation of Healthcare Organizations: Overview of the community acquired pneumonia (CAP) core measurement set (3/22/2002), Available at http://www.jcaho.org/pms/core+measures/cap_overview.htm. Accessed April 24, 2004.

23. Dunbar LM: High-dose, short-course levofloxacin for community-acquired pneumonia: A new treatment paradigm. *Clin Infect Dis* 27(6):752–760, 2003.

24. Hagberg L, Carbon C, van Rensburg DJ, et al.: Telithromycin in the treatment of community acquired pneumonia: A pooled analysis. *Respir Med* 97:625–633, 2003.

25. Houck PM, Bratzler DW, Nsa W, et al.: Timing of antibiotic administration and outcomes for medicare patients hospitalized with community-acquired pneumonia. *Arch Int Med* 164:637–644, 2004.

26. Silber SH, Garrett C, Singh R, et al.: Early administration of antibiotics does not shorten time to clinical stability in patients with moderate-to-severe community-acquired pneumonia. *Chest* 124(5):1798–1804, 2003.

27. Gonzales R, Bartlett JG, Besser RE, et al.: Principles of appropriate antibiotic use for treatment of uncomplicated acute bronchitis: Background. *Ann Emerg Med* 37(6):720–727, 2001.

28. Bent S, Saint A, Vittinghoff E, et al.: Antibiotics in acute bronchitis: A meta-analysis. *Am J Med* 107:62–67, 1999.

29. McCrory DC, Brown C, Gelfand SE, et al.: Management of acute exacerbations of COPD: A summary and appraisal of published evidence. *Chest* 119:1190–1209, 2001.

30. Anthionisen NR, Manfreda J, Warren PW, et al.: Antibiotic therapy in exacerbations of chronic obstructive pulmonary disease. *Ann Int Med* 106:196–204, 1987.

31. Destache CJ, Dewan N, O'Donohue WJ, et al.: Clinical and economic considerations in the treatment of acute exacerbations of chronic bronchitis. *J Antimicrob Chemother* 43(Suppl. A):107–113, 1999.

32. Oliveira EC, Marsk PE, Colice G: Influenza pneumonia: A descriptive study. *Chest* 119:1717–1723, 2001.

33. Kaiser L, Keene ON, Hammond JM, et al.: Impact of zanamivir on antibiotic use for respiratory events following acute influenza in adolescents and adults. *Arch Intern Med* 160:3234–3240, 2000.

34. Centers for Disease Control and Prevention: Revised U.S. surveillance case definition for Severe Acute Respiratory

Syndrome (SARS) and update on SARS cases—United States and Worldwide, December 2003. *Morb Mortal Wkly Rep* 52(49):1202–1206, 2003.

35. Paul S, Gilbert HM, Ziecheck W, et al.: The impact of potent antiretroviral therapy on the characteristics of hospitalized patients with HIV infection. *AIDS* 13:415–418, 1999.

36. Wolff AJ, O'Donnell AE: Pulmonary manifestations of HIV infection in the era of highly active antiretroviral therapy. *Chest* 120(6):1888–1893, 2001.

37. Hirstick RE, Glassroth J, Jordan MC et al.: Bacterial pneumonia in persons infected with the human immunodeficiency virus. *N Engl J Med* 333:845–851, 1995.

38. Perlman DC, el-Sadr WM, Nelson ET, et al.: Variation of chest radiographic patterns in pulmonary tuberculosis by degree of human immunodeficiency virus-related immunosuppression. *Clin Infect Dis* 25(2):242–246, 1997.

39. Avery RK, Long J: Pneumonia in the immunocompromised host without HIV. *Curr Treat Options Infect Dis* 4:249–266, 2002.

40. Hughes WT, Armstrong D, Bodey GP, et al.: 2002 guidelines for the use of antimicrobial agents in neutropenic patients with cancer. *Clin Infect Dis* 34:730-751, 2001.

41. Metlay JP, Schulz R, Li YH, et al.: Influence of age on symptoms at presentation in patients with community-acquired pneumonia. *Arch Intern Med* 157:1453–1459, 1997.

42. Muder RR: Pneumonia in residents of long-term care facilities: Epidemiology, etiology, management and prevention. *Am J Med* 105:319–330, 1998.

43. Johnson JC, Jayadevappa R, Baccash PD, et al.: Nonspecific presentation of pneumonia in hospitalized older people: Age effect of dementia? *J Am Geriatr Soc* 48 (10):1316–1320, 2000.

44. Gleason PP, Meehan TP, Fine JM, et al.: Associations between initial antimicrobial therapy and medical outcomes for hospitalized elderly patients with pneumonia. *Arch Intern Med* 159:2562–2572, 1999.

11

Tuberculosis

Juzar Ali

HIGH YIELD FACTS

1. Tuberculosis (TB) remains the most common infectious cause of death in adults worldwide. Public health measures and effective chemotherapy have substantially reduced the incidence and prevalence of TB in the United States. Nevertheless certain segments of the population remain at increased risk for TB. Some of these segments of the population use the emergency department for their medical emergencies and acute care.

2. TB is defined as a disease caused by members of the *Mycobacterium tuberculosis* complex, which includes *M. tuberculosis*, *M. bovis*, *M. africanum*, and *M. microti*. The cell wall components give the mycobacterium its characteristic staining properties. The organism stains gram positive. The mycolic acid structure confers the ability to resist destaining by acid alcohol after being stained by certain aniline dyes, hence the term acid-fast bacillus (AFB).

3. A tuberculous cavity contains a complex collection of abundant bacilli with its caseous material in its core surrounded by a heterogeneous cellular response of giant cells and lymphocytes and contained at the periphery by low bacillary or a bacillus free zone of encapsulating fibrosis.

4. In general, individuals who become infected with *M. tuberculosis* have approximately a 10% risk for developing active TB during their lifetimes. This risk is greatest during the first 2 years after infection. Immunocompromised persons have a greater risk for the progression of latent TB infection to active TB disease. Immunosuppressive conditions associated with reactivation TB include HIV infection and AIDS, end-stage renal disease and diabetes mellitus (DM), malignancies, chronic immunosuppressive drug use, and age-related immune deficiencies.

5. Early pulmonary TB is asymptomatic with incidental findings noted on chest radiographs. However, when the bacterial load increases, nonspecific constitutional symptoms of fatigue, weight loss, afternoon fevers, and night sweats may set in. As disease burden advances, cough, sputum production, and localized symptoms such as hemoptysis may appear.

6. It is essential that laboratory testing for mycobacteria be performed rapidly and that the results are reported immediately. Logistical delays in this connection are potentially disastrous as they result in delays in diagnosis and treatment. Various lab tests based on clinical mycobacteriology can be performed. Pulmonary TB is diagnosed by visualization of acid-fast bacilli (AFB) on a sputum smear and isolation of the organism from a culture of this sputum.

7. Management and clinical disposition of a TB patient from the ED begins with triaging and identifying potential TB cases, initiating isolation techniques, emphasizing enhanced ventilatory and respiratory control measures, stratifying cases, and establishing disposition parameters. As soon as a patient is known or suspected to have active TB, this information should be reported to the public health department so that appropriate follow-up can be arranged and a community contact investigation can be performed. The health department should be notified well before patient discharge to facilitate follow-up and continuation of therapy. A discharge plan coordinated with the patient, the health department, and the inpatient facility if applicable should be implemented.

CLINICAL SCENARIOS ENCOUNTERED IN THE ED

Multiple case scenarios related directly or indirectly to tuberculosis may be encountered in the ED. They have been listed below and outlined in Fig. 11–1 and the management of these cases will be discussed in this chapter within the pertinent sections. An algorithmic follow-up plan is also suggested.

- *Encounter A*: A 34-year-old man comes to the ED with a history of a blunt injury to his left foot while working on his job. He has had a recent preemployment physical examination which was normal except for a positive PPD reaction. However, he failed to obtain follow-up.

- *Encounter B*: A 23-year-old woman with a previous prenatal follow-up in the OB/Gyn Clinic now comes in with a cough of 3 months duration, fever, chills, night sweats, and fatigue. She had a positive PPD

TB related clinical scenarios encountered in the ED

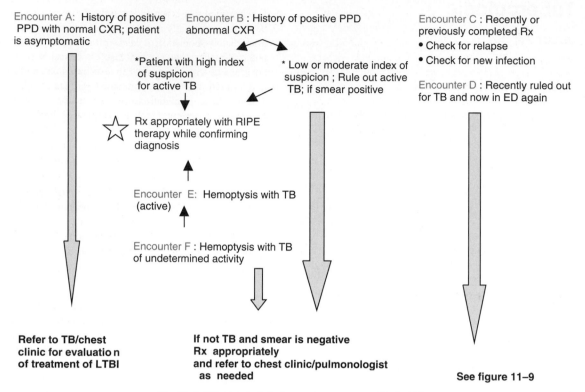

Fig. 11–1. TB related clinical scenarios encountered in the ED.

reaction during that prenatal visit 1 year ago but was not treated.

• *Encounter C*: A 54-year-old man with history of poorly controlled DM has recently been discharged from the TB clinic after completion of treatment for active TB and now comes to the ED with cough, sputum, and low grade fever.

• *Encounter D*: A 45-year-old man is sent from the homeless shelter with a 3 day history of cough, greenish sputum production, and high grade fever. Records show that he was in the ED a month ago with similar complaints.

• *Encounter E*: A 36-year-old man with a history of substance abuse comes to the ED with a moderate amount of hemoptysis, fever, and night sweats. Chest x-ray (CXR) reveals multiple cavitary lesions in the left upper lobe.

• *Encounter F*: A 46-year-old Vietnamese-American man, who is a recent immigrant with past history of TB, comes to the ED with symptoms of mild hemoptysis, nausea, vomiting, and loose stools. He is admitted with a diagnosis of severe gastroenteritis. His CXR reveals old calcified scars in the right upper lung zone.

INTRODUCTION AND EPIDEMIOLOGY

TB remains the most common infectious cause of death in adults worldwide, and the World Health Organization (WHO) has declared it a global emergency (www.who.org). Public health measures and effective chemotherapy have substantially reduced the incidence and prevalence of TB in the United States. Nevertheless certain segments of the population remain at increased risk for TB. These include foreign-born persons from areas with high TB prevalence, homeless persons, or those residing in underserved sections of inner cities, current and former residents of correctional facilities, persons with history of substance abuse, and the elderly in long-term facilities. It is these segments of the population who also potentially use the emergency department for their medical emergencies and acute care. Awareness of the epidemiology of TB in different parts of the world is important in the ER setting. Besides administrative, engineering, and personal control measures, which must be implemented to ensure a successful TB control program in any institution, early identification and management of patients with TB and increased awareness among health care workers at the point of first contact is essential (1, 2). Besides HIV-infected individuals, tuberculosis is increasingly concentrated in persons of lower socioeconomic status. Low income, crowded living conditions, unemployment, and lower educational attainment account for much of the elevated risk for tuberculosis that has been noted among African-, Hispanic-, Asian-, and Native-Americans (3).

Both social and medical factors underlie the emergence of MDR-TB. Multidrug-resistant organisms are created when tuberculosis is treated inappropriately, whether due to prescribing error or to poor compliance with therapy. Tuberculosis occurring in foreign-born persons residing in the United States has played a major role in the resurgence of tuberculosis (4, 5). People originally from Mexico, the Philippines, Vietnam, India, China, Haiti, and South Korea are responsible for approximately two-thirds of the foreign-born cases.

MICROBIOLOGY, IMMUNOLOGY, PATHOGENESIS, AND PATHOPHYSIOLOGY

Microbiology

M. tuberculosis belongs to the genus *Mycobacterium* that includes more than 50 other species, often collectively referred to as nontuberculous mycobacteria. TB is defined as a disease caused by members of the *M. tuberculosis* complex, which includes the tubercle bacillus (*M. tuberculosis*), *M. bovis*, *M. africanum*, and *M. microti*. This genus is distinguished by its cell envelope composed of a core of three macromolecules covalently linked to each other (peptidoglycan, arabinogalactan, and mycolic acids) and a lipopolysaccharide, lipoarabinomannan (LAM), which is thought to be anchored to the plasma membrane (6). These cell wall components give the mycobacterium its

characteristic staining properties. The organism stains positive with Gram stain. The mycolic acid structure confers the ability to resist destaining by acid alcohol after being stained by certain aniline dyes, hence the term AFB.

Worldwide, microscopy to detect AFB (using Ziehl-Neelsen or Kinyoun stain) is the most commonly used procedure to diagnose TB. However, a specimen must contain at least 10^4 colony forming units (CFU)/mL to yield a positive smear (7). Microscopy of specimens stained with a fluorochrome dye, such as auramine O, provides a more sensitive alternative. However, microscopic detection of mycobacteria does not distinguish *M. tuberculosis* from nontuberculous mycobacteria, leading to confusion in diagnosis in areas where atypical TB is endemic. However, once the organism is isolated, its identification as *M. tuberculosis* is based upon morphologic and biochemical characteristics. Nucleic-acid-based detection methods have decreased the dependence upon many of the conventional microbiologic and biochemical tests.

Immunology

The human host serves as the only natural reservoir for *M. tuberculosis*, and the ability of the organism to efficiently establish latent infection has enabled it to spread to nearly one-third of the world's population. From this infected reservoir, eight million new TB cases occur each year and about two million infected patients die annually. Ninety percent of individuals in the general population who become infected with *M. tuberculosis* will never develop clinical disease (8). This observation indicates that the innate and adaptive immune response of the host in controlling such an infection is quite effective. The complete genome sequence of *M. tuberculosis* strain H37Rv has been determined and is annotated (http://www.sanger.ac.uk/Projects/M_tuberculosis/) (9).

The role of cytokines in outcome after *M. tuberculosis* infection is unclear. TNF-alpha is important for proper granuloma formation. Persistently infected mice treated with neutralizing anti-TNF-alpha antibody develop granuloma disorganization. Mice deficient in Interferon-gamma or TNF-alpha receptor are highly susceptible to *M. tuberculosis* infection. Together, multiple cytokine responses determine the disease outcome of the infected host (10). TB is an infection that initiates and requires a cellular immune response for its control. The influence and response of macrophages vary between individuals and even within the same individual from time to time. Unrestricted bacterial multiplication during the initial stages of infection then leads to lymphatic and hematogenous spread with development of delayed hypersensitivity and cell mediated immunity (11). Two to six weeks after infection, T cells that specifically recognize *M. tuberculosis* antigens appear; this response can be demonstrated clinically by the development of a delayed-type hypersensitivity (DTH) response to intradermally injected tuberculin or PPD. The DTH response per se does not correlate with protection against TB, since numerous BCG vaccination trials have demonstrated that disease can occur in those who mount a DTH response. The protective T cell response must be distinguished from the T cell response associated with DTH (12).

Pathogenesis

The pathologic features of TB resulting from tissue hypersensitivity lead to granuloma formation with organization of lymphocytic predominant cellular proliferation with Langhan cell giant cells fibroblasts and capillaries. Classically referred to as "hard" tubercles, this granuloma reflects a well-contained tissue reaction, fibrosis, encapsulation, and scar formation. However, when the antigenic burden and subsequent degree of hypersensitivity are high, cellular organization is diffuse, sparse, and results in tissue necrosis of a variable nature. This causes an exudative caseous response with inherent instability and an enhanced propensity to disseminate. It may also produce a cavity with high bacterial load. A tuberculous cavity therefore contains a complex collection of abundant bacilli with its caseous material in its core surrounded by a heterogeneous cellular response of giant cells and lymphocytes and contained at the periphery by low bacillary or a bacillus-free zone of encapsulating fibrosis (11). The granuloma formation is an important mechanism by the host to control, if not eliminate, the infection. Granuloma formation requires balanced expression of cytokines and chemokines. These observations suggest that a certain level of proinflammatory response induced by *M. tuberculosis* itself is necessary for proper granuloma formation, which is protective both to the host and the bacterium (12). Factors that influence the transmission of TB are outlined in Tables 11–1 and 11–2.

M. tuberculosis is carried in airborne particles, or droplet nuclei, that can be generated when persons who have pulmonary or laryngeal TB sneeze, cough, speak, or sing. The particles are an estimated 1–5 μm in size, and normal air currents can keep them airborne for prolonged time periods and spread them throughout a room or building. Infection occurs when a susceptible person inhales droplet nuclei containing *M. tuberculosis*, and these

Table 11–1. Factors that Influence the Transmission of MTB

Environment factors
Circulation of air in closed spaces
Filtration
Use of UV lights in high traffic areas
Inadequate Ventilation

In an active case	**For contact cases**
• Symptoms especially cough	• Closeness of contact
• Cavitary disease	• Duration of exposure
• Bacterial load; aerosolized source	• Immune status of contact
• Volume of Secretions	• History of previous latent infection
• Initiation and duration of therapy	
• Use of INH-RIF based regimens	
• Compliance and adherence factors	

droplet nuclei traverse the mouth or nasal passages, upper respiratory tract, and bronchi to reach the alveoli of the lungs. Once in the alveoli, the organisms are taken up by alveolar macrophages and spread throughout the body.

Table 11–2. Facts Regarding Source Case and Infectivity in Pulmonary TB

- For infectivity, organisms must have access to environment and must be aerosolized
- A single bacillus in a tiny droplet nucleus is more hazardous than a large number of bacilli in a larger particle
- Coughing is the most effective mechanism for production of droplet nuclei and is equivalent to 5 minutes of loud talking
- A single sneeze may produce 20,000–40,000 droplets, but many are large nonrespirable particles, and thus not infectious
- Thin watery secretions are more easily fragmented into small respirable droplets than is more viscous mucus
- The number of bacilli in solid nodular lesions ranges from 10^2 to 10^{44} CFU/mL whereas in cavitary lesions populations are no the order of 10^7–10^9 CFU/mL

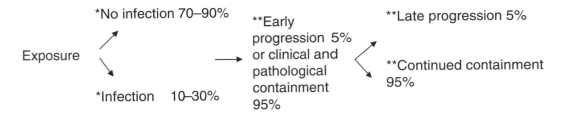

* Depends upon the adequacy of nonimmunologic defenses and transmission factors
** Depends upon adequacy of immunologic host defenses

Fig. 11–2. Host reponse to *M. tuberculosis* infection based on immunologic and nonimmunologic defense factors (adapted from Hopewell and Bloom (12, Chapter 34)).

Usually within 2– weeks to 10 weeks after initial infection with *M. tuberculosis*, the immune response limits further multiplication and spread of the tubercle bacilli; however, some of the bacilli remain dormant and viable for many years. This condition is referred to as latent TB infection. Persons with latent TB infection usually have positive purified protein derivative (PPD)-tuberculin skin-test results, but they do not have symptoms of active TB and they are not infectious. In general, persons who become infected with *M. tuberculosis* have an approximately 10% risk for developing active TB during their lifetimes. This risk is greatest during the first 2 years after infection. Immunocompromised persons have a greater risk for the progression of latent TB infection to active TB disease; HIV infection is the strongest known risk factor for this progression.

Persons with latent TB infection who become coinfected with HIV have approximately an 8–10% risk per year for developing active TB. HIV-infected persons who are already severely immunosuppressed and who become newly infected with *M. tuberculosis* have an even greater risk for developing active TB (Fig. 11–2).

If the innate defense system of the host fails to eliminate this infection, the bacilli proliferate inside alveolar macrophages and kill the cells. The infected macrophages produce cytokines and chemokines that attract other phagocytic cells, including monocytes, other alveolar macrophages, and neutrophils, which eventually form a nodular granulomatous structure called the tubercle. Initial infection with *M. tuberculosis* in an immunocompetent individual usually producies a subpleural lesion called a Ghon focus. In the subapical region this walled-off "cheesy" nodule is referred to as the Simon focus from where reactivation disease may later initiate. Granulomatous involvement of peribronchial and/or

hilar lymph nodes is frequent in primary tuberculosis due to lymphangitic spread from the Ghon focus. The early Ghon focus together with the lymph node lesion constitute the Ghon complex. These lesions undergo healing and over time usually evolve to fibrocalcific nodules. The combination of late fibrocalcific lesions of the lung parenchyma and lymph node which evolved from the Ghon complex is referred to as the Ranke complex (Fig. 11–3).

If the mycobacterial growth continues to remain unchecked, the bacilli may spread hematogenously to produce disseminated TB. Miliary TB describes a disseminated disease with lesions resembling millet seeds. Bacilli can also spread mechanically by erosion of the caseating lesions into the lung airways. It is at this point that the host becomes infectious to others. The chronic disease is characterized by repeated episodes of spontaneous healing by fibrotic changes around the lesions and tissue breakdown. Healing by complete spontaneous eradication of the bacilli is rare.

Reactivation TB results when the persistent mycobacteria in a host suddenly proliferate. While immunosuppression is clearly associated with reactivation TB, it is not clear what host factors specifically maintain the infection in a latent state for many years and what triggers the latent infection to become overt. Immunosuppressive conditions associated with reactivation TB include HIV infection and AIDS, end-stage renal disease and DM, malignancies, chronic immunosuppressive drug use, and age-related immune deficiencies.

In contrast to primary disease, the disease process in reactivation TB tends to be localized; there is little regional lymph node involvement and less caseation. The lesion typically occurs at the lung apices, and disseminated

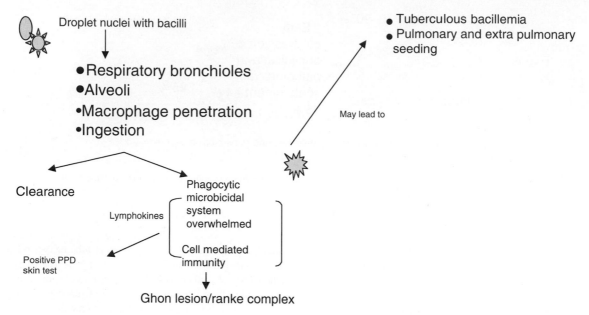

Fig. 11–3. Illustration of the pathogenesis of TB in a nonimmunized host with the the development of the primary complex (Ghon Lesion and Ranke complex).

disease is unusual, unless the host is severely immunosuppressed.

Characteristics of the persons exposed to *M. tuberculosis* that may affect the risk for becoming infected are not as well defined. In general, persons who have been infected previously with *M. tuberculosis* may be less susceptible to subsequent infection. However, reinfection can occur among previously infected persons, especially if they are severely immunocompromised. Vaccination with Bacille of Calmette and Guérin (BCG) probably does not affect the risk for infection; rather, it decreases the risk for progressing from latent TB infection to active TB. Finally, although it is well established that HIV infection increases the likelihood of progressing from latent TB infection to active TB, it is unknown whether HIV infection increases the risk for becoming infected if exposed to *M. tuberculosis*.

Pathophysiology

The pathophysiologic derangement resulting from tuberculosis depends upon its stages of pathogenesis. It also is reflected in its varied clinical presentations. The positive PPD skin tests reflect the delayed hypersensitivity stage with the cellular response. Clinically the patient is usually asymptomatic until the primary TB stage. Post

primary pulmonary TB is usually an asymmetric process clinically showing up as pneumonia with its characteristic radiographic presentation. The highly infectious nature of these lesions with subsequent endobronchial inflammation and ulceration results in pulmonary symptoms of fever, cough, and dyspnea with signs of respiratory insufficiency depending upon the extent of the process. Subsequent healing mechanisms and chronic cavitary and fibrotic foci lead to scarring and restrictive pulmonary physiology with progressive dsypnea, V/Q mismatching, hypoxemia, and respiratory failure. Hemoptysis from cavities and bronchiectactic areas, secondary infections with nontuberculous mycobacteria, or Aspergillus may further amplify the pathophysiologic derangement (13).

CLINICAL PRESENTATION

The clinical presentation of TB varies with the organ system and sites involved (Fig. 11–4). The lungs are the major site for *M. tuberculosis* infection. Pulmonary manifestations of TB include primary, reactivation, endobronchial, and lower lung field infection. Moreover, complications of TB can also involve the lung, including bronchiectasis, hemoptysis, pneumothorax, and necrotizing lung destruction referred to as pulmonary gangrene.

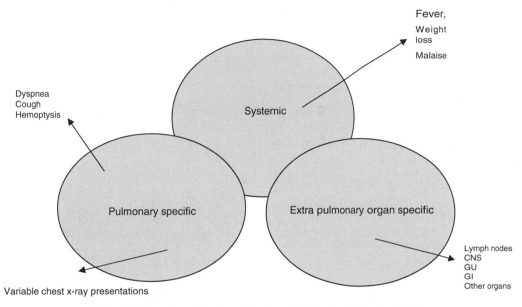

Fig. 11–4. The various clinical manifestations of TB (refer to Figs. 5, 6A–6E).

Primary TB

Fever is the most common symptom, occurring in approximately 70% of patients. It is generally low grade but can be as high as 39°C, and lasts for an average of 14–21 days. It generally resolves in 98% of patients by 10 weeks. Additionally, both pleuritic and nonpleuritic chest pain are common. This pain may be retrosternal and interscapular in location and dull in nature. Other symptoms include fatigue, cough, and generalized arthralgias. The physical examination is usually normal unless there is an associated pleural effusion. The most common abnormality on chest radiography is hilar adenopathy, which can be seen as early as 1 week after skin test conversion and within 2 months in all cases. Associated middle lobe collapse may complicate the adenopathy, presumably because of its anatomic and structural characteristics (14).

Reactivation TB

Reactivation TB represents 90% of adult cases in the non-HIV-infected population and results from reactivation of a previously dormant focus seeded at the time of the primary infection. The apical posterior segments of the lung are frequently involved. The original site of spread may have been previously visible as a small scar called a Simon focus. Early pulmonary TB is asymptomatic with incidental findings noted on chest radiographs. However, when the

bacterial load increases, nonspecific constitutional symptoms of fatigue, weight loss, afternoon fevers, and night sweats may develop. As disease burden advances, productive cough, sputum production (rarely foul smelling), and localized symptoms such as hemoptysis may appear. Chest pain implies pleural involvement. Upper airway signs and symptoms result from highly infectious pulmonary secretions disseminating into the larynx. Dyspnea can occur when patients have extensive parenchymal involvement, pleural effusions, or a pneumothorax. Physical findings of pulmonary TB are not specific and usually are absent in mild or moderate disease. Dullness with decreased fremitus may indicate pleural thickening or effusion. Crackles may be present throughout inspiration or may be heard only after a short cough (posttussive rales). When large areas of the lung are involved, signs of consolidation associated with open bronchi, such as whispered pectoriloquy or tubular breath sounds, may be heard. Distant hollow breath sounds over cavities can be heard and are referred to as amphoric or cavernous breath sounds. Clubbing is uncommon unless TB is associated with severe bronchiectasis.

Atypical clinical presentation

It has been well documented that pulmonary TB differs in elderly patients compared to younger ones, including a longer duration of symptoms before diagnosis and a lower frequency of pulmonary and constitutional symptoms. Fever, sweats, and hemoptysis are less common in the elderly, and these patients are less likely to have cavitary disease or a positive PPD skin test. A nonspecific tuberculous pneumonitis, without typical clinical features of either primary or reactivation TB, can affect the lower lobes. Symptoms in lower lobe TB resemble reactivation disease and are generally either subacute in onset (mean of 12 weeks) or chronic (up to 6 months). Compared to upper lobe TB, consolidation in the lower lobes tends to be more extensive and homogeneous. Cavitation (including large cavities) may be present. This form of TB is frequently misdiagnosed initially as viral or bacterial pneumonia, bronchiectasis, or carcinoma. Furthermore, patients with comorbid conditions such as diabetes, renal or hepatic disease, or those receiving corticosteroids appear most at risk for lower lobe TB. Patients of Asian ethnicity tended to lack symptoms and may be even less likely to report symptoms than other patients (15).

Endobronchial TB

Two mechanisms for developing endobronchial TB have been postulated: direct extension to the bronchi from an adjacent parenchymal focus (usually a cavity) or spread of organisms to the bronchi via infected sputum from a distant site. It is common to find upper lung parenchymal or cavitary disease with bronchogenic spread to the lower lung fields, presumably from pooled infected secretions. Endobronchial disease with primary infection is more often associated with impingement of enlarged lymph nodes on the bronchi. Inflammation results and can be followed by endobronchial ulceration or even perforation. Complications of endobronchial TB can include obstruction, atelectasis (with or without secondary infections), bronchiectasis, and bronchial stenosis. Symptoms include a barking type of cough, often accompanied by sputum production which in some cases may result in production of caseous material from endobronchial lesions or calcific material from extension of calcific nodes into the bronchi (i.e., lithoptysis). Wheezing and hemoptysis can also develop.

TB of undetermined activity

As many as 5% of patients with active TB may present with upper lobe fibrocalcific changes thought to be indicative of healed primary TB. Lesions described by clinicians as "hard" and at times mistakenly thought to represent "inactive, old, healed, scarred disease" may actually represent an active focus. If such patients have any pulmonary symptoms or lack serial films documenting stability of the lesion, they should be evaluated for active TB.

Tuberculoma

Defined as a rounded mass lesion, a tuberculoma can develop during primary infection or when a focus of reactivation TB becomes encapsulated. These lesions rarely cavitate. Since sputum cultures are often negative, fine needle aspiration or open lung biopsy may be necessary for diagnosis.

Complications

Pulmonary complications of TB include hemoptysis, pneumothorax, bronchiectasis, and extensive pulmonary destruction (including pulmonary gangrene). Tuberculosis is thought to account for 5–15% of cases of hemoptysis in the United States, but an increased proportion in countries with higher rates of TB. Although more common with active tuberculosis, hemoptysis may also occur after completion of effective chemotherapy and does not necessarily imply active disease. Many patients with hemoptysis are smear positive and have cavitary disease, but the absence of these findings does not preclude hemoptysis. Bleeding usually is of small volume, appearing as blood-streaked sputum. Massive hemoptysis is a rare complication nowadays and prior to effective chemotherapy, accounted for approximately 5% of deaths from TB. Well described albeit rare, "Rasmussen's aneurysm" causes massive hemoptysis when the disease process extends into the adventitia and media of bronchial arteries, resulting in inflammation and thinning of the vessel wall; this aneurysm subsequently ruptures into the cavity, producing hemoptysis (13, 16). Hemoptysis after the completion of therapy for TB only occasionally represents recurrence of TB. It is most likely due to bronchiectasis, an aspergilloma or other mycetoma invading an old healed cavity (Fig. 11–5), a ruptured broncholith that erodes through a bronchial artery, or any other malignant or nonmalignant inflammatory process.

Pneumothorax results from the rupture of a peripheral cavity or a subpleural caseous focus with liquefaction into the pleural space. Bronchiectasis may develop after primary or reactivation TB. After primary TB, extrinsic compression of a bronchus by enlarged nodes may cause bronchial dilation distal to the obstruction. There may be no evidence of parenchymal TB. In reactivation TB, progressive destruction and fibrosis of lung parenchyma may lead to localized bronchial dilation resulting in what is referred to as "dry" bronchiectasis. If endobronchial

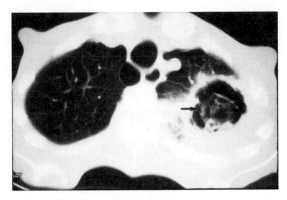

Fig. 11–5. CT scan of the chest showing a mycetoma in an old tuberculous cavity (see arrow).

disease is present, bronchial stenosis may result in distal bronchiectasis. Bronchiectasis is more frequent in the common sites of reactivation TB (apical and posterior segments of the upper lobe), but may be found in other involved areas of the lung. As noted above, bronchiectasis can also be associated with hemoptysis (13).

Pulmonary gangrene

Rarely, TB can cause progressive, extensive destruction of areas of one or both lungs. This is seen especially in primary TB, although occasionally lymph node obstruction of the bronchi with a combination of distal collapse, necrosis, and bacterial superinfection can produce parenchymal destruction. However, destruction more typically results from years of chronic reactivation TB, typically in the absence of continuous or prolonged effective chemotherapy. Symptoms include progressive dyspnea, hemoptysis, and weight loss. The term pulmonary gangrene refers to a more acute destructive process. Patients with this form of TB have rapid progression from a homogeneous, extensive infiltrate to dense consolidation. Development of air-filled cysts which coalesce into cavities is also observed. Necrotic lung tissue may be seen attached to the wall of the cavity. Alternatively, pulmonary gangrene may resemble an intracavitary clot, fungus ball, or the Rasmussen aneurysm. Pathology shows arteritis and thrombosis of the vessels supplying the necrotic lung. While resolution with effective therapy has been reported, mortality is usually high (17).

Extrapulmonary TB

About 80% of all TB is pulmonary. Of the 20% "extrapulmonary group," 30% is pleural disease, 30% involves lymph nodes, and the rest includes genitourinary tract, bone, the central nervous system (CNS), and miliary disease (18). Extrapulmonary signs and findings are localized to the sites of involvement. Symptoms of miliary disease are varied and range from fever and fatigue to multiorgan system involvement. Physical signs such as hepatosplenomegaly, neurologic findings, ascites, and jaundice may be present. PPD may be negative in 50–70% of these cases. CNS tuberculosis, which is not necessarily associated with HIV infection, includes three clinical syndromes: meningitis, intracranial tuberculoma, and spinal tuberculous arachnoiditis.

LABORATORY AND DIAGNOSTIC TESTING

General Considerations

It is essential that laboratory testing for mycobacteria be performed rapidly and the results reported immediately. Logistical delays in this connection are potentially disastrous as they result in delays in diagnosis and treatment. Various lab tests based on clinical mycobacteriology can be performed (Table 11–3).

Skin testing for TB is an epidemiologic tool to assess exposures and should not be performed as a test to include or exclude active pulmonary TB. It is neither sensitive nor specific. Patients with positive reactions may not have active TB, and 20–30% of those with a new diagnosis of active TB have negative reactions. Moreover, the degree of the skin test reaction as measured by induration at the site cannot predict if a patient has active disease (19).

Sputum examination. Pulmonary TB is diagnosed by visualization of AFB on a sputum smear and isolation of the organism from a culture of the sputum. Most laboratories currently use auramine-rhodamine or auramine O to stain the sputum, allowing scanning for fluorescence as opposed to Ziehl-Neelsen stain, which requires more time and labor to identify organisms. Concentrating sputum specimens and obtaining a larger quantity of sputum (≥5 mL) have both been shown to increase the probability of visualizing organisms. Conventional teaching is that sputum specimens should be obtained on three consecutive days and that first morning specimens have the highest yield (20, 21). Gastric aspirates obtained in the morning can also be cultured for MTB and reflect sputum swallowed over the course of the night. However, gastric aspiration for the diagnosis of TB is rarely performed in contemporary practice because there are other methods for directly collecting sputum, and AFB smears cannot be done on gastric aspirates.

Table 11–3. Characteristics of Methodology Used in Clinical Mycobacteriological Diagnosis of TB

Method	Microscopy	Culture	Identification	Drug Susceptibility	Special Tests Such as PCR and RFLP
Advantages	• Rapid • Inexpensive • Detects infectious cases	• "Gold standard" • Newer methods enable rapid results	• Identifies specific agent • DNA probes rapid	• Necessary in certain cases	• PCR: rapid • RFLP: useful for epidemiological purposes and tracing transmission
Disadvantages	Low sensitivity	• Expensive • Requires special skills and labs	• Expensive • Probes limited	Expensive and slow	• Expensive • Complex • Expertise required

Source: Modified and adapted from Hopewell PC, Bloom BR. Tuberculosis and other Mycobacterial Disease Chapter 34 in Murray JF, Nadel JA, Mason RJ, Boushey HA (eds): Textbook of Respiratory Disease, 3rd (ed.) W.B. Saunders Philadelphia.

While the standard recommendations are to send three sputum specimens on different days, several articles have been written questioning the necessity of this practice. Published data indicate that 95% of cases would have been detected with two specimens. A high quality expectorated sputum sample is desirable for smear detection of MTB. Induced sputum is not superior to a good expectorated sample. The yield is generally equivalent for both sputum induction sample and bronchoscopy. The cost of induced sputum is considerably lower than that of bronchoscopy. Both sputum induction and bronchoscopy require TB respiratory precautions for the operators. Based upon the available data, it is reasonable to attempt multiple sputum inductions in a patient undergoing work-up for pulmonary TB who is unable to produce good quality expectorated sputum. Bronchoscopy with lavage should be reserved for the unusual patient in whom sputum induction is unsuccessful or in whom any delay in obtaining specimens is considered dangerous (22, 23). The surrogate marker for infectivity is the smear of sputum, whether expectorated or obtained by induction or bronchoscopy. Patients with three negative smears are generally considered noninfectious.

Imaging. Chest radiography is frequently used to evaluate for the presence of active pulmonary TB, but the sensitivity and specificity of such a determination is low. A number of patterns are suggestive on chest radiography, but none are diagnostic. Unusual radiographic findings are common in HIV-infected patients and in the elderly. Reactivation TB typically involves the apical-posterior segments of the upper lobes (80–90% of patients), followed in frequency by the superior segment of the lower lobes. "Atypical" radiographic patterns for adult TB include hilar adenopathy, sometimes associated with right middle lobe collapse, nodules, and lower zone cavities. These findings are more common in primary TB and probably represent the known increasing incidence of primary TB in adults, rather than "atypical" forms of TB (Figs 11–6A to 11–6E).

Computed tomography (CT) of the head with contrast enhancement can also define the presence and extent of basilar arachnoiditis, cerebral edema and infarction, and the presence and course of hydrocephalus. In two large community-based series hydrocephalus was seen in approximately 75% of patients, basilar meningeal enhancement in 38%, cerebral infarcts in 15–30%, and tuberculomas in 5–10%. Magnetic resonance imaging (MRI) is superior to CT in defining lesions of the basal ganglia, midbrain, and brain stem and for evaluating all forms of suspected spinal TB.

Laboratory findings. Generally normal in early disease, hematologic changes may include a normocytic anemia, leukocytosis, or, more rarely, monocytosis. Hyponatremia may be associated with the syndrome of inappropriate adrenocortical hormone secretion (SIADH) or rarely with adrenal insufficiency. Hypoalbuminemia and hypergammaglobulinemia also can occur as late findings.

Pleural fluid. Classically demonstrating a lymphocytic-predominant exudate, tuberculous pleural effusions are generally thought to represent a delayed-type hypersensitivity reaction to mycobacterial antigens. Thus, the burden

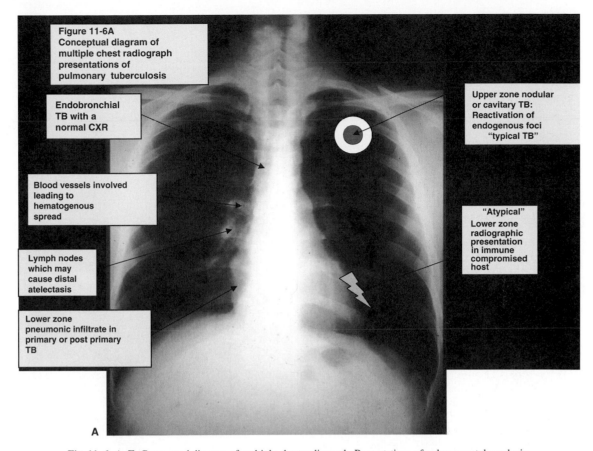

Figure 11-6A Conceptual diagram of multiple chest radiograph presentations of pulmonary tuberculosis

Endobronchial TB with a normal CXR

Upper zone nodular or cavitary TB: Reactivation of endogenous foci "typical TB"

Blood vessels involved leading to hematogenous spread

"Atypical" Lower zone radiographic presentation in immune compromised host

Lymph nodes which may cause distal atelectasis

Lower zone pneumonic infiltrate in primary or post primary TB

A

Fig. 11–6. A–E. Conceptual diagram of multiple chest radiograph. Presentations of pulmonary tuberculosis.

of organisms compared to the amount of fluid is low, and culture is more frequently positive from pleural tissue than from pleural fluid. An AFB smear of pleural fluid is positive in only about 15–20% of cases, but the cultures are positive in 80% to 90% of patients with AIDS who have pleural TB.

CSF. The cerebrospinal fluid (CSF) usually demonstrates lymphocytosis, high protein, and a low glucose. The yield of both smear and culture for MTB increases with a larger volume of CSF. Polymerase chain reaction (PCR) of the CSF may be especially useful in diagnosing tuberculous meningitis, but a negative finding does not exclude the disease. Early in the course of illness, the cellular reaction is often atypical with only a few cells or with polymorphonuclear (PMN) leukocyte predominance. Such cases usually rapidly change to a lymphocytic cellular response with subsequent CSF examination(s). Upon initiation of antituberculous chemotherapy, the CSF of some patients briefly reverts

to a neutrophil-predominant cellular reaction. This CSF profile coupled with an associated transient clinical deterioration refers to a phenomenon known as "therapeutic paradox."

Urine cultures. Although genitourinary TB rarely occurs in the absence of other sites of extrapulmonary disease, it is frequently observed in disseminated TB, even in the absence of pyuria. Because urine samples are easy to obtain and have a good yield for diagnosing disseminated TB, a first morning urine sample on three consecutive days should be collected for mycobacterial culture.

Tissue culture. Patients, especially elderly individuals, may present with failure to thrive or fever of unknown origin and few other localizing symptoms suggesting a diagnosis of miliary or disseminated disease. The tuberculin skin test is only positive in 28–53% of patients in collected series (24). Culture of a variety of fluids is recommended since no one culture (e.g., sputum) is of high yield. Gastric

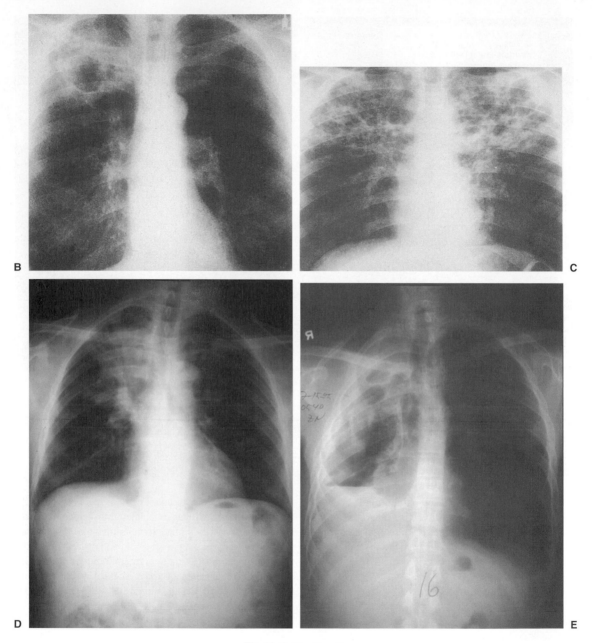

Fig. 11–6. (*Continued*)

aspirates were frequently positive and thus can be considered in patients with a negative sputum smear. Tissue biopsy is also useful, with liver biopsy having the highest yield. Bone marrow biopsies may be positive, but usually only in patients with pancytopenia. Lymph nodes may also be a source of tissue for culture.

MANAGEMENT

The management process begins with steps of triage and identification of potential TB cases, initiating isolation or segregation techniques, emphasizing enhanced ventilatory and respiratory control measures, stratifying cases and establishing disposition parameters (Fig. 11–7). Evaluation should start with a thorough history and physical examination, with attention to epidemiologic risk factors and complaints suspicious for active TB such as persistent (>3 weeks) cough and constitutional symptoms (fever, drenching night sweats, unintentional weight loss). Chest radiography should be performed promptly if any degree of suspicion exists for active TB. PPD testing of the patient provides important supportive data, and although it

must be emphasized that the negative predictive value of this test is inadequate to rule out active TB, it is important to elicit any history of a positive tuberculin skin test and verify its documentation.

Many persons with active TB will first present to an ambulatory care site. Patients who may have active TB must be identified and evaluated promptly in order to minimize exposure of others. Ideally, such patients should be isolated in negative pressure rooms, and a surgical mask (not an N95 mask) should be placed on the patient, who should then be instructed to cover the mouth and nose with tissues when sneezing or coughing. Once a patient is diagnosed with active TB, such precautions should continue until the patient is deemed noninfectious. Any hospitalized patient with significant suspicion of active TB (especially pulmonary or laryngeal) should be placed immediately in a negative pressure isolation room. The diagnosis of pulmonary TB should be pursued with sputum samples for acid-fast smear and subsequent mycobacterial culture. Efforts should be made to collect proper samples. Enhancing general ventilation and/or using air disinfection techniques such as ultraviolet germicidal irradiation, and/or high efficiency particulate air (HEPA) filters will

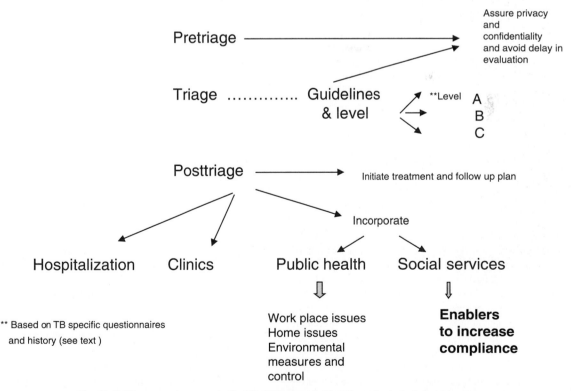

Fig. 11–7. Management process in the ED. TB fast track: identify, evaluate, isolate, and assess.

be of additional benefit in TB control measures at the ED level.

Early identification of patients with active TB is critical. Physicians must be astute in identifying patients who may have active TB, both to benefit the patient and to minimize exposure to health-care workers (HCWs) and to other patients. Early recognition of TB meningitis is also of paramount importance because the clinical outcome depends greatly upon the stage at which therapy is initiated. Empiric antituberculous therapy should be started immediately in suspect cases.

TRIAGE ISSUES

The triage area should be set up to provide the patient with as much privacy as possible. Patients may be reluctant to answer triage questions truthfully when they can be overheard by others, potentially leading to a delay in identifying suspected TB-infected patients. In some emergency departments, a patient score based on risk factors and presenting complaints is developed and used to dictate the need for fast tracking, segregation of TB cases, isolation, and appropriate dispensation (25).

TB transmission is a recognized risk to patients and HCWs in health-care settings. The magnitude of this risk varies significantly depending on facility type, patient population, the prevalence and incidence of infectious TB in the community, occupational group and work area of the HCW, and the effectiveness of the facility's TB control program. The risk of transmission is greater in areas in which care is provided to patients with TB disease before they are identified, properly isolated, and started on appropriate therapy. In addition to providing care to persons with unidentified TB disease, EDs increasingly provide care to those populations most impacted by the TB epidemic such as the urban inner city and medically underserved poor and recent immigrants who may not have health coverage or regular physician follow-up. These patients may wait for long periods under crowded conditions with inadequate room ventilation and potentially increase the risk of transmission to ED staff. Generally the initial ED triage interaction focuses only on patient acuity. As a result, the stable, but infectious, TB patient may be left sitting in the waiting room for a long time. Efforts to identify infectious patients and contain infection should begin as soon as the patient enters the door and approaches the admission or registration desk. When suspected TB-infected patients are identified early in the admission process, these patients can be placed on a "fast-track" for further triaging and possible isolation or masking precautions. Emergency departments that do not have a specific triage tool for this purpose tend to overlook suspected TB-infected patients and triage for acuity only.

Emergency departments present a unique intersection of risk factors. Given these factors, the cornerstone of effective TB control programs in EDs is early identification of patients with infectious TB. After identifying these patients, implementing appropriate isolation and diagnostic procedures are the most important and effective risk reduction activities. An index of suspicion for TB appropriate to the facility, the community, and the client population is an essential component of these practices.

GENERAL TB CONTROL ISSUES IN ED

Nosocomial Transmission

Particular procedures, which can result in the dispersal of droplet nuclei, have been associated with an increased risk of TB transmission. These include endotracheal intubation, bronchoscopy, sputum induction, aerosol treatments, and irrigation/drainage of a tuberculous abscess. Extraordinary precautions are needed when such procedures are performed in the emergency department.

Masking Considerations

Patients who are suspected or known to have infectious TB must be masked until placement in appropriate negative pressure isolation. A regular surgical mask is sufficient to block droplets from escaping into the room air. Masks must be changed if they become difficult to breathe through or damp. Respirators should not be worn by these patients. Some respirators have exhalation valves which allow expired air to escape unfiltered. All increase the work of breathing which can prompt the patient to remove the respirator. Negative pressure is employed to prevent the escape of droplet nuclei. To further this goal, doors must be kept closed, and negative pressure should be verified daily.

Respiratory protection masks should be worn under the following circumstances:

- Persons entering a TB isolation room when the patient is present
- Persons present during a cough-inducing or aerosol-inducing procedure on such patients, such as

bronchoscopy, induced sputum collection, or administration of aerosolized drugs

- Persons in other settings where administrative and engineering controls are unlikely to be protective, for example, in emergency transport vehicles

These devices are designed to filter air before it is inhaled; thus, patients with known or suspected TB should not wear these masks. Instead, when required to be outside TB isolation rooms, such patients should wear surgical masks, which are designed to prevent the respiratory secretions of the person wearing the mask from entering the environment (26, 1).

TREATMENT ISSUES

Recognizing that the aims of treatment of tuberculosis include (1) to cure the individual patient and (2) to minimize the transmission of disease to other persons, TB treatment protocols and their implementation constitute a multidisciplinary exercise. This process may have to be initiated at the ED level with a clear understanding of roles and responsibilities of the public health program and a private physician.

Knowledge of the various drug components of anti-TB therapy and their side effects is imperative for the physician in the emergency department. Generally, rifampin, isoniazid, pyrazinamide, and ethambutol (RIPE) therapy is initially recommended. In special circumstances streptomycin or a quinolone is added to the regimen. Details and doses of therapy are available through various referral Web-based data sources (27, 28, 30). The treatment is divided into two phases that is the induction phase and the maintenance phase with strict adherence to public health protocols and utilization of the direct observed therapy strategy (DOTS).

Moreover, treatment regimes in special situations require attention. These include but are not limited to pregnancy, breast feeding, women using oral contraception, patients with liver disorders (established chronic liver or acute hepatitis), renal failure, and HIV infection. Immediate consultation with the pulmonary/infectious diseases team should be sought in these cases and a multidisciplinary approach implemented (27, 28).

Actively infected individuals who come to the emergency department with treatment interruption warrant special attention. Treatment changes must not be based randomly and addition of new drugs must be made with proper consultation of the specialists. A single new drug must never be added to a failing regimen or a noncompliant patient. These patients require close liaison with the public health department and social services. Medical decision making is dependent upon the immune status of the patient, drug susceptibility, degree of remission, and stage of current disease. Very close follow-up with TB clinic personnel is required and evaluation of the current clinical status and sputum data will dictate resumption of treatment as well as the specific drug regimen (27, 28).

OUTCOME AND DISPOSITION

Clinicians taking care of persons with TB are often asked to assess the contagiousness of the disease. Persons with active, untreated respiratory tract disease (including pneumonia and tracheal infection) are contagious; coughing and singing have been found to increase droplet nuclei production and disease transmission. Successful treatment diminishes this risk. Two weeks of therapy has long been considered sufficient to render a patient noncontagious, although this guideline is somewhat arbitrary.

In general, patients who have suspected or confirmed active TB should be considered infectious if they (a) are coughing, (b) are undergoing cough-inducing procedures, or (c) have positive AFB sputum smears, and if they (a) are not on chemotherapy, (b) have just started chemotherapy, or (c) have a poor clinical or bacteriologic response to chemotherapy. A patient who has drug-susceptible TB and who is on adequate chemotherapy and has had a significant clinical and bacteriologic response to therapy (i.e., reduction in cough, resolution of fever, and progressively decreasing quantity of bacilli on smear) is probably no longer infectious. However, because drug susceptibility results are not usually known when the decision to discontinue isolation is made, all TB patients should remain in isolation while hospitalized until they have had three consecutive negative sputum smears collected on different days and they demonstrate clinical improvement.

Suspected or confirmed cases of TB should be reported promptly to the local public health department in order to expedite contact investigation and to help plan outpatient follow-up. Anti-TB treatment administered during the hospitalization should be directly observed therapy (DOT). Transitioning to outpatient management requires careful planning, including liaison with public health field workers to continue DOT in an uninterrupted manner.

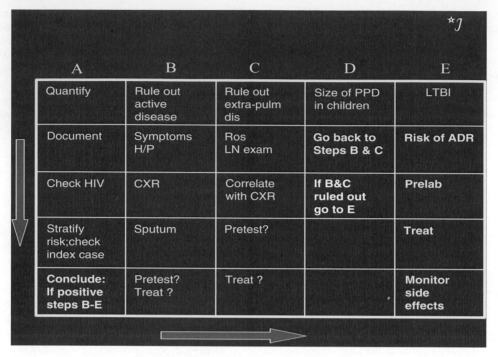

Fig. 11–8. A "positive" PPD: A suggested algorithm.

Discontinuation of TB Isolation

TB isolation can be discontinued if the diagnosis of TB is ruled out. For some patients, TB can be ruled out when another diagnosis is confirmed. If a diagnosis of TB cannot be ruled out, the patient should remain in isolation until a determination has been made that the patient is noninfectious. However, patients can be discharged from the health-care facility while still potentially infectious if appropriate postdischarge arrangements can be ensured. The length of time required for a TB patient to become noninfectious after starting anti-TB therapy varies considerably. Isolation should be discontinued only when the patient is on effective therapy, is improving clinically, and has had three consecutive negative sputum AFB smears collected on different days. Continued isolation throughout the hospitalization should be strongly considered for patients who have MDR-TB because of the tendency for treatment failure or relapse (i.e., difficulty in maintaining noninfectiousness) that has been observed in such cases.

Discharge planning. Cooperation between hospital staff and the local public health department is essential. Discharge to home may be considered once the following conditions are met:

- An outpatient appointment has been arranged with a provider who will manage the TB and plans for DOT has been ensured and assured.

- Case management from the local public health department is involved and agrees with the plan

- The patient is in possession of sufficient anti-TB medication (not just the prescriptions) to last until the outpatient appointment.

A patient may be discharged home while still infectious, provided that the household does not contain members at high risk for active TB (e.g., immunocompromised or age less than 4). While still considered infectious, the patient should stay at home as much as possible and should wear a surgical mask when leaving the home or when receiving visitors.

Coordination with the Public Health Department

As soon as a patient or HCW is known or suspected to have active TB, the patient or HCW should be reported to the public health department so that appropriate follow-up can be arranged and a community contact

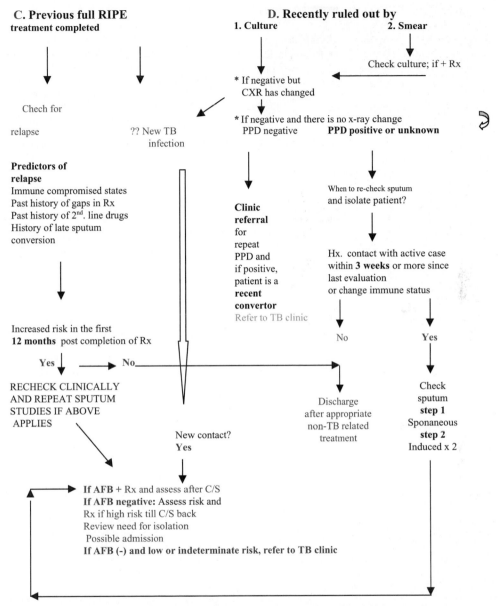

Fig. 11–9. Scenarios c and d as mentioned in the section high yield facts.

investigation can be performed. The health department should be notified well before patient discharge to facilitate follow-up and continuation of therapy. A discharge plan coordinated with the patient or HCW, the health department, and the inpatient facility should be implemented.

DISPOSITION AND OUTCOME OF CASES AS OUTLINED IN SCENARIOS DESCRIBED IN HIGH YIELD FACTS

Encounter A. This case illustrates the need for evaluation for treatment of latent TB infection (LTBI) (Fig. 11–8) previously referred to as "chemoprophylaxis." Indication for this treatment is dependent upon the degree of PPD positivity in relation to the prevalence of disease in a particular group. Isoniazid for 9 months or Rifampin for 4 months is recommended in usual cases. Further details may be obtained through various references quoted (28–30).

Encounter B. This patient has active TB unless proven otherwise. While confirmation of the diagnosis is awaited, it is mandatory to start empirical anti-TB treatment (28, 30).

Encounters C and D. Risks of relapse after completion of therapy depend upon many risk factors. New infection can also occur in areas of high prevalence such as homeless shelters. Extreme vigilance to screening such cases is needed (Fig. 11–9).

Encounters E and F. While hemoptysis does not always imply the presence of active TB, a cavitary lesion in a patient with symptoms and signs suggestive of TB mandates that the diagnosis be ruled out (Fig. 11–9).

SUMMARY

A "cold case" with TB which has been ruled out within the last 3 weeks and with no obvious clinical and CXR changes should be treated appropriately for non-TB related Dx and discharged for follow-up appointment with Pulm/TB clinic and information forwarded to clinics.

REFERENCES

1. CDC: CDC guidelines for preventing the transmission of *Mycobacterium* TB in health-care facilities, 1994. *Morb Mortal Wkly Rep* 43(RR-13), 1994.
2. CDC: Essential components of a tuberculosis prevention and control program. Screening for tuberculosis and tuberculosis infection in high-risk populations. *Morb Mortal Wkly Rep* 44(RR-11), 1995.
3. Cantwell MF, McKenna MT, McCray E, Onorato IM: Tuberculosis and race/ethnicity in the United States. Impact of socioeconomic status. *Am J Respir Crit Care Med* 157:1016, 1998.
4. McKenna MT, McCray E, Onorato I: The epidemiology of tuberculosis among foreign-born persons in the United States, 1986 to 1993. *N Engl J Med* 332:1071, 1995.
5. Talbot EA, Moore M, McCray E, Binkin NJ: Tuberculosis among foreign-born persons in the United States, 1993–1998. *JAMA* 284:2894, 2000.
6. McNeil M, Brennan PJ: Structure, function, and biogenesis of the cell envelope of mycobacteria in relation to bacterial physiology, pathogenesis, and drug resistance: Some thoughts and possibilities arising from recent structural information. *Res Microbiol* 142:451, 1991.
7. Allen BW, Mitchison DA: Counts of viable tubercle bacilli in sputum related to smear and culture gradings. *Med Lab Sci* 49:94, 1992.
8. Comstock GW: Epidemiology of tuberculosis. *Am Rev Respir Dis* 125:8, 1982.
9. Cole ST, Brosch R, Parkhill J, et al.: Deciphering the biology of *Mycobacterium tuberculosis* from the complete genome sequence. *Nature* 393:537, 1998.
10. Orme IM, Cooper AM: Cytokine/chemokine cascades in immunity to tuberculosis. *Immunol Today* 20:307, 1999.
11. Hass DW, Des Prez RM: *Mycobacterium tuberculosis*, in Gerald L Mandell, John E Bennett, Raphael Dolin (eds.): *Principles & Practice of Infectious Diseases*, 4th ed. Chapter 230. Churchill & Livingstone Inc, vol. 2, pp. 2213–2243.
12. Hopewell PC, Bloom BR: Tuberculosis and other mycobacterial disease, in Murray JF, Nadel JA, Mason RJ, Boushey HA (eds.): *Textbook of Respiratory Disease*, 3d ed. Chapter 34 Philadelphia, W.B. Saunders.
13. Ali J: , in Ali J, Summer W, Levitzky M (eds.): *Pulmonary Pathophysiology 2d ed.* Chapters 2, 3. New York, Mcgraw Hill/Lange Series.
14. Krysl J, Korzeniewska-Kosela M, Muller NL, FitzGerald JM: Radiologic features of pulmonary tuberculosis: An assessment of 188 cases. *Can Assoc Radiol J* 45:101, 1994.
15. Miller LG, Asch SM, Yu EI, et al.: A population-based survey of tuberculosis symptoms: How atypical are atypical presentations? *Clin Infect Dis* 30:293, 2000.
16. Conlan AA, Hurwitz SS, Krige L, et al.: Massive hemoptysis. Review of 123 cases. *J Thorac Cardiovasc Surg* 85:120, 1983.
17. Khan FA, Rehman M, Marcus P, et al.: Pulmonary gangrene occurring as a complication of pulmonary tuberculosis. *Chest* 77:76, 1980.
18. Reider HL, Snider DE, Cauthen GM: Extrapulmonary TB in US. *Am Rev Respir Dis* 141:347–351, 1990.
19. Al Zahrani K, Al Jahdali H, Menzies D: Does size matter? Utility of size of tuberculin reactions for the diagnosis of mycobacterial disease. *Am J Respir Crit Care Med* 162:1419, 2000.
20. Peterson EM, Nakasone A, Platon-DeLeon JM, et al.: Comparison of direct and concentrated acid-fast smears to identify specimens culture positive for Mycobacterium spp. *J Clin Microbiol* 37:3564, 1999.
21. Warren JR, Bhattacharya M, De Almeida KN, et al.: A minimum 5.0 ml of sputum improves the sensitivity of acid-fast smear for *Mycobacterium tuberculosis*. *Am J Respir Crit Care Med* 161:1559, 2000.
22. Merrick ST, Sepkowitz KA, Walsh J, et al.: Comparison of induced versus expectorated sputum for diagnosis of pulmonary tuberculosis by acid-fast smear. *Am J Infect Control* 25:463, 1997.

23. Anderson C, Inhaber N, Menzies D: Comparison of sputum induction with fiber-optic bronchoscopy in the diagnosis of tuberculosis. *Am J Respir Crit Care Med* 152:1570, 1995.

24. Kim JH, Langston AA, Gallis HA: TI—miliary tuberculosis: Epidemiology, clinical manifestations, diagnosis, and outcome. *Rev Infect Dis* 12(4):583–590, 1990.

25. A guideline for establishing effective practices: Identifying persons with infectious TB in the emergency department. Francis J Curry National Tuberculosis Center Institutional Consultation Services San Francisco, California, 1998.

26. CDC: Guidelines for preventing the transmission of tuberculosis in health-care settings, with special focus on HIV-related issues. *Morb Mortal Wkly Rep* 39(RR-17), 1990.

27. Blanc L, Chaulet P, Spinal M, et al.: Treatment of TB: Guidelines for national programs Document WHO/CDS/TB/2003. 313 *3d ed.,* 2003. Prepared for the WHO stop TB Department.

28. Core Curriculum on TB: What the Clinician should know *4th ed.* 2000 CDC P Publication.

29. Centers for Disease Control and Prevention: Targeted tuberculin testing and treatment of latent tuberculosis infection. *Morb Mortal Wkly Rep* 49(No.RR-6), 122–124, 2000.

30. CDCP publication. *Am J Respir Crit Care Med* 167:603, 2003.

Glossary of pertinent terms (adapted from CDC/ MMWR publications)

Acid-fast bacilli (AFB): Bacteria that retain certain dyes after being washed in an acid solution. Most acid-fast organisms are mycobacteria. When AFB are seen on a stained smear of sputum or other clinical specimen, a diagnosis of TB should be suspected; however, the diagnosis of TB is not confirmed until a culture is grown and identified as *M. tuberculosis.*

Aerosol: The droplet nuclei that are expelled by an infectious person (e.g., by coughing or sneezing); these droplet nuclei can remain suspended in the air and can transmit *M. tuberculosis* to other persons.

Anergy: The inability of a person to react to skin-test antigens (even if the person is infected with the organisms tested) because of immunosuppression.

Bacillus of Calmette and Guérin (BCG) vaccine: A TB vaccine used in many parts of the world.

BACTEC®: One of the most often used radiometric methods for detecting the early growth of mycobacteria in culture. It provides rapid growth (in 7–14 days) and rapid drug-susceptibility testing (in 5–6 days). When BACTEC® is used with rapid species identification methods, *M. tuberculosis* can be identified within 10–14 days of specimen collection.

Booster phenomenon: A phenomenon in which some persons (especially older adults) who are skin tested many years after infection with *M. tuberculosis* have a negative reaction to an initial skin test followed by a positive reaction to a subsequent skin test. The second (i.e., positive) reaction is caused by a boosted immune response. Two-step testing is used to distinguish new infections from boosted reactions (see two-step testing).

Contact case : A person who has shared the same air with a person who has infectious TB for a sufficient amount of time to allow possible transmission of *M. tuberculosis.*

Directly observed therapy (DOT): An adherence-enhancing strategy in which an HCW or other designated person watches the patient swallow each dose of medication.

DNA probe: A technique that allows rapid and precise identification of mycobacteria (e.g., *M. tuberculosis* and *M. bovis*) that are grown in culture. The identification can often be completed in 2 h.

Droplet nuclei: Microscopic particles (i.e., 1–5 μm in diameter) produced when a person coughs, sneezes, shouts, or sings. The droplets produced by an infectious TB patient can carry tubercle bacilli and can remain suspended in the air for prolonged periods of time and be carried on normal air currents in the room.

Drug resistance, acquired: Resistance to one or more anti-TB drugs that develops while a patient is receiving therapy and which usually results from the patient's nonadherence to therapy or the prescription of an inadequate regimen by a health-care provider.

Drug resistance, primary: Resistance to one or more anti-TB drugs that exists before a patient is treated with the drug(s). Primary resistance occurs in persons exposed to and infected with a drug-resistant strain of *M. tuberculosis.*

Fixed room-air HEPA recirculation systems: Nonmobile devices or systems that remove airborne contaminants by recirculating air through a HEPA filter. These may be built into the room and permanently ducted or may be mounted on the wall or ceiling within the room. In either situation, they are fixed in place and are not easily movable.

Fluorochrome stain: A technique for staining a clinical specimen with fluorescent dyes to perform a microscopic examination (smear) for mycobacteria. This technique is preferable to other staining techniques because the mycobacteria can be seen easily and the slides can be read quickly.

Gastric aspirate: A procedure sometimes used to obtain a specimen for culture when a patient cannot cough up adequate sputum. This procedure is particularly useful for diagnosis in children, who are often unable to cough up sputum.

High-efficiency particulate air (HEPA) filter: A specialized filter that is capable of removing 99.97% of particles $\geq$0.3 mm in diameter and that may assist in controlling the transmission of *M. tuberculosis*. Filters may be used in ventilation systems to remove particles from the air or in personal respirators to filter air before it is inhaled by the person wearing the respirator. The use of HEPA filters in ventilation systems requires expertise in installation and maintenance.

Induration: An area of swelling produced by an immune response to an antigen. In tuberculin skin testing or anergy testing, the diameter of the indurated area is measured 48–72 h after the injection, and the result is recorded in millimeters.

Latent TB infection: Infection with *M. tuberculosis*, usually detected by a positive PPD skin-test result, in a person who has no symptoms of active TB and who is not infectious.

Mantoux test: A method of skin testing that is performed by injecting 0.1 mL of PPD tuberculin containing five tuberculin units into the dermis (i.e., the second layer of skin) of the forearm with a needle and syringe. This test is the most reliable and standardized technique for tuberculin testing (see tuberculin skin test and purified protein derivative (PPD)-tuberculin test).

Multidrug-resistant tuberculosis (MDR-TB): Active TB caused by *M. tuberculosis* organisms that are resistant to more than one anti-TB drug; in practice, often refers to organisms that are resistant to both INH and rifampin with or without resistance to other drugs (see drug resistance, acquired and drug resistance, primary).

M. tuberculosis complex: A group of closely related mycobacterial species that can cause active TB (e.g., *M. tuberculosis*, *M. bovis*, and *M. africanum*); most cases of TB in the United States are caused by *M. tuberculosis*.

Negative pressure: The relative air pressure difference between two areas in a health-care facility.

A room that is at negative pressure has a lower pressure than adjacent areas, which keeps air from flowing out of the room and into adjacent rooms or areas.

Portable room-air HEPA recirculation units: Free-standing portable devices that remove airborne contaminants by recirculating air through a HEPA filter.

Purified protein derivative (PPD)-tuberculin test: A method used to evaluate the likelihood that a person is infected with *M. tuberculosis*. A small dose of tuberculin (PPD) is injected just beneath the surface of the skin, and the area is examined 48–72 h after the injection. A reaction is measured according to the size of the induration. The classification of a reaction as positive or negative depends on the patient's medical history and various risk factors (see Mantoux test).

Purified protein derivative (PPD)-tuberculin test conversion: A change in PPD test results from negative to positive. A conversion within a 2-year period is usually interpreted as new *M. tuberculosis* infection, which carries an increased risk for progression to active disease. A booster reaction may be misinterpreted as a new infection (see booster phenomenon and two-step testing).

Radiometric method: A method for culturing a specimen that allows for rapid detection of bacterial growth by measuring production of CO_2 by viable organisms; also a method of rapidly performing susceptibility testing of *M. tuberculosis*.

Smear (AFB smear): A laboratory technique for visualizing mycobacteria. The specimen is smeared onto a slide and stained, and then examined using a microscope.

Smear results should be available within 24 h. In TB, a large number of mycobacteria seen on an AFB smear usually indicate infectiousness. However, a positive result is not diagnostic of TB because organisms other than *M. tuberculosis* may be seen on an AFB smear (e.g., nontuberculous mycobacteria).

Sputum induction: A method used to obtain sputum from a patient who is unable to cough up a specimen spontaneously. The patient inhales a saline mist, which stimulates a cough from deep within the lungs.

Sputum smear, positive: AFB are visible on the sputum smear when viewed under a microscope.

Persons with a sputum smear positive for AFB are considered more infectious than those with smear-negative sputum.

TB case: A particular episode of clinically active TB. This term should be used only to refer to the disease itself, not the patient with the disease. By law, cases of TB must be reported to the local health department.

TB infection: A condition in which living tubercle bacilli are present in the body but the disease is not clinically active. Infected persons usually have positive tuberculin reactions, but they have no symptoms related to the infection and are not infectious. However, infected persons remain at lifelong risk for developing disease unless preventive therapy is given.

Tuberculosis (TB): A clinically active, symptomatic disease caused by an organism in the *M. tuberculosis* complex (usually *M. tuberculosis* or, rarely, *M. bovis* or *M. africanum*).

Two-step testing: A procedure used for the baseline testing of persons who will periodically receive tuberculin skin tests (e.g., HCWs) to reduce the likelihood of mistaking a boosted reaction for a new infection. If the initial tuberculin-test result is classified as negative, a second test is repeated 1–3 weeks later. If the reaction to the second test is positive, it probably represents a boosted reaction. If the second test result is also negative, the person is classified as not infected. A positive reaction to a subsequent test would indicate new infection (i.e., a skin-test conversion) in such a person.

12

Anaerobic Lung Abscess

John R. Godke
Bennett P. deBoisblanc

HIGH YIELD FACTS

1. The diagnosis of anaerobic lung abscess is entirely clinical with confirmatory sputum culture, blood culture, or other diagnostic test(s) generally unhelpful.

2. The classic radiographic features of an anaerobic lung abscess include a solitary nodule with an "air-fluid" level, a wall thickness of 5–15 mm, a doubling time less than 60 days, and a location either in the superior segment of a lower lobe or in the posterior segment of the right upper lobe.

3. Recommended outpatient therapy of an anaerobic lung abscess is clindamycin or amoxicillin/clavulanate, with prolonged (weeks to months) treatment duration necessary to resolve symptoms and radiographic abnormalities.

4. Metronidazole is *not* considered an optimal therapy for anaerobic lung abscess.

5. Immunocompetent patients with upper lobe cavitary disease and immunocompromised patients with cavities in any location should be placed in respiratory isolation until mycobacterial disease can be excluded.

CASE PRESENTATION

A 44-year-old homeless man presents to the emergency department after falling down a flight of stairs. Although he sustained only minor abrasions and denies any chronic symptoms, an emergency room chest radiograph is abnormal. The patient's past medical history is largely unknown. The patient reports smoking 1–2 packs of cigarettes per day and he drinks alcohol daily.

The patient does not appear acutely ill. Vital signs are normal, with a temperature of 98.4°F, a respiratory rate of 16, and room-air pulse oximetry of 97%. Physical exam reveals a thin, malnourished man with poor dentition. Breath sounds are coarse bilaterally. There is bruising of the left lateral chest wall and a laceration requiring five sutures on the left arm. The chest radiograph is significant for a 3 cm cavity in the posterior segment of the right upper lobe. The cavity is approximately 8 mm at its thickest

point and contains an "air-fluid" level. No evidence of pleural effusion exists and the rest of the chest film is unremarkable. No previous films exist for comparison.

INTRODUCTION/EPIDEMIOLOGY

Introduction and Definition of Anaerobic Lung Abscess

Necrotizing infections of the lung represent an important subset of pneumonia, with unique epidemiology, radiographic presentation, parthenogenesis, and treatment. Broadly speaking, any pyogenic infection of the lung which causes total parenchymal destruction can be labeled as a lung abscess. For close to a century, oral anaerobic organisms have been implicated in the etiology of lung abscesses. Anaerobic microorganisms cause a disease that differs from the necrotizing pneumonia of aerobic microorganisms. Terms like "lung abscess," "putrid lung abscess," and "anaerobic lung abscess" have traditionally defined an anaerobic process. Terms like "lung gangrene" and "necrotizing pneumonia" have traditionally defined an aerobic process. The focus of this chapter will be on the emergency department presentation and management of anaerobic lung abscess. Because all necrotizing lung infections have overlapping characteristics, it is necessary to include some discussion of all clinical entities.

Predisposing Conditions for Anaerobic Lung Abscess

Because anaerobic lung abscess is a complication of aspirated oral flora, conditions that predispose to aspiration are associated with this disease. Several mechanisms can either enhance the volume of aspirated secretions or increase the frequency of aspiration: depressed levels of consciousness, increased reflux of gastric contents, and mechanical obstruction of epiglottic/glottic function. In addition, patients with impaired host immune defense and patients with very high colony counts of oral bacteria (i.e., poor oral hygiene) are at increased risk for lung abscess (1, 2). Recognizing underlying risk factors is the first step toward securing the clinical diagnosis of lung abscess (Table 12–1).

PATHOPHYSIOLOGY/MICROBIOLOGY

The bacteriology of an anaerobic lung abscess can be assumed to be polymicrobial. Although aspirated anaerobes can exist as exclusive pathogens, they frequently coexist with aerobic organisms (2, 3). The bacteriologic profile

Table 12–1. Predisposing Factors for the Development of Anaerobic Lung Abscess

Risk Factor	Examples
Increased risk of aspiration	Depressed level of consciousness • Seizure • General anesthesia • Intoxication with central nervous system depressant • Stroke or encephalopathy Increased reflux of gastric contents • Intractable emesis • Esophageal obstruction or achalasia • Intestinal obstruction Mechanical barrier to epiglottic/glottic function • Nasogastric tube • Endotracheal tube
Impaired host defense	• Human immunodeficiency virus infection • Alcohol abuse • Bronchial obstruction, impaired cough, or ciliary dysfunction
Increased oropharyngeal bacterial counts	• Periodontal disease • Oropharyngeal infection

of the upper aero-digestive system differs from that of the lower one. In the lower digestive tract, the *Bacteroides fragilis* group is a common isolate whereas in the upper aero-digestive tract, anaerobic cocci (i.e., *Peptostreptococcus*), microaerophilic streptococci, *Prevotella* spp., *Porphyromonas* spp., and *Fusobacterium* are the predominate organisms identified by culture (2–6). The *B. fragilis* group has less influence on the pathogenicity of abscesses found within the lung (2, 6, 7).

Aerobic pathogens are commonly isolated from lung abscesses. Nosocomial acquisition of infection, an underlying immunocompromised state, an abscess linked to airway obstruction, and radiographic/clinical evidence of a necrotizing pneumonia increase the likelihood that aerobic organisms exist. *Staphylococcus aureus, Pseudomonas aeruginosa, Klebsiella pneumonia* (and other enteric gram-negative rods), and viridans streptococci can be aerobic pathogens in lung abscess(es) (3, 8).

CLINICAL PRESENTATION

Signs and Symptoms of Anaerobic Lung Abscess

Clinical symptoms of anaerobic lung abscess are rarely specific and overlap with other infectious diseases of the lung. Fever, cough, and sputum production are the most common presenting symptoms (1). The intensity of symptoms is usually less than that encountered with pneumococcal pneumonia. Patients with anaerobic lung abscess do not experience rigors, and severe respiratory impairment (i.e., hypoxemia, dyspnea) is rare. This disease tends to assume an indolent, subacute course and is less incapacitating than traditional community-acquired pneumonia. Most patients describe symptoms with a median duration of 2 weeks prior to emergency department presentation (2). Weight loss and general malaise are common, with weight loss testifying to the chronicity of infection. One symptom is specific to this disease and can provide strong evidence of underlying anaerobic lung abscess: the expectoration of putrid sputum. Unfortunately, the expectoration of putrid sputum occurs in only 50–60% of patients, and its absence does not exclude the diagnosis (2, 9).

Obviously, symptoms alone do not allow the emergency medicine physician to make the clinical diagnosis of anaerobic lung abscess. The clinical presentation of an acute, bacterial, community-acquired pneumonia is usually sufficiently different to allow this diagnosis to be excluded. More indolent pulmonary infections, like pulmonary tuberculosis and chronic fungal infection, are difficult to differentiate based on symptoms. Noninfectious pulmonary disease, like malignancy, can mimic the symptoms of anaerobic lung abscess. A significant

number of patients are asymptomatic and disease is discovered as incidental chest radiograph abnormalities (8). Therefore, identifying patient risk factors and reviewing chest radiographs are very important initial steps toward securing the diagnosis.

Radiographic Findings of Anaerobic Lung Abscess

The hallmark radiographic finding of an anaerobic lung abscess is the pulmonary cavity. A pulmonary cavity can be defined as an air-containing lesion with relatively thick walls (usually >1 mm) or surrounded by infiltrate/mass (10, 11). The emergency medicine physician is often the first to identify this radiographic abnormality, introducing a differential diagnosis that includes anaerobic lung abscess (Table 12–2). Awareness of the differential diagnosis and appreciation of classic abscess radiographic features (Table 12–3) can help physicians make an accurate diagnosis. Chest films are also critical for the recognition of complex disease that would prevent discharge from the emergency room on empiric antimicrobial therapy.

Certain radiographic characteristics of pulmonary cavities can help narrow the differential diagnosis (see Fig. 12–1). Physicians should be careful while identifying

Table 12–2. Differential Diagnosis of Cavitary Lung Disease

	Diagnosis
Infection	**Anaerobic lung abscess**
	Reactivation pulmonary tuberculosis or atypical mycobacterium
	Necrotizing aerobic pneumonia[a]
	Septic emboli[a]
	Fungal or parasitic infection
Malignancy	**Bronchogenic carcinoma**
	Metastatic carcinoma[a]
	Lymphoma
Inflammatory	Wegener granulomatosis[a]
	Lymphomatoid granulomatosis[a]
	Rheumatoid nodules[a]
	Nodular sarcoidosis[a]
Congenital	Pulmonary sequestration
	Congenital cystic adenomatoid malformations[a]
Other	Cavitary pulmonary infarction

Diseases in bold font represent the most common etiologies.
[a]Diseases that classically present as multiple cavitary lesions.

Table 12–3. Radiographic Features of Anaerobic Lung Abscess

Anaerobic Lung Abscess	
Characteristic	**Classic Radiographic Finding**
Number	Solitary
Location	Poster segment, right upper lobe
	Superior segment, right lower lobe
	Basilar segments, right lower lobe
	Superior segment, left lower lobe
	Basilar segments, left lower lobe
Wall thickness and internal contour	5–15 mm; smooth or shaggy
Air-fluid level	Present
Regional adenpoathy or pleural effusion	Not present

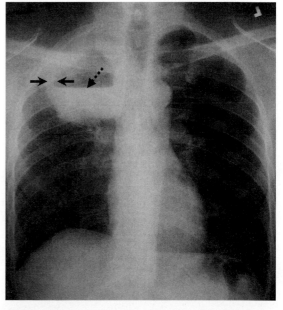

Fig. 12–1. An anterior-posterior chest radiograph of a 48-year-old alcoholic man with a 6-week history of fever, malaise, and cough producing putrid sputum. The film demonstrates a very large (7 cm), solitary cavity in the right upper lung zone. A classic air-fluid level (dashed arrow) is evident. Wall thickness (solid arrows) is 1 cm, with an irregular internal contour. The abnormality was not present on an emergency room chest radiograph taken 4 months prior to this film. This patient was diagnosed and treated for an anaerobic lung abscess.

cavities as single or multiple and localizing cavities, if possible, to a pulmonary segment. The cavity wall thickness, internal wall contour, and cavity contents are important discriminators. If old radiographs are available, lesion growth and "doubling time" can be estimated. Radiographic abnormalities separate from the cavity itself can provide additional clues as to the etiology. The absence of a pulmonary cavity does not exclude the possibility of an early anaerobic infection, but the radiographic presentation of a noncavitary lung abscess will not allow differentiation from other types of pneumonia. Cavitation has been estimated to require 8–14 days after an aspiration event to be visible on the chest radiograph (1, 9).

The classic anaerobic lung abscess is solitary although multifocal disease occurs. Bronchogenic carcinoma, anaerobic lung abscess, and reactivation pulmonary tuberculosis are important considerations in the differential diagnosis of the solitary pulmonary cavity (Table 12–2). Multiple cavitary lesions in a patient with signs and symptoms of active infection raise concern for an aerobic necrotizing pneumonia or septic embolization (12). Because lung abscess results from aspiration of oral flora, gravity-dependent pulmonary segments are the most likely to manifest infection. The posterior segment of the right upper lobe, the superior segment of the right and left lower lobes, and all lower lobe basilar segments are at greatest risk for aspiration-induced infection. These pulmonary segments are involved in 76% of anaerobic lung abscesses (1, 10).

Cavity location has important implications for patient management in the emergency department. Reactivation pulmonary tuberculosis more commonly involves the apical pulmonary segments. Physicians should place symptomatic patients with upper lobe cavitary disease in respiratory isolation until this diagnosis can be excluded. Superior segment and lower lobe cavities are rarely a manifestation of reactivation tuberculosis in patients *known* to be immunocompetent, and respiratory isolation is not always necessary.

Maximum cavity wall thickness has been studied as a differentiating characteristic of the pulmonary cavity. Wall measurement can be used to identify the likelihood that malignancy is the etiology. Anaerobic lung abscess cavities usually have a moderate wall thickness of 5–15 mm. Cavity walls >15 mm thick have a 95% chance of being malignant. Thin-walled cavities, with a maximum thickness of <4 mm, are almost always benign. Wall thickness between 5 mm and 15 mm cannot be used to exclude or include malignancy, with benign and malignant causes equally common (13). The internal contour of the cavity wall is smooth or shaggy in most lung abscesses. A nodular appearance is more typical of malignant lesions (1, 10).

By definition, cavities contain air, but liquid and solid materials can also fill the lumen. A putrid lung abscess evolves through liquefaction necrosis and expulsion of necrotic material through the conducting airways. Liquid and air coexist and present radiographically as an "air-fluid level." The absence of an air-fluid level does not exclude the diagnosis of an anaerobic abscess, but a "dry" abscess is more suggestive of malignancy or fungal/mycobacterial infection. Occasionally, solid material can be seen within a cavity on chest radiographs. Possible causes include coagulated blood (i.e., a cavity with recent hemoptysis), fungal colonization (i.e., a mycetoma or "fungus ball"), and necrotic lung (i.e., a necrotizing pneumonia) (10).

Lesion growth is a characteristic that is used extensively by radiologists and pulmonologists to predict etiology and provide prognostic information. The concept of quantifying growth with chest radiography or computed tomography has been best validated in the evaluation of the pulmonary nodule. Even so, appreciating the natural history of cavitary lung lesions is important, and attempts should always be made to obtain old radiographs when cavities are encountered. Lesion "doubling time" can be defined as the time required for the *volume* of a lesion to double, i.e., when the diameter increases by approximately 125%. Infectious processes tend to have the shortest doubling time, and a lesion doubling in less than 60 days is almost always infectious. Cavitary lesions that are radiographically stable over years often reflect scarred lung parenchyma from prior insult.

LABORATORY/DIAGNOSTIC TESTING

From the perspective of the emergency department physician, lung abscess is a clinical diagnosis. No immediately available confirmatory test exists. Even routine microbiologic assessment is unlikely to be reliable or of high enough yield to justify its pursuit. Therefore, efforts to identify the underlying pathogen(s) should not be pursued in the emergency department. The diagnostic approach should be aimed at excluding alternate diagnoses or identifying possible complicating features of a suspected infection.

Appropriate specimens for the confirmation of an anaerobic pulmonary infection can be obtained, but all are invasive and reserved for refractory or complicated disease. Accepted specimens include transtracheal aspirates, transthoracic needle aspirates, fiberoptic bronchoscopic aspirates with protected brush, and pleural fluid aspirates if the abscess is complicated by an empyema (9). In practice, thoracentesis is the only invasive diagnostic procedure likely to occur in the emergency department setting. Pleural fluid specimens should be obtained using aseptic technique and placed immediately in an anaerobic transport system or anaerobic blood culture bottle system. Refrigeration is *not* recommended; prompt laboratory processing to maximize yield is critical (6).

Sputum staining and culture are felt to have no utility in the identification of anaerobic pathogens due to unavoidable contamination by oropharyngeal flora (6, 9). Blood culture yield is extremely low for anaerobic pathogens, and positive blood cultures occur in <3% of cases (9). Unless an aerobic bacterial infection is suspected, blood cultures should not be drawn in a stable patient who will be discharged on empiric therapy. In contrast, patients who are acutely ill, patients with suspected septic emboli, and patients with necrotizing pneumonia should have blood cultures drawn.

Excluding alternate diagnoses is an important focus of emergency department diagnostic testing. Patients with epidemiologic risks for pulmonary tuberculosis, appropriate symptoms of active infection (i.e., fever, productive cough, weight loss, night sweats), and apical cavitary disease should be placed in respiratory isolation with sputum collection for acid-fast bacilli staining. Sputum staining for fungal pathogens can also be helpful if these pathogens are suspected. Defining the patient's underlying immune status is paramount when considering the differential diagnosis. Serology for human immunodeficiency virus (HIV) infection and T cell subset analysis should be obtained for all patients with risk factors for this disease. Physicians should place every patient with suspected or known HIV infection and cavitary lung disease in respiratory isolation. Reactivation pulmonary tuberculosis is common in HIV infection and can occupy any pulmonary segment (see Chapter 11). If a cavitary pulmonary infarct is suspected, ventilation-perfusion scanning or spiral chest computed tomography is an appropriate diagnostic test. Otherwise, chest computed tomography is not necessary for the emergent diagnosis of anaerobic lung abscess.

Identifying complicating features of anaerobic lung abscess is another important focus of emergency department diagnostic testing. Patients presenting with hemoptysis need evaluation for coagulopathy. Pleural effusions associated with anaerobic abscess or any pulmonary infection require sampling to identify complex effusions and empyema. Overall, cases that are characterized by diagnostic uncertainty or refractory/complicating features will require hospital admission (Table 12–4). Extensive or

Table 12–4. Patients with Anaerobic Lung Abscess who Require Hospital Admission for Evaluation or Treatment

Complicating Feature	Example
1. Severe symptoms	• High fever • Dehydration/prostration • Hypoxemia/respiratory distress • Hemodynamic instability
2. Alternate or coexisting diagnosis possible	• Suspected bronchogenic carcinoma • Suspected tuberculosis or fungal infection • Suspected necrotizing pneumonia (or nonaspiration cavitary process)
3. Abscess requires mechanical drainage or excision	• Empyema • Very large cavities (>6 cm) • Cavities refractory to antibiotic therapy • Hemoptysis
4. Comorbid diseases and noncompliance	• Advanced immune deficiency • Alcohol or drug withdrawal • Uncontrolled seizures or unexplained neurologic disease • Advanced liver, kidney, pulmonary, or cardiac disease

invasive diagnostic testing is not necessary in the emergency department.

MANAGEMENT

Factors that Influence Treatment Decisions

Appropriate therapy for a patient with anaerobic lung abscess who presents to the emergency room is dictated by three important factors. These factors include the bacteriology of the abscess, the severity of presenting illness, and the cost of curative therapy.

The bacteriology of anaerobic lung abscesses has been previously addressed in this chapter (see the section pathophysiology/microbiology). An appreciation of the polymicrobial, anaerobic flora, unique to the upper aerodigestive tract, is necessary to make appropriate treatment decisions. Recognizing potential coinfection with aerobic pathogens is also important. A second factor that influences the choice of therapy is the overall severity of presenting symptoms and the degree of respiratory impairment. A subacute illness with mild-to-moderate symptoms can effectively be managed with empiric oral antibiotics as an outpatient. These patients can be discharged directly from the emergency department with appropriate follow-up. An acute presentation with high fevers, overall prostration, or symptoms that suggest a disease complication (i.e., hemoptysis, hypoxemia, pleural effusion) warrants inpatient therapy with a parenteral antimicrobial agent. Recognizing complicated abscesses that may require bronchoscopic/catheter drainage or surgical excision is important. Hospitalization can also be justified if the diagnosis remains in question. The emergency department physician must be able to identify patients with complicated infection who will require hospital admission and subspecialty consultation (Table 12–4).

Patient compliance and the cost of prolonged outpatient therapy are additional factors which often influence treatment decisions made by physicians in the emergency department setting. Curative oral therapy often requires between 1 and 4 months, and cost can exceed $500 (2, 4, 14).

Antimicrobial Therapy

Until the 1980s, penicillin G was regarded as the treatment of choice for putrid lung abscess (15). The emergence and discovery of penicillin-resistant anaerobes prompted clinical trials to identify a more efficacious agent (5, 7, 16). Anaerobic organisms have the potential to produce beta lactamases, and this production appears to be the predominant mechanism of resistance for oral *Bacteroides* species (3, 14, 17). An appropriate agent would have to demonstrate stability in the presence of anaerobic-associated beta lactamase(s) in order to maximize the treatment efficacy (5, 7).

Clindamycin is now widely recognized to be a drug of choice for anaerobic lung abscess. A member of the lincosamide group of antibiotics, clindamycin is not degraded by anaerobic beta lactamases and inhibits protein synthesis by binding to the 50S ribosomal subunit. Two clinical trials comparing clindamycin to penicillin suggest that this agent produces superior microbiologic and clinic cure rates (5, 7). Between 1977 and 1981, Levison et al. conducted a prospective, randomized, comp arative trial and found that 7 of 15 patients treated with penicillin failed to achieve a cure. No treatment failures occurred in 13 patients treated with clindamycin (p <0.01). Similar results were published by Gudiol et al. in 1990. This single-center, prospective, randomized trial demonstrated treatment failure rates of 44.4% for penicillin and 5.4% for clindamycin (p <0.017).

Clindamycin can be administered as a parenteral or oral agent, allowing sequential treatment for cases that initially require more aggressive therapy. Recommended doses vary: clindamycin, 450–900 mg IV q6 h to 8 h and clindamycin, 300 mg PO tid to qid (4, 5, 7, 18). Dosage reduction is necessary with severe liver impairment. Gastrointestinal intolerance is the most common side effect, with less common precipitation of pseudomembranous enterocolitis possible.

Certain clinical situations exist where clindamycin may have drawbacks. Although early studies isolated *B. fragilis* as a pathogen in 15–20% of lung abscesses, more recent investigations suggest laboratory growth in less than 5% of cases (3, 4, 7, 9, 15). Although considered a minor lung abscess pathogen, *B. fragilis* has developed increasing resistance to clindamycin. An antimicrobial resistance survey for the year 2000 documents clindamycin resistance in 26% of *B. fragilis* isolates (19). Non-*B. fragilis* anaerobes demonstrate lower resistance rates to clindamycin, but rates are higher than the beta lactam/beta lactamase class of antibiotics (i.e., 5% vs. 0%) (3). Clindamycin also demonstrates relatively slow in vitro kill rates for anaerobes (20).

Aerobic gram-negative rods are not included in the antimicrobial spectrum of clindamycin. Aerobic gram-negative rods have been isolated from lung abscesses in patients with multiple medical comorbidities, nosocomial aspiration, and underlying immune deficiency states (3, 8). For these reasons, clindamycin should not be used as monotherapy for critically ill patients with lung abscess and for any patient at risk for aerobic abscess involvement.

Beta lactam/beta lactamase combinations offer the theoretical advantage of broader antimicrobial coverage. These agents are more active than clindamycin against resistant *B. fragilis* group pathogens (<3% resistant) and have very low rates of resistance against the anaerobic family of organisms as a whole (3, 19). Enteric gram-negative-rod coverage is superior to clindamycin for patients at risk for aerobic copathenogenesis.

In practice, efficacy has been shown to be comparable to clindamycin +/− cephalosporin for treatment of lung abscess, achieving a sustained cure in over two-thirds of patients (4). The combination of intravenous and oral amoxicillin-clavulanate therapy achieved a clinical cure in all 35 patients given the drug for anaerobic lung abscess (14). The beta lactam/beta lactamase class and clindamycin are equally tolerated. Oral (amoxicillin/clavulanate) and parenteral (ampicillin/sulbactam; ticarcillin/clavulanate; piperacillin/tazobactam) preparations are available for empiric therapy. Although no firm oral dosing recommendations are available, amoxicillin/clavulanate, 875 mg PO bid to tid is the dose that favorably compares to those used in available reports (4, 14).

Table 12–5. Antibiotic Therapy of Anaerobic Lung Infections (2, 3, 7, 9, 11, 15)

Antibiotic	Dose	Route	Frequency	Note
Clindamycin	300 mg	PO	TID-QID	Outpatient drug of choice; avoid as
	450–900 mg	IV	Q6–8 h	monotherapy in critically ill patients or those with suspected aerobic GNR infection
Amoxicillin-clavulanate	875 mg	PO	bid-tid	Outpatient drug of choice
Cefoxitin	2 g	IV	Q8 h	Hospitalized patients
Ampicillin-sulbactam	3 g	IV/IM	Q6 h	Hospitalized patients
Ticarcillin-clavulanate	3.1 g	IV	Q4–6 h	Hospitalized patients
Piperacillin-tazobactam	3.375–4.5 g	IV	Q6–8 h	Hospitalized patients

Note: The carbapenem class of antibiotics is efficacious with critically ill, life-threatening, anaerobic lung infections. Clindamycin can be combined with agents active against aerobic gram-negative rods (GNR) if a true allergy to penicillin exists with severe infection.

Metronidazole is a novel antimicrobial agent that is almost universally used in the setting of anaerobic infections, especially those linked to the lower gastrointestinal tract. However, its performance in anaerobic infections above the diaphragm is suboptimal, especially if used as monotherapy. Facultative anaerobes and anaerobic cocci are more prominent pathogens in the upper aero-digestive tract. These organisms are less susceptible to the intracellular reduction of metronidazole (2). In a recent report, one quarter of anaerobes isolated from lung abscesses were resistant to metronidazole (3). Treatment failures have been reported for metronidazole, and it should not be considered "first-line" therapy for lung abscess (21, 22). More acceptable therapeutic options for the treatment of anaerobic lung abscess are presented in Table 12–5.

To effect resolution of anaerobic lung abscesses, several months of outpatient therapy are necessary. Treatment cost has plagued physicians, especially when recognizing the patient population at greatest risk. Patients of low socioeconomic status, patients with substance abuse problems, and patients with neurologic disorders are often unable or unwilling to finance the cost of curative therapy. This may force physicians to consider prolonged hospitalization, discharge with little hope for compliance, or prescription of agents thought to be less efficacious (but more affordable) than the current standard of care.

No clear data exist to direct total duration of antibiotic therapy. Expert opinion suggests that treatment should be continued past symptom resolution when the chest radiograph is clear or demonstrates a small, stable scar. Arrangement of appropriate follow-up for long-term therapy is essential if patients are discharged from the emergency department on empiric therapy. Symptom response begins within 3–4 days and complete defervescence usually oc-

curs by day 7–10. Symptoms that persist beyond 2 weeks are indicators of a complex infection (2).

Nonantimicrobial Therapy

Important treatment adjuncts to antimicrobial therapy include postural drainage and reversal of factors that place the patient at increased risk of aspiration (2). Periodontal care, seizure control, nutritional support, and substance abuse counseling are examples of interventions that will reduce the likelihood of recurrence in appropriate patients. Lung abscess can be complicated by empyema if the cavity erodes into the pleural space and by hemoptysis if the cavity erodes into a bronchial artery. In addition, large cavities (>6 cm) can be refractory to antimicrobial therapy and require needle/catheter drainage or surgical excision. An endobronchial survey with bronchoscopy should be considered when suspicion of coexisting malignancy is high or the patient fails to respond to therapy. Pulmonary and surgical consultation may be required for complicated disease.

PROGNOSIS AND CONCLUSION

Despite appropriate treatment, significant mortality remains associated with necrotizing lung infections. Several features of infection portend a worse prognosis: multiple underlying comorbidities, infection with aerobic pathogens (especially *S. aureus*, *K. pneumoniae*, and *P. aeruginosa*), large abscess size, and abscess location in the right lower lobe (23). Mortality has been reported to be as low as 2.4% for uncomplicated, community-acquired lung abscess but appears higher, 15–20%, when all necrotizing lung infections are considered (8, 23).

Emergency medicine physicians play a pivotal role in the diagnosis of anaerobic lung abscess, in the identification of patients who can be managed as outpatients, in the recognition of complicated disease, and in the empiric therapy of all patients with necrotizing lung infections. Initial emergency department management will hopefully continue to improve treatment outcomes and prevent disease recurrence.

CASE OUTCOME

The emergency physician recognized the potential risk of active pulmonary tuberculosis and immediately placed the patient in respiratory isolation. Because the physician suspected an anaerobic lung abscess, oral amoxicillin/ clavulanate, 875 mg po bid, was started. Routine chemistries, a liver profile, and complete blood counts were drawn. Blood cultures and further chest imaging were not deemed necessary prior to consultation with the hospital's pulmonologist. Consent was obtained for serologic HIV testing. Sputum induction with hypertonic saline nebulization was arranged, and an acceptable sputum specimen was collected for acid-fast and fungal staining.

A brief hospital admission course revealed no sputum evidence of pulmonary tuberculosis. An immunodeficiency state was not identified and the patient remained completely stable. A community clinic was contacted to provide antibiotic assistance, and a family member agreed to provide temporary residence. Referral to an area substance abuse clinic was made. The patient was discharged on amoxicillin/clavulanate and achieved a complete symptomatic and radiographic cure over a 4-week period.

REFERENCES

1. Groskin SA, Panicek DM, Ewing DK, et al.: Bacterial lung abscess: A review of the radiographic and clinical features of 50 cases. *J Thorac Imaging* 6(3):62, 1991.
2. Hill MK, Sanders CV: Anaerobic disease of the lung. *Infect Dis Clin N Am* 5(3):453, 1991.
3. Hammond MJ, Potgieter PD, Hanslo D, et al.: The etiology and antimicrobial susceptibility patterns of microorganisms in acute community-acquired lung abscess. *Chest* 108:937, 1995.
4. Allewelt M, Schuler P, Bolcskei L, et al.: Ampicillin+ sulbactam vs. clindamycin +/− cephalosporin for the treatment of aspiration pneumonia and primary lung abscess. *Clin Microbiol Infect* 10:163, 2004.
5. Levison ME, Mangura CT, Lorber B, et al.: Clindamycin compared with penicillin for the treatment of anaerobic lung abscess. *Ann Intern Med* 98:466, 1983.
6. Verma P: Laboratory diagnosis of anaerobic pleuropulmonary infections. *Semin Respir Infect* 15(2):114, 2000.
7. Gudiol F, Manresa F, Pallares R, et al.: Clindamycin vs penicillin for anaerobic lung infections. *Arch Intern Med* 150: 2525, 1990.
8. Mansharamani N, Balachandran D, Delaney D, et al.: Lung abscess in adults: Clinical comparison of immunocompromised to non-immunocompromised patients. *Respir Med* 96: 178, 2002.
9. Bartlett JG: Anaerobic bacterial infections of the lung. *Chest* 91(6):901, 1987.
10. Fraser RG, Pare JA, Fraser RS, et al.: *Diagnosis of Diseases of the Chest*. Philadelphia, W.B. Saunders, 1988.
11. Meholic A, Ketai L, Lofgren R: *Fundamentals of Chest Radiology*. Philadelphia, W.B. Saunders Company, 1996.
12. Ryu JH, Swensen SJ: Cystic and cavitary lung diseases: Focal and diffuse. *Mayo Clin Proc* 78:744, 2003.
13. Woodring JH, Fried AM, Chuang VP: Solitary cavities of the lung: Diagnostic implications of wall thickness. *AJR* 135: 1269, 1980.
14. Fernandez-Sabe N, Carratala J, Dorca J, et al.: Efficacy and safety of sequential amoxicillin-clavulanate in the treatment of anaerobic lung infections. *Eur J Clin Microbiol Infect Dis* 22:185, 2003.
15. Bartlett JG, Gorbach SL: Treatment of aspiration pneumonia and primary lung abscess: Penicillin G vs clindamycin. *JAMA* 234(9):935, 1975.
16. Agger WA, Glasser JE, Rahimi A, et al.: Penicillin-resistant bacteroides melaninogenicus. *JAMA* 248(8):925, 1982.
17. Brook I: Antibiotic resistance of oral anaerobic bacteria and their effect on the management of upper respiratory and head and neck infections. *Semin Respir Infect* 17(3):195, 2002.
18. Gilbert DN, Moellering RC, Eliopoulos GM, et al.: *The Sanford Guide to Antimicrobial Therapy 2004, 34th ed.* Hyde Park, Antimicrobial Therapy, Inc., 2004.
19. Syndman DR, Jacobus NV, McDermott LA, et al.: National survey on the susceptibility of *Bacteroides fragilis* group: Report and analysis of trends for 1997–2000. *CID* 35(Suppl. 1): S126, 2002.
20. Credito KL, Jacobs MR, Appelbaum PC: Time-kill studies of the antianaerobic activity of garenoxacin compared with those of nine other agents. *Antimicrob Agents Chemother* 47(4):1399, 2003.
21. Perlino CA: Metronidazole vs clindamycin treatment of anaerobic pulmonary infection: Failure of metronidazole therapy. *Arch Intern Med* 141:1424, 1981.
22. Sanders CV, Hanna BJ, Lewis AC: Metronidazole in the treatment of anaerobic infections. *Am Rev Respir Dis* 120: 337, 1979.
23. Hirshberg B, Sklair-Levi M, Nir-Paz R, et al.: Factors predicting mortality of patients with lung abscess. *Chest* 115:746, 1999.

13

Infective Endocarditis

Jorge A. Fernandez
Stuart P. Swadron

HIGH YIELD FACTS

1. Infective endocarditis (IE) refers to an infection of the endocardium, and it may involve cardiac valves or papillary muscles and extend into the myocardium.

2. Risk factors include congenital or acquired cardiac lesions, prosthetic heart valves, intravenous drug use (IVDU), indwelling IV access devices, peritoneal or hemodialysis, poor dental hygiene, and immunosuppression.

3. Although the definitive diagnosis of IE is difficult to make in the emergency department (ED), it should be considered in any febrile patient with predisposing risk factors. Three separate sets of blood cultures are recommended prior to the initiation of antibiotics.

4. Transesophageal echocardiography (TEE) is extremely sensitive (>90%) for the diagnosis, whereas transthoracic echocardiography (TTE) is less sensitive (55–65%).

5. Valvular destruction and peripheral embolization are the most frequent complications of IE. Unstable patients may require emergent surgical intervention.

6. Prophylactic antibiotics should be administered 30–60 minutes prior to high-risk procedures in patients at moderate to high risk of developing IE.

CASE PRESENTATION

A 34-year-old Mexican-American man was transported to the ED by ambulance after he was found lying on the street in downtown Los Angeles. He reported to the paramedics that he had been feeling sick during the last several days with flu-like symptoms, diarrhea, and body aches. These symptoms progressively worsened to the point that he was unable to ambulate because of pain and fatigue.

In the ED, both the history and physical examination were difficult to obtain because the patient was extremely uncooperative. On review of systems, he admitted to experiencing fevers, chills, watery diarrhea, and total body pain from head to toe. He denied recent trauma, drug use, pho-

tophobia, visual changes, cough, dysuria, rash, or neurological symptoms. He also denied urinary or bowel incontinence. When asked why he was covered in urine, he reported that he was too weak to move. Importantly, he was unable to specify where he hurt most, and he adamantly denied any history of IVDU.

On physical examination, he appeared uncomfortable but nontoxic, grossly disheveled, with obvious recent urinary incontinence. Vital signs were as follows: heart rate 110, blood pressure 160/90, respiratory rate 22, and oral temperature 100.0°F. Pulse oximetry was 97% on room air. He reported a pain score of 10/10 and requested morphine for analgesia. He was alert and fully oriented, without evidence of trauma. There was no stigmata of IVDU, AIDS, IE, or chronic liver disease. Head and neck examination was normal without nuchal rigidity. Lungs were clear to auscultation and no murmur was detected. The abdomen was diffusely tender but soft without peritoneal signs. Rectal tone was normal with guaiac negative stool. His skin was dirty but without rash. His musculoskeletal exam was notable for total body tenderness to light touch from head to toe, and it was not possible to localize a specific source of his pain. His neurological exam demonstrated symmetrical movement and response to light touch; however, the patient would not cooperate with strength, cerebellar, or gait testing.

Laboratory analysis was as follows: leukocytes 22.4, (poly 82%, lymph 13%, mono 4%, eos <1%, bas <1%), hemoglobin 10.8, platelets 420, C-reactive protein (CRP) 22, and erythrocyte sedimentation rate (ESR) 90. Serum chemistries including creatinine and liver function tests were within normal limits, with the exception of a mildly elevated total bilirubin and lactate dehydrogenase. Urinalysis was also normal. Chest, pelvis, and lumbar spine x-ray films were unremarkable. CT scan of the abdomen and pelvis revealed mild, nonspecific large bowel inflammatory changes without evidence of diverticulitis, appendicitis, or abscess. Blood, urine, and stool cultures were obtained. The patient was started on empiric ceftriaxone and fluid resuscitated for presumed sepsis, he was given morphine sulfate for analgesia, and he was admitted to the inpatient medical service.

INTRODUCTION/EPIDEMIOLOGY

Infective endocarditis refers to any infection involving the endocardium of the heart. It may involve native or prosthetic valves, papillary muscles, or the myocardium itself. More commonly, IE affects the left side of the heart; however, multiple valves may be infected simultaneously on each side of the heart. Although the true incidence of IE is difficult to determine, it has been estimated that approximately 15,000 cases occur annually in the United States. Both age and gender influence the incidence of IE. More males acquire the disease than females, with a ratio of almost 2:1. Because the incidence of acquired cardiac valvular lesions increases with age, the mean incidence of IE is shifting toward the elderly (1). A wide variety of pathogens may cause IE, including gram-positive, gram-negative, anaerobic bacteria, atypical organisms such as *Legionella* and *Rickettsia*, and fungi in susceptible hosts (2).

Historically, the dominant risk factor for IE was rheumatic heart disease (RHD). Because the incidence of RHD has declined in the developed world, other cardiac lesions are now more prevalent. Currently, mitral valve prolapse (MVP) is statistically the most common predisposing condition in developed nations; however, the lifetime risk of IE in patients with MVP remains very low, unless there is associated mitral regurgitation (3). Aortic valvular disease is a common predisposing factor in the elderly population, and these lesions have a higher propensity to become infected (4). In children, the majority of IE cases are attributable to congenital cardiac disorders, such as tetralogy of Fallot, ventricular septal defect, patent ductus arteriosus, or bicuspid aortic valves (3). Patients with prior IE or those with prosthetic heart valves are at particularly high risk of acquiring the disease. It has been estimated that IE affects up to 3% of prosthetic valve recipients within the first 5 years of surgery (5).

Intravenous drug use may result in IE even in the absence of any valvular abnormality, particularly in IVDUs with concomitant HIV infection (6). Although the majority of cases of IE affecting the right side of the heart occur in IVDUs, left-sided IE occurs more commonly in this population (7). Other risk factors for IE include chronic indwelling IV access devices, hemodialysis or peritoneal dialysis, and poor dental hygiene (8). Importantly, each of these scenarios is frequently associated with recurrent, transient bacteremia or fungemia. Finally, patients with HIV infection, diabetes mellitus, organ transplants, and those receiving chemotherapeutic drugs are more likely to develop IE secondary to immuno suppression (9).

PATHOPHYSIOLOGY/MICROBIOLOGY

The key event in the development of IE is the adherence of the infectious agent to the endocardium of the heart. Most frequently, the infection surrounds abnormal cardiac valves, where turbulent blood flow induces local en-

docardial damage. As a result, the pathogen may bind to a matrix of platelets and coagulation factors. Once a vegetation forms, the organism is effectively shielded from cellular immunity (2).

The complications of IE can be classified based upon various mechanisms of disease. Localized spread of infection may cause acute valvular destruction, resulting in either stenotic or regurgitant flow. Furthermore, growth can extend into the myocardium, resulting in ring abscesses or *mural* endocarditis. These can be particularly difficult to diagnose, especially in the absence of vegetations (10). Septic emboli may affect distant sites such as the CNS, lungs, kidneys, spine, or extremities. Immunological abnormalities such as immune-complex glomerulonephritis may also occur.

The progression of IE has traditionally been divided into acute versus subacute. Recently, the utility of that classification has been questioned (6). Although a variety of factors influence the time course over which complications manifest, disease progression may vary independently of each. Such factors include the type of pathogen, the immune status of the patient, and the side of the heart involved. In general, IE presents more acutely with virulent bacteria such as *Staphylococcus aureus*, when the left side of the heart is involved, and in immunosuppressed patients (7).

The microbiology of IE varies in different populations and settings. In the general population, *S. aureus*, including oxacillin-resistant strains, and coagulase negative *staphylococci* now collectively account for a greater number of cases than the viridans group of *streptococci*, including *Streptococcus sanguis*, *Streptococcus bovis*, and *Streptococcus mutans*. Enterococci, including vancomycin-resistant strains, are also increasingly recognized as causative organisms in the general population (1). Among IVDUs, *S. aureus* overwhelmingly predominates; however other pathogens, including gram-negative bacilli and fungi, are sometimes implicated (11).

Nosocomial cases of IE are most commonly attributable to contamination of indwelling IV devices or as a result of an invasive procedure. The causative organism in general will correspond to the location of the device or procedure. For example, *staphylococci* species most frequently cause IE in dialysis patients, viridans *streptococci* are most commonly implicated after oral or dental procedures, and gram-negative organisms most often cause IE after gastrointestinal or genitourinary procedures (3).

The so-called culture-negative IE represents approximately 5% of cases. This diagnosis is rarely made in the ED because the organisms responsible are less likely to produce fever and more likely to require special media or immunological testing for definitive diagnosis. Various causes of culture-negative IE include *Bartonella* species, the HACEK organisms, *Legionella*, *Chlamydia*, and fungi (2). Fungal endocarditis remains a rare yet significant cause of IE because these cases are notoriously difficult to treat with mortality rates approaching 60% (12).

CLINICAL PRESENTATION

Patients with *acute* IE appear septic, with fever, chills, tachycardia, and/or tachypnea. In severe cases, septic shock with multiorgan system failure may occur. Endocarditis should be included on the differential diagnosis in any case of sepsis, particularly in the presence of a cardiac murmur or in a patient with risk factors. Unfortunately, in busy EDs, cardiac murmurs can be difficult to auscultate and may be missed (13).

In patients with *subacute* IE, nonspecific symptoms predominate. As a result, subacute disease can be more difficult to diagnose and is frequently mislabeled a "viral syndrome," "acute gastroenteritis," or "bronchitis." Often, patients with subacute IE experience intermittent fever, malaise, anorexia, or weight loss. However, fever may be absent in a significant number of cases (1). Other complaints may include headache, cough, diarrhea, arthralgias, myalgias, or back pain. Splenomegaly may be noted. A cardiac murmur may be absent, especially in patients with right-sided disease (11).

Frequently, the clinical picture of IE is clouded by the presence of its complications. However, if recognized as such, they may actually facilitate the diagnosis and prompt the appropriate work-up. The complications of IE differ depending upon whether the process affects the right or left side of the heart.

Right-sided IE may result in either tricuspid or pulmonic valvular stenosis or incompetence, which may lead to elevated jugular venous pressure, hepatosplenomegaly, and peripheral edema. Septic pulmonary emboli frequently complicate right-sided IE, which can cause acute respiratory distress, hypoxia, and possibly hemoptysis. Multilobar pneumonia and/or lung abscess can also develop and in practice, right-sided endocarditis with secondary pulmonary infiltrates is often mistaken for a severe pneumonia with sepsis. Rarely, patients with right-sided IE may present with systemic emboli secondary to patent foramen ovale (11).

Left-sided IE may cause either mitral or aortic valve stenosis or incompetence. Acute outflow obstruction rarely occurs, and if so, may result in syncope and sudden death (14). More commonly, regurgitant flow occurs and causes pulmonary hypertension and edema, resulting in dyspnea on exertion, orthopnea, and paroxysmal nocturnal dyspnea. Right-sided cardiac failure may eventually develop. In cases of acute valvular incompetence, pulmonary edema may accompany cardiogenic shock. In these cases, the actual diagnosis may be confused with septic shock and acute respiratory distress syndrome, especially if murmurs are not audible.

Systemic emboli affecting virtually any organ system may complicate the clinical picture in left-sided IE. CNS emboli may cause a variety of neurological symptoms, including acute hemiplegia, amaurosis fugax, cerebellar dysfunction, or altered mental status. Meningitis, encephalitis, and brain abscesses may develop. Mycotic aneurysms may develop anywhere in the body and cause signs and symptoms resulting from either compression of adjacent structures or acute aneurysmal rupture (15). Septic emboli may also cause osteomyelitis or epidural abscesses of the cervical, thoracic, or lumbar spine. Quadriplegia, paraplegia, or cauda equina syndrome may develop, depending on the level of cord involvement. Septic arthritis, usually involving the axial skeleton, is rarely seen in IE. Renal, splenic, or mesenteric embolism also rarely occurs. Finally, embolism to peripheral extremities may completely obstruct large arteries (causing the hallmark syndrome of pain, pallor, paresthesias, paralysis, and pulselessness) or smaller arterioles and capillaries, leading to purpuric and necrotic lesions.

Immunological abnormalities may also occur in patients in IE. Most often, immune-complex glomerulonephritis presents as renal insufficiency with white cell casts, proteinuria, and microscopic hematuria. Other less frequent findings include subungual splinter hemorrhages and petechiae (of the palate, conjunctiva, or beneath the finger nails). Notably, the "classic" stigmata of IE are seen in less than 25% of patients (16). These include *Roth spots* (exudative lesions on the retina), *Janeway* lesions (painless erythematous lesions on the palms and soles), and *Osler nodes* (painful violet lesions on the fingers or toes).

Patients with mural endocarditis or ring abscesses have similar signs, symptoms, and complications as those with valvular infections. Additionally, ring abscesses may cause conduction abnormalities, including fascicular, bundle branch, or complete heart blocks. Acute pericarditis is rarely seen in cases of transmural IE. In severe cases, cardiac rupture or tamponade may occur (17).

LABORATORY/DIAGNOSTIC TESTING

The differential diagnosis of IE is vast, including a variety of systemic infectious, rheumatologic, cardiovascular, or neurological disorders. A correct diagnosis may be particularly difficult if a complication of the disease over-shadows the unifying diagnosis. Furthermore, subacute IE frequently causes vague, nonspecific symptoms.

The Duke criteria, based upon various clinical, laboratory, and echocardiographic data, have been used since 1994 as the standard for diagnosing IE (18) (see Table 13–1). Various follow-up studies have demonstrated the accuracy of these criteria (19, 20). Unfortunately, many of the data elements required to apply the Duke criteria are not readily available in the ED; therefore, the diagnosis usually cannot be made definitively. As a result, the emergency physician must rely heavily on clinical suspicion alone. Unfortunately, the costs and risks are substantial if the disease is either underdiagnosed or overdiagnosed (1).

Blood culture remains the most important diagnostic test in the ED for the diagnosis of IE. Studies have demonstrated that the sensitivity of blood culture increases dramatically if at least 5 mL of blood is obtained per vial. Ideally, at least three separate sets of blood cultures (aerobic, anaerobic, and fungal) should be drawn prior to the initiation of empiric antibiotics in order to achieve optimal sensitivity and specificity. Microbiologists advocate drawing each set at least 1 h apart, preferably timed with documented fever; however, antibiotics should not be delayed in patients who are acutely ill. In these patients, the time interval between each set of blood cultures should be shortened to 20 minutes or less. Unfortunately, the majority of culture-negative IE cases actually result from antibiotic administration in the ED prior to obtaining sufficient cultures (2).

Aside from blood cultures, most other laboratory or radiographic testing in the ED is either insensitive or non-specific for IE. Leukocytosis may be absent in immuno-suppressed patients or in subacute disease. C reactive protein and ESR levels are generally elevated, though nonspecific. In subacute disease, chronic normocytic anemia is frequently accompanied by splenomegaly; however, these findings are also not specific. In cases with immune-complex glomerulonephritis, hematuria, proteinuria, and casts will be seen. With pulmonary involvement or severe sepsis, ABG analysis may reveal a metabolic acidosis and respiratory alkalosis with or without hypoxia. Chest x-ray may demonstrate multilobar infiltrates in cases of right-sided IE. In cases with CNS involvement, lumbar puncture may reveal elevated leukocytes and protein, which could represent meningitis, epidural abscess, or brain abscess. However, cranial CT or MRI should be performed before lumbar puncture in patients with a decreased level of consciousness, focal neurological deficits, or papilledema on funduscopic examination. Unfortunately, positive results on any of the above investigations may lead the emergency physician astray from the diagnosis of IE.

EKG findings in IE vary tremendously. Virtually any cardiac rhythm may be seen in the disease; however, the most frequent is sinus rhythm. Right heart strain patterns may be seen with acute septic pulmonary emboli. Changes consistent with acute myocardial infarction may be seen in rare cases of coronary embolism or aneurysms. Finally, third-degree heart block should raise the suspicion of a myocardial ring abscess.

Echocardiography is the most important imaging technique in establishing the diagnosis of IE and for assessing associated valvular dysfunction. Recently, the American College of Cardiology and the American Heart Association (AHA) published recommendations concerning echocardiography in the setting of suspected IE (21a). Unfortunately, the sensitivity of TTE remains poor despite improving technology; however, it is the initial modality employed at most centers. If the TTE is negative, TEE can be performed with much better sensitivity and specificity. Nevertheless, TEE may still miss very small vegetations, small ring abscesses, or mural endocarditis (10). In cases where IE is strongly suspected despite a normal TEE, other diagnostic techniques may be employed, such as molecular methods, cardiac angiography, or nuclear scans, but these techniques are outside the scope of standard emergency medicine practice.

MANAGEMENT

Antimicrobials remain the mainstay of medical therapy for IE. In communities and hospitals with a high prevalence of oxacillin-resistant *S. aureus* (ORSA), a suitable empiric regimen consists of vancomycin, 15 mg/kg every 12 h, *and* gentamicin, 1 mg/kg every 8 h. In those areas *without* a high prevalence of resistant organisms, nafcillin or oxacillin *and* penicillin G or ampicillin should replace vancomycin; gentamicin should also be administered (11). Again, it is preferable to obtain three separate sets of blood cultures prior to the administration of empiric antibiotics. Moreover, if the patient is not acutely ill, many experts advocate withholding empiric antibiotics until culture results are available. Drugs for atypical bacteria or fungi should be held in most cases in the ED setting unless the causative organism is already known. The duration and type of antimicrobial therapy vary depending on the responsible organism and valve involved. In general, treatment is required for between 2 and 6 weeks. Recently, a variety of outpatient regimens have been developed; however, this is a decision that can be deferred to the admitting physician.

Recently, the AHA published guidelines for administering IE prophylaxis (3) (see Tables 13–2 and 13–3).

Table 13–1. Duke Criteria for Bacterial Endocarditis

Major criteria
1. Positive blood culture for infective endocarditis
   Typical microorganism for infective endocarditis from two separate blood cultures
   Viridans streptococci[a], *S. bovis*, HACEK group, *or*
   Community-acquired *S. aureus* or enterococci, in the absence of primary focus, *or*
   Persistently positive blood culture, defined as recovery of a microorganism consistent with infective
      endocarditis from:
      Blood cultures drawn more than 12 h apart, *or*
      Two of three or a majority of four or more separate blood cultures, with first and last drawn at least 1 h apart

2. Evidence of endocardial involvement
   Positive echocardiogram for infective endocarditis
   Oscillating intracardiac mass, on valve or supporting structures, or in the path of regurgitant jets, or on implanted
      material, in the absence of an alternative anatomic explanation, *or*
      Abscess, *or*
      New partial dehiscence of prosthetic valve, *or*
      New valvular regurgitation (increase or change in preexisting murmur not sufficient)
Minor criteria
1. Predisposition: predisposing heart condition or intravenous drug use
2. Fever (38.0°C [100.4°F])
3. Vascular phenomena: major arterial emboli, septic pulmonary infarcts, mycotic aneurysm, intracranial hemorrhage,
   conjunctival hemorrhages, Janeway lesions
4. Immunologic phenomena: glomerulonephritis, Osler nodes, Roth spots, rheumatoid factor
5. Microbiologic evidence: positive blood culture but not meeting major criterion as noted previously[b] or
   serologic evidence of active infection with organism consistent with infective endocarditis
6. Echocardiogram: consistent with infective endocarditis but not meeting major criterion as noted previously

Definite endocarditis
Pathologic criteria
   Microorganisms: demonstrated by culture or histology in a vegetation, or in a vegetation that has embolized,
      or in an intracardiac abscess, *or*
   Pathologic lesions: vegetation or intracardiac abscess present, confirmed by histology showing active endocarditis
Clinical criteria, using definitions provided in Table 13–2
   Two major criteria, *or*
   One major and three minor criteria, *or*
   Five minor criteria
Possible endocarditis
Findings consistent with endocarditis that do not meet criteria for "definite" or for "rejected"
Endocarditis rejected
   Firm alternative diagnosis that explains manifestations of endocarditis, *or*
   Resolution of manifestations of endocarditis after 4 or fewer days of antibiotic therapy, *or*
   Absence of pathologic evidence of endocarditis at surgery or autopsy after 4 or fewer days of antibiotic therapy

[a]Including nutritional variant strains.
[b]Excluding single positive cultures for coagulase-negative staphylococci and organisms that do not
cause endocarditis.
HACEK = *Haemophilus parainfluenzae, Haemophilus aphrophilus, Actinobacillus actinomycetem-
comitans, Cardiobacterium hominis, Eikenella corrodens,* and *Kingella kingae.*
Source: Adapted with permission from (18).

Table 13–2. Cardiac Conditions and Endocarditis Prophylaxis

Endocarditis prophylaxis recommended

High-risk category

Prosthetic cardiac valves, including bioprosthetic and homograft valves

Previous bacterial endocarditis

Complex cyanotic congenital heart disease (e.g., single ventricle states, transposition of the great arteries, tetralogy of Fallot)

Surgically constructed systemic-pulmonary shunts or conduits

Moderate-risk category

Congenital cardiac malformations other than those listed in the high-risk and negligible-risk categories

Acquired valvular dysfunction (e.g., rheumatic heart disease)

Hypertrophic cardiomyopathy

Mitral valve prolapse with valvular regurgitation and/or thickened leaflets

Endocarditis prophylaxis not recommended

Negligible-risk category (no greater risk than the general population)

Isolated secundum atrial septal defect

Surgical repair of atrial septal defect, ventricular septal defect, or patent ductus arteriosus (without residua beyond 6 months)

Previous coronary artery bypass graft surgery

Mitral valve prolapse without valvular regurgitation

Physiologic, functional, or innocent heart murmur

Previous Kawasaki disease without valvular dysfunction

Previous rheumatic fever without valvular dysfunction

Cardiac pacemakers (intravascular and epicardial) and implanted defibrillators

Source: Adapted with permission from (21b).

In general, prophylaxis is recommended prior to certain high-risk procedures in moderate to high-risk patients. Unfortunately, in the ED it is often difficult to risk stratify patients accurately by this system. Furthermore, the majority of procedures listed as high risk are not performed in the ED, and few studies have investigated the risk of IE associated with common ED procedures (22, 23). A prudent policy would be to consider a high-risk patient *anyone* with a history of endocarditis, known cardiac lesion, or audible murmur. In these patients, single-dose oral or intravenous antibiotics should be administered 30 minutes to 1 h prior to high-risk procedures. High-risk procedures in the ED include urethral catheterization in the setting of a known urinary tract infection (UTI), nasotracheal intubation, and upper gastrointestinal endoscopy, when sclerotherapy of esophageal varices is anticipated. Routine prophylaxis is *not* recommended for orotracheal intubation, urethral catheterization in the absence of a UTI, or for incision and drainage of uncomplicated abscesses (3, 22, 23).

The emergency physician should be prepared to manage the vast array of potential complications of IE. *Cardiac arrhythmias or blocks* should be treated according to the American Heart Association guidelines and possible cardiology consultation. If the diagnosis of *acute valvular regurgitation or rupture* is entertained, an emergent echocardiogram should be obtained. Prompt immediate mobilization of a cardiothoracic surgical team in conjunction with a cardiologist should occur and the patient is stabilized with mechanical ventilation and vasoactive agents. In severe cases, intraaortic balloon pump placement may be necessary as a bridge to cardiothoracic surgery.

Hemorrhagic stroke or *subarachnoid hemorrhage* secondary to ruptured mycotic aneurysms should be recognized rapidly and prompt emergent neurosurgical consultation. *Ischemic stroke* should also prompt specialist consultation; in the setting of endocarditis, an increased risk of hemorrhagic transformation may complicate management (1, 17). Importantly, *peripheral embolism* should *not* be treated with heparin, except in patients with another obvious indication, because anticoagulants have shown to be ineffective in preventing recurrent embolization in IE (1). However, local thrombolytics may be useful in cases of acute arterial thromboembolism, in conjunction with interventional radiology and vascular surgeon consultation. Complications such as *acute renal failure*

Table 13–3. Endocarditis Prophylaxis in Various Procedures

Dental Procedures

Endocarditis prophylaxis recommended[a]

Dental extractions

Periodontal procedures

Dental implant placement and reimplantation of avulsed teeth

Endodontic (root canal) instrumentation or surgery only beyond the apex

Subgingival placement of antibiotic fibers or strips

Initial placement of orthodontic bands (but not brackets)

Intraligamentary local anesthetic injections

Prophylactic cleaning of teeth or implants, where bleeding is anticipated

Endocarditis prophylaxis not recommended

Restorative dentistry (operative and prosthodontic),

Local anesthetic injections (nonintraligamentary)

Intracanal endodontic treatment (postplacement and buildup)

Placement of rubber dams

Postoperative suture removal

Placement of removable prosthodontic or orthodontic appliances

Oral impressions

Fluoride treatments

Oral radiographs

Orthodontic appliance adjustment

Shedding of primary teeth

Other Procedures

Endocarditis prophylaxis recommended

Respiratory tract

Tonsillectomy and/or adenoidectomy

Surgical procedures that involve respiratory mucosa

Bronchoscopy with a rigid bronchoscope

Gastrointestinal tract[d]

Sclerotherapy for esophageal varices

Esophageal stricture dilation

Endoscopic retrograde cholangiography with biliary obstruction

Biliary tract surgery

Surgical procedures that involve intestinal mucosa

Genitourinary tract

Prostatic surgery

Cystoscopy

Urethral dilation

Endocarditis prophylaxis not recommended

Respiratory tract

Endotracheal intubation

Bronchoscopy using a flexible bronchoscope, with or without biopsy

Tympanostomy tube insertion

Gastrointestinal tract

Transesophageal echocardiography[e]

Endoscopy with or without gastrointestinal biopsy[e]

Genitourinary tract

Vaginal hysterectomy[e]

Vaginal delivery[e]

Cesarean section

In uninfected tissue:

Urethral catheterization

Uterine dilatation and curettage

Therapeutic abortion

Sterilization procedures

Insertion or removal of intrauterine devices

Other procedures

Cardiac catheterization, including balloon angioplasty

Coronary stents and implanted cardiac pacemakers and defibrillators

Incision or biopsy of surgically scrubbed skin

Circumcision

---

[a]Prophylaxis is recommended for patients with high- and moderate-risk cardiac conditions.

[b]Procedures include the restoration of decayed teeth (placement of fillings) and the replacement of missing teeth

[c]Based on clinical judgment, antibiotic use may be indicated for selected circumstances in which significant bleeding may occur

[d]Prophylaxis is recommended for high-risk patients and is optional for medium-risk patients.

[e]Prophylaxis is optional for high-risk patients.

Source: Adapted with permission from (21b).

or thrombosis may rarely require emergent hemodialysis and possibly urological consultation. In many community hospitals, it may be necessary to transfer the patient to a referral center for appropriate surgical care once the patient is stabilized (24).

The most common indication for cardiothoracic surgical intervention in IE is *cardiac failure*. Multiple studies have demonstrated improved mortality in patients with moderate to severe heart failure when medical therapy is combined with surgical valve repair or replacement (1). Ideally, surgery should be performed early in patients with IE and cardiac failure, because hemodynamic instability greatly increases perioperative mortality (25). Therefore, emergency physicians should routinely consult cardiothoracic surgeons in addition to cardiologists for patients with IE and significant signs of failure. Other common indications for cardiothoracic surgery in the medical and surgical literature include persistent infection, enlarging vegetations, myocardial abscesses, prosthetic valve infections, or recurrent embolization despite appropriate medical therapy (26). In these cases, cardiothoracic surgical consultation may be obtained either emergently or urgently depending on the stability of the patient.

DISPOSITION

In general, any patient with suspected IE should be admitted for appropriate work-up and therapy. Patients with severe complications may require admission to a monitored setting. In certain low-risk cases, well-appearing reliable patients may be discharged after drawing appropriate blood cultures and/or echocardiography. However, that decision should be made in conjunction with the patient's primary physician or cardiologist. Several studies have attempted to risk stratify febrile IVDUs in the ED (27–29). Unfortunately, most reveal that physicians are *unable* to reliably predict which febrile IVDUs have IE. Therefore, routine admission of these patients should be strongly considered.

CASE OUTCOME

Unfortunately, this patient did not have a favorable outcome. Within several hours, he developed a temperature of 103.2° and stool incontinence. Reassessment by the subsequent EP on duty revealed severe point tenderness of the lumbar spine, diminished rectal tone, and mild lower extremity weakness. An emergent MRI was obtained, which revealed a large L2-4 epidural abscess with cauda equina syndrome. The patient was taken to the operating room

emergently for neurosurgical decompression. All blood cultures and intraoperative cultures grew ORSA. While in the hospital, TTE demonstrated nonspecific changes of the aortic valve. Subsequent TEE revealed small vegetations of the aortic valve with mild regurgitant flow. Only after a positive HIV test did the patient admit to former IVDU. He remained in the hospital for 7 days on IV vancomycin and was subsequently transferred to a skilled nursing facility for continued IV antibiotics and physical therapy. Despite these interventions, the patient remained permanently stool incontinent and unable to ambulate without assistance.

REFERENCES

1. Mylonakis E, Calderwood SB: Infective endocarditis in adults. *N Engl J Med* 345(18):1318–1330, 2001.
2. Towns ML, Reller LB: Diagnostic methods current best practices and guidelines for isolation of bacteria and fungi in infective endocarditis. *Infect Dis Clin North Am* 16(2): 363–376, ix–x, 2002.
3. Dajani AS et al.: Prevention of bacterial endocarditis: Recommendations by the American Heart Association. *Clin Infect Dis* 25(6):1448–1458, 1997.
4. Gersony WM et al.: Bacterial endocarditis in patients with aortic stenosis, pulmonary stenosis, or ventricular septal defect. *Circulation* 87(2 Suppl): I121–I126, 1993.
5. Agnihotri AK et al.: The prevalence of infective endocarditis after aortic valve replacement. *J Thorac Cardiovasc Surg* 110(6):1708–1720; discussion 1720–1724, 1995.
6. Wilson LE et al.: Prospective study of infective endocarditis among injection drug users. *J Infect Dis* 185(12):1761–1766, 2002.
7. Mathew J et al.: Clinical features, site of involvement, bacteriologic findings, and outcome of infective endocarditis in intravenous drug users. *Arch Intern Med.* 155(15):1641–1648, 1995.
8. Strom BL et al.: Risk factors for infective endocarditis: Oral hygiene and nondental exposures. *Circulation* 102(23): 2842–2848, 2000.
9. Cabell CH et al.: Changing patient characteristics and the effect on mortality in endocarditis. *Arch Intern Med* 162(1): 90–94, 2002.
10. Daniel WG et al.: Improvement in the diagnosis of abscesses associated with endocarditis by transesophageal echocardiography. *N Engl J Med* 324(12):795–800, 1991.
11. Brown PD, Levine DP: Infective endocarditis in the injection drug user. *Infect Dis Clin North Am* 16(3):645–665, viii–ix, 2002.
12. Ellis ME et al.: Fungal endocarditis: Evidence in the world literature, 1965–1995. *Clin Infect Dis* 32(1):50–62, 2001.
13. Delaney KA: Endocarditis in the emergency department. *Ann Emerg Med* 20(4):405–414, 1991.

14. Vongpatanasin W, Hillis LD, Lange RA: Prosthetic heart valves. *N Engl J Med* 335(6):407–416, 1996.

15. Tsao JW et al.: Mycotic aneurysm presenting as Pancoast's syndrome in an injection drug user. *Ann Emerg Med* 34(4 Pt 1):546–549, 1999.

16. Bayer AS: Infective endocarditis. *Clin Infect Dis* 17(3): 313–320; quiz 321–322, 1993.

17. Sexton DJ, Spelman D: Current best practices and guidelines. Assessment and management of complications in infective endocarditis. *Infect Dis Clin North Am* 16(2):507–521, xii, 2002.

18. Durack DT, Lukes AS, Bright DK: New criteria for diagnosis of infective endocarditis: Utilization of specific echocardiographic findings. Duke Endocarditis Service. *Am J Med* 96(3):200–209, 1994.

19. Sandre RM, Shafran SD: Infective endocarditis: Review of 135 cases over 9 years. *Clin Infect Dis* 22(2):276–286, 1996.

20. Dodds GA et al.: Negative predictive value of the Duke criteria for infective endocarditis. *Am J Cardiol* 77(5):403–407, 1996.

21a. Cheitlin MD et al.: ACC/AHA/ASE 2003 Guideline Update for the Clinical Application of Echocardiography: Summary article. A report of the American College of Cardiology/American Heart Association Task Force on Practice Guidelines (ACC/AHA/ASE Committee to Update the 1997 Guidelines for the Clinical Application of Echocardiography). *J Am Soc Echocardiogr* 16(10):1091–1110, 2003.

21b. Dajani AS, Taubert KA, Wilson W, et al.: Prevention of bacterial endocarditis. Recommendations by the American Heart Association. *JAMA* 277:1794–1801, 1997

22. Bobrow BJ et al.: Incision and drainage of cutaneous abscesses is not associated with bacteremia in afebrile adults. *Ann Emerg Med* 29(3):404–408, 1997.

23. Cannon LA, et al.: The incidence of bacteremia associated with emergent intubation: Relevance to prophylaxis against bacterial endocarditis. *Ohio Med* 86(8):596–599, 1990.

24. Calder KK, Severyn FA: Surgical emergencies in the intravenous drug user. *Emerg Med Clin North Am* 21(4):1089–1116, 2003.

25. Alexiou C, et al.: Surgery for active culture-positive endocarditis: Determinants of early and late outcome. *Ann Thorac Surg* 69(5):1448–1454, 2000.

26. Olaison L, Pettersson G: Current best practices and guidelines indications for surgical intervention in infective endocarditis. *Infect Dis Clin North Am* 16(2):453–475, xi, 2002.

27. Marantz PR, et al.: Inability to predict diagnosis in febrile intravenous drug abusers. *Ann Intern Med* 106(6):823–828, 1987.

28. Young GP, et al.: Inability to validate a predictive score for infective endocarditis in intravenous drug users. *J Emerg Med* 11(1):1–7, 1993.

29. Samet JH, et al.: Hospitalization decision in febrile intravenous drug users. *Am J Med* 89(1):53–57, 1990.

14

Myocarditis and Pericarditis

Jorge A. Martinez
Melissa A. McKay

MYOCARDITIS

High Yield Facts

- The most common cause of myocarditis is viral infection.

- Most cases of myocarditis are clinically insignificant and self-limited.

- Severe cases of myocarditis present with acute heart failure, arrhythmias, and conduction blocks.

- The pathophysiology of myocarditis is the result of invasion of the myocardium by the causative agent in conjunction with the associated inflammatory response.

- The management of myocarditis consists of bed rest, restriction of physical activity, removal of the precipitating agent or control of the systemic disease process, and continuous follow-up.

Case Presentation

A 24-year-old male presents to the emergency department with a complaint of worsening shortness of breath and heart palpitations. The patient states that he recently got over a "cold" in which he had fever, chills, weakness, and shortness of breath with exertion. He claims that the "cold" caused him to miss a week of work. He admits that he has not recuperated because he is still tired and weak with worsening shortness of breath.

Physical examination reveals a well developed, well nourished male who is tachypneic but not in distress. His vital signs are temperature of 98.9°, blood pressure of 180/62, pulse of 118 beats per minute, and respiratory rate of 30 per minute. Pulse oximetry is 96% oxygen saturation on room air. His pupils are round and reactive to light and his extraocular movements are normal. His mucous membranes are moist and pink. His neck is supple with venous distension at 60°. He has rales bilaterally in both lung bases that do not clear with coughing. Pulses are

strong bilaterally with an occasional extrasystole. His first and second heart sounds are normal. There is a third heart sound and an occasional extrasystole, but no murmurs. His abdomen is nondistented and nontender with normal bowel sounds and no organomegaly. He has trace pedal edema of his feet and ankles.

He is placed on a cardiac monitor, which demonstrates sinus tachycardia at a rate of 110 beats per minute, occasional premature ventricular complexes, and a five beat run of ventricular tachycardia. Chest x-ray shows cardiomegaly, Kerley B lines, and interstitial markings in the lungs. Electrocardiogram (ECG) reveals sinus tachycardia and occasional PVCs. Cardiac enzymes are normal. He is admitted to the intensive care unit with acute heart failure. He responds well to an angiotensin converting enzyme inhibitor, a diuretic, and vasodilators. He is transferred to telemetry after 2 days, where he remains stable without further episodes of heart failure or arrhythmias.

Introduction/Epidemiology

Generally, myocarditis is a subtle disease and most cases are asymptomatic or associated with vague and nonspecific symptoms. However, in some cases the initial presentation is acute heart failure, arrhythmias, conduction block, or sudden death. Myocarditis is the result of myocardial inflammation and necrosis, which can cause substantial destruction of the myocardium and cytoskeleton of the heart. While most cases of myocarditis are due to viral infection, numerous bacteria and protozoa also cause myocarditis. Systemic diseases, such as uremia and the Kawasaki disease, and connective tissue diseases, such as systemic lupus erythematosus and rheumatoid arthritis, cause myocarditis. The disease also results from exposure to certain toxins, heavy metals, medications, hypersensitivity reactions, and radiation. Doxorubicin, a cancer chemotherapy agent, is a well-known cause of myocarditis. Zidovudine, an antiretroviral used to treat acquired immunodeficiency syndrome (AIDS), may precipitate myocarditis. Lithium and acetaminophen are directly toxic to the myocardium. Alcohol, cocaine, and amphetamines are associated with myocarditis. Hypersensitivity reactions involving hydrochlorothiazide, penicillin, ampicillin, methyldopa, and sulfamethoxazole may instigate myocarditis (Table 14–1).

The inflammatory changes in the myocardium include infiltration of mononuclear cells with concomitant myocardial necrosis. It is postulated that the pathological changes of myocarditis are the result of direct invasion of the infecting agent coupled with the intrinsic immune response to the cellular invasion (1). Typically, myocardial

Table 14–1. Causes of Myocarditis

Infections: viral, bacteria, fungus, protozoa, parasites, spirochetes, rickettsia

Collegen vascular diseases: rheumatoid arthritis, systemic lupus erythematosus, Reiter syndrome, Sjögren syndrome, sarcoidosis, giant cell arteritis

Systemic diseases: uremia, serum sickness, rheumatic fever, Kawasaki disease

Medications: doxorubicin, zidovudine, lithium, acetaminophen

Hypersensitivity reactions: penicillin, ampicillin, methyldopa, sulfamethoxazole, hydrochlorothiazide, toluene, acetazolamide, reserpine

Heavy metals: lead, arsenic, iron, copper

Toxins: alcohol, cocaine, amphetamines, cobalt

Radiation therapy

Pregnancy

Cardiac transplant rejection

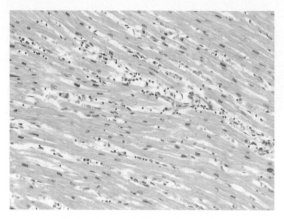

Fig. 14–1. Myocarditis—microscopic.

Pathophysiology/Microbiology

The inflammatory process in myocarditis is typically diffuse, involving the entire myocardium. Occasionally the inflammation may be focal and patchy. Lymphocytic infiltration, which varies in extent and severity, and concomitant myocardial necrosis are classic findings microscopically (Fig. 14–1). Diffuse myocardial necrosis and subsequent interstitial fibrosis may lead to disorganization of the heart's cytoskeleton leading to ventricular dilation and dysfunction. In rare cases the inflammatory process involves the valves and pericardium. Three mechanisms have been proposed for myocardial damage in infectious myocarditis. First, the organism produces a toxin that is directly toxic to the myocardium. Bacteria that produce such toxins are *Corynebacterium diphtheria* and *Shigella dysenteriae*. Second, the organism invades the myocyte and destroys it. Third, the elicited inflammatory response promotes myocardial cell destruction.

Most studies dealing with the pathophysiology of myocarditis have examined the effect of cardiotropic viral agents in animal myocardium. These studies suggest that a threefold mechanism causes myocardial damage. The first mechanism involves the invasion of the myocardium by cardiotropic virus. The virus replicates in the myocardial cells causing myocytolysis and necrosis (1, 3). Viral replication causes myocyte necrosis within 4 days of viral invasion. (4) In the second phase the immune system's response to viral invasion induces natural killer cells (NKCS) which migrate into the myocardium and interact with viral-infected myocytes (4). Normally, NKCs inhibit viral replication, clear viral particles from the myocardium, and eliminate infected myocytes. In doing so, they release proinflammatory cytokines, including interlukin-1B, tumor necrosis factor, interferon, interlukin-2B, and perforin into the myocardial

inflammation is diffuse; however, it may be patchy and localized. Patients with diffuse myocardial involvement present with malignant arrhythmias or acute heart failure. In addition, bradycardia or high degree atrioventricular conduction blocks, the result of inflammation of the cardiac conduction system, cause weakness, fatigue, dizziness, or syncope. Sudden death may be the result of malignant ventricular arrhythmias. Continued myocardial inflammation and necrosis result in ventricular dilation and failure and ultimately nonischemic dilated cardiomyopathy (NDC). The Myocarditis Treatment Trial found that the mortality rate from myocarditis was 20% at 1 year and 56% at 4.3 years (2).

The true incidence of myocarditis is unknown because the vast majority of cases are asymptomatic. Furthermore, aside from overt heart failure, arrhythmia, or conduction block, there are no characteristic signs and symptoms of myocarditis. Usually, the successful diagnosis of myocarditis is based on the recognition of cardiac symptoms associated with systemic illnesses, physical agents, or microorganisms known to cause myocarditis. Myocarditis should be excluded in young patients who present with new-onset heart failure, arrhythmias, conduction disturbances, or symptoms consistent with acute pericarditis or myocardial infarction following viral illness. It should also be considered in children who develop cardiac symptoms after exanthematous viral diseases or when tachycardia is out of proportion owing to fever. Finally, myocarditis should be suspected in patients with chest pain and elevated cardiac enzymes in the absence of coronary artery disease.

cells (1, 4). Tumor necrosis factor activates endothelial cells, enhances the release of cytokines, promotes inflammatory cell infiltration, and has a negative inotropic effect on the heart (4). Interferon inhibits viral replication within the myocardial cell, while perforin promotes the destruction of myocardial cells (1, 4). Occasionally, despite the NKCs' actions, the virus continues to replicate in the myocardium causing progressive destruction of myocardial cells with cardiac dysfunction (1). Pauschinger et al. (5) examined the myocardium of 45 patients with myocarditis and left ventricular dysfunction and found that 22% had active enteroviral RNA replication in the myocardium. Wessely et al. studied viral replication in cardiac myocytes and found that the presence of viral genetic material induced disruption of cardiac filaments and the cardiac cytoskeleton (6). Other studies have demonstrated that malnutrition, increasing age, and continued physical activity in the face of ongoing cardiotropic viral replication are associated with increased cardiac necrosis, cardiac dysfunction, and mortality (1). The third mechanism of myocardial damage is due to the infiltration of T lymphocytes into the myocardium with localized antibody response against viral and myocardial antigens. Cytotoxic T lymphocytes infiltrate the myocardium subsequent to the viral invasion (3). These T lymphocytes play a major role in clearing viral particles from the myocardium: however, they may also damage myocardial cells. It is postulated that some myocardial membrane antigens are similar to viral antigens. Thus, while destroying viral particles, T lymphocytes cross react with myocardial cell antigens and destroy myocardial cells (1, 4). In one study of coxsackie B myocarditis myocardial inflammation and damage was reduced if CD4+ and CD8+ T lymphocytes were not found in myocardial tissue (7).

Nitric oxide synthase, released during viral invasion of the myocardial cells, is proposed as an important cause of myocardial necrosis. In the normal heart, nitric oxide, derived from nitric oxide synthase, is produced by endothelial cells. Nitric oxide is essential for myocardial relaxation, diastolic function, excitation-contraction coupling, and beta-adrenoreceptor responsiveness (1). In myocarditis an isoform of nitric oxide synthase generates nitric oxide and perioxynitrite, a free radical, which causes myocardial depression, apoptosis, necrosis, and may promote ventricular dilation (8).

Finally, persistent viral RNA in the myocardium has been linked to autoantibody formation against myocardial cell antigens. Sole and Liu (9) demonstrated that the amino acid sequence of the coxsackie B and the beta myosin heavy chain protein in cardiac myocytes are 50% similar. Other studies have shown that autoantibodies react with adenine nucleotide translator, cardiac myosin, B-adrenoreceptors, and myocardial structures including mitochondria, myolemma, and sarcolemma (4). Autoantibody reactions to myocardial antigens worsen ventricular systolic and diastolic functions (10). Intramyocardial antialpha myosin antibodies are associated with a worse prognosis because patients without the antibodies have improved left ventricular systolic and diastolic functions (10).

Nonischemic dilated cardiomyopathy is the result of continued deterioration of ventricular function and concurrent dilation of the ventricles. Several studies suggest that NDC is due to progressive autoimmune mechanisms. NDC is associated with persistent viral RNA in myocardial tissue despite the resolution of inflammation (8). Fujioka et al. (11) demonstrated enteroviral RNA in 35% of NDC patients. Other studies identified the enteroviral genome in 5–50% of patients with NDC (3). Enteroviral protease disrupts the cardiac cytoskeleton resulting in ventricular dilation (12). Mouse hearts with full-length copy of the coxsackie B genome have cardiac cytoskeleton changes and abnormal excitation-contraction coupling typical of NDC (13). Patients with myocarditis or NDC have a mortality rate of 26% if they have persistent enteroviral genome in the myocardium versus a 3% mortality rate if they do not (3). Furthermore, a genetic predisposition to develop NDC may exist (14).

The majority of cases of myocarditis are caused by cardiotropic viruses (1). In the United States and Europe the most common cause of viral myocarditis is the enterovirus coxsackie B, which accounts for up to 50% of cases (15). The incidence of coxsackie B myocarditis increases in warm weather when the virus's activity peaks. Commonly, in adults coxsackie B myocarditis is subclinical with a benign course. On the other hand, neonatal myocarditis, most frequently caused by coxsackie B, is severe with an abrupt onset of respiratory distress, tachycardia, cyanosis, jaundice, diarrhea, temperature instability, and poor peripheral circulation. Echocardiography usually demonstrates left or biventricular function dysfunction. Infants with coxsackie B myocarditis frequently have concurrent meningoencephalitis, pneumonia, hepatitis, or pancreatitis. The mortality rate of isolated coxsackie B myocarditis in infants is 30–50%. It is higher when other organs systems are involved (16). Other cardiotropic viruses implicated in myocarditis include echovirus, adenovirus, poliovirus, herpes simplex virus, hepatitis C virus, Epstein-Barr virus, varicella zoster, rubella, rubeola, mumps, and parvovirus B19. Myocarditis is also caused by numerous bacterial pathogens, *Mycoplasma pneumoniae*, rickettsia, and parasites. Enterocolitis caused by *Campylobacter jejuni* may be associated with concurrent myocarditis (17) (Table 14–2).

Table 14–2. Myocarditis—Infectious Organisms

Virus: coxsackie B, influenza, echovirus, influenza, Epstein-Barr virus, hepatitis A, hepatitis C, herpes simplex, herpes zoster, human immunodeficiency virus, paramyxovirus, rubella, parvovirus, poliovirus, cytomegalovirus, mumps, yellow fever, smallpox

Bacteria: *C. diphtheria, Escherichia coli, Haemophilus influenzae, L. pneumophila, M. tuberculosis, M. pneumoniae, Neisseria gonnorrhoeae, Neisseria meningitidis, Salmonella typhi, Serratia marcescens, Shigella dysenteriae, Staphylococcus aureus, S. pneumoniae, Vibrio cholera*

Fungus: Actinomyces, Aspergillus, Blastomyces, Candida, Coccidioides, Cryptomyces, Histoplamosis, Mucormyces, Nocardia, Sporothrix

Protozoa: *T. gondii, T. cruzi*

Parasites: *Echinococcus granulosus, Paragonimus westermani, T. spiralis, Visceral larval migrans, Wuchereria bancrofti,* Shistosoma

Spirochetes: *Borrellia burgdorferi, Treponema pallidum,* Leptosporia

Rickettsia: *Coxiella burnetii, Rickettsia rickettsii, Rickettsia tsutsugamushi*

Diphtheria, caused by *C. diphteriae,* is rare in the United States. However, it remains a common cause of myocarditis in underdeveloped countries. Clinically, diphtheria presents as fever, nasopharyngitis, and edematous mucous membranes. A posterior pharyngeal pseudomembrane, caused by an exotoxin, may obstruct the upper airway causing respiratory distress. Myocarditis is caused by the same exotoxin, which is toxic to the myocardium and conduction system, and causes a dilated, hypocontractile heart and severe conduction blocks. Treatment includes support of the respiratory and cardiac systems; high-dose intravenous penicillin (or erythromycin if the patient is allergic to penicillin); and diphtheria antitoxin.

Lyme disease is a tick-borne disease caused by the spirochete *Borrelia burgdorferi.* Cardiac involvement occurs in approximately 10% of patients infected and usually within 3 weeks of onset of erythema migrans. Atrioventricular and bundle branch block are common manifestations of Lyme myocarditis. Dysrhythmias and left ventricular failure may also occur. Temporary pacing for high degree atrioventricular block and aggressive treatment of heart failure are essential. Lyme disease is diagnosed by a

history of exposure to an endemic area, classic skin eruptions of erythema migrans, and positive serological testing for the spirochete. Lyme myocarditis is treated with high dose intravenous penicillin, amoxicillin, or ceftriaxone.

Chagas disease is caused by the hemoflagellate protozoa *Trypanosoma cruzi,* which is transmitted by the bite of the reduviid insect. Chagas disease is the most common cause of myocarditis and heart disease in Central and South America. There are three phases of Chagas disease: the acute phase, a prolonged latent phase, and a chronic phase. The diagnosis is usually confirmed by positive serological tests for the protozoa. If the patient receives treatment during the acute or latent phase, major cardiac damage can be averted. The antitrypanosomal agents used to treat Chagas disease are nifurtimox for 60–90 days or benznidazole for 60 days. Treatment is not effective in the chronic phase.

Patients with acute Chagas disease develop an acute pancarditis, the result of intense myocardial inflammation instigated by trypanosoma pseudocysts within the myocardium. Most cases of acute Chagas disease are subclinical. However, some patients have symptoms including fever, facial or unilateral palpebral edema (Romana sign), and swelling and induration of the site of reduviid bite (chagoma). Significant cardiac symptoms develop in only 1% of patients infected, but the mortality rate is 10% (18).

Patients remain infected with the protozoa during the latent phase of the disease, which lasts for 15–20 years. The continuous inflammatory process results in myocardial necrosis and fibrosis with interspersed myocardial hypertrophy (18). Although the inflammatory process is widespread, the major effect of the inflammation is on the conduction system and apex of the left ventricle. The anterior fascicle of the left bundle and the right bundle are most commonly involved. However, the inflammation may involve the atrioventricular node, resulting in complete heart block, or the sinus node, resulting in bradycardia. Inflammation of the apex of the left ventricle leads to apical aneurysm with mural thrombus formation. Inflammation may also involve the autonomic nervous system resulting in variable and uncontrolled heart rates.

Chronic Chagas disease is the end result of inflammatory destruction of the myocardium and cardiac conduction system with heart failure being the predominate feature. Nonetheless, only 30–40% of chronic Chagas-disease patients develop anatomic cardiac abnormalities and only 10–20% develop overt cardiac symptoms (18). The ECG demonstrates right bundle branch, the left anterior fascicle block, or both in 80% of patients (18). Complete heart block or bradycardia may be present.

Pulmonary and peripheral embolism may be the result of mural thrombi.

Because Chagas disease is subclinical for most of its natural history, criteria have been established to confirm the diagnosis. Importantly, all four criteria must exist for the diagnosis to be made. The criteria include a history of residence where Chagas disease is endemic; an unequivocally positive serologic test for the protozoa; a clinical syndrome compatible with Chagas heart disease; and no evidence of another cardiac disorder that could cause the clinical manifestations (18).

Toxoplasmosis myocarditis, caused by *Toxoplasma gondii*, is a common cause of myocarditis in immunocompromised patients. Humans become infected with *T. gondii* by ingesting contaminated water or food, particularly raw or undercooked meat. Less common sources of transmission include organ and bone marrow transplants and blood transfusions. Usually in the immunocompetent host, *T. gondii* infection is subclinical and self-limited. However, in the immunocompromised patient it is a serious and life-threatening disease that commonly involves the brain and the heart. *T. gondii* is the most common infectious agent causing myocarditis in patients with AIDS (19). Hofman et al. (20) conducted autopsies on 182 patients with human immunodeficiency virus (HIV) infection over a 4-year period. They found *T. gondii* in the myocardium of 21 patients. Six of the 21 patients had diffuse myocarditis and 8 of the 21 patients had focal myocarditis (20). Typical manifestations of toxoplasmosis myocarditis include heart failure, dysrythmias, bundle branch block, and pericarditis. *T. gondii* myocarditis is fatal if left untreated. Antimicrobial treatment includes a regimen of pyrimethamine, folinic acid, and sulfadiazine. Clindamycin or clarithromycin may be substituted for sulfadiazine in patients with sulfa allergy.

Trichinosis is the result of the ingestion of the cysts of the roundworm *Trichinella spiralis*. The cysts are found in undercooked contaminated meat, usually pork or wild game. After the cysts are ingested, the larvae invade skeletal muscle, and occasionally, the myocardium. The cysts invoke an inflammatory response composed mainly of eosinophils. Clinical manifestations include fever, myalgia, muscle tenderness, and periorbital edema. Cardiac symptoms, usually chest pain, dysrhythmias, atrioventricular conduction block, and heart failure, develop within 2–3 weeks of cyst ingestion. The diagnosis of trichinosis is based on clinical symptoms, along with positive serological studies, or visualization of the cysts in muscle tissue on biopsy. Peripheral eosinophilia is a characteristic finding. Treatment with antihelmintic drugs mebendazole, thiabendazole, or albendazole is essential. Death

from trichinosis is usually due to cardiac dysfunction. In one series *T. spiralis* cysts were found at autopsy in the myocardium of 94% of patients who died from trichinosis (21).

Human immunodeficiency virus is a common cause of myocarditis worldwide. Changes in the myocardium consistent with myocarditis have been found in 46% of AIDS patients at autopsy (22). HIV-1 RNA has been found in the myocardium of patients with AIDS. Proposed mechanisms of myocarditis include direct invasion of the myocardium by HIV, concomitant systemic infection with another organism, and invasion of the myocardium by opportunistic organisms (23). Several studies suggest that HIV causes myocardial damage either through a direct toxic effect on the myocardial cell or through an "innocent bystander" mechanism (19). Barbaro et al. evaluated 952 asymptomatic AIDS patients with echocardiography to assess the incidence of dilated cardiomyopathy. Seventy-six of the 952 patients had findings consistent with dilated cardiomyopathy. Endomyocardial biopsy was performed on all 76 patients. The HIV nucleus was found in the myocardium of 58 of the 76 patients. Furthermore, 36 of the 58 patients met biopsy criteria for myocarditis. Six of the 36 patients had a second cardiotropic virus, including coxsackie B, cytomegalovirus, and Epstein-Barr virus in the myocardial cells. The authors concluded that myocarditis in HIV infections was due to direct toxicity of HIV or due to an autoimmune process induced by the HIV virus in association with other cardiotropic viruses (24). The innocent bystander mechanism proposes that HIV causes the release of toxic enzymes, or lymphokines, as it replicates in myocardial lymphocytes and macrophages. These enzymes and lymphokines damage the myocardial cell membrane allowing the HIV to enter the cell and destroy it (19).

Clinical Presentation

The clinical presentation of myocarditis is varied. Most cases of myocarditis are clinically silent with vague complaints and few signs, symptoms, or physical findings to suggest the diagnosis. Thus, a high degree of suspicion is necessary to make the diagnosis. In all suspected cases of myocarditis, a thorough history and physical examination are essential. Sixty percent of patients have a history of preceding "flu-like" symptoms related to an upper respiratory or gastrointestinal viral illness, while 35% complain of chest pain and 18% have fever (1). Other common symptoms include anorexia, chills, headache, fatigue, weakness, myalgia, and arthralgia. Chest pain is usually nonspecific and, in the absence of cardiac manifestations, may suggest pneumonia, pleurisy, pericarditis, pulmonary embolus, or cardiac ischemia. In addition, the patient may have systemic signs and symptoms related to the causative systemic illness, physical agent, or infectious organism.

In severe cases of myocarditis the physical examination reveals clinical manifestations consistent with cardiac dysfunction. Patients with left ventricular heart failure typically complain of dyspnea, fatigue, cough, orthopnea, and paroxysmal nocturnal dyspnea. On physical examination there may be crackles, rhonchi, or wheezes in the lungs. Third and fourth heart sounds are not uncommon. Ventricular dilation may give rise to mitral or tricuspid regurgitation with holosystolic murmurs. Signs of right heart failure include peripheral edema, jugular venous distension, hepatomegaly, and ascites. Infants and children may appear anxious, listless, or in respiratory distress. Palpitations, fatigue, weakness, dizziness, dyspnea, decreased exercise tolerance, syncope, and hemodynamic instability may be the result of arrhythmias, such as atrial fibrillation, ventricular tachycardia, sinus bradycardia, or high-degree atrioventricular node blockade. Patients may have symptoms, clinical manifestations, and electrocardiographic changes suggestive of acute myocardial infarction (AMI) (25). Myocarditis has been found to be a cause of sudden death in adults less than 40 years old and young athletes (4).

Myocarditis is classified as fulminant or nonfulminant (26). Fulminant myocarditis is characterized by sudden, severe hemodynamic compromise requiring the use of high doses of vasopressors, left ventricular assist devices, or extracorporeal membrane oxygenation. Fulminant myocarditis is frequently fatal (27). Nonfulminant myocarditis, commonly referred to as acute myocarditis, is an afebrile illness with an insidious onset of heart failure over weeks to months. Nonfulminant myocarditis is usually hemodynamically stable or requires only low doses of vasopressors (27).

If patients with fulminant myocarditis survive the initial catastrophic event, they are more likely to regain normal ventricular function than those with nonfulminant myocarditis. Rockman et al. (28) demonstrated that recovery in fulminant myocarditis is maximized if the systemic circulation can be supported long enough for myocardial function to recover. McCarthy et al. found that 93% of patients with fulminant myocarditis were alive without a heart transplant after 1 year while only 85% of nonfulminant myocarditis patients were still alive. Furthermore, patients with fulminant myocarditis were less likely to require heart transplantation (27). Importantly, myocarditis patients who undergo heart transplant have a decreased survival at 1 year compared to patients receiving heart transplants for other reasons. They also have earlier transplant rejections with rejection rates twice that of other transplant recipients (29).

Laboratory/Diagnostic Testing

At present there are no noninvasive diagnostic tests to establish the diagnosis of myocarditis. In most cases of myocarditis laboratory tests are normal or demonstrate only mild, nonspecific abnormalities. Diagnostic tests used in the evaluation of myocarditis include complete blood count, erythrocyte sedimentation rate, blood cultures, viral titers, cardiac enzymes, ECG, and chest x-ray. The erythrocyte sedimentation rate is elevated in 60% of cases, while 24% of cases have leukocytosis (1). Viral titers and bacterial blood cultures are frequently negative for the causative agent. Elevated viral titers indicate a recent viral infection but are not pathognomonic for acute myocarditis. Elevated creatinine kinase occurs in 12% of myocarditis patients (1, 4). In one series 30% of patients with coxsackie myocarditis had elevated serum creatinine kinase and troponin I levels (30). The Myocarditis Treatment Trial found elevated Troponin I levels in 34% of patients with biopsy proven myocarditis compared to 11% with negative biopsies (31).

Likewise, there are no specific ECG findings in myocarditis. Common findings include sinus tachycardia, nonspecific ST-T wave changes, QT prolongation, low voltage, transitory Q waves, atrial or ventricular dysrhythmias, and atrioventricular block. ST segment elevation may be the result of concurrent pericarditis. In addition, ST segment elevation suggestive of AMI has been described (25). Importantly, reciprocal ST segment depression seen in AMI does not occur in myocarditis. Up to 20% of patients with myocarditis have atrioventricular conduction block or left bundle branch block (1). In most cases complete heart block is transient and rarely requires permanent pacing. However, new-onset left and right bundle branch blocks may persist after myocarditis has resolved. Supraventricular and ventricular arrhythmias may occur. The frequency of sudden death secondary to severe conduction block or malignant arrhythmias is not known. One study of 162 subjects under 40 years of age who died suddenly found that myocarditis accounted for 22% of deaths under 30 and 11% of deaths between 30 and 40 years (32). Thus, myocarditis should be considered in young patients with new onset ventricular arrhythmias and a history of recent viral infection.

Typical imaging studies used to evaluate myocarditis include chest x-ray and echocardiography. Chest x-ray findings range from normal cardiac silhouette and lung fields to cardiomegaly, pulmonary vascular congestion, pulmonary edema, and pleural effusion. Echocardiography demonstrates ventricular function and dimensions, valve function, and the presence of ventricular aneurysm and mural thrombi. Echocardiographic findings are not uniform because of the variability in cardiac inflammation. Diffuse myocardial inflammation leads to diastolic and systolic ventricular dysfunction and dilation of the ventricles. Focal myocardial inflammation is associated with regional, segmental wall abnormalities. Cardiac catheterization and coronary angiography are often used to rule out other causes of cardiac disease, but offer no advantage over echocardiography in diagnosing myocarditis.

Endomyocardial biopsy (EMB), using the Dallas criteria, is the gold standard for diagnosing myocarditis. According to the Dallas criteria, myocarditis is present if the EMB demonstrates myocardial necrosis or degeneration, or both, in addition to adjacent inflammatory infiltrate with or without fibrosis in the absence of significant coronary artery disease. Borderline myocarditis is present if the inflammatory infiltrate is sparse or myocardial damage is not apparent. Myocarditis does not exist if the biopsy specimen fails to show intramyocardial inflammation or myocyte necrosis (33). The preferred site for EMB is the right ventricular septum because of increased risk of embolic stroke associated with left ventricular EMB. The role of EMB in diagnosing myocarditis is controversial because of a lack of prospective data addressing its utility to confirm the diagnosis. The diagnostic accuracy of EMB in myocarditis ranges from 0% to 80% (4). Nonetheless, EMB is appropriate in patients with a rapidly deteriorating cardiac function or when heart failure is refractory to medical management. Due to the potentially patchy inflammation in myocarditis, multiple tissue samples may be necessary to establish the diagnosis. While the presence of inflammatory cells and myocyte necrosis confirms the diagnosis, the absence of these findings does not necessarily exclude it because of the potential for patchy involvement and rapid clearance of inflammatory cells (34).

Several other diagnostic tests have been proposed to diagnose myocarditis, although their utility at present is limited. Gallium scanning demonstrates myocardial inflammation; however its sensitivity and specificity in diagnosing myocarditis is unknown. Antimyosin scintigraphy uses Indium-111 antimyosin antibodies to bind to exposed myosin in damaged myocardial cells, thereby visualizing myocardial necrosis. Antimyosin uptake in myocarditis is usually diffuse, faint, and heterogeneous. Conversely, in myocardial infarction intense antimyosin uptake is localized to the region of the involved coronary artery. A normal antimyosin scan effectively rules out myocarditis (35). Detection of viral or bacterial genome by polymerase chain reaction (PCR) may identify the specific pathogen causing myocarditis. With PCR a single DNA or RNA fragment is replicated into millions of strands allowing specific DNA or RNA of a particular virus or bacteria to be identified. Myocardial tissue, pericardial fluid, or other body fluids may be utilized to extract the genetic material necessary to perform PCR.

Management

The treatment of viral myocarditis consists of bed rest and continued monitoring for the development, or worsening, of cardiac manifestations. Antiviral agents are not currently recommended. Bacterial, fungal, and protozoal causes of myocarditis should be identified promptly and treated with appropriate antimicrobial agents. Basic principles in the treatment of myocarditis are supportive care, bed rest, and avoidance of physical exertion. Strenuous activity or exercise during viremia promotes myocardial inflammation. Animal models demonstrate that reducing physical activity leads to better outcomes. Restricting physical activity during the febrile phase of the illness, during active systemic infection, and during acute heart failure reduces cardiac workload and minimizes myocardial inflammation (36). A return to physical activity, especially competitive sports, should only be allowed on a gradual basis with continuous monitoring for evidence of cardiac decompensation. Athletes with myocarditis should refrain from moderate to vigorous activity for no less than 6 months. They must have normal cardiac function and no evidence of arrhythmia before returning to competition (37). Cardiac symptoms should be addressed. Furthermore, specific steps to neutralize or remove the causative agent or control the systemic illness precipitating myocardial inflammation should be instituted. Alcohol and tobacco, which aggravate myocardial inflammation, should be eliminated.

Heart failure should be managed according to conventional guidelines using the same medications and dietary principles as ischemic heart failure. Angiotensin converting enzyme inhibitors are essential. Spirinolactone and loop diuretics are also beneficial. Beta-adrenoreceptor blockers at low doses may be added after the acute episode of heart failure has been stabilized. Digoxin should be used at low doses because high doses augment the release of proinflammatory cytokines and increase mortality (8). Cardiogenic shock and refractory heart failure should be treated with inotropic and vasodilator agents along with mechanical circulatory support with intra-aortic balloon pump, extracorporeal membrane oxygenation, or an external left ventricular assist device. Ventricular assist devices should be used liberally because most patients with myocarditis are young with normal-sized, but hypocontractile left ventricles. Several reports describe the successful use and removal of ventricular support devices once the viral agent has cleared the myocardium and myocardial function has begun to return to baseline (4).

Although conduction blocks are usually transient, severe conduction blocks, such as Mobitz Type II or third degree heart block, should undergo cardiac pacing. Tachyarrhythmias should be converted expeditiously because the rapid ventricular rate may induce or aggravate heart failure. If cardioversion is not feasible, the ventricular rate should be controlled. There are no controlled studies dealing with antiarrhythmic agent use in myocarditis. Thus, their use should follow the same guidelines as those for ischemia-induced arrhythmias. Caution is essential when using these agents because most are negative inotropes and can aggravate heart failure. Complex ventricular arrhythmias should be treated aggressively with the appropriate antiarrhythmic agents, as well as correcting precipitating factors, such as hypoxia and electrolyte imbalance. For unknown reasons 15% of myocarditis patients develop abnormalities of the coagulation pathway with resulting mural thrombus and systemic or pulmonary thromboembolism (1). Therefore, all patients with ventricular dysfunction require systemic anticoagulation.

The treatment of myocarditis with antiviral agents is controversial. In animal models of coxsackie B3 myocarditis ribivarin and alpha-interferon reduced the severity of myocardial lesions and mortality. The greatest effect was when the medications were initiated prior to viral inoculation or early in the course of the disease (38). In a study of mice with coxsackie myocarditis those treated with ribivarin had longer survival intervals than those receiving placebo (39). In 22 myocarditis patients treated with interferon for 24 weeks, the viral genome was cleared from the myocardium and there were decreased left ventricular end-diastolic and end-systolic diameters in all 22 patients. Fifteen of the 22 patients had an increase in left ventricular ejection fraction (40).

Immunosuppressive therapy has been suggested for biopsy-proven myocarditis. Twenty uncontrolled studies evaluated the use of prednisone alone, prednisone and azathioprine, prednisone and cyclosporine, and anti-CD3 monoclonal antibody to treat myocarditis. Immunosuppressive agents resulted in rapid reduction in myocardial inflammation without an equivalent improvement in ventricular dysfunction (41). Three controlled trials studied prednisone and cyclosporine in the treatment of

myocarditis and nonischemic dilated cardiomyopathy. Again, there was a decrease in myocardial inflammation without improvement in ventricular function or decrease in mortality. Thus, the present consensus is that immunosuppressive agents offer no clinical benefit in the treatment of myocarditis (41).

Disposition

All patients with suspected myocarditis should have a formal cardiology consultation in the emergency department. New onset cardiac manifestations such as heart failure, conduction block, arrhythmias, or systemic thromboembolism should be treated aggressively and admitted to a telemetry unit. Clinical outcome of myocarditis varies from complete resolution of symptoms to progressive ventricular dysfunction and dilation with severe heart failure. No method or tests exist at present that can accurately determine which patient will improve and which will deteriorate. Most asymptomatic cases of myocarditis resolve spontaneously without sequella. Patients who develop cardiac manifestations have a higher likelihood of cardiac decompensation and death. Patients with fulminant myocarditis have a worse acute clinical course than nonfulminant myocarditis, but a lower long-term mortality rate than nonfulminant myocarditis. Fifty percent of myocarditis patients will develop NDC within 6 months of its onset (1). However, 30% of these patients will undergo spontaneous improvement of ventricular function (34). Progressive heart failure is the most common cause of death. Complications such as arrhythmias and mural thrombus formation are more likely as left ventricular function deteriorates. Hypotension and cardiogenic shock are associated with a poorer prognosis and higher mortality rate.

All myocarditis patients should be followed closely by a cardiologist at regular intervals. Echocardiography should be employed liberally to evaluate ventricular function and size and to search for ventricular aneurysm, mural thrombus, and pericardial effusion. Arrhythmias, their response to antiarrhythmic therapy, and conduction blocks can be followed with Holter monitoring.

Case Outcome

While in the telemetry unit, the patient underwent an echocardiogram which demonstrated diffuse left ventricular hypokenesis and an ejection fraction of 40%. Continuous cardiac monitoring showed occasional premature ventricular complexes but no atrial or ventricular arrhythmias. The angiotensin converting enzyme inhibitor and spirinolactone were continued, and a low-sodium diet was instituted. He was discharged home 4 days after admission. His medications and diet were continued and he was put at strict bed rest. During that time, he had no shortness of breath, chest pain, palpitations, or dyspnea with exertion. He was seen by a cardiologist at 2 weeks where his physical examination and echocardiogram were unchanged since discharge. His medications and diet were continued and he was allowed to return to work on a limited basis, but restricted from participating in strenuous activities. Over a 6-month period he had no further exacerbations of heart failure, extrasystoles, or arrhythmias. Repeat echocardiogram at 6 months showed normal left ventricular dimensions and function with an ejection fraction of 58%. His medications were discontinued and he was allowed to return to work on a full-time basis and to exercise normally.

PERICARDITIS

High Yield Facts

- Viral and idiopathic are the most common forms of pericarditis.
- The clinical presentation of pericarditis consists of chest pain with a pericardial friction rub.
- Pericarditis is associated with characteristic diffuse ST segment elevation on electrocardiogram.
- Pericarditis may be associated with pericardial effusion, which can cause hemodynamic instability if pericardial tamponade develops.
- Purulent pericarditis must be treated aggressively with intravenous antibiotics and pericardial drainage.
- All patients with pericarditis must be admitted to a telemetry unit for treatment and hemodynamic monitoring.

Case Presentation

A 42-year-old female presents to the emergency department with a complaint of fever, chills, chest and back pain, and shortness of breath. She claims that the chest pain is worse when she lies supine, and sometimes radiates to between her shoulders. She has a history of community-acquired pneumonia diagnosed 7 days ago. She did not finish taking her antibiotics. She explains that she still has a cough with chills and a fever of 100° to 102°. On physical examination she is awake and alert, but quiet with an intermittent cough. Her temperature is 102.6° orally, pulse is 130 beats per minute, blood pressure is 90/46, and

respiratory rate is 32 per minute. Her head and neck examinations are normal. On auscultation she has occasional rales and rhonchi in the left upper lobe, which clear when she coughs. Her heart sounds are distant and there are no third or fourth heart sounds or murmurs. There is a soft one-component friction rub best heard at the left sternum. Her abdominal, genital, and extremity examinations are normal.

She is placed on a cardiac monitor, which demonstrates sinus tachycardia. An ECG shows sinus tachycardia with 2-mm diffuse ST segment elevation in the limb and precordial leads. Chest x-ray reveals cardiomegaly and an infiltrate in the left upper lobe. Complete blood count has an elevated white blood count of 18,000 with 80 neutrophils, 5 lymphocytes, 13 bands, and 2 monocytes. An echocardiogram demonstrates a pericardial effusion without evidence of pericardial tamponade. She is admitted to the intensive care unit where she is started on intravenous ceftriaxone and azithromycin, for community-acquired pneumonia, and oral nonsteroidal antiinflammatory agents (NSAIDs) for a presumptive diagnosis of viral pericarditis.

Introduction/Epidemiology

Pericarditis is defined as inflammation of the pericardial sac surrounding the heart and origins of the great vessels (42). It is viral or idiopathic in origin in more than 80% of cases (43). Other causes of pericarditis include neoplasms; connective tissue diseases, including systemic lupus erythematosus and rheumatoid arthritis; metabolic disorders, such as uremia; radiation; trauma; myocardial infarction; postcoronary artery bypass surgery; and certain medications, particularly hydralazine, procainamide, dantrolene, and methysergide. Infectious causes include viruses, bacteria, including *Mycobacterium tuberculosis* (TB), mycoplasma, parasites, HIV, and fungi, such as Histoplasmosis, Aspergillosis, Candida, Blastomycosis, Coccidioides, and Cryptococcosis (Table 14–3).

Clinically, pericarditis may be silent, it may present as chest pain with distinctive physical and laboratory findings, or it may present as severe hemodynamic instability due to pericardial tamponade. Normally, the clinical manifestations of pericarditis are confined to the pericardium. However, symptoms and clinical manifestations related to the causative organism or precipitating factor may predominate. Constrictive pericarditis is a complication of purulent pericarditis caused by bacteria, TB, and fungi.

Purulent pericarditis is not as common as it was in the preantibiotic era. Before the antibiotic era, the most common cause of purulent pericarditis was *Streptococcus pneumoniae*, along with other gram-positive organisms.

Table 14–3. Causes of Pericarditis

Idiopathic

Infection: virus, bacteria, fungus, rickettsia, toxoplasmosis

Medications: procainamide, hydralazine, isoniazid, reserpine, methysergide, dantrolene

Trauma: blunt and penetrating chest trauma, postcoronary artery bypass surgery

Malignancy: mesothelioma, lymphoma, leukemia, melanoma, metastatic carcinoma

Myocardial infarction: postmyocardial infarction pericarditis, Dressler syndrome

Systemic illness: connective tissue diseases, rheumatic fever, sarcoidosis, systemic lupus erythematosus, inflammatory bowel disease, scleroderma, polyarteritis nodosa, uremia, hypothyroidism, Reiter syndrome, rheumatoid arthritis, serum sickness

Radiation

However, in the antibiotic era the spectrum of organisms has changed with gram-negative bacteria, "atypical" bacteria (e.g., *M. pneumoniae*, *Chlamydia pneumoniae*, and *Legionella pneumophila*), and fungi being common causative agents (44). Infectious causes of pericarditis are listed in Table 14–4.

Pathophysiology/Microbiology

The pericardium consists of a fibrous outer parietal layer and a thin inner visceral layer. The fibrous pericardium surrounds the heart and attaches to the diaphragm, sternum, and mediastinum. The thin, inner serous layer lies

Table 14–4. Infectious Causes of Pericarditis

Virus: coxsackie, echovirus, adenovirus, Epstein-Barr virus, influenza, herpes zoster, human immunodeficiency virus, parvovirus B19, paramyxovirus

Bacteria: *S. aureus, S. pneumoniae, N. meningitidis, H. influenzae, S. typhi, M. tuberculosis, M. pneumoniae, C. pneumoniae, L. pneumophila, P. aeruginosa, E. coli, Klebsiella pneumoniae*, Proteus, Rickettsia, *T. pallidum*

Fungus: Aspergillus, Blastomycosis, Histoplasmosis, Coccidioides, Candida, Nocardia

Parasites: *Entamoeba histolytica, T. gondii*, Echinococcus

---

adjacent to the surface of the heart. The potential space between the fibrous and serous layers of the pericardium contains approximately 15–60 mL of serous fluid, which allows the heart to move freely in the pericardial sac. The pericardium functions to protect the heart from direct injury and to limit the spread of infection or inflammation from adjacent structures.

An increase in the fluid volume within the pericardial sac is known as pericardial effusion. Importantly, the rapidity of fluid accumulation, as well as the amount of fluid in the pericardial sac, affects the hemodynamic function of the heart. Approximately 120 mL of pericardial fluid can gradually accumulate in the pericardial sac without significantly increasing the intrapericardial pressure. However, a rapid accumulation of fluid results in a dramatic, sudden increase in intrapericardial pressure, which compresses the heart and impedes filling of the right atrium and ventricle. The result is decreased cardiac output with systemic hypotension, a condition called pericardial tamponade.

Purulent pericarditis is a lethal form of pericarditis, occurring most commonly in children and immunocompromised individuals. If untreated, the mortality rate is nearly 100%. Nonetheless, immediate treatment with intravenous antibiotics and pericardial drainage is still associated with a mortality rate of 40% (45). Purulent pericarditis results from the direct extension of a pulmonary or mediastinal infection to the pericardium, or from hematogenous seeding of the pericardium during bacteremia (46). It is most commonly related to thoracic surgery, empyema, bacterial endocarditis, pneumonia, pericardial effusion, hemodialysis, and bacteremia.

The onset of purulent pericarditis may be acute with rapid progression to pericardial tamponade or it may be insidious (47, 48). Because of its varied clinical onset, a high index of suspicion is necessary to make the diagnosis. Clinical findings in purulent pericarditis include fever, chills, dyspnea, tachypnea, cough, weakness, and tachycardia out of proportion to fever. Chest pain and friction rubs are not common. Nonetheless, chest pain may be sudden or gradual in onset with radiation to the back, neck, left shoulder, or arm. Signs of systemic infection may predominate over localized signs and symptoms of pericarditis.

Sagrista-Sauleda et al. reviewed 33 cases of purulent pericarditis in a community hospital over a 20-year period. They noted that these patients did not have classic findings of pericarditis, that is, chest pain and pericardial rub. Fifteen of the 33 patients had pericardial tamponade. The most common cause of purulent pericarditis was pneumonia, with empyema being the second most common cause. The most common organisms involved were streptococci, pneumococci, and staphylococci. The diagnosis was usually made after the onset of pericardial tamponade or at autopsy (49). Several case reports have described the atypical clinical presentation of and variety of organisms causing purulent pericarditis. Arsura et al. described four cases of purulent pericarditis which were initially misdiagnosed as septic shock. Classic symptoms of pericarditis occurred in only 50% of patients. Clinical findings consistent with pericardial tamponade were subtle or absent in all four patients. The authors concluded that purulent pericarditis does not exhibit classic clinical signs and symptoms of pericarditis; therefore a high index of suspicion is necessary to assure diagnosis (50). Purulent pericarditis has been described in a postpartum patient due to Group F streptococcus (48) and in a colon cancer patient due to Group G streptococcus (51). Donnelly et al. reported a case series where the presentation of purulent pericarditis in children was consistent with an acute abdomen (52).

M. tuberculosis is a common cause of purulent pericarditis worldwide and a major cause of pericarditis in immunocompromised individuals. TB pericarditis results from the retrograde spread of peribronchial, peritracheal, or mediastinal lymph nodes; military TB; or seeding from the lungs, spine, or sternum (53). Less than half of patients with TB pericarditis have pulmonary TB (54). Typical findings in TB pericarditis include chest pain, fever, night sweats, weight loss, and tachycardia. The purified protein derivative skin test is negative in up to 30% of patients. In addition, chest x-ray demonstrates a pleural effusion in 50% of patients (53). Most cases of TB pericarditis have a concurrent pericardial effusion. In one series three of nine patients with TB pericarditis presented initially with pericardial tamponade (54).

In TB pericarditis aspiration of pericardial effusion is essential to prevent pericardial tamponade and to obtain fluid for culture and stain. However, cultures and stains of pericardial effusion are positive for TB in only 30–75% of patients (54). TB cultures must be followed for at least 6 weeks. TB pericarditis is treated with the same medications as used for pulmonary TB and resolution occurs in 80% of patients (54). Complications of TB pericarditis include caseous and constrictive pericarditis, which are more common in longstanding and untreated TB pericarditis. Furthermore, 30–50% of patients who receive treatment after 2–4 months of the onset of TB pericarditis develop constrictive pericarditis (54). Concurrent administration of steroids with antituberculous medications may decrease the incidence of constrictive pericarditis. Even with effective antituberculous therapy the mortality rate for TB pericarditis is 20–40% (53).

Clinical Presentation

Patients with viral and idiopathic pericarditis usually present with a myriad of symptoms including chest pain, dyspnea, dysphagia, cough, and fever. However, it may be subclinical and asymptomatic. Often, patients with bacterial, TB, or HIV pericarditis have systemic signs and symptoms which overshadow those of the pericarditis. Importantly, pericardial effusion is a common finding in pericarditis. If the pericardial effusion adversely affects the heart's mechanical function, the initial presentation of pericarditis may be hemodynamic instability from pericardial tamponade.

Pericarditis is usually diagnosed through a history of chest pain in conjunction with characteristic physical findings and ECG changes. The chest pain of pericarditis is typically substernal and radiates to the neck, the left trapezius area, scapula, or shoulder. It may be sharp or dull. It varies from mild to severe in intensity, and is usually aggravated by motion, cough, and respiration. The chest pain is most severe when the patient is supine and is relieved when the patient sits up and leans forward. It may be confused with pleurisy, pulmonary embolism, and acute myocardial infarction. The most prominent physical finding in pericarditis is the pericardial friction rub. The typical friction rub consists of three components during the cardiac cycle: ventricular systole (systolic), early diastole (diastolic), and atrial contraction (presystolic). However, the systolic component is most commonly heard (55). The friction rub may be transient or it may wax and wane. Its intensity may vary with change of position. It is best appreciated with the patient sitting down and leaning forward or in the hands-and-knees position. Generally, it is a "scratchy" or "leather-like" sound that is best heard with the diaphragm of the stethoscope along the left lower sternal border or at the apex. It can be distinguished from a cardiac murmur by the way it changes from beat-to-beat and with changes of position.

Physical findings of pericardial effusion include muffled heart sounds and an increased area of cardiac dullness. Ewart sign, found in large pericardial effusions, consists of dullness and bronchial breathing between the tip of the left scapula and the vertebral column. It is due to compression of the left lower lung by the pericardial effusion. If the pericardial effusion accumulates rapidly, it may precipitate pericardial tamponade. An acute increase of fluid within the pericardial sac causes an increase in pressure in the intrapericardial sac. This increased pressure compresses the atria and ventricles, especially the right atrium and ventricle, impeding their ability to fill with blood. Encumbered atrial and ventricular filling causes a reduction in stroke volume and cardiac output with corresponding systemic hypotension. Clinical findings of pericardial tamponade include hypotension, tachycardia, anxiety, distended jugular veins, muffled heart sounds, change in mental status, and pulsus paradoxus. Elevated right atrial venous pressure causes jugular venous distension. Pulsus paradoxus is present when the systolic blood pressure falls by more than 10 mm Hg during inspiration. In severe cases, the blood pressure may disappear completely with inspiration. Pulsus paradoxus is not specific for pericardial tamponade because it also occurs in chronic obstructive pulmonary disease, bronchial asthma, pulmonary embolism, right ventricular infarction, and shock.

Constrictive pericarditis is a common complication of purulent pericarditis. Clinical findings are the result of chronically elevated cardiac filling pressures, depressed cardiac output, and venous congestion. In most cases patients have symptoms of chronic left and right heart failure. Symptoms of left heart congestion include tachypnea, exertional dyspnea, orthopnea, paroxysmal nocturnal dyspnea, and cough. Chronic fatigue and weakness result from low cardiac output and corresponding low blood pressure. Symptoms related to venous congestion of the gastrointestinal tract, which include dyspepsia, anorexia, postprandial fullness, and increased abdominal girth, are common. Visceral congestion adversely affects the gastrointestinal tract's ability to absorb nutrients leading to weight loss and body-wasting. Passive congestion of the liver leads to hepatic dysfunction. The characteristic physical presentation of patients with constrictive pericarditis is a swollen abdomen, edematous lower extremities contrasted by a cachectic and wasted upper torso. Examination of the neck reveals elevated jugular veins with a prominent Y decent. Elevated venous pressure causes peripheral edema, jugular venous distension, and ascites. Other physical findings include decreased pulse pressure, dullness in the base of the lungs due to pleural effusions, hepatomegaly, Kussmaul sign, and occasionally, a pericardial knock. The Kussmaul sign is the loss of the normal inspiratory decrease in the jugular venous pressure with inspiration. In severe constrictive pericarditis, the jugular venous pulse paradoxically increases with inspiration. A pericardial knock is an early diastolic sound heard best on inspiration. It is high-pitched and occurs before the third heart sound. It is due to the abrupt halt of ventricular filling by the rigid pericardium.

Laboratory/Diagnostic Testing

Common laboratory tests used in diagnosing the cause of infectious pericarditis include a complete blood count with differential, erythrocyte sedimentation rate, cardiac enzymes, protein purified derivative, bacterial and fungal blood cultures, viral titers, HIV blood tests, antinuclear antibody, and rheumatoid factor. Echocardiogram, chest x-ray, and ECG are also essential components of the evaluation. In viral pericarditis the white blood count is only slightly elevated, if at all. In purulent pericarditis the white blood count is significantly elevated with a shift to the left and immature polymorphonuclear cells. The erythrocyte sedimentation rate is elevated in both viral and purulent pericarditis. Viral titers are not helpful in the initial stages of pericarditis because they take days to weeks before elevating. Although not routinely obtained aspirated pericardial fluid should be cultured for virus, bacteria, fungi, and mycobacteria. Fungal and mycobacteria cultures may take up to 6 weeks or more before the organism can be identified, if they result in growth of the organism at all.

The chest x-ray in pericarditis may be normal or it may suggest causes of infectious pericarditis, such as pneumonia, empyema, or TB. Substantial pericardial effusion may cause an enlarged cardiac silhouette. Pericardial effusion should be suspected when the cardiac silhouette enlarges in serial chest x-rays, especially if the lung fields remain clear. Pericardial calcification is suggestive of constrictive pericarditis.

Sinus tachycardia is usually present on ECG in pericarditis. Importantly, the ECG in pericarditis undergoes several distinctive phases due to the effects of the pericardial inflammation on the epicardial surface of the heart. There is no propensity for a specific phase to be seen in the emergency department. Therefore, in suspected pericarditis the ECG should be evaluated for all three phases. In phase 1 there is diffuse ST segment elevation with upward concavity in all leads except leads AVR and V1 (Fig. 14–2). ST segment depression may be present in leads AVR and V1. PR segment depression, which is characteristic of pericarditis, occurs in the limb leads, while reciprocal PR segment elevation occurs in lead AVR. In phase 2 the ST segments and PR segments return to normal and T waves flatten. Finally, in phase 3, the ST segments become isoelectric and diffuse T wave inversion develops. If there is an associated pericardial effusion, the ECG may have low voltage complexes, which is the result of the fluid between the heart and the electrode. Electrical alternans, with alternating P wave, QRS complexes, and T waves, is due to the swinging of the heart in pericardial effusion. Atrial fibrillation may occur due to inflammatory irritation of the atria. Ventricular dysrhythmias are uncommon.

ECG changes associated with pericarditis can be differentiated from those of AMI. In pericarditis ST segments are elevated at the J point and are rarely greater

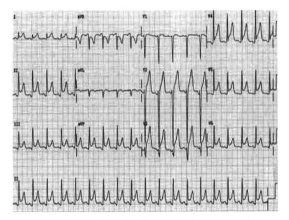

Fig. 14–2. Electrocardiogram: Pericarditis (phase 1).

than 5 mm. Furthermore, the ST segments retain their normal concavity, while they are dome-shaped in AMI. Importantly, ST segment elevations are diffuse in pericarditis, whereas in AMI they are limited to the anatomic area involved. Finally, ST segment elevation and T wave inversion rarely occur simultaneously in pericarditis. PR segment depression is almost exclusively associated with pericarditis, while QT prolongation and sustained ventricular arrhythmias are uncommon.

Echocardiography is utilized to visualize the pericardium and fluid within the pericardial sac. In most cases of pericarditis the pericardium appears normal. Therefore, echocardiography is used mainly to locate pericardial effusion and display its size, extent, and hemodynamic effect. Echocardiography may demonstrate the heart swinging within the pericardial effusion. Right atrial and ventricular collapse during diastole is diagnostic of pericardial tamponade. A dilated inferior vena cava without inspiratory collapse also suggests pericardial tamponade. On occasion pericardial thickening and calcification associated with constrictive pericarditis may be seen.

Computed tomography (CT) may assist in diagnosing pericarditis. Because CT exhibits the pericardium in 2 mm cuts, it can demonstrate inflammation induced pericardial thickening, pericardial effusion, and pericardial calcification associated with constrictive pericarditis. CT imaging for pericarditis is limited by the need for contrast media, exposure to ionizing radiation, and in difficulty differentiating intrapericardial fluid from thickened pericardium. Conversely, magnetic resonance imaging (MRI) provides anatomic detail of the pericardium, including pericardial effusion, without contrast or ionizing radiation. MRI is inferior to CT in demonstrating pericardial calcification.

The evaluation of purulent pericarditis includes a complete blood count, blood cultures, erythrocyte sedimentation rate, chest x-ray, and echocardiogram. The white blood count shows a shift to the left with elevated polymorphonuclear white blood cells and immature bands. The erythrocyte sedimentation rate is elevated. The chest x-ray usually demonstrates cardiomegaly, as well as the causative process, such as pneumonia or empyema. Echocardiogram typically exhibits a pericardial effusion, which may be associated with pericardial tamponade.

Management

Because the most common infectious cause of pericarditis is viral the principal treatment is NSAIDs which usually suppresses clinical manifestations within 24 h. Antibiotics are not indicated. In cases where NSAID are not effective, steroids can be administered for 1 to 2 weeks. If symptoms recur after steroids are tapered, they can be reinstituted and maintained for 1–2 months with a gradual taper. If multiple relapses occur despite steroids, immunosuppressive therapy may reduce the necessity for long-term steroid therapy. Idiopathic pericarditis recurs in 15–32% of cases (56).

All patients with suspected purulent pericarditis should be started immediately on an empiric regimen of intravenous vancomycin, a third-generation cephalosporin, and an aminoglycoside. If TB is the suspected cause, a four drug regime with isoniazid, rifampin, pyrazinamide, and ethambutol should be instituted. Emergent pericardiocentesis in the emergency department may be required to address pericardial tamponade and to acquire fluid for culture and sensitivities. Adequate drainage of the pericardium is essential. If the purulent effusion reaccumulates or is too thick to aspirate, surgical pericardiotomy or pericardial window is necessary. All patients with purulent pericarditis must be admitted to an intensive care unit where antibiotic treatment should be guided by pericardial aspirate cultures and sensitivities.

Special Circumstances—HIV

Pericardial involvement accounts for 60% of all cardiac pathology in HIV infections (57). More than 25% of AIDS patients have pericardial effusions, usually small and asymptomatic (58). Several mechanisms have been proposed as the cause of HIV pericardial disease including a direct effect of HIV on the pericardium; viral, bacterial, fungal or TB seeding of the pericardium during systemic infection; invasion of the pericardium by opportunistic microorganisms; or the consequence of concurrent neoplastic process. Small to moderate pericardial effusions usually resolve spontaneously. Conversely, 9% of AIDS patients with pericarditis and pericardial effusion develop pericardial tamponade requiring pericardiocentesis or surgical drainage. All HIV patients with pericarditis and symptomatic pericardial effusion should be extensively evaluated for mycobacteria infection. However, in many cases systemic anergy and low culture yields make the diagnosis difficult to establish. Pericardial effusion associated with HIV infection predicts a poorer prognosis at 6 months (58).

The treatment of HIV pericarditis is directed toward eliminating or controlling the causative agent. All AIDS patients should be on appropriate antiretroviral therapy. Purulent pericarditis should be aggressively treated with intravenous antibiotics and pericardial drainage. Opportunistic organisms and malignancies, especially Kaposi sarcoma and Non-Hodgkin lymphoma, should be excluded as causes of pericarditis.

Disposition

All patients with pericarditis require urgent cardiology consultation in the emergency department. Hemodynamically stable pericarditis should be admitted to a telemetry bed with continuous monitoring of cardiac rhythm and vital signs. A recent report, however, describes successful outpatient management for patients with pericarditis who do not have any of the following clinical poor prognostic indicators; temperature > 38°C, subacute onset (symptoms developing over 2 weeks), immunodepression, trauma, oral anticoagulant therapy, myopericarditis, severe pericardial effusion (> 2 cm on echocardiography), or cardiac tamponade (59). If the patient has no poor prognostic indicators and is determined to be a candidate for outpatient therapy, the emergency physician should arrange discharge only in consultation with a cardiologist.

Anticoagulants should be avoided or discontinued because they can precipitate intrapericardial hemorrhage with resultant pericardial tamponade. If pericardial tamponade is present, pericardiocentesis is essential in order to remove intrapericardial fluid, reduce intrapericardial pressure, and restore blood pressure. Unstable pericardial tamponade unresponsive to pericardiocentesis requires immediate cardiothoracic surgery consultation for thoracotomy and pericardiotomy.

Case Outcome

In the intensive care unit the patient's vital signs continued to deteriorate with a blood pressure of 74/66, pulse of 134 beats per minute, respirations at 32 per minute,

and oral temperature of 103°. An echocardiogram demonstrated a large pericardial effusion with right atrial and ventricular collapse. Immediate pericardiocentesis was performed with the removal of 65 cc of exudative fluid. Her vital signs improved to a blood pressure of 102/76, pulse of 104 beats per minute, and respirations at 24 per minute. She was continued on intravenous ceftriaxone. In addition, vancomycin and gentamicin were added to her antibiotic regimen. Repeat echocardiogram exhibited decreased pericardial effusion with full distension of the right atrium and ventricle during diastole. Gram stain of the exudative fluid showed gram-positive diplococci in chains. Culture and sensitivities of the pericardial aspirate grew *S. pneumoniae*, which was sensitive to penicillin and third-generation cephalosporins. In response intravenous ceftriaxone was continued and vancomycin and gentamicin were discontinued. Repeat echocardiogram in 24 h revealed a reaccumulation of pericardial fluid, but no collapse of the right atrium. The patient underwent a surgical pericardiotomy for drainage of the pericardial sac. Over the next 4 days her temperature normalized and vital signs improved. She was transferred to telemetry where a subsequent echocardiogram failed to show any residual pericardial effusion. She was discharged home on outpatient antibiotic therapy 8 days after admission.

REFERENCES

1. Kearney MT, Cotton JM, Richardson PI, et al.: Viral myocarditis and dilated cardiomyopathy: Mechanisms, manifestations, and management. *Postgrad Med J* 77(903):4–10, 2001.

2. Mason JW, O'Connell JB, Herskowitz A (The Myocarditis Treatment Trial Investigators): A clinical trial of immunosuppressive therapy for myocarditis. *N Engl J Med* 333(5):269–275, 1995.

3. Pathak SK, Kukreja RC, Hess M: Molecular pathology of dilated Cardiomyopathies. *Curr Probl Cardiol* 21(2):99–144, 1996.

4. Feldman AM, McNamara D: Myocarditis. *N Engl J Med* 343(19):1388–1398, 2000.

5. Pauschinger M, Doerner A, Kuehl U, et al.: Enteroviral RNA replication in the myocardium of patients with left ventricular dysfunction and clinically suspected myocarditis. *Circulation* 99(7):889–895, 1999.

6. Wessely R, Henke A, Zell R, et al.: Low-level expression of a mutant coxsackieviral cDNA induces a myocytopathic effect in culture: An approach to the study of enteroviral persistence in cardiac myocytes. *Circulation* 98:450–457, 1998.

7. Opavsky MA, Penninger J, Aitken K, et al.: Susceptibility to myocarditis is dependent on the response of alphabeta T lymphocytes to coxsackie viral infection. *Circ Res* 85(6):551–558, 1999.

8. Batra AS, Lewis AB: Acute myocarditis. *Curr Opin Pediatr* 13(3):234–239, 2001.
9. Sole MJ, Liu P: Viral myocarditis: A paradigm for understanding the pathogenesis and treatment of dilated cardiomyopathy. *J Am Coll Cardiol* 22(4 Suppl. A):99A–105A, 1993.
10. Lauer B, Schannwell M, Kuhl U, et al.: Antimyosin autoantibodies are associated with deterioration of systolic and diastolic left ventricular function in patients with chronic myocarditis. *J Am Coll Cardiol* 35(1):11–18, 2000.
11. Fujioka S, Kitaura Y, Ukimura A, et al.: Evaluation of viral infection in the myocardium of patients with idiopathic dilated cardiomyopathy. *J Am Coll Cardiol* 36(6):1920–1926, 2000.
12. Badorff C, Lee GH, Lamphear BJ, et al.: Enteroviral protease 2A cleaves dystrophin: Evidence of cytoskeletal disruption in an acquired cardiomyopathy. *Nat Med* 5(3):320–326, 1999.
13. Wessely R, Klingel K, Santana LF, et al.: Transgenic expression of replication-restricted enteroviral genomes in heart muscle induces defective excitation-contraction coupling and dilated cardiomyopathy. *J Clin Invest* 102(7):1444–1453, 1998.
14. Baig MK, Goldman JH, Caforio AL, et al.: Familial dilated cardiomyopathy: Cardiac abnormalities are common in asymptomatic relatives and may represent early disease. *J Am Coll Cardiol* 31(1):195–201, 1998.
15. Baboonian C, Davies MJ, Booth JC, et al.: Coxsackie B viruses and human heart disease. *Curr Top Microbiol Immunol* 223:31–52, 1997.
16. Modlin JF: Enteroviruses: Coxsackieviruses, echoviruses, and newer enteroviruses, in Long SS (ed.): *Principles and Practice of Pediatric Infectious Disease, 2ded*. New York, Churchill Livingstone; 2000.
17. Cunningham C, Lee CH: Myocarditis related to *Campylobacter jejuni* infection: A case report. *BMC Infect Dis* 3(1):16, 2003.
18. Hagar JM, Rahimtoola SH: Chagas' heart disease. *Curr Probl Cardiol* 20(12):825–924, 1995.
19. Michaels AD, Lederman RJ, MacGregor JS, et al.: Cardiovascular involvement in AIDS. *Curr Probl Cardiol* 22(3):109–148, 1997.
20. Hofman P, Drici MD, Gibelin P, et al.: Prevalence of toxoplasma myocarditis in patients with the acquired immunodeficiency syndrome. *Br Heart J* 70(4):376–381, 1993.
21. Compton SJ, Celum CL, Lee C, et al.: Trichinosis with ventilatory failure and persistent myocarditis. *Clin Infect Dis* 16(4):500–504, 1993.
22. DeCastro S, Migliau G, Silvestri A, et al.: Heart involvement in AIDS: A prospective study during various stages of the disease. *Eur Heart J* 13(11):1452–1459, 1992.
23. Barbaro G, Fisher SD, Lipshultz SE: Pathogenesis of HIV-associated cardiovascular complications. *Lancet Infect Dis* 1(2):115–124, 2001.
24. Barbaro G, DiLorenzo G, Grisorio B: Incidence of dilated cardiomyopathy and detection of HIV in myocardial cells of HIV-positive patients. *N Engl J Med* 339(16):1093–1099, 1998.
25. Dec GW Jr., Waldman S, Southern J, et al.: Viral myocarditis mimicking acute myocardial infarction. *J Am Coll Cardiol* 20(1):85–89, 1992.
26. Lieberman EB, Hutchins GM, Herskowitz A, et al.: Clinicopathologic description of myocarditis. *J Am Coll Cardiol* 18(7):1617–1626, 1991.
27. McCarthy RE 3rd, Boehmer JP, Hruban RH, et al.: Long-term outcome of fulminant myocarditis as compared with acute (nonfulminant) myocarditis. *N Engl J Med* 342(10):690–695, 2000.
28. Rockman HA, Adamson RM, Dembitsky WP, et al.: Acute fulminant myocarditis: Long-term follow-up after circulatory support with left ventricular assist device. *Am Heart J* 121(3 Pt 1):922–926, 1991.
29. Brown CA, O'Connell JB: Myocarditis and idiopathic dilated cardiomyopathy. *Am J Med* 99(3):309–314, 1995.
30. Dec GW Jr., Palacios IF, Fallon JT, et al.: Active myocarditis in the spectrum of acute dilated cardiomyopathies. Clinical features, histologic correlates, and clinical outcome. *N Engl J Med* 312(14):885–890, 1985.
31. Smith SC, Ladenson JH, Mason JW, et al.: Elevations of cardiac troponin I associated with myocarditis. Experimental and clinical correlates. *Circulation* 95(1):163–168, 1997.
32. Drory Y, Turetz Y, Hiss Y: Sudden unexpected death in persons less than 40 years of age. *Am J Cardiol.* 68(13):1388–1392, 1991.
33. Aretz HT: Myocarditis: The Dallas criteria. *Hum Pathol* 1987;18(6):619–624.
34. Lewis AB: Late recovery of ventricular function in children with idiopathic dilated cardiomyopathy. *Am Heart J* 138 (2 Pt 1):334–338, 1999.
35. Narula J, Khaw BA, Dec GW Jr., et al.: Brief report: Recognition of acute myocarditis masquerading as acute myocardial infarction. *N Engl J Med* 328(2):100–104, 1993.
36. Ilback NG, Fohlman J, Friman G: Exercise in coxsackie B3 myocarditis: Effects on heart lymphocyte subpopulations and the inflammatory reaction. *Am Heart J* 117(6):1298–1302, 1989.
37. Brennan FH Jr., Stenzler B, Oriscello R: Diagnosis and management of myocarditis in athletes. *Curr Sports Med Rep* 2(2):65–71, 2003.
38. Matsumori A, Tomioka N, Kawai C: Protective effect of recombinant alpha interferon on coxsackievirus B3 myocarditis in mice. *Am Heart J* 115(6):1229–1232, 1988.
39. Kishimoto C, Crumpacker CS, Abelmann WH: Ribavirin treatment of murine coxsackievirus B3 myocarditis with analyses of lymphocyte subsets. *J Am Coll Cardiol* 12(5):1334–1341, 1988.
40. Kuhl U, Pauschinger M, Schwimmbeck PL, et al.: Interferon-beta treatment eliminates cardiotropic viruses and improves left ventricular function in patients with myocardial persistence of viral genomes and left ventricular dysfunction. *Circulation* 107(22):2793–2798, 2003.
41. Heart Failure Society of America: HFSA guidelines for management of patients with heart failure caused by left

ventricular systolic dysfunction–pharmacological approaches. *Pharmacotherapy* 20(5):495–522, 2000.

42. Goyle KK, Walling AD: Diagnosing pericarditis. *Am Fam Physician*. 66(9):1695–1702, 2002.

43. Soler-Soler J, Permanyer-Miralda G, Sagrista-Sauleda J: A systematic diagnostic approach to primary acute pericardial disease. The Barcelona experience. *Cardiol Clin* 8(4):609–620, 1990.

44. Ho JS, Flamm SD, Cook PJ: Purulent and constrictive pericarditis arising from a staphylococcal lumbar infection. *Tex Heart Inst J* 28(3):212–214, 2001.

45. Maisch B, Seferovic PM, Ristic AD, et al.: Guidelines on the diagnosis and management of pericardial diseases. *Euro Heart J* 25:587–610, 2004.

46. Rubin RH, Mollering RC: Clinical, microbiologic, and therapeutic aspects of purulent pericarditis. *Am J Med* 59(10):68–78, 1975.

47. Goodman LJ: Purulent pericarditis. *Curr Treat Options Cardiovasc Med* 2(4):343–350, 2000.

48. Snyder RW, Braun TI: Purulent pericarditis with tamponade in a postpartum patient due to Group F streptococcus. *Chest* 115:1746–1747, 1999.

49. Sagrista-Sauleda J, Barrebas JA, Permanyer-Miralda G, et al.: Purulent pericarditis: Review of a 20-year experience in a general hospital. *J Am Coll Cardiol* 22(6):1661–1665, 1993.

50. Arsura EL, Kilgore WB, Strategos E: Purulent pericarditis misdiagnosed as septic shock. *South Med J* 92(3):285–288, 1999.

51. Kim NH, Park JP, Jeon SH, et al.: Purulent pericarditis caused by group G streptococcus as an initial presentation of colon cancer. *J Korean Med Sci* 17(4):571–573, 2002.

52. Donnelly LF, Kimball TR, Barr LL: Purulent pericarditis presenting as acute abdomen in children: Abdominal imaging findings. *Clin Radiol* 54(10):691–693, 1999.

53. Gultekin F, Bakici MZ, Elaldi N, et al.: Tuberculous pericarditis: A report of three cases. *Curr Med Res Opin* 17(2):142–145, 2001.

54. Permanyer-Miralda G, Sagrista-Sauleda J, Soler-Soler J: Primary acute pericardial disease: A prospective series of 231 consecutive patients. *Am J Cardiol* 56(10):623–630, 1985.

55. Spodick DH: Pericardial rub. Prospective, multiple observer investigation of pericardial friction in 100 patients. *Am J Cardiol* 35(3):357–362, 1975.

56. Fowler NO: Recurrent pericarditis. *Cardiol Clin* 8(4):621–626, 1990.

57. Yunis NA, Stone VE: Cardiac manifestations of HIV/AIDS: A review of disease spectrum and clinical management. *J Acquir Immune Defic Syndr Hum Retrovirol* 18(2):145–154, 1998.

58. Kaul S, Fishbein MC, Seigel RJ: Cardiac manifestations of acquired immune deficiency syndrome: A 1991 update. *Am Heart J* 122(2):535–544, 1991.

59. Imazio M, Demichelis B, Parrini I, et al. Day-hospital treatment of acute pericarditis: A management program for out-patient therapy. *J Am Coll Cardiol* 2004, 43(6):1042–1046.

COLOR PLATES

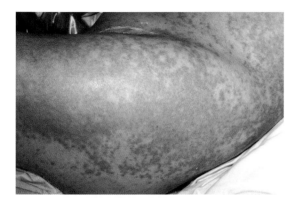

PLATE 1 Myocarditis—microscopic.

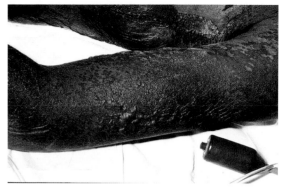

PLATE 4 In this patient with TEN, dusky-colored lesions cover over 50% of the body surface area. The lesions are progressing to bullae, and some have already begun to slough, exposing the dermis underneath.

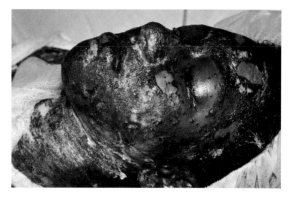

PLATE 5 Extensive epidermal necrosis, as well as oral and conjunctival involvement, is seen in this TEN patient.

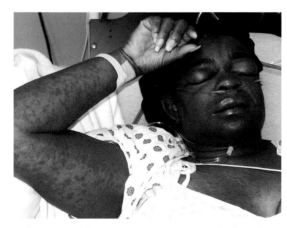

PLATE 2 An exanthematous drug eruption (also known as a morbilliform or measles-like eruption).

PLATE 3 DRESS syndrome due to trimethoprim/sulfamethoxazole. An exanthematous eruption involves the upper extremities and trunk. Edema of the face, most noticeable in the eyelids and lips, is a hallmark of this disease.

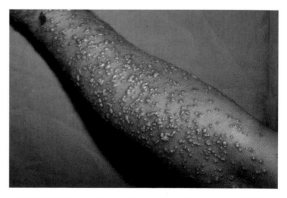

PLATE 6 A pustular eruption such as that seen in AGEP.

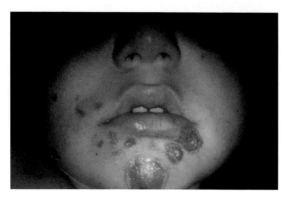

PLATE 7 Streptococcal impetigo. Honey-colored crusts of the face.

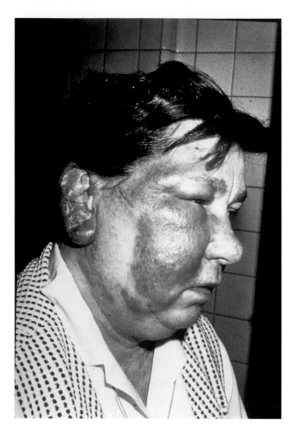

PLATE 9 Erysipelas due to group A streptococcus on a female's face.

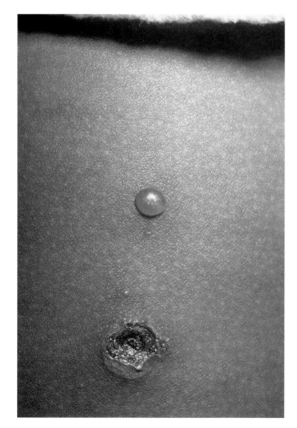

PLATE 8 Bullous impetigo, with an early vesicle and later lesion showing a crust formation.

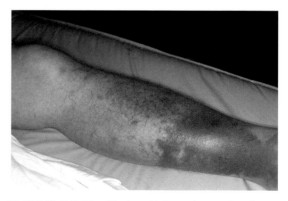

PLATE 10 Cellulitis of the leg with hemorrhage and erythematous border.

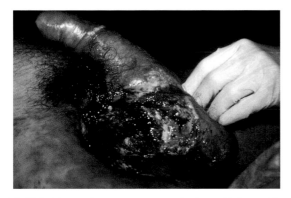

PLATE 11 Fournier gangrene. A mixed aerobic/anaerobic infection.

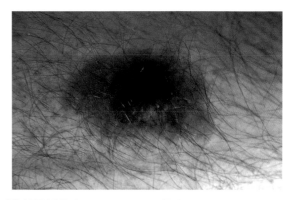

PLATE 14 Ecthyma gangrenosum. Ecthyma gangrenosum due to bacteremia from *P. aeruginosa*. Central necrotic eschar with surrounding erythema.

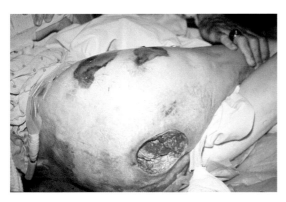

PLATE 12 A mixed aerobic and anaerobic infection involving the fascia.

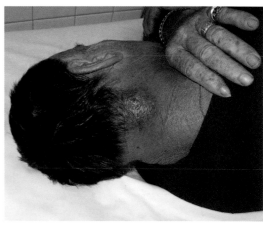

PLATE 15 Carbuncle.

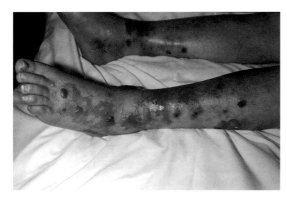

PLATE 13 *V. vulnificus*. Hemorrhagic and bullous skin lesions of the feet and lower legs, also showing hemorrhagic necrosis of the dorsum of the left foot.

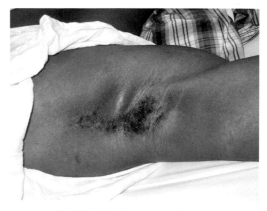

PLATE 16 Subcutaneous abscess.

4

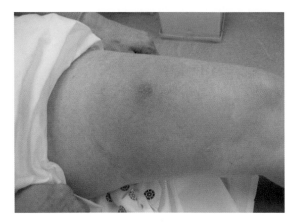

PLATE 17 Subcutaneous abscess with surrounding cellulitis.

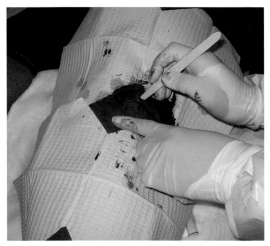

PLATE 18 Incision and drainage.

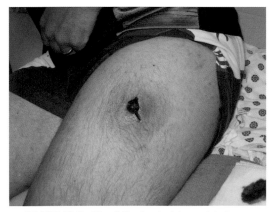

PLATE 19 Packing following incision and drainage.

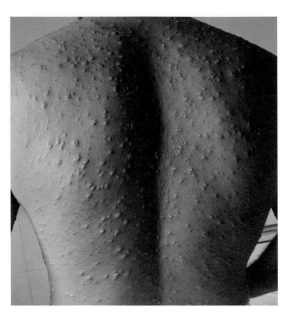

PLATE 20 Varicella (Sugathan Paramoo, MD, Dermatlas; http://www.dermatlas.org).

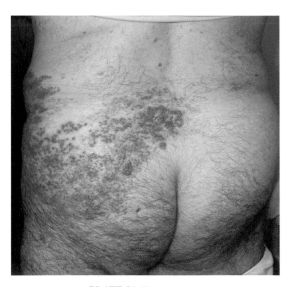

PLATE 21 Herpes zoster.

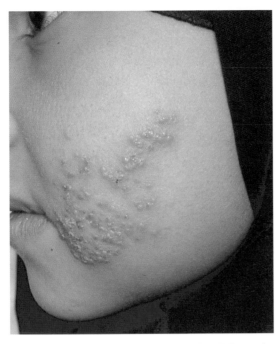

PLATE 22 Herpes simplex virus (Yahia Albaili, MD, Dermatlas; http://www.dermatlas.org).

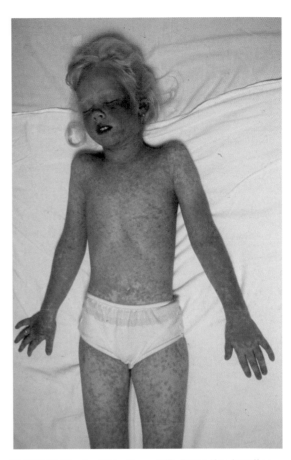

PLATE 24 Measles (Peter Rowe, MD, Dermatlas; http://www. dermatlas.org).

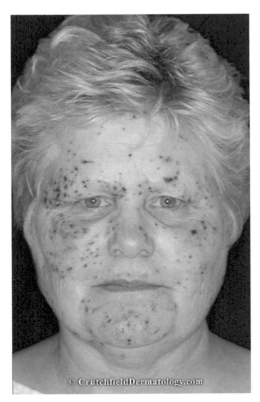

PLATE 23 Eczema herpeticum (contributor Charles Crutchfield, MD).

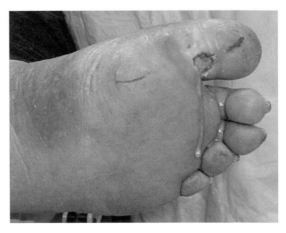

PLATE 25 Example of diabetic foot ulcer.

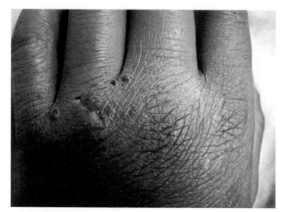

PLATE 26 Image reproduced with permission from EMed-Home.com: www.EMedHome.com.

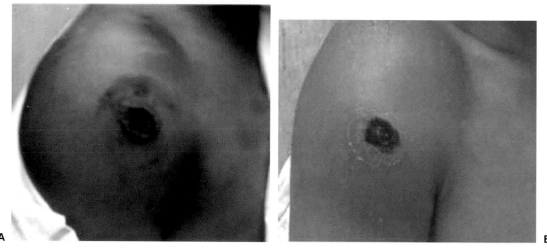

A   B

PLATE 27 (A) Ulcer and vesicle ring and (B) black eschar. *Source:* Courtesy of the Centers for Disease Control (Public Domain).

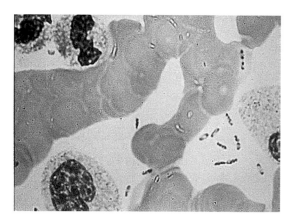

PLATE 28 Wayson stain of *Yersinia pestis*. Note the characteristic "safety pin" appearance of the bacteria. *Source:* Courtesy of Centers for Disease Control and Prevention (Public Domain).

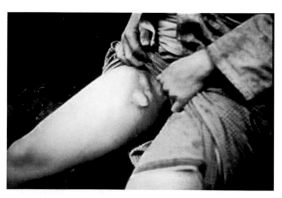

PLATE 29 Inguinal buboes in patient with bubonic plague. *Source:* Courtesy of Centers for Disease Control and Prevention (Public Domain).

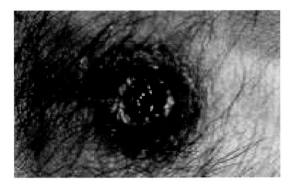

PLATE 30 Cutaneous ulcer of tularemia. *Source:* Courtesy of William Beisel, M.D., Colonel, Medical Corps, U.S. Army (Ret).

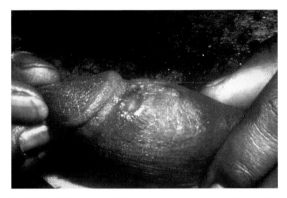

PLATE 31 Primary syphilis chancre or ulcer (from Martin DH, Mroczkowski TF: Dermatologic manifestations of STDs other than HIV. *Infect Dis Clin North Am* 8:535, 1994, permission pending).

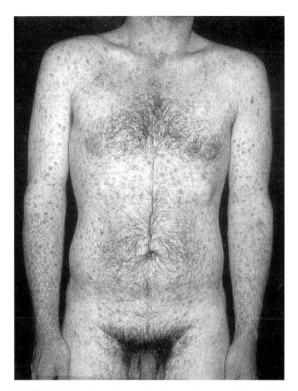

PLATE 32 Maculopapular rash of secondary syphilis (CDC STD slide file).

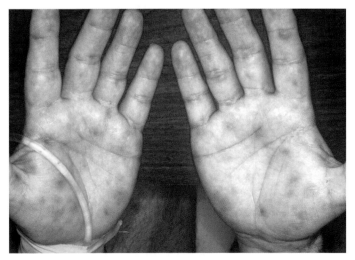

PLATE 33. Secondary syphilis—rash of the palms (from Martin DH, Mroczkowski TF: Dermatologic manifestations of STDs other than HIV. *Infect Dis Clin North Am* 8:538, 1994, permission pending).

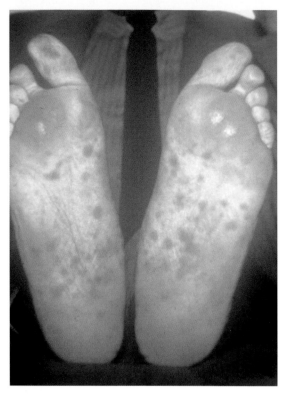

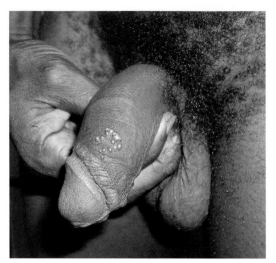

PLATE 36 Genital herpes (provided courtesy of Stephanie N. Taylor, MD).

PLATE 34 Secondary syphilis—rash of soles (CDC STD slide file).

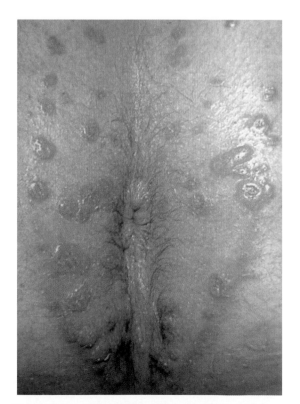

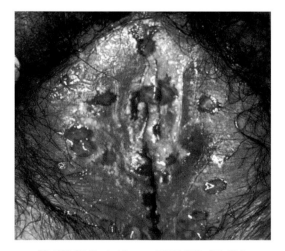

PLATE 37 Genital herpes (CDC STD slide file).

PLATE 35 Secondary syphilis—condyloma LATA (CDC STD

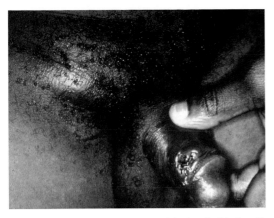

PLATE 38 Chancroid—ulcer with right inguinal buboe (from Martin DH, Mroczkowski TF: Dermatologic manifestations of STDs other than HIV. *Infect Dis Clin North Am* 8: 550, 1994, permission pending).

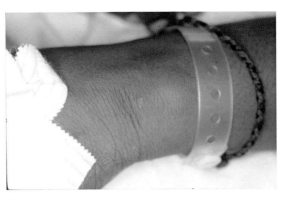

PLATE 41 Disseminated gonococcal infection (provided courtesy of Stephanie N. Taylor, MD).

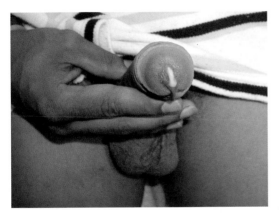

PLATE 39 Gonococcal urethritis (provided courtesy of Stephanie N. Taylor, MD).

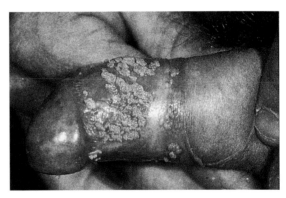

PLATE 42 Genital warts (CDC STD slide file).

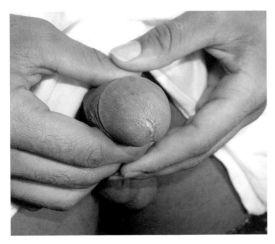

PLATE 40 Nongonoccocal urethritis (provided courtesy of Stephanie N. Taylor, MD).

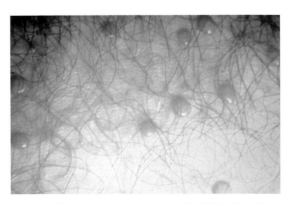

PLATE 43 Molluscum contagiosum (CDC STD slide file).

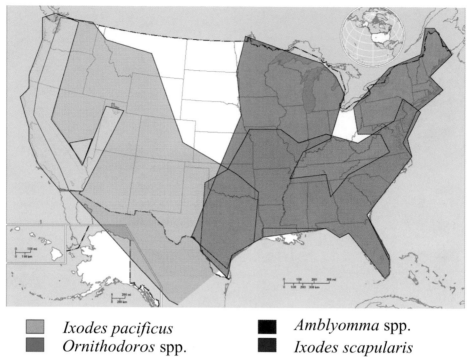

▨	*Ixodes pacificus*	■	*Amblyomma* spp.
▨	*Ornithodoros* spp.	▨	*Ixodes scapularis*

PLATE 44 **(A)** Geographic distributions for the major genera of ticks that are responsible for human disease.

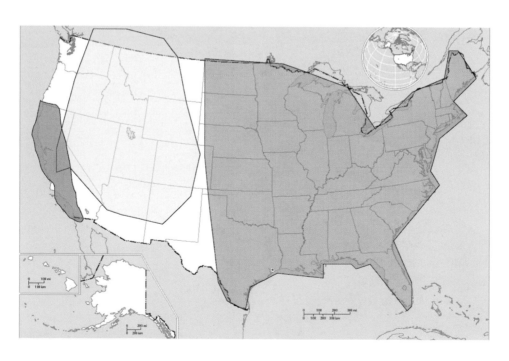

☐ *Dermacentor andersoni* ■ *Dermacentor variabilis*

PLATE 44 **(B)** (*Continued*)

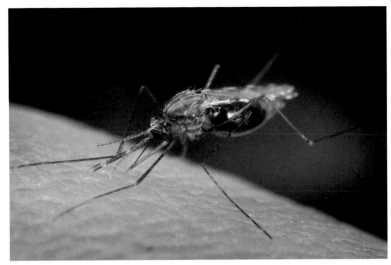

PLATE 45 Night-biting Anopheles mosquito responsible for malaria transmission (see "mosquito" TIFF).

Malaria
(Plasmodium spp.)

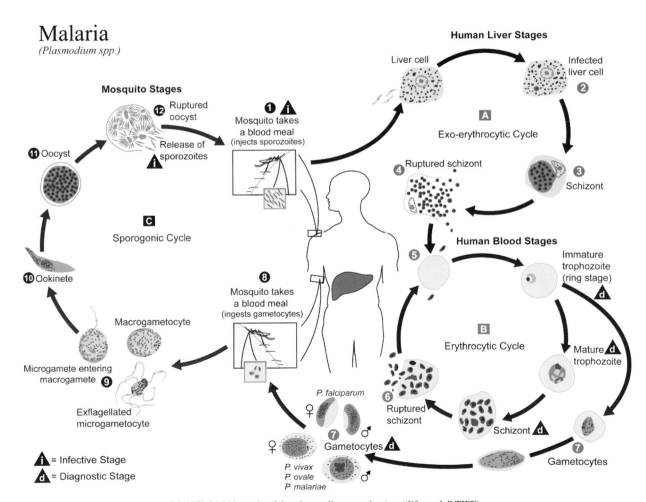

PLATE 46 Life cycle of the plasmodium species (see "life cycle" TIFF).

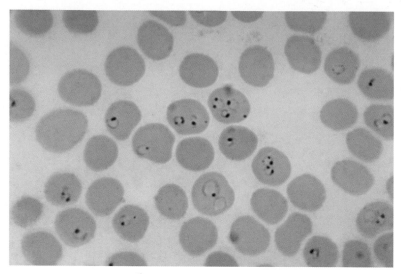

PLATE 47 Large intraerythrocytic parasite load seen in a patient infected with falciparum malaria (see multiple ring forms TIFF).

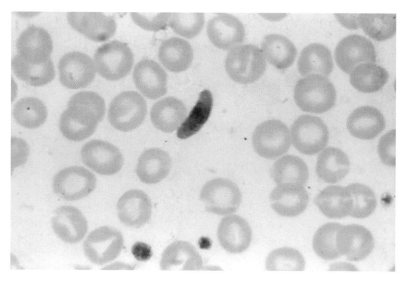

PLATE 48 Microgametocyte seen on thin smear, indicative of falciparum malaria infection (see "microgametocyte" TIFF).

15

Hepatitis

Jan M. Shoenberger

HIGH YIELD FACTS

1. Viral hepatitis is a widely prevalent disease caused by a variety of etiologic agents.

2. The clinical presentation of viral hepatitis infections covers a wide spectrum and patients may even be asymptomatic.

3. The emergency physician has a public health responsibility to begin the process of identifying potentially infectious patients, report confirmed viral hepatitis, and to help prevent transmission through education and vaccination.

4. Postexposure prophylaxis should be initiated in the emergency department when warranted.

CASE PRESENTATION

A 48-year-old man presents with mild right upper quadrant pain. He states that he has had "yellow eyes" for 3 days. He has experienced nausea for 1 week as well as several episodes of vomiting and subjective fevers. On further questioning, he admits to light colored stools and dark urine. He has no significant past medical or surgical history and is not taking any medications. He does admit to unprotected sex recently with an intravenous drug user but denies any illicit drug use himself. No household contacts have similar symptoms.

He is ambulatory and appears uncomfortable. His blood pressure in 137/90, his pulse 85, his respiratory rate is 20 and his temperature is 99.0°F. On physical examination, he is noted to have scleral icterus and mild right upper quadrant tenderness on palpation without guarding or rebound. Rectal examination reveals light colored stool that is guaiac negative.

Initial laboratory studies revealed a normal complete blood cell count and a normal chemistry panel. His total bilirubin level was 9.0. Serum aspartate aminotransferase (AST) and alanine aminotransferase (ALT) were 1519 and 1757, respectively.

INTRODUCTION/EPIDEMIOLOGY

Most cases of acute hepatitis of an infectious etiology are caused by one of the hepatitis viruses. This group includes hepatitis A virus (HAV), hepatitis B virus (HBV), hepatitis C virus (HCV), hepatitis D virus (HDV), or hepatitis E virus (HEV) (1). Hepatitis G virus has recently been described (2) but evidence suggests that it is not pathogenic and is not responsible for cases of non-A-E hepatitis.

Hepatitis A virus is transmitted through the fecal-oral route either by ingestion of contaminated food or water or by direct contact with an infected individual (3). It is highly prevalent in densely populated areas with poor sanitation. In 2001, approximately 10,000 new cases were reported to the Centers for Disease Control (CDC) (4); however, this number is an underestimate and the CDC estimates that there were at least 45,000 acute clinical cases. It is believed that 31.3% of the population has been infected at one time or another.

Hepatitis A often causes large outbreaks due to the viral shedding from an asymptomatic host. In late 2003, there was a widely publicized outbreak in Pennsylvania that was linked to green onions that had been served at a Mexican restaurant. The onions were grown in Mexico and handled by a carrier without appropriate hygiene. Approximately 555 infected persons were identified and 3 deaths occurred (5).

Hepatitis B virus is transmitted by percutaneous and more rarely by body fluid exposures. Infection results in acute and chronic disease states. Ninety percent of children infected at birth will go on to be chronically infected but only 5–10% of adults will progress to chronic infection. Fulminant hepatic failure will occur in 0.5–1% of patients with a case fatality rate of almost 80%. Almost 8000 new cases were reported to the CDC in 2001 and 78,000 new infections were estimated to have occurred in that year. It is estimated that approximately 1.25 million people in the United States were chronically infected as of 2001 (4). The incidence of new infections has been on the decline since the widespread use of the recombinant hepatitis B vaccine was instituted. The vaccine was introduced in 1982. It is estimated that 16,000 HBV infections among children in the United States have been prevented each year since routine childhood immunization was implemented (6).

Hepatitis C virus is responsible for more than 80% of non-A, non-B hepatitis. It is transmitted percutaneously and sexually. Before testing was available, it caused many cases of post-transfusion hepatitis. In 2001, the CDC estimated there to be 30,000 new cases and 2.7 million chronically infected patients in the United States (4). At least 85% of patients will progress to chronic infection, and HCV-associated zliver disease is the most common indication for liver transplantation among adults. Two studies examining prevalence among patients in the emergency departments in urban teaching hospitals showed a 17–18% positivity rate for HCV antibodies in random samplings (7, 8).

Infection with hepatitis D virus only occurs in the setting of HBV infection. It is transmitted percutaneously. Approximately 4% of acute HBV cases are thought to involve co-infection with HDV. HDV is most prevalent in Mediterranean countries, the Middle East, and northern Africa. Persons vaccinated against HBV are additionally protected from HDV.

Hepatitis E virus is similar to HAV in that it is transmitted through the fecal-oral route. It has been the cause of several epidemics in underdeveloped countries such as rural Mexico. It is thought to be uncommon in the United States and most cases have occurred in travelers returning from endemic areas (9).

PATHOPHYSIOLOGY/MICROBIOLOGY

Hepatitis A virus is a picornavirus and the only natural hosts are primates. There is only one serotype and infection is thought to result in lifelong immunity. The incubation period is approximately 28 days (time of exposure to symptom onset). The viral shedding occurs during the 14 days that precede the onset of jaundice and infectivity declines during the week after symptom onset. Therefore, patients will pass the virus without knowing they are infected. No chronic infection state exists.

Hepatitis B is a hepadnavirus and is the only member of that family that infects humans. It is a DNA virus and there are seven genotypes. The hepatitis B virus contains a core protein (HBcAg) as well as a surface coat protein (HBsAg). The hepatitis B e antigen (HBeAg) is a protein that is produced by the virus in the secretory process but the function of the protein is not well understood. Interestingly, the HBV replication cycle is not directly harmful to the cells it infects. This correlates with the fact that many HBV carriers are asymptomatic and do not have extensive liver injury despite ongoing viral replication at high levels. Immunological research has shown that it is the patient's immune response itself that causes much of the liver injury (10).

Hepatitis C is a flavivirus and is composed of single stranded RNA. It contains structural proteins, a core protein, envelope proteins, and nonstructural proteins. There are several different genotypes but genotype 1 is the most common type in the United States.

CLINICAL PRESENTATION

Hepatitis A infection causes a spectrum of clinical diseases from asymptomatic infection to fulminant hepatitis. Asymptomatic or anicteric infection is common in children. Less than 10% of children under the age of 6 years with HAV infection will be jaundiced (3). Among young adults with HAV, 76–97% will have symptoms and 40–70% will experience jaundice (11).

Typically, symptomatic HAV infection begins with nonspecific symptoms such as low-grade fever, nausea, vomiting, diarrhea, myalgias, anorexia, and malaise. Symptoms such as jaundice, light-colored stools, dark urine, right upper quadrant pain, or general abdominal discomfort might follow in a few days or be present at onset. Physical examination may reveal abdominal tenderness or hepatomegaly. Splenomegaly is present in approximately 10% of patients. Unusual physical findings include peripheral edema, asterixis, or ascites and these would suggest that the disease course is quite severe and the prognosis is poor. For the majority of cases with mild symptoms, the duration is in the range of several weeks.

Hepatitis B and C infections can also clinically present with the same constitutional symptoms. Additionally, it should be noted that a wide variety of extrahepatic symptoms are known to be associated with these two infections. Polyarthralgia and polyarthritis may be seen during the prodromal period of HBV infection. The symptoms mostly involve the small joints of the hands and frequently precede the onset of jaundice (12). At least 36 extrahepatic disease manifestations have been reported to be associated with HCV infection (13). Thirty-eight percent of patients with HCV will experience symptoms of at least one extrahepatic manifestation during their illness. The most common manifestations are renal disease (glomerulonephritis), neuropathy, lymphoma, and Sjogren-syndromelike symptoms with or without mixed cryoglobulinemia. Porphyria cutanea tarda has also been linked to HCV (14). Most of these diseases are immunological and chronic HCV infection seems to be necessary for their development.

Associations between HCV infection and various ocular syndromes have been described and this may be the presenting complaint in the emergency department. Patients may present with a dry eye syndrome similar to the Sjogren syndrome or an ischemic retinopathy caused by

Table 15–1. Differential Diagnosis of Acute and Chronic Hepatitis

Viral causes
    Hepatitis A, B, C, D or E
    Epstein-Barr virus
    Cytomegalovirus
    Herpes simplex virus
    Varicella-Zoster virus
Other causes
    Drug-induced—idiosyncratic reaction or overdose
    Liver abscess
    Autoimmune hepatitis
    Alcoholic hepatitis
    Toxic hepatitis (carbon tetrachloride, benzene, mushroom poisoning)
    Parasitic infections (toxoplasmosis)
    Secondary syphilis
    Wilson disease

either an HCV-induced vasculitis or treatment with interferon (15).

A feature of the natural history of HBV infection is the association with hepatocellular carcinoma. It has been demonstrated that patients who are chronically infected with HBV have a risk of developing hepatocellular carcinoma that is 100 times higher than the risk for noncarriers (16). The role of HBV is incompletely understood in the exact pathogenesis of hepatocellular carcinoma. HCV infection similarly results in an increased risk for development of primary hepatocellular carcinoma and cirrhosis.

Clinical manifestations of chronic hepatitis vary widely. Patients may demonstrate mildly elevated aminotransferase levels without any clinical symptomatology. Alternatively, they may experience a rapidly progressive illness with fulminant hepatic failure. Most commonly, patients experience fatigue and mild abdominal pain. Stigmata of cirrhosis may be seen in those patients who have progressed to end-stage liver disease.

The differential diagnosis of acute hepatitis includes a wide variety of causes other than viral causes (see Table 15–1).

LABORATORY/DIAGNOSTIC TESTING

Identification of the causative agent in infectious hepatitis is important for public health reasons. It is true, however, that we often cannot determine the exact cause of the hepatitis in one emergency department visit. The practicing emergency physician must possess a solid understanding of the appropriate serologic tests that should be ordered.

The IgM antibody to HAV (IgM anti-HAV) is detectable 5–10 days before the onset of symptoms and is usually undetectable within 6 months. This antibody is the classic marker of acute hepatitis A infection. The sensitivity and specificity of commercially available IgM anti-HAV tests is over 95%. IgG anti-HAV, which reflects immune status of the host, will begin to rise at approximately 4 weeks after exposure and reach peak levels at 12 weeks after exposure.

There are quite a few serologic markers of hepatitis B infection. HBsAg is a surface protein and appears in the serum of infected patients as early as 1–2 weeks after exposure. This is the protein that is used in recombinant vaccines. The antibody to HBsAg (anti-HBs) usually appears 2–4 months after an attack of acute HBV infection that resolves. That means that usually HBsAg is no longer detectable at that point. This antibody is also the marker of successful vaccination. Hepatitis B immune globulin is derived from serum with high anti-HBs titers.

Antibody to hepatitis B core antigen (anti-HBc) appears right away after infection and persists indefinitely. It can be used as evidence that the patient has been infected in the past or is currently infected with HBV. High titers of IgM anti-HBc are found in patients with acute disease and may be the only marker of acute infection if HBsAg is no longer detectable. HBeAg is a soluble protein derived from the core particle and its presence correlates with a high replication rate. Serum that is positive for HBeAg is highly infectious. Anti-HBe will appear weeks to months after HBeAg is no longer detectable.

Diagnosing HCV infection requires detection of HCV viral load, positive antibody testing, and possibly elevated alkaline phosphatase at 6 months postexposure. The test is an enzyme-linked immunosorbent assay (ELISA) and uses several viral antigens. Also available is a recombinant immunoblot assay (RIBA). HCV RNA assays including quantitative and qualitative versions are used in the management of chronically infected patients.

Liver enzyme measurements along with bilirubin will be helpful. Typically, serum AST and ALT will rise to greater than 300 IU/L and, occasionally, 1,000–3,000 IU/L. Generally, ALT will be higher than AST. Bilirubin levels can range from moderate to markedly elevated. Both total and direct bilirubin will rise. Alkaline phosphatase levels should be normal to mildly elevated. Prothrombin time (PT) is useful in assessing the synthetic capacity of the liver. Elevated PT is a poor prognostic sign. It is the serologic testing, however, that will aid in identifying the specific etiologic agent.

Table 15–2. Serologic Tests in Hepatitis Infections

Antibody/ Antigen	Significance
IgM anti-HAV	IgM antibody to hepatitis A virus. Indicates acute HAV infection
IgG anti-HAV	IgG antibody to hepatitis A virus. Past exposure to HAV. Lasts for patient's lifetime. Indicates immunity
HBsAg	Hepatitis B surface antigen. Probably appears as early as 1–2 weeks after infection. Associated with acute or chronic infection. Can be negative late in course of acute disease
Anti-HBs	Antibody to surface antigen. Indicates acute or past infection. Marker of immunization
Anti-HBc	Antibody to core protein. Present in acute or chronic infection. Will also be positive in patients who have been exposed to the virus in the past but have "cleared" the infection
IgM anti-HBc	IgM antibody to core protein. Marker of acute infection. May be the only marker of acute infection if HBsAg is negative
HBeAg	Hepatitis e antigen. Positive serum is highly infectious and represents high levels of circulating virus. Can be positive in acute or chronic infection
Anti-HBeAg	Antibody to e antigen. Appears weeks to months after HBeAg is no longer detectable
Anti-HDV	Antibody to hepatitis D virus. Positive test reflects superinfection with HDV. HBsAg will usually be present as well
Anti-HCV	Antibody to hepatitis C virus. Acute, past, or chronic infection

Imaging will generally not be helpful in the diagnosis of viral hepatitis. Ultrasound imaging of the abdomen in cases of chronic hepatitis will generally reveal variable degrees of hepatomegaly with or without splenomegaly. The contour of the liver may appear irregular and evidence of portal hypertension or cirrhosis may be present.

Differentiating between the different viral etiologies is virtually impossible based on symptomatology alone. How then is the emergency physician to differentiate between them when the serologic antibody tests will not be available for 24 h? Historical elements will be helpful in this differentiation. Hepatitis A should be suspected when a patient presents with symptoms of hepatitis but has no risk factors for percutaneous or body-fluid transmission. IgM anti-HAV should be positive, confirming acute HAV infection. Certainly, the remainder of the hepatitis panel should be sent as well (HBsAg, anti-HBs, anti-HBc, and anti-HCV) (see Table 15–2).

MANAGEMENT

Patients experiencing the acute symptoms of hepatitis should receive symptomatic treatment. The most common complications from an acute infection are dehydration and/or electrolyte imbalance from vomiting. This can be corrected with fluid administration and antiemetics may be employed. No therapies have proven useful in shortening the disease process.

Treatments do exist for chronic HBV and HCV. This is an active area of clinical research. Traditionally, interferon alfa-2b has been used in the treatment of chronic hepatitis B. About 30% of patients who were able to tolerate the therapy had a successful response (17). Patients undergoing this treatment may present to the ED with symptoms due to side effects of the treatment. Interferon causes influenza-like symptoms (fever, malaise, myalgias, headache, and arthralgia). Fatigue can be quite pronounced. It can also cause granulocytopenia, leukopenia, and thrombocytopenia.

Recently, lamivudine was introduced as a therapy for HBV infection. It is a nucleoside analogue that inhibits viral DNA synthesis and was approved in 1998 for use in chronic HBV infection. This drug was initially used for HIV suppression alone but was found to be useful when used in the setting of co-infection with HIV and HBV. The patients had major declines in HBV viremia. It is administered orally at a dose of 100 mg/day and is well tolerated.

Chronic hepatitis C is also treated with interferon. In 1998, the combination of interferon alfa-2b and ribavirin became standard therapy based on two landmark studies.

The two in combination resulted in a significant decrease in viral burden. Approximately 40% of patients treated for 1 year with combination therapy had sustained decreases in viral load 6 months after completion of treatment (18).

Emergency department management must include consideration of public health issues when faced with a patient with acute viral hepatitis. Viral hepatitis is reportable and the appropriate forms must be submitted. Immunoprophylaxis should be offered for the patient's household and personal contacts in the case of acute hepatitis A. Postexposure prophylaxis with immunoglobulin is more than 85% effective in preventing hepatitis A if administered within 2 weeks after exposure (19). If the 2-week time period has passed, immunoglobulin is not indicated. Specific indications for postexposure prophylaxis include nonimmune persons (1) who have had household or sexual contact with an HAV-infected patient during the time when the patient was likely to be infectious (2 weeks before onset of illness to 1 week after onset) and (2) whose last contact was in the previous 2 weeks. The postexposure prophylactic dose of immunoglobulin is 0.02 mL/kg given intramuscularly in one dose. If the exposed person has received a dose of hepatitis A vaccine more than 1 month previously or has a history of laboratory confirmed HAV infection, immunoglobulin is not indicated.

Food service workers with HAV can expose other workers and immunoglobulin should be given to all other food service workers in the same establishment if they have never been vaccinated or infected. Patients with HAV who handle food must not return to work while they are potentially infectious. Hepatitis A vaccine has never been compared to immunoglobulin for use in postexposure prophylaxis in any controlled trial and thus, the CDC still recommends immunoglobulin only.

Hepatitis A vaccine is only recommended in certain populations (see Table 15–3). One of the most common indications for vaccination is travel to an endemic area. Travelers to regions where hepatitis A is endemic should begin their vaccination series (which consists of two vaccinations) 4 weeks prior to travel. If the traveler misses this window, immunoglobulin can be used for passive protection.

Recommendations for HBV postexposure management include initiation of the hepatitis B vaccine series to any susceptible, unvaccinated person who sustains an exposure to possibly infected blood or body fluid. This includes many different scenarios including occupational exposures and sexual assault victims (21). In addition, consideration must be given to adding hepatitis B

immunoglobulin (HBIG) to the treatment regimen (see Table 15–4) (20).

Postexposure management after possible exposure to HCV is controversial. No definitive studies have shown that immunoglobulin administration is effective. Antiviral agents are not FDA-approved for this indication. There have been some studies to suggest that treatment with interferon alfa started early in the course of acute HCV infection may prevent the development of chronic infection (22). The most prudent plan for these exposed individuals would be early referral for evaluation of treatment options.

DISPOSITION

Most patients with viral hepatitis will not require hospital admission. Reasons for admission include intractable vomiting or significant fluid and electrolyte imbalances that require prolonged correction. Patients with any evidence of fulminant disease such as prolonged PT, hepatic encephalopathy, or marked edema should be admitted and possibly referred to a transplantation center (23).

Patients with possible HAV infection need counseling regarding hygiene, utensil cleaning, and modes of transmission. In patients with suspected acute HBV, HCV, or HDV infection, advice regarding sexual protection should be given. In addition, treatment for household contacts in the setting of hepatitis A should be considered (see previous section). Alcohol use should be terminated until all signs of liver injury have resolved. It has also been suggested that no acetaminophen should be taken until the acute hepatitis has resolved (24).

Table 15–3. Indications for Hepatitis A Vaccination

Men who have sex with men
Illegal drug users (injection drug users or not)
Patients with chronic liver disease
Patients with clotting-factor disorders
People who work in research laboratories dealing with hepatitis A virus
Persons traveling to or working in countries with intermediate to high rates of hepatitis A endemicity (vaccination should be started 1 month before travel)
Persons who live in communities with high rates of hepatitis A (American Indian, Alaskan Native, Pacific Islander, and some religious communities)
Children living in communities with high rates of hepatitis A

Table 15–4. Postexposure Prophylaxis for Hepatitis B

Nature of Exposure	Source	Exposed Patient	
		Never Been Vaccinated	**Vaccinated**
Percutaneous or Mucosal	HBsAg positive	HBIG and Vaccine	Anti-HBs titer neg: HBIG and vaccine Anti-HBs titer pos: no treatment Anti-HBs titer unk: test for titer
	HBsAg negative	Vaccine only	No treatment
	Unknown status	Vaccine only	Anti-HBs titer neg: if high-risk source, treat as if HBsAg pos Anti-HBs titer pos: no treatment Anti-HBs titer unk: test for titer

Notes:
(1) HBsAg is hepatitis B surface antigen.
(2) Hepatitis B immune globulin (HBIG); dose is 0.06 mL/kg intramuscularly.
(3) Anti-HBs is antibody to hepatitis B surface antigen.
(4) An adequate antibody titer is $\geq$ 10 mIU/mL.
(5) neg = negative; pos = positive; unk $\geq$ unknown.
Source: Modified from (20).

Patients with acute hepatitis who are able to tolerate oral liquids may be discharged home with close follow-up. They should be seen within 1 week by their primary care provider. If they do not have access to one, the emergency physician should provide such follow-up for public health reasons or, alternatively, have them follow-up with a public health clinic.

CASE OUTCOME

The patient was hospitalized secondary to protracted vomiting and poor clinical appearance. Serologic tests were as follows: IgM anti-HAV ($-$), IgM anti-HBc ($-$), HBsAg ($-$), HBcAg ($+$), anti-HCV ($+$). This patient was determined to have had past exposure to hepatitis B but an acute hepatitis C infection. His liver enzymes peaked on day 3 and began trending downward with clinical improvement. He was discharged on day 5 with follow-up in hepatology clinic.

REFERENCES

1. Keefe EB: Acute viral hepatitis. ACP Medicine Online. November 2001. Norris Medical Library, USC. Los Angeles. 20 May 2004.http://www.acpmedicine.com
2. Alter MJ, Gallagher M, Morris TT, et al.: Acute non A-E hepatitis in the United States and the role of hepatitis G virus infection. *N Eng J Med* 336:741–746, 1997.
3. Fiore AE: Hepatitis A transmitted by food. Food safety. *Clin Infect Dis* 38:705–715, 2004.
4. Centers for Disease Control. 20 May 2004. CDC August 2002 data. http://www.cdc.gov/ncidod/diseases/hepatitis/resource/PDFs/disease_burden2002.pdf
5. Centers for Disease Control and Prevention. Hepatitis A outbreak associated with green onions at a restaurant-Monaca, Pennsylvania. *MMWR Morb Mortal Wkly Rep* 52:1155–1157, 2003.
6. Alter MJ: Epidemiology and prevention of hepatitis B. *Semin Liver Dis* 23:39–46, 2003.
7. Brillman JC, Crandall CS, Florence CS, et al.: Prevalence and risk factors associated with hepatitis C in ED patients. *Am J Emerg Med* 20:476–480, 2002.
8. Kelen GD, Green GB, Purcell RH, et al.: Hepatitis B and hepatitis C in emergency department patients. *N Engl J Med* 326:1399–1404, 1992.
9. Centers for Disease Control and Prevention: Hepatitis E among US travelers, 1989–1992. *MMWR Morb Mortal Wkly Rep* 42:1, 1993.
10. Chisari FV, Ferrari C: Hepatitis B virus immunopathogenesis. *Annu Rev Immunol* 13:29–60, 1995.
11. Lednar WM, Lemon SM, Kirkpatrick JW, et al.: Frequency of illness associated with epidemic hepatitis A infections in adults. *Am J Epidemiol* 122:226–233, 1985.
12. Chi ZC, Ma SZ: Rheumatologic manifestations of hepatic diseases. *Hepatobiliary Pancreat Dis Int* 2:32–37, 2003.
13. Agnello V, De Rosa FG: Extrahepatic disease manifestations of HCV infection: Some current issues. *J Hepatol* 40:341–352, 2004.
14. Mayo MJ: Extrahepatic manifestations of hepatitis C infection. *Am J Med Sci* 325:135–148, 2003.

15. Zegans ME, Anninger W, Chapman C, et al.: Ocular manifestations of hepatitis C virus infection. *Curr Opin Ophthalmol* 13:423–427, 2002.

16. Beasley RP: Hepatitis B virus: The major etiology of hepatocellular carcinoma. *Cancer* 61:1942–1956, 1988.

17. Ganem D, Prince AM: Hepatitis B infection—natural history and clinical consequences. *N Engl J Med* 350:1118–1129, 2004.

18. McHutchison JG, Gordon SC, Schiff ER, et al.: Interferon alfa-2b alone or in combination with ribavirin as initial treatment for chronic hepatitis C. *N Engl J Med* 339:1485–1492, 1998.

19. Winokur PL, Stapleton JT: Immunoglobulin prophylaxis for hepatitis A. *Clin Infect Dis* 14:580–586, 1992.

20. Centers for Disease Control and Prevention: Updated U.S. Public Health Service Guidelines for the Management of Occupational Exposures to HBV, HCV and HIV and Recommendations for Postexposure Prophylaxis. *Morb Mortal Wkly Rep* 50(RR11):1–42, 2001.

21. Mein JK, Palmer CM, Shand MC, et al.: Management of acute adult sexual assault. *Med J* 178:226–230, 2003.

22. Quin JW: Interferon therapy for acute hepatitis C viral infection—a review by meta-analysis. *Aust N Z J Med* 27:611–617, 1997.

23. Sass DA, Shakil AO: Fulminant hepatic failure. *Gastroenterol Clin North Am* 32:1195–1211, 2003.

24. Lentschener C, Ozier Y: What anaesthetists need to know about viral hepatitis. *Acta Anaesthesiol Scand* 47:794–803, 2003.

16

Hepatobiliary Infections

Robert L. Trowbridge

HIGH YIELD FACTS

1. The diagnosis of acute cholecystitis is often difficult to establish and may depend on a combination of historical, physical, laboratory, and radiology findings.

2. Ascending cholangitis is a medical/surgical emergency and requires consideration of immediate drainage of the biliary tree and prompt institution of appropriate antimicrobial therapy.

3. Many patients with acute cholecystitis are not infected, but empiric antibiotics are generally indicated as it is difficult to differentiate infected from noninfected patients.

4. Cephalosporins may not provide adequate coverage for organisms causing infections of the biliary tree.

CASE PRESENTATION

An otherwise healthy 53-year-old man presents to the Emergency Department with an 8-h history of abdominal pain. The pain, which is centered in the epigastrium and right upper quadrant, began shortly after eating a large meal and has progressively worsened since onset. He admits to mild nausea and anorexia, but denies emesis, fever, or diarrhea. He has had similar but less severe episodes of pain in the past for which he had not sought medical attention. The previous episodes of pain have never lasted longer than an hour.

On exam, he appears to be in moderate distress and has a temperature of 38.2°C, a heart rate of 110 beats per minute, and a normal blood pressure. He has moderate tenderness to palpation in the epigastric region and right upper quadrant. Additionally, there is guarding in the right upper quadrant but no rebound tenderness. Murphy sign is positive and the remainder of the abdomen is firm but not rigid. Rectal examination reveals no tenderness.

Laboratory studies reveal a modest leukocytosis with normal serum chemistries, including liver function studies. Amylase and lipase levels are also normal. Plain films of the abdomen reveal a nonspecific bowel gas pattern, and no free air is noted.

INTRODUCTION/EPIDEMIOLOGY

Cholelithiasis is exceedingly common, affecting over 20 million people in the United States alone (1). Although the majority of patients with cholelithiasis remain asymptomatic, up to 5% may present with complicated disease including acute cholecystitis, choledocholithiasis, and ascending cholangitis (2, 3). Such clinical syndromes constitute a frequent reason for presentation to the emergency department, with acute cholecystitis being the cause of discomfort in up to 9% of patients presenting with abdominal pain (4, 5). Despite its frequency, however, acute cholecystitis remains a difficult diagnosis to establish on clinical grounds alone and most patients with suspected acute cholecystitis undergo some form of radiologic testing before the diagnosis is made. Complications are not uncommon and include ascending cholangitis and pyogenic liver abscess. Treatment of all hepatobiliary infections is usually multifaceted with decompression of the biliary tree and appropriate antimicrobial therapy both playing important roles (6).

PATHOPHYSIOLOGY/MICROBIOLOGY

Acute Cholecystitis/Ascending Cholangitis

The gallbladder is an oblong pouch positioned on the underside of the right lobe of the liver and is connected to the biliary tree by the cystic duct. The duct is usually 3–4 cm in length and anastamoses with the common hepatic duct just distal to the convergence of the right and left hepatic ducts to form the common bile duct. The common bile duct then merges with the main pancreatic duct and empties into the second part of the duodenum through the ampulla of Vater (7). A great deal of variability in ductal structure, however, is present and anatomic variants may be present in up to 20% of individuals (8). The gallbladder, which itself consists of a thin mucosal layer overlaid with smooth muscle, serves as a reservoir for bile which is produced by the liver. Bile serves to aid in digestion of fatty foods and ingestion of an appropriate meal prompts release of cholecystokinin, which stimulates contraction of the smooth muscle in the gallbladder wall and the subsequent expulsion of the stored bile into the digestive tract (9).

Cholelithiasis results when there is an imbalance between the three basic constituents of bile: cholesterol, lecithin, and conjugated bile salts. Normally the bile salts and lecithin aid micelle formation, which prevents precipitation of the ordinarily insoluble cholesterol. An excess of cholesterol microcrystals, among other factors, however, may result in production of a nidus for stone formation (9). Although most stones in the United States are cholesterol-based, stones may also form in specific clinical situations including pigment overproduction (10). Most patients with cholelithiasis remain asymptomatic; however, approximately 10–25% will develop biliary colic and 2–5% acute cholecystitis (2, 7, 9, 11, 12).

Biliary colic results when a stone transiently blocks the flow of bile from the gallbladder to the intestines. The usual inciting event in acute cholecystitis, however, is impaction of the stone in the cystic duct (6). In a small percentage of patients, cholelithiasis is not present and obstruction of the cystic duct is thought to result from biliary sludge, biliary stasis, or thrombosis of the cystic artery (13). Yet none of these processes alone is sufficient to cause acute cholecystitis, as it appears that gallbladder irritation and inflammation from concurrent infection, lysolecithin, or other mediators must also be present. Infection is not present in all patients with acute cholecystitis, as over 50% of patients have no pathologic or microbiologic evidence of infection at the time of surgery (14). It is impossible, however, to determine which patients are infected prior to surgery. Organisms most frequently isolated from infections of the biliary tree are *Escherichia coli*, *Klebsiella*, *Enterobacter*, and *Enterococcus* species; anaerobic bacteria have also been implicated in acute cholecystitis (Table 16–1) (14).

Choledocholithiasis occurs when stones migrate down the cystic duct and lodge in the common bile duct (9). If nonobstructive, they may be little more than an incidental finding in the patient with acute cholecystitis. A stone causing obstruction of the common bile duct, however, can lead to a number of serious complications including ascending cholangitis (spread of the infection into the proximal biliary tree) and gallstone pancreatitis. Ascending cholangitis, while most commonly secondary to biliary stone disease, may occur in any situation in which there is an obstruction to biliary flow. Sclerosing

Table 16–1. Causative Organisms in Acute Cholecystitis and Ascending Cholangitis

---

E. coli (41%)
Enterococcus (12%)
Klebsiella (11%)
Enterobacter (9%)
Proteus (5%)
Clostridium (5%)
Other bacteria (16%)

Source: Adapted from (14).

cholangitis, biliary strictures, and cholangiocarcinoma may all predispose the patient to ascending cholangitis (15, 16).

Pyogenic hepatic abscesses occur most frequently as a sequela of ascending cholangitis but are also associated with diverticulitis and appendicitis. A substantial number of hepatic abscesses, however, are of unclear etiology (17). The microbiology of pyogenic hepatic abscesses reflects the underlying process. Gut organisms are most commonly isolated when concomitant cholangitis is present while there is an increased frequency of anaerobic infections with preexisting appendicitis and diverticulitis. Polymicrobial infections are not uncommon (17, 18).

Amebic liver abscesses occur with hematogenous dissemination of intestinal infection with *Entamoeba histolytica*, usually in patients returning from or native to endemic areas. Men are affected in disproportionally higher numbers, as are elderly and immunocompromised patients (19, 20).

CLINICAL PRESENTATION

Acute Cholecystitis

Many patients with acute cholecystitis present with the acute onset of right upper quadrant pain associated with nausea and vomiting (21). Epigastric pain may also be present and a minority of patients have no pain. Some patients describe an antecedent history of biliary colic, but this is not universal (22). Additional symptoms may include fever, chills, and anorexia. Physical exam often reveals right upper quadrant tenderness with rebound and guarding being present less frequently. Murphy sign, or inspiratory arrest with palpation of the right upper quadrant, has often been described in the setting of acute cholecystitis (21), although the finding is neither sensitive nor specific (23). In fact, none of the components of the history or physical examination are particularly powerful in establishing or excluding the diagnosis of acute cholecystitis (Table 16–2) (24). In most patients with acute cholecystitis, the pain subsides within 24 h although gallbladder perforation with resultant peritonitis may also occur (21). Patients with this complication often exhibit peritoneal signs on exam and may be profoundly ill, especially in the setting of medical comorbidities.

Patients with biliary colic, in contrast to those with acute cholecystitis, have less severe pain that is usually brief in duration and not associated with evidence for systemic inflammation (25). It often follows the intake of a meal with high fat content.

Table 16–2. History and Physical in the Diagnosis of Acute Cholecystitis

Finding	Sensitivity	Specificity
Nausea	0.77	0.36
Emesis	0.71	0.53
Anorexia	0.65	0.50
RUQ pain	0.76	0.82
Fever	0.35	0.80
Murphy sign	0.54	0.90
Guarding	0.45	0.70
Rebound	0.30	0.68

Source: Adapted from (20).

Ascending Cholangitis

Ascending cholangitis, often associated with choledocholithiasis and obstruction of the common bile duct, has traditionally been linked to Charcot triad of fever and chills, right upper quadrant pain, and jaundice. Although all three criteria are present in a minority of patients with ascending cholangitis, the presence of the triad should strongly raise the clinical suspicion of this severe infection. Patients may also demonstrate confusion, lethargy, rigors, and other signs and symptoms of sepsis (15).

Hepatic Abscess

In contrast to the presentation of acute cholangitis, patients with pyogenic liver abscesses may present with relatively mild symptoms. Many patients will have only nonspecific symptoms including fever, chills, weight loss, anorexia, and nausea and a significant percentage will not have abdominal pain. The physical exam is similarly nonspecific although some patients may demonstrate right upper quadrant tenderness and a palpable liver (17, 18). Patients with amebic liver abscess, however, tend to present with right upper quadrant pain and fever of more acute onset. Most have had symptoms for less than 2 weeks and patients are often younger than those with pyogenic liver abscess (26). An enlarged liver, often with point tenderness, is a frequent physical finding. It is difficult, however, to distinguish between amebic and pyogenic liver abscesses on the basis of history and physical findings; only a small percentage of patients with amebic liver abscess will have concomitant diarrhea (19, 20, 26).

LABORATORY/DIAGNOSTIC TESTING

Acute Cholecystitis/Ascending Cholangitis

The diagnosis of acute cholecystitis is often difficult to make on the basis of history and physical findings alone and most patients will require directed laboratory and radiology testing. Routine laboratory studies, however, have limited utility because of poor sensitivity and specificity for acute cholecystitis (Table 16–3) (24, 27). The main utility of such testing may be in assessing the likelihood of alternate diagnoses. Leukocytosis is common as are elevations in the transaminases (AST, ALT) and alkaline phosphatase; however, none of these are associated with a likelihood ratio of greater than 2.0. Hyperbilirubinemia may occasionally be present, but a normal bilirubin level is a common finding in acute cholecystitis (28). Lack of an elevated bilirubin level, however, is strong evidence against the presence of common bile duct obstruction as most patients with significant obstruction have elevated bilirubin levels. Such patients may also have strikingly elevated transaminases, although this elevation is usually transient. Amylase and lipase may be elevated with concomitant gallstone pancreatitis, but are usually normal in acute cholecystitis and ascending cholangitis. Blood cultures are usually negative in acute cholecystitis, but may be positive in patients with ascending cholangitis and should be obtained in most patients.

Given the limitations of the clinical exam and routine laboratory testing, most patients with suspected acute cholecystitis undergo some form of abdominal imaging (9). Plain films, although useful in assessing for intraabdominal catastrophe and intestinal obstruction, are not helpful in making the diagnosis of acute cholecystitis. The most commonly performed initial test for acute cholecystitis has become the right upper quadrant (RUQ) ultrasound (29). Fast, widely available, and relatively inexpensive, RUQ ultrasound is associated with a sensitivity of 88% (95% CI: 74–100%) and specificity of 80% (95%

Table 16–3. Laboratory Testing in the Diagnosis of Acute Cholecystitis

Finding	Sensitivity	Specificity
Leukocytosis	0.63	0.56
Elevated bilirubin	0.45	0.63
Elevated AST or ALT	0.38	0.62
Elevated alkaline phosphatase	0.45	0.52

Source: Adapted from (20).

CI: 62–98%) for acute cholecystitis (30). It is also the best initial test in assessing for biliary ductal dilation and common bile duct obstruction as is commonly seen with ascending cholangitis. In addition, because imaging includes the liver and pancreas, information regarding alternate diagnoses (e.g., hepatic and pancreatic masses, pancreatitis) may be obtained.

Nuclear medicine scans, including the HIDA scan, are an alternative to ultrasound but are not as universally available and do not provide information regarding alternate diagnoses (31). They are, however, associated with better test characteristics than the RUQ ultrasound with a sensitivity of 97% (95% CI: 96–98%) and a specificity of 90% (95% CI: 86–95%) (30). They are often used as a second line test when there is a strong clinical suspicion for biliary tract disease but no ultrasonographic evidence of acute cholecystitis.

Computed tomography of the abdomen, although very useful for other abdominal processes that may be confused with acute cholecystitis, has poor test characteristics for the diagnosis of acute biliary disease. It should not be considered a first-line test in patients with suspected acute cholecystitis, although it performs remarkably well in diagnosing the complications of disease including hepatic abscess and gallbladder perforation with abscess formation (32). It may also be useful in the diagnosis of underlying disorders that predispose one to ascending cholangitis, including malignancy.

Given the limitations of the clinical exam and history as well as the laboratory and radiology testing available, the approach to a patient with suspected acute cholecystitis must be individualized. The most immediate question to be addressed is whether the clinical likelihood of disease is sufficiently high as to require radiographic assessment. No simple algorithms or risk scores exist to aid in this decision-making process, although experienced clinicians likely use a combination of clinical and laboratory features to make this decision (24). Subsequently, if the radiology results do not correlate with the clinical impression, the clinician must strongly consider further testing (i.e., pursuing nuclear medicine scan after a negative ultrasound in a patient thought to have a high likelihood of disease) given the imperfect test characteristics of the available tests.

Hepatic Abscess

Pyogenic liver abscesses are more likely to be associated with abnormal liver function studies than acute cholecystitis. Serum alkaline phosphatase is elevated in over 70% of cases with AST/ALT and bilirubin each being abnormal

50% of the time. Approximately 50% of patients will have positive blood cultures (17). Amebic abscesses are often associated with an abnormal ALT but the alkaline phosphatase is usually normal. A majority of patients (80%) will have serum antibodies to *E. histolytica* at the time of presentation (19, 26).

Imaging usually establishes the presence of an abscess and both ultrasound and computed tomography are helpful in establishing the diagnosis. Radiology findings, however, are nonspecific.

MANAGEMENT

Acute Cholecystitis

The majority of patients with acute cholecystitis will improve with conservative therapy inclusive of bowel rest and analgesics (11). Meperidine has traditionally been considered the opioid of choice because of concerns regarding morphine-induced constriction of the Sphincter of Oddi. The clinical significance of this observation, however, is unclear. Although many patients with acute cholecystitis do not harbor infection (14), it is difficult to differentiate infected patients from those with "sterile" cholecystitis and empiric antimicrobial therapy in all patients with acute cholecystitis is reasonable. There exists, however, no clear and convincing evidence that antibiotics are beneficial in this setting. Therapy should be directed toward typical gut organisms and reasonable choices include ampicillin plus gentamicin and the penicillin/beta-lactamase inhibitor combinations (piperacillin-tazobactam, ticarcillin-clavulanate) (Table 16–4). Cephalosporins are frequently prescribed for this indication, but they do not cover enterococcus, which may be responsible for up to 12% of infections (14). Several studies have suggested that despite this shortcoming, cephalosporins may be effective in this setting (33). The duration of antimicrobial therapy for acute cholecystitis is poorly defined with most patients receiving a

Table 16–4. Antimicrobial Therapy for Acute Cholecystitis and Ascending Cholangitis

---

Ampicillin (2 g IV q4 h) plus gentamicin (4–6 mg/kg IV once daily)
Piperacillin-tazobactam (3/0.375 g every 6 h)
Ticarcillin-clavulanate (3.1 g every 4–6 h)
If penicillin allergic: Ciprofloxacin 500 mg IV every 12 h, consider adding metronidazole

---

7–10-day course if evidence of infection is noted at the time of surgery.

Although most patients will improve with conservative treatment, the risk of recurrent attack is substantial at 10% within 1 month and 30% within 1 year. Most patients should thus undergo cholecystectomy within several days of presentation (6, 34, 35). In the patient with severe disease who is otherwise at low risk for perioperative complication, emergent cholecystectomy may be indicated. Patients at high risk for perioperative morbidity or mortality on the basis of medical comorbidities, however, may be treated more conservatively with consideration given to percutaneous cholecystostomy with continued antimicrobial therapy if improvement does not occur. Percutaneous cholecystostomy should also be considered in the septic or unstable patient who may be too ill to tolerate cholecystectomy (36, 37).

Choledocholithiasis/Ascending Cholangitis

If nonobstructive, choledocholithiasis may be an incidental finding in the setting of acute cholecystitis and not require emergent therapy. Precholecystectomy ERCP, however, will likely be necessary in most such cases. Preoperative ERCP or intraoperative ductal exploration should be strongly considered in the setting of jaundice (bilirubin >2 mg/dL), a dilated common bile duct (>6 mm), or known choledocholithiasis (as demonstrated most frequently on RUQ ultrasonography) (9).

Patients with choledocholithiasis and ascending cholangitis are often substantially more ill than those with acute cholecystitis and require more aggressive and immediate treatment (6). Such patients, who usually present with fever and jaundice, represent a medical emergency and many patients will require immediate decompression of the biliary tree which is most commonly achieved via ERCP (6, 15, 38, 39). Antimicrobial therapy consisting of agents similar to those used for acute cholecystitis should also be started immediately. Biliary cultures should be taken at the time of drainage to help tailor antimicrobial therapy. Duration of therapy in ascending cholangitis is usually more prolonged than that for acute cholecystitis, with most patients completing a 10–14-day course of therapy.

Pyogenic Hepatic Abscess

Most patients require drainage of the abscess coupled with appropriate antimicrobial therapy (40, 41). Percutaneous aspiration, guided by CT or ultrasound, followed by catheter drainage is the procedure of choice in most patients. Needle aspiration without catheter placement may be possible in some patients while others require an open or laparoscopic drainage procedure. The choice of antimicrobial therapy depends on the suspected source of origin of the abscess. Those with a biliary source should be treated as for cholangitis while those with a suspected colonic source can be treated with a third-generation cephalosporin and metronidazole (40, 41). Duration of therapy is controversial with most advocating at least 2 weeks of parenteral antibiotics with a total course of 4–6 weeks.

Amebic Liver Abscess

In contrast to those with pyogenic liver abscesses, most patients with amebic abscesses will respond to antimicrobial therapy alone (19, 20). Metronidazole (750 mg PO three times daily for 7–10 days) effects a cure in the majority of patients. If the patient is toxic-appearing upon presentation, cyst aspiration may result in significant improvement in symptoms. Percutaneous drainage should also be considered in patients with large abscess cavities (greater than 5 cm) or left sided abscesses and those with a poor response to drug therapy. After completing therapy with metronidazole, all patients should also receive a course of iodoquinol (650 mg PO three times daily for 20 days) or paromomycin (25–35 mg/kg/day PO divided into three daily doses for 7–10 days) to treat the intraluminal phase of the parasite (19, 42).

DISPOSITION

Patients with acute cholecystitis, liver abscess, and ascending cholangitis are typically admitted to the hospital, the latter often in an intensive care unit setting. Patients with biliary colic, however, are treated in the outpatient setting, usually with elective cholecystectomy. All patients with biliary colic, however, should be carefully educated regarding the possibility of acute cholecystitis and other complications and instructed to seek medical attention immediately for such symptoms.

CASE OUTCOME

The patient underwent RUQ ultrasound, which revealed several small gallstones but no evidence to suggest acute cholecystitis. Given the relatively high clinical suspicion for acute cholecystitis, the patient was admitted and begun on bowel rest, intravenous fluids, and piperacillin-tazobactam. The following day, a HIDA scan was performed which revealed a lack of filling of the cystic duct, consistent with acute cholecystitis. A laparoscopic cholecystectomy was performed 2 days after admission and an inflamed "boggy" gallbladder was removed. The patient recovered uneventfully, completing a 7-day course of antimicrobial therapy.

REFERENCES

1. Everhart JE, Khare M, Hill M, Maurer KR: Prevalence and ethnic differences in gallbladder disease in the United States. *Gastroenterology* 117:632–639, 1999.
2. Friedman GD: Natural history of asymptomatic and symptomatic gallstones. *Am J Surg* 165:399–404, 1993.
3. Thistle JL, Cleary PA, Lachin JM, Tyor MP, Hersh T: The natural history of cholelithiasis: The National Cooperative Gallstone Study. *Ann Intern Med* 101:171–175, 1984.
4. Powers RD, Guertler AT: Abdominal pain in the ED: Stability and change over 20 years. *Am J Emerg Med* 13:301–303, 1995.
5. Brewer BJ, Golden GT, Hitch DC, Rudolf LE, Wangensteen SL: Abdominal pain. An analysis of 1,000 consecutive cases in a University Hospital emergency room. *Am J Surg* 131:219–223, 1976.
6. Lillemoe KD: Surgical treatment of biliary tract infections. *Am Surg* 66:138–144, 2000.
7. Ahrendt SA PH: Biliary tract, in Townsend CM BR, Evers BM, Mattox KL (eds.): *Sabiston Textbook of Surgery.* Philadelphia, W. B. Saunders, 2001.
8. Lamah M, Karanjia ND, Dickson GH: Anatomical variations of the extrahepatic biliary tree: Review of the world literature. *Clin Anat* 14:167–172, 2001.
9. Johnson CD: ABC of the upper gastrointestinal tract. Upper abdominal pain: Gall bladder. *BMJ* 323:1170–1173, 2001.
10. Schubert TT: Hepatobiliary system in sickle cell disease. *Gastroenterology* 90:2013–2021, 1986.
11. Mulagha E, Fromm H: Acute cholecystitis. *Curr Treat Options Gastroenterol* 2:144–146, 1999.
12. McSherry CK, Ferstenberg H, Calhoun WF, Lahman E, Virshup M: The natural history of diagnosed gallstone disease in symptomatic and asymptomatic patients. *Ann Surg* 202:59–63, 1985.
13. Kalliafas S, Ziegler DW, Flancbaum L, Choban PS: Acute acalculous cholecystitis: Incidence, risk factors, diagnosis, and outcome. *Am Surg* 64:471–475, 1998.
14. Csendes A, Burdiles P, Maluenda F, Diaz JC, Csendes P, Mitru, N: Simultaneous bacteriologic assessment of bile from gallbladder and common bile duct in control subjects and patients with gallstones and common duct stones. *Arch Surg* 131:389–394, 1996.
15. Sinanan MN: Acute cholangitis. *Infect Dis Clin North Am* 6:571–599, 1992.
16. Boey JH, Way LW: Acute cholangitis. *Ann Surg* 191:264–270, 1980.
17. Silen W. *Cope's Early Diagnosis of the Acute Abdomen.* New York, Oxford University Press, 2000.
18. Gunn A, Keddie N. Some clinical observations on patients with gallstones. *Lancet* 2:239–241, 1972.
19. Adedeji OA, McAdam WA: Murphy's sign, acute cholecystitis and elderly people. *J R Coll Surg Edinb* 41:88–89, 1996.
20. Trowbridge RL, Rutkowski NK, Shojania KG: Does this patient have acute cholecystitis? *JAMA* 289:80–86, 2003.
21. Berger MY, van der Velden JJ, Lijmer JG, de Kort H, Prins A, Bohnen AM: Abdominal symptoms: Do they predict gallstones? A systematic review. *Scand J Gastroenterol* 35:70–76, 2000.
22. Lindenauer SM, Child CGd: Disturbances of liver function in biliary tract disease. *Surg Gynecol Obstet* 123:1205–1211, 1966.
23. Dunlop MG, King PM, Gunn AA: Acute abdominal pain: The value of liver function tests in suspected cholelithiasis. *J R Coll Surg Edinb* 34:124–127, 1989.
24. Reiss R, Deutsch AA: State of the art in the diagnosis and management of acute cholecystitis. *Dig Dis* 11:55–64, 1993.
25. Shea JA, Berlin JA, Escarce JJ, et al.: Revised estimates of diagnostic test sensitivity and specificity in suspected biliary tract disease. *Arch Intern Med* 154:2573–2581, 1994.
26. Johnson H, Jr., Cooper B: The value of HIDA scans in the initial evaluation of patients for cholecystitis. *J Natl Med Assoc* 87:27–32, 1995.
27. Fidler J, Paulson EK, Layfield L: CT evaluation of acute cholecystitis: Findings and usefulness in diagnosis. *AJR Am J Roentgenol* 166:1085–1088, 1996.
28. Yellin AE, Berne TV, Appleman MD, et al.: A randomized study of cefepime versus the combination of gentamicin and mezlocillin as an adjunct to surgical treatment in patients with acute cholecystitis. *Surg Gynecol Obstet* 177:23–29; discussion 35–40, 1993.
29. Rutledge D, Jones D, Rege R: Consequences of delay in surgical treatment of biliary disease. *Am J Surg* 180:466–469, 2000.
30. Lo CM, Liu CL, Fan ST, Lai EC, Wong J: Prospective randomized study of early versus delayed laparoscopic cholecystectomy for acute cholecystitis. *Ann Surg* 227:461–467, 1998.
31. Davis CA, Landercasper J, Gundersen LH, Lambert PJ: Effective use of percutaneous cholecystostomy in high-risk surgical patients: Techniques, tube management, and results. *Arch Surg* 134:727–731; discussion 731–732, 1999.
32. Melin MM, Sarr MG, Bender CE, van Heerden JA: Percutaneous cholecystostomy: A valuable technique in high-risk patients with presumed acute cholecystitis. *Br J Surg* 82:1274–1277, 1995.
33. Lai EC, Mok FP, Tan ES, et al.: Endoscopic biliary drainage for severe acute cholangitis. *N Engl J Med* 326:1582–1586, 1992.
34. Chijiiwa K, Kozaki N, Naito T, Kameoka N, Tanaka M: Treatment of choice for choledocholithiasis in patients with acute obstructive suppurative cholangitis and liver cirrhosis. *Am J Surg* 170:356–360, 1995.

Peritonitis: Primary SBP and Secondary Peritonitis

Lynne McCullough
Sunil Shroff

HIGH YIELD FACTS

- A low threshold for performing paracentesis and ruling out spontaneous bacterial peritonitis is the key to early diagnosis and treatment of spontaneous bacterial peritonitis (SBP), a potentially fatal infection.

- Bedside inoculation of at least 10 ml of ascitic fluid into both aerobic and anaerobic culture bottles increases the yield of positive cultures following paracentesis.

- Up to one in five patients with advanced liver disease who are admitted for gastrointestinal hemorrhage has spontaneous bacterial peritonitis on admission.

- Albumin administration (1.5 g/kg of body weight) in the setting of both large volume therapeutic paracentesis (>5 L) and in patients with cirrhosis and SBP reduces the incidence of subsequent renal impairment for both and mortality in the latter.

- Antibiotics are only an adjunct to the definitive surgical treatment of secondary peritonitis.

CASE PRESENTATION

A 65-year-old male with a history of advanced liver disease secondary to both alcohol and hepatitis C, is Childs–Pugh Class B, and is brought in by his wife for decreased level of alertness and mild confusion, low-grade temperatures, and complaints of diffuse abdominal discomfort for the past 2 days. He has no vomiting, change in his stools, urinary, or pulmonary symptoms. He has not been recently hospitalized and has no history of gastrointestinal hemorrhage or spontaneous bacterial peritonitis. On presentation, the patient reports only malaise and anorexia. His medications include spironolactone and furosemide. On examination, he has a temperature of 99°F, a pulse of 105 bpm, blood pressure of 103/74 mmHg, and is mildly tachypneic at a rate of 22 breaths/minute. He is alert and

oriented, but is slow to answer questions. His exam is remarkable only for mild tachycardia, a distended and diffusely tender abdomen to palpation with moderate ascites elicited by a fluid wave and 2+ pedal edema.

INTRODUCTION

Spontaneous bacterial peritonitis is the most well described infectious complication of advanced liver disease and heralds the onset of a precipitous worsening in a cirrhotic patient's prognosis. From its first description in the early 1970s when in-hospital mortality approached 90%, the mortality rate has been reduced to around 20% through the widespread use of paracentesis leading to earlier recognition, as well as the prompt use of safer and more appropriate antibiotics (1, 2). Patients with ascites secondary to cirrhosis have a 10% annual risk of ascitic fluid infection (3, 4) and the probability is even higher in patients with more severe hepatic dysfunction and low ascitic fluid protein concentration (<1 g/dL) (5, 6).

Ascitic fluid infection has been estimated to range from 7% to 30% in cirrhotic patients who are hospitalized for any reason (7–9), with approximately 20% of those admitted for gastrointestinal hemorrhage already infected at the time of admission (10). For those patients who survive an initial bout of SBP, the 1-year cumulative recurrence rate is 70% and the probability of survival to 1 year is 30% (1, 2). In patients undergoing peritoneal dialysis (CAPD), peritonitis is also quite common. It accounts for two-thirds of peritoneal catheter loss and one-third of patients returning to hemodialysis (11). Fortunately, its incidence has declined precipitously from 4–5 episodes per patient per year to less than 0.5 episode per patient per year over the past 20 years. Much of this decline has been attributed to better patient education, improved catheter techniques, and antibiotic prophylaxis.

Although primary bacterial peritonitis is commonly an infectious complication of ascitic fluid in patients with advanced cirrhosis, or in those undergoing peritoneal dialysis, it has been described in other clinical settings as well. Peritoneal carcinomatosis or tuberculous peritonitis may masquerade as SBP, at least initially. Furthermore, primary bacterial peritonitis may also be identified in the setting of heart failure or nephrotic syndrome, though far less frequently (4). In contrast to primary bacterial peritonitis, which is a diffuse bacterial infection that occurs without the loss of digestive integrity or a surgically identifiable source, peritonitis can also occur as a secondary complication of normal microbes in the digestive tract that contaminate the otherwise sterile peritoneal cavity. Secondary peritonitis is an acute process of diffuse peritoneal inflammation, most commonly following perforation of a hollow abdominal viscus. Alternatively, contamination of the peritoneum may occur in the setting of blunt or penetrating trauma, postoperatively, or secondary to pancreatic or renal inflammation and necrosis (12).

PATHOPHYSIOLOGY

Primary Spontaneous Bacterial Peritonitis

The presence of ascites is a prerequisite for the development of spontaneous bacterial peritonitis, thus, advanced liver disease is the main predisposing factor (1, 13). From animal studies, it has been shown that colonic gram-negative bacteria colonize the small intestine in cirrhosis and bacterial overgrowth occurs (9). Subsequently, the gut becomes more permeable to translocation of the bacteria across the intestinal wall and into intestinal and mesenteric lymph nodes (MLNs). Several factors contribute to the increased permeability of the gut including higher concentrations of bacteria present in the intestines leading to increased bacterial endotoxin concentrations, as well as structural abnormalities created by vascular congestion (due to portal hypertension) and intestinal wall edema (1, 9, 14). From MLNs, bacteria may enter the bloodstream (leading to septicemia), the lymphatic system, or the ascitic fluid. Cirrhotic patients have compromised humoral and cellular bacterial systems characterized by decreased serum levels of complement factors, impaired chemotaxis and poor function and phagocytic activity of neutrophils. The liver also contains stationary macrophages, known as Kupfer cells, and in the presence of intra- and extra-hepatic shunts, bacteria can bypass these important components of immunity resulting in prolongation of bacteremia and higher rates of distant seeding, including ascitic fluid.

Transient bacterascites develops and in the absence of adequate complement proteins and peritoneal macrophage activity, opsonization does not occur and bacterial overgrowth ensues leading to spontaneous bacterial peritonitis (4). Thus, SBP is the result of failure of the intestine to contain bacteria and failure of the immune system to kill the bacteria once they arrive in the ascitic fluid.

Secondary Peritonitis in the Cirrhotic with Ascites

The vast majority of patients with cirrhosis, ascites, and peritoneal infection have spontaneous bacterial peritoni-

tis. However, a very small subset may develop peritonitis secondary to bacterial contamination of the peritoneum as a result of intraabdominal viscus perforation, acute inflammation of an intraabdominal organ, or previous surgical procedures (15). Due to the origins of secondary peritonitis it is typically polymicrobial, and a delayed diagnosis in patients at risk for SBP as well.

Peritonitis in Patients Undergoing Peritoneal Dialysis (CAPD/APD)

The average CAPD patient performs 1200 exchanges a year. The high frequency of dialysate exchanges, combined with the routine loss of activated macrophages with each exchange, the decreased activity of peritoneal defenses secondary to a hyperosmolor, hyperglycemic and acidic dialysate, and a catheter which bridges a sterile and nonsterile environment, places the CAPD patient at significant risk for peritonitis. The most common route of peritoneal contamination in CAPD patients is touch or luminal contamination during dialysate exchanges by pathogenic skin flora. Other sources include, in descending order of frequency, periluminal catheter (exit-site) infections, transmural contamination from the abdominal viscera, female genital tract leak, and hematogenous contamination.

CLINICAL PRESENTATION

Spontaneous Bacterial Peritonitis

The clinical presentation of SBP in cirrhotics with ascites is quite varied depending on the stage at which it is diagnosed. Typically, the presentation of SBP is more subtle than that of patients who have surgical peritonitis in the absence of ascites. Patients with SBP commonly present in the early stages of development with mild and insidious symptoms, the most common of which are fever (69%) and abdominal pain (59%). Even a low-grade temperature in a cirrhotic patient can herald the onset of a serious infection, as these patients are not infrequently hypothermic at baseline.

Although diffuse and significant abdominal pain are the hallmarks of peritonitis, in cirrhotics, it may be just a mild change from their baseline discomfort associated with the tense stretching of the abdominal wall with large volume ascites. Interestingly, rigidity is not commonly elicited as the ascites typically present prevents contact of the visceral and parietal peritoneal surfaces needed to stimulate the spinal reflex that results in rigidity. Other nonspecific signs and symptoms are quite common and include anorexia or nausea, abdominal tenderness (49%), vomiting and diarrhea (32%), the development of hepatic encephalopathy (54%), an ileus (30%), hypotension (21%), and hypothermia (17%) (1).

Up to one-third of patients with SBP can be essentially asymptomatic. A frequently overlooked sign of SBP is a very mild deterioration in mental status, detectable only by a spouse or other primary caregiver. It is important to note that such subtle changes do not correlate well with ammonia levels (16). Occasionally, a cirrhotic patient may present to the ED with no clinical signs or symptoms, but with the referral of "abnormal screening laboratory values." These may include an unexplained leukocytosis, azotemia, or metabolic acidosis. Such findings in a cirrhotic with ascites should prompt an evaluation and paracentesis to rule out SBP as the precipitant (1, 4).

Peritonitis and CAPD

Another group of patients prone to develop secondary peritonitis are those who are undergoing continuous peritoneal dialysis. These patients can present anywhere along the continuum from very mild and subtle signs of peritoneal inflammation, much like SBP, with low-grade temperature and abdominal pain or with frank and classic peritonitis characterized by marked abdominal tenderness or rigidity, fever, and hypotension (11).

CAPD patients with peritonitis will commonly have cloudy dialysis effluent and complain of abdominal tenderness. Cloudy effluent is the most consistent finding present in 94–100% of all cases of CAPD-associated peritonitis (17, 18). Other symptoms such as fever, nausea/vomiting, or diarrhea are only present in less than half of the cases (19).

Secondary Peritonitis in the Cirrhotic Patient

An important feature in the differential diagnosis of peritonitis in the cirrhotic with ascites is to distinguish primary SBP from secondary peritonitis due to a surgically treatable cause. This distinction cannot usually be made only on clinical signs and symptoms. Initially, the patient with ascites who appears to have SBP will be started on appropriate antibiotic therapy and will not have a typical response. They may have persistent fever, leukocytosis, and abdominal pain. Radiologic imaging and repeat paracenteses with characteristic findings (see below in Diagnosis) are frequently required to confirm the presence of a surgically treatable cause.

Secondary Peritonitis in the Noncirrhotic Patient

In noncirrhotic patients, the severity of abdominal pain on clinical presentation will depend on the inciting process. There may be localized findings in the area of the inciting event initially, as with a perforated diverticulitis, or the symptoms may be vague, and visceral, as is typically the case in appendicitis. As the infection spreads to the peritoneal cavity, pain increases, and the abdominal exam becomes progressively more remarkable. The patient may lie motionless, in the fetal position (to decrease the stretch on the peritoneal nerve fibers) and the exam may demonstrate significant voluntary or involuntary guarding of the anterior abdominal wall musculature. Later findings will include rebound tenderness, and most patients will be febrile.

LABORATORY/DIAGNOSTIC TESTING

Spontaneous Bacterial Peritonitis

As many patients with SBP will have little or no clinical signs or symptoms on presentation, the diagnosis cannot be made on clinical criteria alone. Emergency physicians must have a very low threshold for performing a diagnostic paracentesis to rule out the possibility of peritoneal infection. The diagnosis of spontaneous bacterial peritonitis is defined as an ascitic fluid infection without a surgically treatable intraabdominal source. The variants of ascitic fluid infection are not particularly useful in the acute phase of treatment or diagnosis (see Table 17–1), with the exception of monomicrobial nonneutrocytic bacterascites (MNB) that occurs in patients with clinical symptoms of peritonitis, but without the threshold PMN value needed for treatment. Based on the frequency with which symptomatic patients with MNB progress to SBP, empiric antibiotic treatment may help prevent serious morbidity and mortality (20) (see Table 17–2).

Paracentesis

This diagnostic and therapeutic procedure should be performed in any cirrhotic patient with ascites who has signs or symptoms of peritoneal inflammation, has a gastrointestinal hemorrhage, is being admitted to the hospital, develops hepatic encephalopathy, or has a laboratory deterioration in hepatic or renal function (see Table 17–3). Physicians have been traditionally reluctant to perform paracentesis because of a fear of complications, resulting in a historically higher mortality rate. In a prospective,

Table 17–1. Ascitic Fluid Infection Definitions and Characteristics

Type of AF Infection	AF PMN Count	Clinical Symptoms	Culture	Tx	Other
Spontaneous bacterial peritonitis	$\geq$250/mm^3	Yes	+	Abx	Monomicrobial
Culture negative neutrocytic ascities (CNNA)	$\geq$250/mm^3	Yes	–	Abx	Monomicrobial[a]
Monomicrobial nonneutrocytic bacterascites (MNB)	<250/mm^3	Yes	+	Yes	
Monomicrobial nonneutrocytic bacterascites (MNB)	<250/mm^3	No	+	No	Resolves without treatment
Secondary peritonitis	$\geq$250/mm^3	Yes	+	Yes[b]	Polymicrobial[c]
Polymicrobial bacterascites	<250/mm^3	+/–	+/–	+/–	Polymicrobial[d]

[a]CNNA: consider other possible causes such as pancreatitis, tuberculous peritonitis or peritoneal carcinomatosis.
[b]Treatment is defined by cause and includes antibiotics, drainage, or laparotomy.
[c]Secondary peritonitis cannot be distinguished solely by clinical symptoms, but usually meets two of the three following criteria: total protein >1 g/dL, glucose of <50 mg/dL and a lactate dehydrogenase level of >225 U/mL.
[d]Occurs as the result of an inadvertent puncture of the intestines during paracentesis (rate of ~1/1000 paracenteses).
Source: Adapted from (2).

observational study by Runyon, he demonstrated that paracentesis can be safely performed when ascitic fluid is identified by ultrasound or by percussion, a narrow needle is used, and abdominal wall scars are avoided (21). Paracentesis can be performed in the midline inferior to the umbilicus, or in the left lower quadrant, 2 finger breadths cephalad and 2 finger breadths medial to the anterior superior iliac spine, or in an area of a collection of ascitic fluid identified by ultrasound (22).

Although it is the practice of some clinicians to give blood products (platelets or FFP) routinely to correct commonly present coagulopathy before performing paracentesis, these decisions are not data driven and since bleeding is sufficiently uncommon, the prophylactic administration of blood products is not recommended in the

2004 American Association for the Study of Liver Diseases' Practice Guidelines (23).

Ascitic Fluid Analysis

Following the successful acquisition of peritoneal fluid, it must be sent to the laboratory for analysis. The most important test to perform is the cell count and differential, which can be sent in a red-topped tube, or the container provided in a commercially available paracentesis kit. In addition, cultures should be performed. Ideally, 10 ml of the fluid should be inoculated into each of the aerobic

Table 17–2. Predisposing Factors for the Development of SBP

- Severity of liver disease: Child-Pugh class C > B
- Previous episode of spontaneous bacterial peritonitis
- Ascitic fluid total protein level <1 g/dL
- Gastrointestinal hemorrhage
- Iatrogenic factors: urinary bladder and intravascular catheters

Source: Adapted from (2) and (9).

Table 17–3. Indications for Paracentesis

- Cirrhotic patients with ascites and clinical signs and symptoms of infection
- Cirrhotic patients with ascites who develop a deterioration in clinical status or laboratory values (azotemia, leukocytosis, acidosis) from baseline
- Patients with new onset ascites in cirrhosis
- On admission to hospital for a cirrhotic patient with ascites
- In patients who develop other complications of cirrhosis, such as encephalopathy or gastrointestinal hemorrhage

Source: Adapted from (9).

Table 17–4. Ascitic Fluid Analysis

Routine	Optional	Unusual	Not Helpful
Cell count and differential	Glucose	AFB smear and culture	pH
Total protein	LDH	Cytology	Lactate
Culture in culture bottles[a]	Amylase	Bilirubin	Cholesterol
Albumin concentration		Triglyceride concentration	Fibronectin
Gram stain[b]			

[a] 10 mL in each aerobic and anaerobic culture bottle at the bedside.
[b] The bacterial concentration is typically too low to give a positive Gram stain in SBP. If positive and polymicrobial consider secondary peritonitis.

and anaerobic culture bottles at the bedside to increase the yield. In the emergency department, these are the only studies that are needed to make a clinical decision; however, the specialist who will be caring for the patient may want a few additional studies. An albumin concentration is helpful in determining the serum ascites albumin gradient (SAAG) as this has been demonstrated to be superior to the older exudate-transudate concept in the differential diagnosis of the cause of ascites, as well as in decision making regarding treatment strategy (24). The total protein can be useful in identifying those patients at greater risk for peritoneal infection and begun on prophylaxis. A gram's stain is of great utility when positive, although the typical concentration of bacteria is too low to generate a positive Gram stain in most patients, and empiric antibiotics should be started based on symptoms and cell count (see Table 17–4).

Peritonitis in CAPD

Two of the following must be present for a diagnosis of peritonitis (26):

- Cloudy dialysis effluent with WBC count >100 cells/mm^3 (with >50% consisting of PMNs)—present in 98% of cases
- Abdominal pain—present in approximately 75% of cases
- Positive culture from dialysate

As in SBP, the Gram stain is rarely positive. However, a positive Gram stain in this setting is 85% predictive of eventual culture results and more importantly can lead to early identification of fungal peritonitis. Furthermore, the finding of Gram-positive cocci and Gram-negative rods together is suggestive of a perforated viscus (27).

Amylase levels may be helpful in patients with an atypical course or where secondary peritonitis is being considered. Amylase levels are typically very low (<8 IU/L) in patients with peritoneal dialysis associated peritonitis or asymptomatic patients and a level greater than 50 IU/L is suggestive of intraabdominal pathology (28). Peritoneal fluid culture should be obtained from the first cloudy effluent. Large volumes of effluent are preferred and can be centrifuged down to manageable volume or a minimum of 10 mL should be placed in each blood culture bottle, a more feasible option in the emergency department. After 24–48 h, positive cultures will be seen in 70–90% of patients. There is no utility in obtaining peripheral blood cultures unless bacteremia or sepsis is suspected.

Secondary Peritonitis

The evaluation and diagnostic approach for otherwise well patients who spontaneously develop peritonitis differs from those who suffer trauma or either have an accumulation of ascitic fluid secondary to cirrhosis or are undergoing CAPD, and subsequently develop secondary peritonitis. In previously well patients, or in those who have suffered blunt or penetrating trauma, once the diagnosis of secondary peritonitis is suspected, a surgeon must be promptly notified, and definitive imaging, such as CT scan (ideally with both water soluble oral and IV contrast), must be ordered. When perforation is suspected as the etiology, a 3 view abdominal series to rule out free air would be the first study of choice. Although this approach may be used for patients with cirrhosis and ascites, or those undergoing CAPD, secondary peritonitis is a rare complication. In this population, it is more commonly diagnosed outside of the ED, by a polymicrobial Gram stain or the growth of multiple organisms in the culture, or suspected in a patient who has a poor response to standard therapy for primary peritonitis and increasing PMNs on a repeat paracentesis.

MANAGEMENT

Spontaneous Bacterial Peritonitis

Patients with ascitic fluid PMN counts greater than 250 cells/mL should receive empiric therapy. In addition to these patients, those who have convincing signs and symptoms of infection (fever, abdominal pain, or unexplained encephalopathy) should also receive empiric antibiotics until culture results return, as they may have monomicrobrial nonneutracytic bacterascites.

Antibiotics

The mainstay of empiric therapy has been cefotaxime or a similar third-generation cephalosporin and is recommended by the AASLD (23). In a randomized controlled trial by Felisart (29), cefotaxime was demonstrated to be superior to ampicillin and tobramycin in terms of survival (85% vs. 56%), incidence of nephrotoxicity (0% vs. 5%), and subsequent superinfection (0% vs. 16%). Furthermore, cefotaxime covers 95% of common flora and covers the three most common isolates *Escherichia coli*, *Klebsiella pneumoniae*, and pneumococci. A minimum of 2 g of cefotaxime every 12 h achieves adequate ascitic fluid levels, but dosing should be adjusted for renal function (see Table 17–5). Treatment for 5 days has been shown to be as efficacious as 10 days and is now the minimum current recommendation (23, 30).

Oral treatment may be considered in a subset of patients with SBP. A randomized controlled trial demonstrated equivalent efficacy of oral ofloxacin when compared with intravenous cefotaxime. However, there were notable exclusion criteria which included recent antibiotic therapy (within 2 weeks), gastrointestinal bleeding, serum creatinine level >3 mg/dL, grade II or greater hepatic encephalopathy, shock, and ileus. As a result, only 61% of patients presenting with SBP could be included in the trial (31). While oral therapy is not yet the standard

Table 17–5. Cefotaxime Dosing for Renal Insufficiency

Creatinine	Cefotaxime Dose
<1.5	2 g every 12 h
1.5–2.0	1.5 g every 12 h
2.1–2.5	1 g every 12 h
>2.5	1 g every 24 h

Source: Rimola et al. 1995.

of care, this trial demonstrated that low risk patients with SBP may be treated as outpatients in the future.

Albumin

Deterioration in renal function is the most sensitive predictor of in-hospital mortality in patients with SBP (31). Cirrhotic patients with ascites have marked activation of their renin-angiotensin system, thought to be secondary to decreased intravascular volume, and thus effective arterial blood volume seen by the kidneys. A single randomized control trial of cefotaxime without intravenous albumin compared with cefotaxime with intravenous albumin found a substantial decrease in mortality, 29% vs. 10%, the lowest hospitalized mortality reported in SBP. Until further studies evaluate this treatment, intravenous albumin treatment is warranted as used in the study, 1.5 g/kg within 6 h of diagnosis and 1 g/kg on hospital day 3 (33).

Prophylaxis

Norfloxacin or trimethoprim/sulfamethoxazole should be given for 7 days to patients with cirrhosis and gastrointestinal hemorrhage as norfloxacin has been found to reduce bacterial infections in these patients (34, 35). Furthermore, cirrhotic patients with ascitic total protein levels less than or equal to 1 g/dL or prior history of SBP should receive daily norfloxacin or trimethoprim/sulfamethoxazole while hospitalized (23).

Peritoneal Dialysis

The recommendations for empiric therapy from the International Society for Peritoneal Dialysis (ISPD) have evolved since the late 1980s to reflect growing concern for resistance to vancomycin and preservation of residual renal function. Residual renal function has been demonstrated to be an independent predictor of survival in CAPD patients and should be preserved as much as possible. Aminoglycosides, in particular, lead to a rapid decline of residual renal function and should not be used in patients with residual urine output greater than 100 mL per day (36). The most current ISPD recommendations for empiric therapy can be found in Table 17–6.

In known fungal peritonitis, a combination of fluconazole and flucytosine are recommended by the ISPD. This combination is less toxic than amphotericin B and found to be as efficacious in retrospective studies. The dose for fluconazole is 200 mg orally or intraperitoneally, each day and that for flucytosine is a loading dose of 2 g orally followed by 1g each day (27). Clearance of fungal infection is rare and often leads to catheter removal (26).

Table 17–6. Empiric Initial Therapy for Peritoneal Dialysis Related Peritonitis

	Residual Urine Output	
Antibiotic	<100 mL/day	>100 mL/day
Cefazolin or cephalothin	1 g/bag (or 15 mg/kg/bag) qD	20 mg/kg/bag qDay
Ceftazidime	1 g/bag qD	20 mg/kg/bag qDay
Gentamicin, tobramycin, netilmycin	0.6 mg/kg/bag qDay	Not recommended
Amikacin	2 mg/kg/bag	Not recommended

Source: Adapted from (27).

Secondary Peritonitis

Bacterial Gram stain and cultures in secondary peritonitis are most commonly polymicrobial, with the source of peritoneal contamination containing progressively higher numbers of bacteria as one goes down the alimentary tract, and the greatest concentration of bacteria in the terminal colon. The best outcomes for secondary peritonitis are created by timely, aggressive surgical treatment combined with short courses of appropriate antimicrobial therapy (37). Antibiotics are therefore, in the ED, a critical adjunct in the treatment of bacterial secondary peritonitis. A regimen that covers gram-positive and gram-negative facultative and obligate anaerobes (*E. coli* and *Bacteroides fragilis* are most common) is recommended. There are several therapeutic combinations recommended in the literature, all with excellent efficacy, probably because the primary management of this condition is surgical. For community-acquired bacteria, a second-generation cephalosporin (i.e., cefotetan, cefoxitin) or ampicillin-sulbactam is adequate; however, third-generation cephalosporins offer additional gram-negative coverage. Other acceptable regimens would include the addition of metronidazole to the cephalosporin, the combination of ciprofloxacin and clindamycin, or the use of piperacillin-tazobactam, meropenem or imipenem-cilastatin in hospital acquired or severe cases (12, 38).

DISPOSITION

Peritonitis, whether primary or secondary in origin, can be associated with significant morbidity in the form of concomitant multisystem organ failure, as well as mortality. With very few exceptions, all patients with peritonitis will be admitted to the hospital for parenteral antibiotics in the case of SBP or bacterial infection in patients undergoing CAPD. There may be a small subset of well appearing patients with SBP, who may be treated as outpatients with ofloxacin (see the section Management). All cases of secondary peritonitis will require definitive surgical management to clear the bacterial infection and, therefore, require admission to the hospital as well.

CASE OUTCOME

In a search for the source of our patients' mental status decline, laboratory studies, including a complete blood cell count, electrolytes, coagulation panel, urinalysis and an ammonia level, were sent to the lab. The patient underwent diagnostic paracentesis after identification of a suitable area of ascitic fluid. The ascitic fluid was sent for cell count with differential, Gram stain and culture. The patient received intravenous normal saline in a 500 cc bolus. Approximately 2 h later, the lab returned the results which demonstrated a decline in his baseline creatinine to 2.4, a normal white blood cell count, thrombocytopenia, abnormal coagulation studies with an INR of 1.5, and a normal urinalysis and ammonia level. His ascitic fluid had 350 PMNs/mm^3 and his Gram stain was negative for any bacteria. Based on the PMN count being $\geq$250/mm^3, empiric cefotaxime was initiated at a dose of 1 g every 12 h, adjusted for his renal function (see Table 17–5). In an effort to decrease his overall morbidity and mortality, an initial dose of albumin at 1.5 g per kilogram was also given in the emergency department and the patient was admitted to the liver transplant service for further management and to await culture results.

REFERENCES

1. Garcia-Tsao G: Current management of the complications of cirrhosis and portal hypertension: variceal hemorrhage, ascites and spontaneous bacterial peritonitis. *Gastroenterology* 120:726–748, 2001.
2. Such J, Runyon BA: State-of-the-art clinical article: Spontaneous bacterial peritonitis. *Clin Infect Dis* 27:669–676, 1998.

3. Navasa M, Rodes RA: Bacterial infections in liver disease [review]. *Semin Liver Dis* 17(4):323–333, 1997.
4. Hillebrand DJ, Runyon BA: Clinical experience: Spontaneous bacterial peritonitis: Keys to management. *Hosp Pract* 35(5):87–90, 96–98, 2000.
5. Runyon BA: Low protein concentration is predisposed to spontaneous bacterial peritonitis. *Gastroenterology* 91: 1343–1346, 1986.
6. Andreu M, Sola R, Sitges-Serra A: Risk factors for spontaneous bacterial peritonitis in cirrhotic patients with ascites. *Gastroenterology* 104:1133–1138, 1993.
7. Gines P, Cardenas A, Arroyo V: Management of cirrhosis and ascites [Review]. *N Engl J Med* 350(16):1646–1654, 2004.
8. Hoefs JC, Canawatti HN, Sapico FL, et al.: Spontaneous bacterial peritonitis. *Hepatology* 2:399–407, 1982.
9. Guarner C, Soriano G: Spontaneous bacterial peritonitis. *Semin Liver Dis* 17(3):203–217, 1997.
10. Rimola A, Garcia-Tsao G, Navasa M: Diagnosis, treatment and prophylaxis of spontaneous bacterial peritonitis: A consensus document. International Ascites Club [Review]. *J Hepatol* 32(1):142–153, 2000.
11. Troidle L, Gorban-Brennan N, Kilger A: Renal research institute symposium: Continuous peritoneal dialysis-associated peritonitis: A review and current concepts. *Semin Dial* 16(6):428–437, 2003.
12. Wittmann DH, Schein M, Condon RE: Management of secondary peritonitis. *Ann Surg* 224(1):10–18, 1996.
13. Runyon BA: Early events in spontaneous bacterial peritonitis [Comment]. *Gut* 53(6):782–784, 2004.
14. Cirera I, Bauer TM, Navasa M: Bacterial translocation of enteric organisms in patients with cirrhosis. *J. Hepatol.* 34(1): 32–37, 2001.
15. Runyon BA, Hoefs JC: Ascitic fluid analysis in the differentiation of spontaneous bacterial peritonitis from gastrointestinal tract perforation into ascitic fluid. *Hepatology* 4:447–450, 1984.
16. Eichler M, Bessman SP: A double-blind study of the effect of ammonium infusion on psychological functioning in cirrhotic patients. *J. Nerv Ment Dis* 134:539, 1962.
17. Koopmans JG, Boeschoten EW, Pannekeet MM, et al.: Impaired initial cell reaction in CAPD-related peritonitis. *Perit Dial Int* 16(Suppl. 1):S362-S367, 1996.
18. Fenton S, Wu G, Cattran D, et al.: Clinical aspects of peritonitis in patients on CAPD. *Peri Dial Bull* 1(Suppl. 1):S4–S7, 1981.
19. Voinescu CG, Khanna R: Peritonitis in peritoneal dialysis. *Int J Artif Organs* 25(4):249–260, 2002.
20. Runyon BA: Monomicrobial nonneutrocytic bacterascites: A variant of spontaneous bacterial peritonitis. *Hepatology* 12(4):710–715, 1990.
21. Runyon BA: Paracentesis of ascitic fluid, a safe procedure. *Archiv Intern Med* 146:2259–2261, 1986.
22. Sakai H, Mendler MH, Runyon BA: The left lower quadrant is the best site for paracentesis: An ultrasound evaluation [abstract]. *Hepatology* 36:525A, 2002.
23. Runyon BA: AASLD practice guideline. Management of adult patients with ascites due cirrhosis. *Hepatology* 39(3):841–856, 2004.
24. Runyon, et al. The serum-ascites albumin gradient is superior to the exudate-transudate concept in the differential diagnosis of ascites. *Ann Intern Med* 117:215–220, 1992.
25. Runyon BA: Management of adult patients with ascites due to cirrhosis. *Hepatology* 39(3):841–856, 2004.
26. Teitelbaum I, Burkart J: Core curriculum in nephrology: Peritoneal dialysis. *Am J Kidney Dis* 42(5):1082–1096, 2003.
27. Keane W, Bailie G, Boeschoten E, et al.: ISPD guidelines/recommendations: Adult peritoneal dialysis-related peritonitis treatment recommendations: 2000 Update. *Perit Dial Int* 20:396–411, 2000.
28. Caruana RJ, Burkart J, Segraves D, Smallwood S, Haymore J, Disher B: Serum and peritoneal fluid amylase levels in CAPD. Normal values and clinical usefulness. *Am J Nephrol* 7:169–172, 1987.
29. Felisart J: Cefotaxime is more effective than is ampicillin-tobramycin in cirrhosis with severe infections. *Hepatology* 5(3):457–462, 1985.
30. Runyon BA: Short-course vs. long course antibiotic treatment of spontaneous bacterial peritonitis: A randomized controlled trial of 100 patients. *Gastroenterology* 100:1737–1742, 1991.
31. Navasa M: Randomized comparative study of oral ofloxacin versus intravenous cefotaxime in spontaneous bacterial peritonitis. *Gastroenterology* 111:1011–1017, 1996.
32. Follo A: Renal impairment after spontaneous bacterial peritonitis in cirrhosis: Incidence, clinical course, predictive factors and prognosis. *Hepatology* 20:1495–1501, 1994.
33. Sort P: Effect of intravenous albumin on renal impairment and mortality in patients with cirrhosis and spontaneous bacterial peritonitis. *N Engl J Med* 341:403–409, 1999.
34. Soriano G: Norfloxacin prevents bacterial infection in cirrhotics with gastrointestinal hemorrhage. *Gastroenterology* 103:1267–1272, 1992.
35. Bernard B: Antibiotic prophylaxis for the prevention of bacterial infections in cirrhotic patients with gastrointestinal bleeding: A meta-analysis. *Hepatology* 29:1655–1661, 1999.
36. Shemin D., Maaz D, St. Pierre D, et al.: Effect of aminoglycoside use on residual renal function in peritoneal patients. *Am J Kidney Dis* 34(1):14–20, 1999.
37. Bosscha K, van Vroonhoven TJMV, van der Werken C: Surgical management of severe secondary peritonitis. *Br J Surg* 86:1371–1377, 1999.
38. Farber MS, Abrams JH: Antibiotics for the acute abdomen. *Surg Clin N Am* 77(6):1395–1417, 1997.

18

Infectious Diarrhea

Tamara L. Thomas
Elizabeth Lynch

HIGH YIELD FACTS

1. Initial ED treatment for infectious diarrhea should focus on fluid resuscitation and correcting electrolyte imbalances.

2. Two types of patients may be considered for empiric antimicrobial therapy without additional evaluation: (1) those in whom bacterial diarrhea is suspected due to clinical features, dysentery, or the presence of occult blood or fecal leukocytes in stool samples and (2) patients in whom diarrhea has lasted for 2 weeks or longer and *Giardia* is suspected.

3. Historically, antimotility agents have not been recommended for patients who were thought to have dysentery due to the theoretical possibility of prolonging the disease state. However, recent research suggests that disease is not prolonged when an antibiotic is added to the antimotility agent.

4. Strategies that improve the cost effectiveness of stool cultures include selective testing for the most likely pathogen, a 3-day rule for hospital inpatients, and screening for inflammatory diarrhea.

5. Predictive factors for a positive stool culture include severe diarrhea, high fever, dysentery, positive fecal leukocytes, lactoferrin, or positive hemoccult stools.

CASE PRESENTATION

A 32-year-old male presents with a 3-day history of watery diarrhea. He complains of abdominal cramping and chills but denies nausea or vomiting. He is uncertain whether he has had blood in his stools and has not measured his fever. The patient feels generally weak and is dizzy when he stands. He has not traveled recently and has no ill contacts. His past medical history is negative with no history of being immunocompromised. He is married with two children and denies drug use. His vital signs are: temperature 101.8; pulse 120; respirations 20; and blood pressure 130/78. Laboratory data show an elevated white blood cell count of 18,000.

Electrolytes are normal except for a CO_2 of 18. Urinalysis is positive only for a trace of ketones. Stool is positive for occult blood. The following questions need to be answered.

1. What is the treatment priority?

2. Should this gentleman be presumptively treated with antibiotics?

3. Should stool cultures be sent?

INTRODUCTION

Diarrhea profoundly impacts worldwide health and is a significant cause of morbidity and mortality. In a review of 31 studies from selected countries an estimated 2.1 million childhood deaths attributed to diarrhea occurred in the world, primarily in developing countries (1). Diarrhea remains the third leading cause of death in children under 5 and accounts for more than 15% overall mortality (2).

In the United States, more than 200 million cases of diarrheal illness occur annually. Gastrointestinal illness rates, measured in extensive prospective studies over the past 50 years, range from 1 to 1.9 illnesses per person annually in the general population (3–5). Infectious diarrhea is one of the most common diagnoses in general practice with 73 million physician consultations, 1.8 million hospitalizations, and 500 deaths each year (6–9). It may account for up to 5% of U.S. emergency department visits (10).

It has been estimated that half of the annual 99 million adult patients with acute gastroenteritis or diarrhea in the United States had their activities restricted for more than a full day, 8.2 million consulted a physician, 250,000 people were hospitalized, 7.9 million saw a physician yet were not hospitalized, and more than 90 million experienced illness without seeking medical attention (5). The Center for Disease Control estimates that in the United States 76 million contract foodborne illnesses annually accounting for 325,000 hospitalizations and more than 5000 deaths (11, 12). In addition, health experts estimate that the yearly cost incurred in all foodborne diseases in the United States is $5–$6 billion in direct medical expenses and lost productivity. Infections with the bacteria *Salmonella* alone account for $1 billion yearly in both direct and indirect medical costs (13).

EPIDEMIOLOGY

Diarrheal illness is a problem worldwide, with substantial regional variation in the prevalence of specific pathogens, the availability of diagnosis and treatment, and the degree of prevention achieved.

The extremes of age are at higher risk for diarrhea illness. Twenty million episodes of diarrhea, 200,000 hospitalizations, and 400 deaths occur in children under 5 years annually. Morbidity and mortality of diarrhea is higher in the elderly than in other age groups (in the United States). Children also remain at higher risk for complications of diarrhea including fluid and electrolyte abnormalities. Diarrhea is a higher risk for those exposed to children and infants in the day care setting, immunosuppressed patients, travelers to developing regions, homosexual males, as well as those with potential exposure to contaminated water and food. Many diarrhea-causing organisms are easily transmitted through food or water and from one person to another (3). In addition, infectious diarrhea outbreaks are transmitted through foods, water, unpasteurized milk, chickens and eggs, fish contamination (particularly raw shellfish), and undercooked beef or pork.

Since immunocompromised patients are susceptible to enteric pathogens, patients with AIDS, on cancer chemotherapy, or with IgA deficiency are at higher risk for developing diarrhea. Patients with underlying medical diseases such as ulcerative colitis and Crohn disease experience more severe illness with diarrhea than normal hosts. Since gastric acid decreases the number of ingested pathogens, H2 blockers and proton pump inhibitors may increase the risk for developing diarrhea. While antacids reduce the stomach's acid barrier they are used intermittently and the stomach acid is probably intact when the food is ingested.

PATHOPHYSIOLOGY AND CLINICAL PRESENTATION

While the definition for acute diarrhea varies, it can be defined practically as an increased number of stools of decreased form (from the normal) lasting less than 14 days. A decrease in consistency and an increase in frequency of bowel movements to greater than or equal to three stools per day has often been used as a definition for epidemiological investigations (14). Additional associated signs and symptoms can include nausea, vomiting, abdominal pain and cramps, fever, bloody stools, tenesmus (constant sensation of urge to move bowels), and fecal urgency (6). Diarrhea can be characterized as acute or chronic. Diarrhea lasting as long as 14 days is considered persistent and that lasting more than a month is chronic diarrhea. The majority of diarrhea is classified as infectious (>80%) which is divided into two syndromes: inflammatory and nonin-

Table 18–1. Infectious Diarrhea—Common Agents (15)

Inflammatory	Noninflammatory
Bacteria	
C. jejuni	*V. cholerae*
Shigella	Enterotoxigenic *E. coli*
Nontyphi *Salmonella*	Foodborne
Enterohemorrhagic and	*S. aureus*
enteroinvasive *E. coli*	*Bacillus cereus*
C. difficile	
Parasites	
Entamoeba histolytica	*Giardia lamblia*
	C. parvum
Viruses	
	Rotavirus
	Calicivirus (includes Norwalk)
	Enteric adenovirus

flammatory. Inflammatory diarrhea is usually accompanied by abdominal pain, tenesmus, bloody (or hemoccult positive) stool, and fever. Organisms in inflammatory diarrhea can disrupt the mucosal lining of the colon (both macroscopically and microscopically). Noninflammatory diarrhea is usually a milder syndrome of symptoms that can include nausea, vomiting, abdominal cramping, and watery stools. Stools do not typically contain blood and polymorphonuclear cells although dehydration can occur. Organisms and toxins affect the small intestine more than the colon and typically do not disrupt the normal colonic mucosa. Although the greatest pathology is usually seen with those agents that cause invasive, inflammatory disease, any infectious agent can be associated with morbidity and mortality (Table 18–1).

Viruses cause the majority of infectious diarrhea followed by bacterial and parasitic organisms. The most commonly diagnosed virus-causing diarrhea in the United States is rotavirus, which accounts for the largest percentage of childhood diarrhea cases. It has seasonal peaks in the winter and spring and usually is managed supportively at home. Other viral agents contributing to diarrheal disease include Norwalk virus, enteric adenovirus, and hepatitis A. Common bacterial organisms causing diarrhea in the United States include *Campylobacter jejuni, Shigella* species, *Salmonella,* and *Yersinia enterocolitica.* Less common agents include *Clostridium perfringens, Staphylococcus aureus, Vibrio cholerae,* and *Vibrio parahaemolyticus.* Shigella species is made of four antigenic groups of 40 serotypes. In the United States,

Table 18–2. Common Diarrhea-Causing Agents

	Incubation Period (days)	Duration (days)	Transmission	Antibiotic
C. jejuni	1–7	7–10	Contaminated meats, milk products, water, exposure to infected pets	• Usually supportive • Erythromycin Tetracycline Aminoglycoside
Shigella	1–3	4–10	Fecal-oral route, contaminated food, water, or milk	• TMP-SMX, ampicillin, tetracycline
Salmonella	6 h to 2 days		Fecal-oral route, contaminated water and foods (poultry)	• Supportive • Occasional ampicillin, chloramphenicol, or TMP-SMX in patients susceptible to bacteremia
Y. enterocolitica	4–10	Usually 2 weeks but can be prolonged	Contaminated food or water, human/animal carriers	• Supportive • Antibiotics in severe cases
Enteropathogenic and invasive *E. coli*	1–3	1–2		• Supportive • BSS seem • TMP-SMX or ciprofloxacin in severe cases
E. histolytica			Travel associated, fecal-oral	• Antimicrobial agents necessary
C. difficile		Consider in patients with >3 days hospitalizations		• Vancomycin • Metronidazole • Ion-exchange resin cholestyramine
Travelers' diarrhea	1–4	3–4	Contaminated food/water	• Supportive • BSS may be helpful • Ciprofloxain

Shigella sonnei most commonly causes dysentery, which can range from mild to severe illness. *Salmonella enteritidis* includes 1700 serotypes, which can include an acute gastroenteritis, a carrier state, bacteremia, or an abscess syndrome. *Campylobacter* is responsible for both international and U.S. diarrhea disease. *Y. enterocolitica* is usually self-limited and may present with a mesenteric adenitis. Most diarrheal diseases due to parasites occur with protozoal infections (Table 18–2).

Emergency Infections Program Food borne Diseases Active Surveillance Network (FoodNet) collects data on 10 foodborne diseases (*Campylobacter*, shiga toxin-producing *E. coli* 0157, *Listeria monocytogenes*, *Salmonella*, *Shigella*, *Vibrio*, *Y. enterocolitica*,

Cryptosporidium parvum, Cyclospora cayetanensis, and cases of hemolytic-uremic syndrome) in nine U.S. sites. Preliminary surveillance data for 2002 reported a total of 16,580 laboratory-diagnosed cases of the 10 surveyed infections. Of the bacterial pathogens, *Salmonella* had the highest incidence (12).

EVALUATION AND MANAGEMENT

Most cases of diarrhea are managed at home by the patient or a family member and do not require medical attention. Medical care should, however, take place for a subset of patients. These patients include the very young or elderly, the immunocompromised, those with recent travel or antibiotic use, and patients with more severe or prolonged illness.

The history and physical exam alone rarely provide enough information to establish a definite diagnosis of acute diarrhea. However, the history assists in developing a differential diagnosis and focused work-up. Initial ED treatment should focus on fluid resuscitation and correcting electrolyte imbalances. Fluid resuscitation aims to restore fluid losses and prevent further dehydration. Most patients can be orally rehydrated.

In otherwise healthy adults with acute diarrhea, sports drinks, diluted fruit juices, and other flavored soft drinks accompanied by saltine crackers, broth, and soup are sufficient for rehydration (6). Alternatively, a homemade oral rehydrating solution (ORS) can be prepared by alternating two separate glasses, the first containing 8 ounces of orange juice, or other potassium-containing fruit juice, one-half teaspoon honey or corn syrup, and a pinch of table salt. The second glass should contain 8 ounces clear water and one-quarter teaspoon of baking soda (6). Elderly

or immunocompromised patients should consume solutions containing sodium (45–75 mEq/L), such as Pedialyte or Rehydralyte (6). In children who are not dehydrated, 100 mL/kg of ORS should be given over 24 h. However, children are least likely to take ORS, due to the salty taste. If stool output is modest and the child continues to take age-appropriate foods and fluids are encouraged, ORS may be unnecessary (16). If mild dehydration is noted, fluid correction of 50 mL/kg should be given in the first 4 h in addition to replacing ongoing losses. Moderate dehydration requires 100 mL/kg during the first 4–6 h as well as replacement (16, 17). Ongoing losses are replaced with 10 mL/kg of ORS for each episode of diarrhea. Additionally, the volume of any emesis should be estimated and replaced as well. Rehydration status should be monitored frequently (every hour) and ongoing losses should be calculated and added into the remaining volume. Solutions similar to the World Health Organization's rehydration therapy are recommended. Table 18–3 compares various commercially available solutions.

More severely dehydrated patients, or patients unable to tolerate oral fluids, will require intravenous therapy and hospitalization. Initial fluid choices are normal saline or Ringer lactate. Adults may receive an initial 500 mL–1 L bolus and then be reassessed. Pediatric patients should be given 20 mL/kg normal saline or the Ringer lactate over 1 h. This may be repeated, and patients should be monitored closely during the rehydration phase.

Medications

Antimicrobial

Empiric antimicrobial therapy for infectious diarrhea is controversial (3, 6, 19). Two types of patients may be considered for empiric antimicrobial therapy without

Table 18–3. Oral Rehydration Solutions and Commonly Consumed Fluids (18)

	CHO (g/dL)	Na$^+$ (mEq/L)	K$^+$ (mEq/L)	Cl$^-$ (mEq/L)	Base (mEq/L)	mOsm/kg H$_2$O
Infalyte	3	50	25	45	30	200
Pedialyte	2.5	45	20	35	30	250
Rehydralyte	205	75	20	65	30	310
WHO/UNICEF ORS	2	90	20	80	30	310
Gatorade[a]	5.9	21	2.5	17	–	377
Apple juice[a]	11.9	0.4	26	–	–	700
Orange juice[a]	10.4	0.2	49	–	50	654
Ginger ale[a]	9	3.5	0.1	–	3.6	565

[a]Not recommended for ORT except as indicated in text.

additional evaluation: (1) those in whom bacterial diarrhea is suspected due to clinical features, dysentery, or the presence of occult blood or fecal leukocytes in stool samples and (2) patients in whom diarrhea has lasted for 2 weeks or longer and *Giardia* is suspected (6). The usual recommended therapy for adult patients with suspected bacterial diarrhea (fever greater than 38.5°C or >101.3°F, plus grossly bloody stools, hemoccult positive stools, or leukocyte- or lactoferrin-positive stools) is a quinolone antimicrobial for 3–5 days (6, 20). In these patients, antibiotics decreased both the length and severity of illness (21). Traveler's diarrhea, with enterotoxicogenic *E. coli* most often implicated, should also be treated with quinolone antibiotics for 1–5 days duration. Patients with persistent diarrhea suggestive of *Giardia* may be started on metronidazole for a 7-day course. The American Academy of Pediatricians advises against empiric administration of antimicrobial agents for children with acute diarrhea (16).

Patients not begun on empiric antimicrobial therapy should await culture results. The most common bacterial causes of community-acquired infectious diarrhea are *C. jejuni*, non-typhi *Salmonella* species, *Shigella* species, and the enterohemorrhagic *E. coli* O157:H7 (22).

Patients with culture-proven *Campylobacter* may be treated with erythromycin or azithromycin to shorten the duration of the illness (6). Quinolone antibiotics may be used if the organism has been shown to be sensitive. Resistance to quinolones is increasing in *Campylobacter* infections worldwide.

Nontyphi *Salmonella* infections are usually self-limited and do not require antibiotic therapy, which can prolong fecal shedding of the organism and also may increase the incidence of relapse (6, 22) Selected patients should be considered for treatment with a quinolone, including those with fever and evidence of systemic infection, dysentery, or underlying immunosuppression. Additionally, because bacteremia can occur in 2–14% of cases, patients with an aortic aneurysm, prosthetic heart valve, vascular graft, or orthopedic prosthesis should be treated to decrease the risk of localized extra-intestinal infection (6).

Treatment for shigellosis is recommended, both in order to shorten the illness and to decrease the potential for person-to-person spread. The treatment of choice for infections acquired in the United States is trimethoprim/sulfamethoxiazole (TMP/SMX). If the infection is acquired during travel, a quinolone is recommended, due to TMP resistance (6).

Hemolytic uremic syndrome (HUS) has been linked to infections with cytotoxin producing strains of *E. coli*, especially *E. coli* 0157:H7, and *Shigella*. Although HUS can occur at any age, it is most common before the second decade of life. About 90% of cases of pediatric HUS are associated with *E. coli* enterocolitis (23). Previous studies have suggested that antibiotic administration might lead to release of toxins from the killed organisms and subsequent increased incidence of HUS (19, 21). Children infected with *E. coli* O157:H7 presented earlier in their course and were more likely to have blood in their stool and abdominal tenderness than those with non-Shiga toxin producing *E. coli* (24). However, retrospective reviews of antibiotic therapy during the Sakai (Japan) outbreak of *E. coli* O157:H7 suggest that the use of oral fluoroquinolones to treat diarrheal illnesses is associated with a lower incidence of HUS, absence of Shiga toxin in the gut, and eradication of *E. coli* from the gut (25, 26). These authors suggest that the use of suitable quinolone antibiotics can prevent the development of *E. coli* O157:H7-associated HUS. In the United States, quinolones are not routinely recommended for children <12 years. The Center for Disease Control does not currently recommend antimicrobial therapy for *E. coli* 0157:H7.

Table 18–4 lists the antimicrobial therapy of choice and duration of treatment for different pathogens.

Other Medications

Biotherapeutic agents show promise in the treatment of infectious diarrhea. With potential antibiotic resistance due to empiric treatment, new strategies for treatment are emerging. A largely unexplored area is the use of living therapeutic organisms—biotherapeutic agents. These agents have the potential advantages of providing multiple mechanisms of action, lowering dependence on antibiotics, and decreasing cost and in addition are easily tolerated by patients. Future needs are to identify which types of infectious diarrhea respond to biotherapeutic agents as well as to conduct systematic placebo trials (27).

Symptomatic relief of diarrhea is promoted by drugs such as kaolin/pectin, anticholingerics, activated charcoal, lactobacillus preparation, and hydrophilic agents, which have shown no significant benefit in many diarrhea studies (28, 29). Attapulgite, a nonabsorbable magnesium aluminum silicate, has shown positive results by giving stool form but does not decrease stool frequency, cramps, or illness length (30). Bismuth subsalicylate (BSS) decreased the number of unformed stools by almost 50% and shortened duration of illness in several placebo-controlled studies (30, 31). BSS has also been show to have some antibacterial activity which adds value to its use as a prophylactic agent in travelers' diarrhea (32, 33). Caution should be used in children due to the large salicylate exposure and risks of toxicity or the Reyes syndrome. BSS

Table 18–4. Antimicrobial Therapy for Common Infectious Agents

Infectious Agent	Antibiotic of Choice	Alternate Regimen	Duration of Treatment
B. cereus	Usually none needed, if severe vancomycin, clindamycin	Fluoroquinolones	3 days
C. jejuni	Azithromycin, erythromycin	Fluoroquinolones if susceptible, tetracycline, aminoglycoside	3–5 days
C. difficile	Metronidazole	Vancomycin	10–14 days
C. perfringens	Metronidazole	Doxycycline	7 days
C. parvum	Nitazoxanide	Paromycin + azithromycin	3 days (in AIDS patients use alt regimen for 4 weeks)
E. histolytica	Paromycin	Diloxanide furoate	10 days
Enterotoxigenic *E. coli*	Ciprofloxacin	Azithromycin	1–5 days
E. coli O157:H7	None—may increase risk of HUS		
G. lamblia	Metronidazole	Tinadazole, paromycin	7 days
L. monocytogenes	Ampicillin	TMP/SMX	
Norwalk agent	Bismuth subsalicylate (not in peds or AIDS)	None	Until symptoms resolve
Rotavirus	None		
S. enteritidis	Ciprofloxacin	Azithromycin	3 days (treatment may increase shedding and risk of relapse); treat patients with indwelling devices and grafts
Shigella sp.	TMP/SMX	Azithromycin (fluoroquinolone if acquired during travels)	3 days
S. aureus	None		
V. cholerae	Ciprofloxacin	Doxycycline, TMP/SMX	1 dose 3 days
V. parahaemolyticus	None		
Y. enterocolitica	Ciprofloxacin	TMP/SMX	3 days

is not recommended in the immunocompromised patient because of the excessive dosing used in persistent diarrhea and possible development of bismuth encephalopathy.

Antimotility drugs are the most common medications directed toward treating symptoms. They facilitate intestinal absorption by slowing intraluminal flow of liquid. While frequent bowel movements and painful abdominal cramping may be treated with antimotility agents, these agents have historically been avoided due to the possibility of prolonging the disease course of invasive enteropathogens. Patients with bloody diarrhea treated with diphenyoxlate alone had a longer disease course than did placebo-treated patients. However, recent research shows that disease is not prolonged when an antibiotic is added to loperamide (34–37). One randomized, double-blinded, placebo-controlled trial compared ciprofloxacin and loperamide with ciprofloxacin and placebo in adult dysentery patients and found that the ciprofloxacin/loperamide group had a decreased number of stools and a shorter duration of illness. The loperamide group had no complications (37). There still appear to be some questions about antimotility agents in certain patient groups and there may be some geographic variations in practice. In patients with enterohemorrhagic *E. coli* (EHEC) infection, antimotility agent use might facilitate hemolytic uremic syndrome (38) or worsen neurologic symptoms (39). Some authorities do not recommend or feel there are insufficient data for antimotility agent use in young children (40, 41). Others believe loperamide to be safe in children greater than 2 years of age unless they have an indication of an invasive organism(42). Loperamide in children younger than 2 years of age was reported to cause drowsiness but showed a decrease in stool volume in the sickest children admitted to hospital with dehydration requiring intravenous therapy (40).

Loperamide is the most commonly recommended agent for symptomatic diarrhea treatment due to safety and an expected efficacy in which stool is reduced by about 80% (34). Loperamide is rapidly absorbed and acts faster than BSS preparations (31, 34). Studies evaluating the combination of an antibiotic and loperamide (with each agent dosed as usual) show superior results compared to either agent alone (34, 36). In one study, over half of the subjects had no further unformed stools when combination therapy was initiated (34). Diphenoxylate plus atropine, a prescription drug, is less effective than loperamide with more side effects. Recently a new calmodulin inhibitor, Zaldaride, was reported as useful in decreasing the duration of diarrhea from an average of 42 h in untreated subjects to an average of 20 h (35, 36). Loperamide continues to be recommended for diarrhea of uncertain etiology. In refractory cases of AIDS-induced diarrhea, octreotide, a synthetic cyclic octapeptide analog of somatostatin, may be effective (6).

Diagnostic Testing

Most acute diarrhea episodes are self-limited and since they do not require medical care, diagnostic testing is rarely helpful in the emergency setting. However, the lack of a specific diagnosis can delay appropriate management and treatment of many infections. While the patient's history and clinical findings give important clues, an organism-specific diagnosis is necessary for some pathogens. As resistant microbe strains increase, treatment failures will become more common. In addition an organism-specific diagnosis allows antimicrobial therapy to be used more judiciously. Fecal leukocytes, lactoferrin, or hemoccult blood tests can be useful for screening patients with moderate to severe infectious diarrhea because they can support empiric therapy in febrile patients

and when negative may eliminate the need for stool culture (6).

Who should be tested? Consensus guidelines published by both the American College of Gastroenterology and the Infectious Diseases Society of America review strategies to develop cost-effective diagnostic approaches for infectious diarrhea (3, 6). Fecal leukocytes, lactoferrin or occult blood are found in diarrhea patients with diffuse colonic inflammation (43, 44). The most commonly identified pathogens in patients with a positive test result include *Shigella, Salmonella, Campylobacter, Aeromonas, Yersinia*, noncholera *Vibrio*s, and *Clostridium difficile* (43, 44).

Fecal Leukocytes

A positive Wright stain has a sensitivity of 82% and specificity of 83% for presence of a bacterial pathogen (45). Loeffler methylene blue and Gram stain may also be used for direct microscopic examination of fecal specimens. A positive test is three or greater leukocytes in at least four fields. A positive test suggests colon inflammation and an invasive diarrhea. This may help to guide the decision of which patients should receive antibiotics.

Bacterial Stool Culture

Patients experiencing severe diarrhea, an oral temperature $>101.3°F$ ($38.5°C$), bloody stool, stools containing hemoccult blood, leukocytes or lactoferrin, or nontreated diarrhea that has been persistent should received a stool culture (6). Predictive factors for a positive stool culture include severe diarrhea, high fever, dysentery, positive fecal leukocytes, lactoferrin, or positive hemoccult stools.

U.S. studies show that stool studies are often inappropriately ordered resulting in excessive medical costs (46). Due to the low sensitivity for detecting pathogens, each positive routine stool culture costs the laboratory about $950–$1200 (depending on the number of samples tested and tests run per sample) (46). This impressive cost results from the relative insensitivity of the test for the most likely pathogens and the poor selection of specimens being cultured (3).

Strategies that improve the cost effectiveness of stool cultures include selective testing for the most likely pathogen, a 3-day rule for hospital inpatients, and screening for inflammatory diarrhea. To decrease costs and increase yields, diagnostic testing should be limited to those with a high pretest probability of bacterial disease such as toxic or severely dehydrated children, immunocompromised patients, and those with >3 days of symptoms. Other scenarios that may require testing include suspected outbreaks, prolonged diarrheal illness, and immunosuppressed patients.

Stool culture usefulness has been questioned. In a 1996 survey of FoodNet (Foodborne Diseases Active Surveillance Network) clinical laboratories, 233,212 stool specimens for *Salmonella* and *Shigella* estimated crude yield estimates of 0.9% for Salmonella and 0.6% for Shigella. *Campylobacter* and *E. coli* 0157 gave crude yield estimates of 1.4% and 0.3%, respectively. Other reports show similar culture yields, from 1.5 to 2.9% (3). Most labs routinely culture for three common bacterial enteropathogens: *Salmonella, Shigella,* and *Campylobacter.* A number of bacterial enteropathogens are not detected in routine stool cultures and should be tested for in certain epidemiologic circumstances. Some of these pathogens include *E. coli* 0157:H7 and other Shigatoxin producing *E. coli, V. cholerae,* other noncholera *Vibrios,* and some Y*ersinia* (3, 6, 47, 48). *E. coli* 0157:H7 can be detected by stool culture using specialized media but the other diarrheagenic *E. coli* are only detected by research laboratories. A 1996 survey found physicians were more likely to request a stool culture for patients with AIDS, bloody stools, fever, recent travel to a developing country, diarrhea for 13 days, or those receiving intravenous rehydration. Twenty-eight percent of physicians were unsure for which specific organisms stool cultures were tested, suggesting a need for education (49).

Ova and Parasites

Ova and parasites (O and P), while less studied than routine stool cultures, are not felt to be cost effective for acute diarrhea in the United States. O and P have a low sensitivity since many parasites are fastidious and organism shedding is intermittent. Multiple samples may need to be obtained to achieve a positive result. However, parasitic causes may need to be investigated if diarrhea is persistent. Recent travel to Russia (*Cryptosporidium* and *Giardia*), Nepal (*Cyclosporine*), or mountainous areas *(Giardia)* should raise suspicion for potential parasitic illness. Intestinal amebiasis usually does not exhibit numerous fecal leukocytes due to uninflamed mucosa between ulcerations and due to the lytic effect of exotoxins produced by the organism. In day care centers outbreaks, *Giardia* and *Cryptosporidium* are common causes of diarrhea. Homosexual males may be infected with parasites (*Giardia* and *Entamoeba histolytica*). Recently, direct immunofluorescence

antibody tests have been shown to improve the sensitivity for detecting *Entamoeba, Giardia,* and *Cryptosporidium.* Immunofluorescent antibody tests and diagnostic enzyme immunoassays add sensitivity, specificity, speed, and cost over ova and parasite tests (15).

C. difficile Toxin Assay

C. difficile toxin can be tested by tissue culture assay or enzyme immunoassay and should be tested in patients who have recently used antibiotics (within last 2 weeks) or had a recent hospitalization. *C. difficile* assay has a 10% false negative rate and may be unavailable to emergency physicians (test usually take 24 h) (50).

Other Diagnostic Tests

Lactoferrin is an indirect measure of leukocytes and has shown promise as a screening test for invasive diarrhea. Yong et al. found fecal lactoferrin test to be more sensitive (75%) than methylene blue microscopy (40% sensitivity) (51). Other potentially useful but less used diagnostic tests include enzyme immunoassays for viruses and parasites, electron microscopy for virus identification, and flexible sigmoidoscopy for biopsy and histology. Investigation into virus pathologies is not routinely indicated since there is no specific treatment for these agents. An effective rotavirus vaccine was available briefly until it was associated with an increased risk of intussusception.

PREVENTION

Many diarrheal diseases can be prevented by simple hand washing (soap and water) and safe food preparation techniques. Immunocompromised people (chemotherapy patients, immunocompromised, those on steroids and other immunosuppressive therapies) are more susceptible to infections with a variety of enteric pathogens. This group is at an increased risk for infections from *L. monocytogenes* and should avoid soft cheeses, raw dairy products, and unheated deli meats. Those with chronic liver disease are at an increased risk for infection due to *Vibrio vulnificus* often contracted from raw shellfish and should avoid them. Pregnant women should avoid undercooked meats to avoid potential infection from *Toxoplasma gondii* or *L. monocytogenes,* both of which are associated with miscarriage. Several vaccines are available for typhoid and may be recommended to the U.S. traveler with potential exposure. Cholera vaccines are available outside the

United States. Rotavirus vaccine, although effective, is not currently available due to complications.

CONCLUSION

Infectious diarrhea remains a significant cause of morbidity in the United States. Epidemiological factors are important to the patient's history in directing a focused workup. The majority of treatment is supportive; however, empiric treatment is indicated in several circumstances. Treatment in the ED should concentrate on rehydration. Strategies for diagnostic testing should focus on cost-effective and selective testing for the most likely pathogen, a 3-day rule for hospital inpatients, and screening for inflammatory diarrhea. Patients experiencing severe diarrhea, an oral temperature $>101.3°F$ ($38.5°C$), bloody stool, stools containing hemoccult blood, leukocytes or lactoferrin, or nontreated diarrhea that has been persistent should be tested.

CASE OUTCOME

For this gentleman treatment priority was fluid balance and he was intravenously rehydrated with 2 L of normal saline with subsequent improvement of his orthostatic symptoms. Since he has a suspected bacterial diarrhea (due to clinical features and the presence of occult blood in the stool) he is a candidate for presumptive antibiotic treatment. Alternatively, with 3 days of symptoms and positive culture predictors (severe diarrhea, high fever, dysentery, and positive hemoccult stools) a decision was made as to whether he would be presumptively treated or cultures obtained. After rehydration, this patient was presumptively treated with ciprofloxacin for 5 days.

REFERENCES

1. Child Health Epidemiology Reference Group. Department of Child and Adolescent Health, World Health Organization, 2002. www.who.int/
2. World Health Report 2003. Shaping the future. http://www.who.int/whr/en/. Accessed April 24, 2004.
3. Guerrant RL, Van Gilder T, Steiner TS, et al: Practice guidelines for management of infectious diarrhea. *Clin Infect Dis* 32(3):331–351, 2001.
4. Feldman R, Banatvala N: The frequency of culturing stools from adults with diarrhoea in Great Britain. *Epidemiol Infect* 113:41–44, 1994.
5. Garthwright W, Archer D, Kvenberg J: Estimates of incidence and cost of intestinal infectious diseases in the United States. *Public Health Rep* 103:107–115, 1988.
6. DuPont HL; Guidelines on acute infectious diarrhea in adults. *Am J Gastroenterol* 92(11):1962–1975, 1997.
7. Herikstadt H, Vergia D, Hadler J, et al.: Population-based estimate of the burden of diarrheal illnesses: Food Net 1996–1997. 1st International Conference on Emerging Infectious Disease (Atlanta), March 1998.
8. LeClere FB, Moss JA, Everhart HE, et al.: Prevalence of major digestive disorders and bowel symptoms. A989, *Adv Data* 212:1–15, 1992.
9. Mead PS, Slutsker L, Dietz V, et al.: Food-related illness and death in the United States. *Emerg Infect Dis* 607–625, 1999.
10. Gough JE, Clement PA: *Diarrhea in Marx: Rosen's Emergency Medicine: Concepts And Clinical Practice*. St. Louis, Mosby, Inc, 2002, pp 200–207.
11. Center for Disease Control Website. Preliminary FoodNet data on the incidence of foodborne illnessesselected site, United States, 2002. http://www.cdc.gov/mmwr/preview/mmwrhtml/mm5215a4.htm Accessed on April 15, 2004.
12. FoodNet Working Group: Preliminary FoodNet data on the incidence of foodborne illnesses-selected sites, United States, 2002. *Morb Mortal Wkly Rep* 52:3410.343, 2003.
13. National Institute of Allergy and Infectious Diseases (NIAID): Food borne disease fact sheet 2002 http://www.niaid.nih.gov/factsheets/foodbornedis.htm Accessed on April 15, 2004.
14. Guerrant RL, Shield DS, Thorson SM, et al.: Evaluation and diagnosis of acute infectious diarrhea. *Am J Med* 78:91–98, 1985.
15. Turgeon DK, Fritsche TR: Laboratory approaches to infectious diarrhea. *Gastroenterol Clin* 30:693–707, 2001.
16. American Academy of Pediatrics: Practice parameter: The management of acute gastroenteritis in young children. *Pediatrics* 97(3):424–435, 1996.
17. Ramaswamy K, Jacobson K: Infectious diarrhea in children. *Gastroenterol Clin* 30(3):611–624, 2001.
18. Gunn VL, Nechyba C (eds.): *Johns Hopkins: The Harriet Lane Handbook: A Manual for Pediatric House Officers, 16th ed.* St. Louis, Mosby, Inc, 2002.
19. American Medical Association, Centers for Disease Control and Prevention, Center for Food Safety and Applied Nutrition, Food and Drug Administration Food Safety and Inspection Service, US Department of Agriculture: Diagnosis and management of foodborne illnesses: A primer for physicians. *Morb Mortal Wkly Rep Recomm Rep* 50(RR-2):1–69, 2001.
20. Brown T: Commentary on acute infectious gastroenteritis. *Ann Emerg Med* 42:420–422, 2003.
21. Gore J, Surawicz C: Severe acute diarrhea. *Gastroenterol Clin* 32(4):1249–1267, 2003.
22. Procop GW: Gastrointestinal infections. *Infect Dis Clin NA* 15(4):1073–1108, 2001.
23. Besser RE: *Escherichia coli* O157:H7 gastroenteritis and the hemolytic uremic syndrome: An emerging infectious disease. *Annu Rev Med* 50:355–367, 1999.

24. Klein EJ, Stapp JR, Clausen CR, et al.: Shiga toxin-producing *Escherichia coli* in children with diarrhea: A prospective point-of-care study. *J Pediatr* 141(2):172–177, 2002.
25. Higami S: Retrospective analysis of the relationship between HUS incidence and antibiotics among patients with *Escherichia coli* O157 enterocolitis in the Sakai outbreak [abstract]. *Kansenshogaku Zasshi* 72(3):266–272, 1998.
26. Shiomi M: Effect of early oral fluoroquinolones in hemorrhagic colitis due to *Eschericia coli* O157:H7. *Pediatr Int* 41(2):228–232, 1999.
27. Elmer GW, McFarland LV: Biotherapeutic agents in the treatment of infectious diarrhea. *Gastroenterol. Clin.* 30:837–854, 2001.
28. National Institute of Health Consensus Development Conference: Travelers' diarrhea. *JAMA* 253:2700–2704, 1985.
29. Center for Disease Control and Prevention Website. www.cdc.gov/foodnet/pub/CID/2004sup.htm Accessed on April 15, 2004.
30. Adachi JA, Backer HD, DuPont HL: Infectious diarrhea from wilderness and foreign travel, in Auerbach PS (ed.): *Wilderness Medicine.* St. Louis, Mosby Inc, 2001; pp 1237–1250.
31. Steffen R: Worldwide efficacy of bismuth subsalicylate in the treatment of travelers' diarrhea. *Rev Infect Dis* 12(Suppl. 1): S80–S86, 1990.
32. Cornick NA, Silva M, Gorbach SL: In vitro antibacterial activity of bismuth subsalicylate. *Rev Infect Dis* 12(Suppl. 1): S9–S10, 1990.
33. Graham D, Estes M, Gentry L: Double-blind comparison of bismuth subsalicylate and placebo in the prevention and treatment of enterotoxigenic *Escherichia coli*. *Gastroenterology* 85(5):1017–1022, 1983.
34. Johnson PC, Ericsson CD, DuPont HL et al.: Comparison of loperamide with bismuth subsalicylate for the treatment of acute travelers' diarrhea. *JAMA* 255(6):757–760, 1986.
35. DuPont HL, Ericsson CD, Mathewson JJ et al.: Zalaride maleate, an intestinal calmodulin inhibitor, in the therapy of travelers' diarrhea. *Gastroenterology* 104:709–715, 1993.
36. Ericsson CD, DuPont HL, Mathewson JS: Single dose of loxacin plus loperamide compared with a single dose or three days of ofloxacin in treatment of travelers' diarrhea. *J Travel Med* 4:3–7, 1997.
37. Murphy G, Bodhidatta L, Echeverria P, et al.: Ciprofloxacin and loperamide in treatment of bacillary dysentery. *Ann Intern Med* 118:582–586, 1993.
38. Cimolai N, Carter J, Morrison B, et al.: Risk factors for the progression of *Escherichia coli* 0157:H7 enteritis to hemolytic-uremic syndrome. *J Pediatr* 116:582–592, 1990.
39. Cimolai N, Morrison B, Carter J: Risk factors for central nervous system manifestations of gastroenteritis-associated hemolytic-uremic syndrome. *Pediatric* 90:616–621, 1992.
40. Motala C, Hill ID, Mann MD, et al.: Effect of loperamide stool output and duration of acute infectious diarrhea in infants. *J Pediatr* 117:467–471, 1990.
41. Group Diarrhea and Dehydrating Diseases: Loperamide in acute diarrhea in childhood: Results of a double-blind placebo controlled multicenter clinical trial. *BMJ* 298:1263–1267, 1984.
42. Rose SR: *International Travel Health Guide, 7th ed.* Northampton MA, , Travel Medicine, Inc., 1996.
43. Harris J, DuPont H, Hornick R: Fecal leukocytes in diarrheal illness. *Ann Intern Med* 76:696–703, 1972.
44. McNeely W, DuPont H, Mathewson J, et al.: Occult blood versus fecal leukocytes in the diagnosis of bacterial diarrhea. A study of U.S. travelers to Mexico and Mexican children. *Am J Trop Med Hyg* 55:430–433, 1996.
45. DuBois D, Binder L, Nelson B: Usefulness of stool Wright's stain in the emergency department. *J Emerg Med* 6:483, 1988.
46. Koplan JP, Fineberg HV, Ferraro MJB, et al.: Value of stool cultures. *Lancet* 2:413–416, 1980.
47. Morris J Jr., Black R: Cholera and other Vibrioses in the United States. *N Engl J Med* 312:343–350, 1985.
48. Lee L, Taylor J, Carter G, et al.: *Yersinia enterocolitica* 0:3: An emergency cause of pediatric gastroenteritis in the United States. *J Infect Dis* 163:66–63, 1991.
49. Hennessy TW, Marcus R, Deneen V: Survey of physician diagnostic practices for patients with acute diarrhea: Clinical and public health implications. *Clin Infect Dis* 38(Suppl. 3): S203–S211, 2004.
50. Bartlett JG: Clinical practice—antibiotic-associated diarrhea. *N Engl J Med* 346(5):334–339, 2002.
51. Yong WH, Mattia AR, Ferraro MJ: Comparison of fecal lactoferrin latex agglutination assay and methylene blue microscopy for detection of fecal leukocytes in *Clostridium difficile*-associated disease. *J Clin Microbiol* 32:1360, 1994.

19

HIV-Associated Gastrointestinal Infections

Andrew Nevins
Mark Holodniy

HIGH YIELD FACTS

1. Gastrointestinal (GI) symptoms represent the most common presentation of HIV-infected patients to the emergency department.

2. Diarrhea and abdominal pain are seen in the majority of HIV-infected patients at some time during infection and can be the result of HIV-associated or non-HIV-associated infectious or noninfectious causes (particularly HIV-specific medications).

3. Opportunistic infections (OIs) (i.e., cytomegalovirus, mycobacterium avium complex, cryptosporidiosis) affecting the GI tract are unlikely in patients with CD4 counts >200/mm^3. Thus, it is important to know the patient's HIV immunologic status (i.e., asymptomatic with high CD4 counts versus AIDS) in determining the differential diagnosis of GI infections.

4. Abdominal imaging studies, such as ultrasound or computed tomography (CT) scans, can reveal significant pathology, but are not specific for GI infections in HIV-infected patients.

CASE PRESENTATION

A 47-year-old woman presents to the emergency department with increasing diarrhea and lower abdominal pain over the last week. She denies any nausea or vomiting, but states she feels like she has had a fever. She describes the pain as being intermittently crampy with some bloating. She was diagnosed with HIV and hepatitis C virus (HCV) infection 3 years ago. Her CD4 count at the time of diagnosis was 68/mm^3. She has been receiving a highly active antiretroviral therapy (HAART) regimen consisting of nelfinavir (Viracept®), ddI (Videx EC®), and 3TC (Epivir®) for the last 2 years. Her last known CD4 count was 240/mm^3, but she admits that her adherence to her HAART regimen has been poor at times. She usually has 2–3 loose brown stools per day, which are controlled with

oral loperamide as needed. She states that her stool frequency has increased to 5–6 stools per day and that they are now watery in consistency. She has not noticed any blood in her stool. She denies any recent travel or new medications, and has two cats at home. She has had no recent sexual contact and denies any injection drug use for the last 2 years.

In the emergency department her examination is significant for a temperature of 101.3°F and orthostatic hypotension. She has maxillary wasting and truncal obesity suggestive of lipodystrophic changes secondary to HAART. Oropharyngeal exam is significant for oral thrush along the right buccal mucosa and posterior pharynx. Her abdominal exam reveals hyperactive bowel sounds, a soft abdomen, and moderate suprapubic and left lower quadrant tenderness to deep palpation. A pelvic exam demonstrates vaginal candidiasis, but is otherwise normal and no cervical motion or adnexal tenderness is appreciated. There is no stool found upon digital rectal examination, but rectal-associated secretions are positive for trace occult blood.

INTRODUCTION/EPIDEMIOLOGY

As described earlier in Chapter 8, HIV infection affects millions of people worldwide. Gastrointestinal symptoms are reported by over 90% of patients at some time during their disease. Many of these symptoms are associated with HIV infection itself or with medications for HIV treatment; however, with advancing HIV disease and development of AIDS, significantly more gastrointestinal infections are found. Overall, in developed countries, there has been a significant reduction in AIDS-associated OIs of the GI system because of HAART and the use of chronic antimicrobial prophylaxis such as trimethoprim-sulfamethoxazole (TMP-SMX) and azithromycin against OIs. However, since more than one-third of patients are chronically coinfected with HCV or hepatitis B virus (HBV) as a consequence of similar transmission mechanisms, new challenges present in the management of these patients.

PATHOPHYSIOLOGY/MICROBIOLOGY

Many pathogens can affect the gastrointestinal system, resulting in infection anywhere from the oral cavity to the anus. Some can be seen throughout the GI tract, whereas others localize to specific organs or luminal sites within the GI tract. Some are common primarily among HIV-infected patients, particularly in whom profound immune

Table 19–1. Common Infectious Etiologies Causing Gastrointestinal Disease in HIV-Infected Individuals

	Oral/Esophageal	Intestinal	Anorectal	Hepatobiliary/Pancreatic
Bacteria	Group A streptococcus	*C. difficile*	*N. gonorrhea*	*E. coli* *Klebsiella* spp.
	N. gonorrhea	Salmonella spp.	*Chlamydia trachomatis*	*Proteus* spp.
	T. pallidum	Shigella spp. Campylobacter *E. coli* spp. MAC MTB	*T. pallidum*	*Bacteroides fragilis* *Bartonella* spp. MAC
Viruses	HSV-1, HSV-2 CMV EBV HPV	CMV Adenoviruses Rotaviruses Noroviruses Coronaviruses	HPV HSV CMV	Hepatitis C Hepatitis B Hepatitis A CMV EBV
Fungi	*C. albicans* Other *Candida* spp.			
Parasites		*G. lamblia* *E. histolytica* *C. parvum* *I. belli* *C. cayetanensis* *Microsporidia* spp. (*Enterocytozoon bieneusi* 90%) *T. gondii*		*E. histolytica* *C. parvum* *Microsporidia* spp.

HSV = herpes simplex virus, CMV = cytomegalovirus, HPV = human papilloma virus, MTB = *M. tuberculosis,* MAC = Mycobacterium avium-intracellulare complex.

suppression is present, while other infections are seen commonly in non-HIV-infected patients as well as HIV-infected patients. Multiple concomitant infections are possible. Most acute infections are the result of fecal-oral contact or contact with contaminated food or water. Once ingested, organisms localize in various locations where disease is established. Disease can result simply from attachment, or enteroinvasion, with resultant damage to mucosal cells, ulcerative disease and subsequent blood stream infections (i.e., *Salmonella* species), or from toxin-mediated disease (i.e., *Shigella, Clostridium difficile, Escherichia coli*). Other infections result from sexual transmission through oral or anal receptive activities (i.e., *Neisseria gonorrhea*, syphilis, human papilloma virus (HPV), *Chlamydia*) or fecal-oral transmission (i.e., *Shigella, Entamoeba histolytica*). Fungal overgrowth (primarily *Candida albicans*) is common in the setting of immune suppression. Some infections are acquired during childhood and reactivated when profound immune system

suppression is present (i.e., herpes viruses, toxoplasmosis). The most common pathogens causing gastrointestinal infections in HIV-infected individuals are summarized in Table 19–1.

CLINICAL PRESENTATION

Oral/esophageal Disease

Fifty percent or more of HIV-infected patients have some kind of significant oral pathology. Common presentations to the emergency department are complaints of pain in the oral cavity, sore throat, or difficulty or pain with swallowing. One of the most common diseases found in those patients not on HAART is oral hairy leukoplakia (OHL), which is manifested by submucosal lesions, generally found along the lateral aspects of the tongue, that are white in color and do not scrape away with pressure from a tongue blade. OHL lesions are most likely a relatively benign lesion thought to be the result of Epstein-Barr virus (EBV) infection. These should be distinguished from oral yeast infections which are also a common infection in the oral cavity. Yeast infections, or "thrush," are usually caused by *C. albicans*, although other *Candida* species have also been implicated. Oral examination may reveal white plaque-like lesions on an erythematous base along the buccal mucosa, tongue, or posterior pharynx; however, *Candida* infections can be primarily erythematous or pseudomembranous as well. In contrast to OHL lesions, those secondary to yeast scrape off easily with a tongue blade.

Another major presentation of oral lesions is ulcerative disease due to HSV, CMV, or other viruses or *Candida* species; HIV during primary infections; and aphthous ulcers of uncertain etiology. Many of these often painful ulcerative lesions start as vesicles and can appear anywhere in the oral cavity with varying numbers and can be shallow or deep. Noninfectious causes include HIV medications such as dideoxycytidine (ddC, Hivid®), although this agent is rarely used today.

In patients with obvious oral thrush and in whom symptoms of dysphagia or odynophagia are elicited, a presumptive diagnosis of *Candida* esophagitis can be made. Although oral thrush can be seen in HIV-infected patients with less advanced disease (i.e., >200 CD4 cells/mm^3), *Candida* esophagitis is more likely to be seen in patients with AIDS (i.e., <200 CD4 cells/mm^3). However, spread of yeast down the oropharynx may also be a result of medication noncompliance and/or infection with non-*albicans* species which may not be susceptible to fluconazole, usually the first-line antifungal treatment for thrush. Furthermore, fluconazole-resistant *C. albicans* species have been reported. Other symptoms of esophagitis can include nonspecific retrosternal chest pain, gastrointestinal bleeding, nausea, and vomiting. Other pathogens causing esophagitis in AIDS patients, and which are more likely to cause ulcerative disease, include cytomegalovirus (CMV), herpes simplex virus (HSV), *Mycobacterium avium-intracellulare* complex (MAC), and, rarely, *Mycobacterium tuberculosis* (MTB). These additional pathogens are more common in patients with lower (<200/mm^3) CD4 counts and can also occur in combination with *Candida* species. Other rare infectious causes include *Nocardia* species, *Bartonella* species, *Pneumocystis carinii*, *Cryptosporidium parvum,* and *Leishmania* species. Idiopathic esophageal ulceration is a term used when no other pathogen or cause other than HIV infection can be found in patients with advanced AIDS. Finally, noninfectious causes, particularly gastrointestinal lymphoma, may present with these symptoms as well.

Sore throat or pharyngitis is usually associated with an erythematous posterior pharynx, enlarged tonsils, fever, adenopathy, and, possibly, an exudative discharge. Although pathogens such as *Streptococcus pyogenes* (group A streptococcus) are most commonly associated with this clinical syndrome, other pathogens such as HSV, *Candida* species, and sexually transmitted diseases such as *N. gonorrhea* and *Treponema pallidum* (the causative agent of syphilis) can also produce these findings in HIV-infected patients. Furthermore, HPV infection in the oral cavity can be manifested by flat or verrucous warts anywhere in the oropharynx. Thus, it is important to obtain a complete sexual history in any patient with oral symptoms in order to include these pathogens in the differential diagnosis of infectious pharyngitis.

Finally, it is important to note that pain in the oral cavity may be the result of gingivitis, necrotizing gingivo-periodontitis, or abscess formation. Many HIV-infected patients have poor dentition and poor oral hygiene as the result of a lack of dental care.

Abdominal Pain

Abdominal pain can be diffuse or localized, chronic or acute, and may be accompanied by diarrhea or constitutional symptoms such as fever. In the pre-HAART era, patients were more likely to have an opportunistic infection or AIDS-associated malignancy as a cause of abdominal pain when compared to HIV-infected patients presenting today (1). Many cases seen today are of unknown etiology or are the result of gastroenteritis/diarrheal syndromes or gastritis/dyspepsia syndromes. However, it is still important to consider the stage of HIV disease (most recent CD4 count) and whether patients are receiving HIV treatment or OI antimicrobial prophylaxis when determining the differential diagnosis of abdominal pain.

In considering infectious etiologies, patients who complain of epigastric pain accompanied by nausea, vomiting, or reflux symptoms are as likely to have a benign gastritis as an infectious gastroenteritis, although the latter should always be excluded. Infectious gastritis in AIDS patients has been associated with a number of etiologies including CMV, syphilis, toxoplasmosis, and *Cryptosporidium*. None of these infectious etiologies has any specific findings, however. *Helicobacter pylori* also causes gastritis-associated symptoms although with less frequency in HIV-infected patients compared to uninfected patients (2). Pancreatitis can also cause these symptoms and in addition to the above infectious agents has also been reported in AIDS patients to be caused by *Cryptococcus neoformans*, MAC, MTB, and *Aspergillus* species. An important noninfectious cause to consider is medication-associated pancreatitis, which may be secondary to didanosine (ddI, Videx®), TMP-SMX (Septra®, Bactrim®), or pentamidine (Pentam®), for example. A lactic acidosis syndrome associated with nausea, vomiting, abdominal pain, and elevated serum lactate levels has been described in association with the HIV medication class known as nucleoside reverse transcriptase inhibitors (NRTI, i.e., d4T, stavudine, Zerit®). In patients receiving these medications who present with significant abnormal abdominal findings and in whom serum lactic acid levels are markedly increased (>5 mmol/L), HIV medications should be discontinued, as the case fatality rate with continued HIV medication utilization is high. In addition, the NRTI abacavir (ABC, Ziagen®, and a component of Trizivir®) has been associated with a hypersensitivity reaction in about 5% of patients, which can be manifested by fever, rash, nausea, vomiting, diarrhea, and/or abdominal pain. Patients should not be rechallenged with these HIV medications.

Diarrhea

An important distinction should be made between small bowel and large bowel diarrhea, as these are often associated with different causative etiologies. Large volume, watery diarrhea, often with associated cramps, bloating, and nausea, suggests a small bowel etiology. Common bacterial pathogens such as *E. coli* are less likely to cause such symptoms, while parasitic infections such as *Giardia lamblia*, *C. parvum*, *Isospora belli*, *Cyclospora cayetanensis*, and *Microsporidia* spp. (i.e., *Encephalitozoon intestinalis*, *Enterocytozoon bieneusi*, *Encephalitozoon hellem*) are more frequently causative. It is important to determine the patient's immune status, as patients with AIDS and low CD4 counts are more likely to develop such parasitic infections than those with higher CD4 counts. Infections causing localized terminal ileitis may also present with symptoms suggestive of small bowel pathology, including *Yersinia* sp., MAC, MTB, and CMV.

In contrast, more frequent, small volume diarrhea suggests large bowel pathology. Hematochezia and tenesmus are common associated findings. There does remain considerable overlap in regard to clinical symptoms, however. Coliform bacteria such as *E. coli*, as well as those causing dysentery (i.e., *Campylobacter jejuni*, *Salmonella* sp., *Shigella* sp., *Yersinia enterocolitica*), are common etiologies in this setting. *C. difficile* colitis should always be considered in the differential diagnosis of large bowel diarrhea, particularly among those patients taking antibiotics for prophylaxis against opportunistic infections. Mycobacteria, particularly MAC, should be considered as

well. MAC-associated intestinal infection typically occurs in patients with CD4 counts less than 50/mm^3 and is usually associated with fever, abdominal pain, lymphadenopathy, other systemic complaints, and mycobacteremia. Among opportunistic parasites, *E. histolytica* may cause large bowel diarrhea, although most other parasites tend to cause small bowel pathology. Amoebic colitis should be considered in patients who present with either microscopically detectable (occult) or gross blood in the stool.

Viral gastroenteritis, due to rotavirus or adenovirus for example, can occur among patients with appropriate exposure. Hepatitis viruses, particularly hepatitis A, may cause an acute diarrheal illness as well. In the pre-HAART era, cytomegalovirus infection of the gastrointestinal tract was a common presenting opportunistic infection, manifested by large bowel diarrhea, often bloody in nature, with associated fever and abdominal pain. While less common nowadays, it is always important to consider CMV in the differential diagnosis of diarrhea, particularly among those patients with CD4 counts less than 100/mm^3.

The extensive and diverse differential diagnosis of diarrhea and abdominal pain illustrates the critical importance of eliciting a thorough epidemiologic history from patients who present with these symptoms. A history including recent food or other ingestions, travel history, animal and water exposures, sick contacts, sexual contacts, and close contact with children in day care settings may point to a particular pathogen in this setting.

In the instances in which no pathogen can be identified, there is often evidence of impaired epithelial barrier function but no evidence of active ion secretion or malabsorption (3). It is important to remember that HIV itself may be an indirect diarrheal pathogen. AIDS enteropathy causes diarrhea in HIV-infected patients who lack an identifiable pathogen. Gastrointestinal malignancies such as lymphoma may cause diarrhea and abdominal pain as well.

Medications are a common cause of diarrhea in patients with HIV disease, especially HIV-1 protease inhibitors such as nelfinavir (Viracept®). The diarrhea is often self-limited, lasting for 2–4 weeks after the initiation of medication. However, some patients have loose stools or frank diarrhea for a prolonged period of time. Small bowel bacterial overgrowth may also cause diarrhea and malabsorption of fats, carbohydrates, and vitamin B12.

Anorectal Disease

Anorectal disease is common in HIV-infected patients, particularly among sexually active individuals and those practicing receptive anal intercourse. The most common clinical presentations of anorectal disease are rectal pain, pain or difficulty with defecation, mass or swelling, bloody stool/bright red blood per rectum, or a purulent discharge. Much anorectal disease is ulcerative in nature, which is often the result of HSV infections, although other viral infections such as CMV may cause similar findings. Sexually transmitted infections such as gonorrhea, chlamydia, and syphilis must also be considered, and are often, but not always, associated with a discharge; routes of sexual transmission in these circumstances include unprotected anal intercourse and oral-fecal contact. Anorectal warts secondary to HPV are also common in this patient population. Kaposi sarcoma, secondary to human herpes virus-8 (HHV-8) infection, remains a distinct possibility, particularly among homosexual men who have a higher seroprevalence of this sexually acquired pathogen. Finally, much ulcerative disease in the anorectum remains idiopathic in nature and may be the result of medication (such as analgesic suppositories), trauma, or unidentified infectious pathogens.

Hepatobiliary Disease

Most infectious syndromes affecting the hepatobiliary tract are associated with right upper quadrant pain, often with accompanying fever, nausea, and vomiting. Many bacteria, most notably mycobacteria including MTB and MAC, can cause an acute hepatitis-like picture although they are more often associated with mass-like hepatic lesions. Though uncommon, bacillary angiomatosus secondary to *Bartonella* infection can present with abdominal pain, abnormal liver function tests, and multiple hepatic vascular lesions on abdominal imaging. Some parasitic infections, in the appropriate epidemiologic context, can cause a similar yet usually more indolent clinical presentation. For example, amoebic liver abscesses, caused by the protozoan *E. histolytica*, can cause singular or multiple liver abscesses and abnormal liver function tests, often evolving in a subacute course, while pyogenic liver abscesses more often present with acute abdominal pain and fever.

Many viruses including not only the hepatitis viruses A, B, and C, but also cytomegalovirus and other herpes viruses such as EBV can cause acute hepatic injury and hepatitis. Acute hepatitis in patients with HIV infection often follows a different clinical course when compared with HIV-negative patients. HIV-positive patients who are subsequently infected with hepatitis A, for example, may experience a longer duration of often-subtle symptoms and have a viremia that is twice as long, yet transaminases

are often not as elevated compared with HIV-negative patients (4). Men who have sex with men are at particular risk for both acute hepatitis A and hepatitis B infections, and these diagnoses should always be considered in the setting of abdominal pain and abnormal transaminases.

The impact of an acute hepatitis syndrome in HIV-infected patients is even more pronounced among those who are coinfected with other hepatitis viruses. Indeed, due to similar transmission mechanisms, 30–50% of HIV-infected patients are chronically infected with hepatitis C and up to 10% are chronically infected with hepatitis B (5, 6). Furthermore, although rare, triple infection with HIV, hepatitis C, and hepatitis B has been reported (7). In these circumstances, the hepatitis disease progression is quicker and other infections can follow a more severe course (8). It is of utmost importance that HIV-infected patients be vaccinated against hepatitis A and hepatitis B, if not previously infected. Coinfected patients also demonstrate a more rapid progression to cirrhosis and thereby have an increased risk for hepatocellular carcinoma as well (9).

Furthermore, with the initiation of antiretroviral therapy, patients with advanced HIV infection may develop an immune reconstitution inflammatory syndrome (IRIS) involving the chronic hepatitides, similar to those seen involving MAC infection and central nervous system processes. Those patients who are coinfected with either hepatitis C or hepatitis B may demonstrate increased transaminases resembling an acute hepatitis and clinical deterioration with the initiation of HAART, despite an overall improvement in immune system function (10, 11).

Hepatic toxicity has been reported in HIV-infected patients being treated with drugs from all three major classes of antiretroviral medications (12). Such toxicity can occur through a variety of mechanisms, including direct hepatic injury, mitochondrial toxicity, steatohepatitis, and lipodystrophy syndromes (13). Most cases involve only asymptomatic elevations in transaminases, although severe and sometimes life-threatening liver disease may occur, notably involving the HIV-1 protease inhibitor class of medications. Ritonavir (Norvir®) is a potent inhibitor of cytochrome P450 enzymes and the use of full-dose ritonavir as part of a HAART regimen poses the greatest risk of drug-induced liver injury (14). Ritonavir can also significantly affect drug concentrations and hence hepatotoxic potential of many classes of medications. The use of ritonavir in combination with lopinavir (Kaletra®) or at reduced dose as part of a so-called boosted protease inhibitor regimen may also result in liver injury. Indinavir (Crixivan®) and the newer protease inhibitor atazanavir (Reyataz®) can cause a usually asymptomatic indirect hyperbilirubinemia without an associated transaminitis. Other classes of antiretroviral medications or medications used in the treatment of HCV (ribavirin and interferon-alpha) and HBV (lamivudine, 3TC, Epivir® and adefovir, Herpsera®) are associated with hepatotoxicity, particularly when given in combination with a protease inhibitor (15). In addition, the NNRTI nevirapine (Viramune®) has been associated with rare instances of liver failure (16). It is important to note that these side effects may be seen both with the initiation of antiretroviral therapy and after such therapy has been ongoing. Furthermore, these effects are often more severe in patients coinfected with hepatitis C (17).

Biliary disease occurs with a greater incidence among HIV-infected individuals. Although many cases of cholecystitis and cholangitis are secondary to cholelithiasis and biliary sludge, those occurring in the absence of stone disease (acalculous cholecystitis) may be a more common manifestation in the setting of HIV disease. The biliary tract is normally void of bacteria; those organisms causing acute biliary infection are usually the same as the normal intestinal flora in healthy individuals. In those infected with HIV and who have AIDS, however, opportunistic pathogens such as *Cryptosporidium*, other gastrointestinal parasites (i.e., *Microsporidia* spp., *Cyclospora*, *Isospora*), CMV, and MAC may cause acalculous cholecystitis. Antiretroviral medications such as indinavir may also cause a similar clinical picture. In patients with advanced AIDS who present with right upper quadrant or midepigastric pain, cholestasis, and symptoms of cholangitis, particularly those with advanced disease, the diagnosis of AIDS cholangiopathy should be considered. This condition is most commonly the result of papillary stenosis and is often secondary to infection with *Cryptosporidium*, CMV, and *Microsporidia* species.

LABORATORY/DIAGNOSTIC TESTING

Oral ulcerations or suppurative pharyngitis in HIV-infected patients can be due to many different etiologies. Bacterial or viral culture of material obtained from these lesions will reveal the diagnosis in most cases. If vesicular or ulcerative lesions are present, vesicular fluid or ulcerative material can be applied on a glass slide and a subsequent Tzanck smear can reveal multinucleated giant cells suggestive of herpes virus infection (primarily HSV, VZV); this material or fluid can also be sent for herpes virus direct fluorescent antibody (DFA) or PCR assays. Alternatively, a Gram stain can reveal bacterial or fungal pathogens. Gram-negative intracellular diplococci (gonococcus), or gram-positive cocci in long chains (group A streptococcus) or gram-positive budding yeast (*Candida* sp.), can all be visualized easily with this inexpensive slide test. Syphilis testing of infected material by dark field microscopy or fluorescent antibody testing should also be obtained. In most cases of oral thrush, no diagnostic tests are necessary unless treatment failure is suspected in those patients previously known to have had and been treated for oral or esophageal candidiasis. In patients with dysphagia, odynophagia and presumptive esophagitis, routine laboratory tests or imaging studies, such as chest radiography or barium swallow, are usually not helpful in establishing the diagnosis. Endoscopy with direct visualization, biopsy, and culture are the preferred means of making a diagnosis.

In patients with abdominal pain, acute drug-induced or infectious pancreatitis can usually be ruled out with normal serum amylase and lipase levels. Serologic evaluation of hepatic function should be obtained as well. Acute viral hepatitis usually results in serum transaminase (AST/SGOT, ALT/SGPT) levels greater than 1000 IU/ml. Patients with chronic HBV or HCV rarely have elevated transaminases more than five times the upper limit of normal and usually with an ALT predominance. Biliary disease, on the other hand, usually results in increased LDH, alkaline phosphatase, and bilirubin levels, more so than elevated transaminase levels. An elevated alkaline phosphatase in AIDS patients may be suggestive of hepatobiliary MAC infection. Noninfectious causes of hepatic enzyme elevations are primarily medication-associated and include hyperbilirubinemia (usually no greater than $5\times$ upper limit of normal) with the protease inhibitors indinavir and atazanavir, and elevated transaminases (usually no greater than $5\times$ upper limit of normal) with nevirapine, for example.

Plain films of the abdomen are usually not helpful in the evaluation of HIV-infected patients with abdominal pain. Abdominal ultrasonography of the hepatobiliary system is recommended to evaluate for stone disease and biliary ductal dilation, although this procedure is usually insufficient to fully evaluate for choledocholithiasis and colonic disease. Furthermore, unless symptoms are clearly isolated to the abdominal right upper quadrant, full abdominal ultrasonographic evaluation is preferred, as additional pathology, including intraabdominal abscesses and splenic and renal pathology, can often be detected. Computerized tomography of the abdomen and pelvis may provide better anatomic visualization (including the pancreas and colonic wall) (18) although ultrasound is usually sufficient for most pathology in the liver, gall bladder, and spleen. In summary, these imaging modalities can reveal

Table 19–2. Recommended Stool Studies in the Evaluation of Diarrhea in the HIV-Infected Patient

Fecal leukocyte count
Routine Gram stain and culture
Sorbitol screen for *E. coli* O157:H7
C. difficile toxin assay × 2
Ova and parasite examination
Modified acid fast stain for detection of MAC, *Isospora*, and *Cryptosporidium*
DFA stain for *Cryptosporidium*
DFA stain for *Giardia*
Weber modified trichrome stain for detection of *Microsporidium* spp.

Notification of the microbiology laboratory will help to facilitate the performance of the appropriate examinations. DFA = direct fluorescent antibody, MAC = Mycobacterium avium-intracellulare complex.

significant pathology; however, there are no specific findings for HIV-specific GI infections.

In patients with diarrhea, basic stool studies should be obtained (Table 19–2) which include stool for bacterial culture (which will detect not only *C. jejuni*, *Shigella* spp., and *Salmonella* spp. but also less common bacterial pathogens such as *Aeromonas hydrophila* and *Plesiomonas shigelloides,* depending on the laboratory), a sorbitol screen for *E. coli* (particularly *E. coli* serotype O157:H7, which is usually performed with the routine stool culture), ova and parasite examination, and *C. difficile* toxin assay. In addition, DFA stains for *Giardia* and *C. parvum* and acid fast stains for MAC and Isospora (which will also be able to detect *Cryptosporidium* and *Cyclospora*) should be obtained. To detect Microsporidia spp., a Weber modified trichrome stain should be used to evaluate the stool specimen. When sending stool samples for gastrointestinal parasites, notify the laboratory to ensure that appropriate evaluation will be performed for *Cryptosporidium, Microsporidium* spp., *Isospora*, and *Cyclospora*. Again, such opportunistic pathogens are less likely in patients with higher CD4 counts (>200/mm³).

For patients with diarrhea and fever, routine blood cultures and blood cultures specific for mycobacteria (i.e., MAC) should also be obtained.

In a comprehensive study of chronic diarrhea in patients with AIDS, more pathogens were identified by stool exam than by endoscopy (19). In most emergency department situations, only one stool sample will be available for laboratory evaluation. However, most sources recommend at least two, and preferably three, independently collected

stool specimens in order to improve diagnostic yield (20). Therefore, multiple samples should be sent for evaluation if possible.

Endoscopic evaluation with esophagogastroduodenoscopy (EGD), flexible sigmoidoscopy, or colonoscopy most frequently occurs either after admission to the hospital or on an outpatient basis, and is less commonly performed in the emergency department setting. HIV-infected patients with severe diarrhea, fever, dysentery, or chronic symptoms with weight loss, particularly those with CD4 counts less than 200/mm³, should be referred to a gastroenterologist for endoscopy. Endoscopy has a particularly high diagnostic yield among patients with AIDS with esophageal symptoms refractory to empiric antifungal therapy and can be used to obtain a small bowel biopsy for severe diarrhea or upper gastrointestinal bleeding (21). In the diagnosis of suspected small bowel-associated diarrhea, the yield of EGD is improved the more distal the biopsy site (22). In the diagnostic evaluation of large bowel diarrhea, colonoscopy is superior to flexible sigmoidoscopy (23).

Anoscopy may facilitate anorectal cytologic examination in screening for squamous cell carcinoma in patients with anal warts secondary to HPV infection. This easily performed inexpensive procedure can also significantly aid in the diagnosis of sexually acquired proctitis and proctocolitis (24). Patients presenting with hematochezia should undergo anoscopy to evaluate for distal sources of bleeding, including hemorrhoids. Anoscopy also facilitates direct visualization and microbiologic sampling of distal ulcerative lesions, which should be evaluated for gonorrhea and chlamydia, preferably by molecular methods (PCR) rather than culture, and with a Tzanck preparation or PCR for HSV. Dark-field microscopic examination and serologic antibody evaluation for syphilis should be considered as well.

MANAGEMENT

For HIV-infected patients with lesions consistent with oral candidiasis, a trial of oral fluconazole is reasonable, with close medical follow-up after discharge from the emergency department. For patients already on prophylactic fluconazole, however, it is imperative that samples be obtained for both pathology and microbiology, as alternative antifungal medication may be required. Similarly, an EGD is imperative for patients with esophageal symptoms to exclude nonfungal etiologies, particularly for those patients with CD4 counts less than 200/mm³.

Treatment options for esophageal candidiasis include fluconazole, itraconazole, amphotericin products, and the newer triazole antifungal voriconazole (VFend®), although this determination should be made in consultation by an infectious diseases specialist or, preferably, the patient's primary HIV health care provider. Acyclovir is the treatment of choice for HSV esophageal ulcerations. Ganciclovir is the preferred treatment for infections due to CMV.

Although only a minority of HIV-infected people with abdominal pain have an opportunistic infection causing this symptom (1), the clinician should nevertheless have a low threshold for surgical consultation, as the presenting symptoms may be subtle despite advanced pathology. This is particularly relevant for patients with AIDS and with concomitant fever. In addition, AIDS patients with baseline leukopenia may not demonstrate the elevated neutrophil counts that are commonly associated with infectious processes.

The cornerstone of therapy for patients presenting with diarrhea is appropriate rehydration, whether it be by oral or intravenous route. Whereas empiric antibiotics are appropriate in the treatment of traveler's diarrhea, shigellosis, *C. difficile*, and, if administered early, *Campylobacter* infection, antibiotics may increase the duration of shedding of *Salmonella* and may increase the risk of complications in shiga-like toxin producing *E. coli* infections (25). Therefore, the risk of these adverse events must be weighed against the potential benefits of therapy. In general, the immunocompromised state afforded by HIV infection poses enough risk to probably justify empiric antibiotics in most cases of bloody diarrhea with or without concomitant fever. Empiric treatment with a fluoroquinolone antibiotic (e.g., ciprofloxacin, Cipro®), or in children with TMP-SMX, is reasonable. However, given the increasing incidence of fluoroquinolone-resistant organisms such as *Campylobacter* (with rates reaching as high as 80% in parts of southern Asia), immunocompromised (or severely ill) patients might include the substitution of TMP-SMX for a fluoroquinolone and perhaps a macrolide antibiotic such as erythromycin or azithromycin. In addition, while the treatment duration for normal hosts is generally 3–5 days, HIV patients, particularly those with AIDS, may require up to 2 weeks of treatment (26). With the extensive list of possible etiologies and increasing antimicrobial resistance profiles, obtaining appropriate stool samples for culture and sensitivity is of paramount importance.

For patients who have been receiving antibiotic therapy, either as prophylaxis or treatment, therapy with oral metronidazole may be appropriate after *C. difficile* toxin assays (at least two) have been sent to the laboratory. This can be discontinued should the results be negative.

Parasitic infections may be more likely in patients with diarrhea and lower CD4 counts (less than 200 cells/mm^3). However, antiparasitic therapy is generally not required prior to confirming a diagnosis. Specific therapy (as seen in Table 19–3) varies depending on the particular pathogen, and may include metronidazole for giardiasis, TMP-SMX for isosporiasis and cyclosporiasis, or albendazole for microsporidiosis, for example.

Ganciclovir is the initial treatment of choice for CMV colitis, although this should be initiated only after an appropriate workup including colonoscopy with biopsy.

Although HPV-induced anal warts can regress with antiretroviral therapy, the initiation of medications for HIV should begin as per the discretion of the patient's primary HIV provider and/or an infectious diseases specialist. Cryotherapy has also been effective in the treatment of these lesions and can usually be performed on an outpatient basis.

Most hepatobiliary infections require surgical evaluation or percutaneous drainage, as antibiotics alone are insufficient to completely resolve abscesses and biliary inflammation. Endoscopic retrograde cholangiopancreatography (ERCP) with sphincterotomy is useful in the management of AIDS cholangiopathy and papillary stenosis (27). Hepatic toxicity secondary to antiretroviral medications or those used to treat hepatitis C often requires cessation of the offending agent(s). This discontinuation should not be undertaken, however, without the knowledge of the patient's primary HIV provider and/or an infectious diseases specialist. It is imperative that all antiretroviral medications be discontinued at the same time, so as to minimize the risk of drug resistance. Some infections might require long-term antimicrobial treatment or prophylaxis depending on the stage of disease, CD4 count, and the specific infection in question. Continuation or discontinuation of such regimens should be left to HIV- or infectious disease experts.

DISPOSITION

Most patients do not require admission to the hospital unless they have signs of an acute abdomen; significant esophagitis symptoms with poor oral intake; evidence of

Table 19–3. Recommended Therapy for Culture-Positive Infectious Diarrhea in HIV-Infected Patients

Organism	Treatment	Duration
E. coli	FQ (ciprofloxacin, 500 mg po bid or levofloxacin, 500 mg po qd); TMP-SMX ds (180/800) po bid if susceptible	1–3 days
Shigatoxin producing *E. coli* (O157:H7)	Role of antibiotics unclear; avoid antimotility agents	
Shigella	FQ (ciprofloxacin, 500 mg po bid or levofloxacin, 500 mg po qd); TMP-SMX ds (160/800) po bid if susceptible	7–10 days
Campylobacter	Erythromycin, 500 mg po bid	At least 5 days, may require longer duration
Salmonella	FQ (ciprofloxacin, 500 mg po bid or levofloxacin, 500 mg po qd); TMP-SMX ds (180/800) po bid if susceptible	14 days, or longer if relapsing
C. difficile	Metronidazole, 250 mg po q6h or 500 mg po q8h	7–10 days
MAC	Clarithromycin, 500 mg po q12h + ethambutol, 15 mg/kg po qd ± rifabutin, 300 mg po qd (azithromycin may be substituted for clarithromycin but is less effective)	Months to years, depending on clinical and radiological response, followed by suppressive therapy
CMV	Ganciclovir, 5 mg/kg iv bid	At least 21 days
Cryptosporidium	Paromomycin, 500 mg po q8h; HAART is most effective therapy. Consider nitazoxanide, 100 mg oral suspension bid	14–28 days, then bid if needed
Isospora	TMP-SMX ds (160/800) po bid	7–10 days, followed by three times weekly for patients with AIDS
Cyclospora	TMP-SMX ds (160/800) po bid	7–10 days, followed by three times weekly for patients with AIDS
Microsporidium spp.	Albendazole 400 mg po bid; *E. bieneusi* infections require treatment with fumagillin 20 mg po q8h	21 days
G. lamblia	Metronidazole, 500–750 mg po q8h	7–10 days
E. histolytica	Metronidazole, 500–750 mg po q8h + Iodoquinol, 650 mg po q8h or Paromomycin, 500 mg po q8h	5–10 days 21 days 7 days

CMV = cytomegalovirus; MAC = Mycobacterium avium-intracellulare complex; FQ = fluoroquinolone; HAART = highly active antiretroviral therapy; TMP-SMX = trimethoprim-sulfamethoxazole.

significant fluid loss or dehydration; or are AIDS patients with abdominal pain and fever. For those patients who have previously established care with an HIV specialist, review of the patient's past medical and medication administration history may be instrumental in helping guide evaluation and management. For those patients who have not established such care, referral to an HIV specialist or clinic should be made. HIV-infected patients should never leave an emergency department setting without appropriately scheduled outpatient follow-up.

CASE OUTCOME

Intravenous fluids were started in the emergency department. Routine laboratory tests were drawn, including blood cultures for routine bacteria and MAC and sent to the laboratory. Stool studies including evaluation for white blood cells, routine pathogen culture, DFA stains for *Giardia* and *Cryptosporidium* and AFB smear were also sent. Routine laboratory testing revealed the following abnormalities: WBC 3.0 (neutrophils 78%, bands 4%, lymphocytes 15%), hemoglobin of 10.1 g/dL, platelet count of 130,000/ mm^3, serum potassium of 3.0 mEq/L, ALT of 97 U/L, AST of 45 U/L, amylase of 180 U/L, lipase of 95 U/L, and an alkaline phosphatase of 180 U/L. Stool evaluation revealed a few white blood cells and the urinalysis was unremarkable.

Because of fever, diarrhea, dehydration, and presumed AIDS, the patient was admitted for further workup. The patient was started empirically on intravenous ciprofloxacin for presumptive bacterial diarrhea and fluconazole for oral and vaginal candidiasis. She felt somewhat better the following day, but several diarrheal episodes of brown and watery stool associated with mucous, fever to 101°F, and abdominal pain in the left lower quadrant were noted. An abdominal CT scan revealed numerous 1–2 cm retroperitoneal and para-aortic lymph nodes. Liver and spleen were of normal size and texture, and the descending colon was moderately thickened. A flexible sigmoidoscopy procedure was performed revealing multiple shallow ulcerations and diffuse inflammation in the rectosigmoid area. Biopsy and cultures were submitted. The following day stool culture for routine bacterial pathogens and two ova and parasite examinations were reported as negative. Routine blood cultures were still negative. T- cell subsets revealed a CD4 cell count of 71/mm^3 (and a CD8 count of 383/mm^3). An AFB smear of stool revealed rare acid-fast bacilli. On hospital day 3, rectal biopsy results indicated an infectious ulcerative colitis consistent with mycobacterial disease. Tissue culture and blood cultures were subsequently positive for MAC.

Ciprofloxacin was discontinued and oral clarithromycin and ethambutol for disseminated MAC infection and oral TMP-SMX for PCP prophylaxis were initiated. The patient's temperature and abdominal pain resolved within 2 days. She was discharged with the aforementioned medications as well as oral fluconazole and a follow-up appointment with the HIV clinic to reinitiate HAART.

REFERENCES

1. Yoshida D, Caruso JM: Abdominal pain in the HIV infected patient. *J Emerg Med* 23(2):111–116, 2002.

2. Chiu HM, Wu MS, Hung CC, Shun CT, Lin JT: Low prevalence of *Helicobacter pylori* but high prevalence of cytomegalovirus-associated peptic ulcer disease in AIDS patients: Comparative study of symptomatic subjects evaluated by endoscopy and CD4 counts. *J Gastroenterol Hepatol* 19(4):423–428, 2004.

3. Stockmann M, Fromm M, Schmitz H, Schmidt W, Riecken EO, Schulzke JD: Duodenal biopsies of HIV-infected patients with diarrhea exhibit epithelial barrier defects but no active secretion. *AIDS* 12(1):43–51, 1998.

4. Ida S, Tachikawa N, Nakajima A, et al.: Influence of human immunodeficiency virus type 1 infection on acute hepatitis virus infection. *Clin Infect Dis* 34(3):379–385, 2002.

5. Sulkowski MS, Mast EE, Seeff LB, Thomas DL: Hepatitis C virus infection as an opportunistic disease in persons infected with human immunodeficiency virus. *Clin Infect Dis* 30(Suppl. 1):S77–S84, 2000.

6. Nunez M, Puoti M, Camino N, Soriano V: Treatment of chronic hepatitis B in the human immunodeficiency virus-infected patient: Present and future. *Clin Infect Dis* 37(12): 1678–1685, 2003.

7. Brenner B, Back D, Ben-Porath E, Hazani A, Martinowitz U, Tatarsky I: Coinfection with hepatitis viruses and human immunodeficiency virus in multiply transfused patients. *Isr J Med Sci* 30(12):886–890, 1994.

8. Matthews G, Bhagani S: The epidemiology and natural history of HIV/HBV and HIV/HCV co-infections. *J HIV Ther* 8(4):77–84, 2003.

9. Verucchi G, Calza L, Manfredi R, Chiodo F: Human immunodeficiency virus and hepatitis C virus coinfection: Epidemiology, natural history, therapeutic options and clinical management. *Infection* 32(1):33–46, 2004.

10. Bonacini M: Liver injury during highly active antiretroviral therapy: The effect of hepatitis C coinfection. *Clin Infect Dis* 38(Suppl. 2):S104–S108, 2004.

11. Stone SF, Lee S, Keane NM, Price P, French MA: Association of increased hepatitis C virus (HCV)-specific IgG and soluble CD26 dipeptidyl peptidase IV enzyme activity with hepatotoxicity after highly active antiretroviral therapy in human immunodeficiency virus-HCV-coinfected patients. *J Infect Dis* 186(10):1498–1502, 2002.

12. Dieterich D: Managing antiretroviral-associated liver disease. *J Acquir Immune Defic Syndr* 34(Suppl. 1):S34–S39, 2003.

13. Kontorinis N, Dieterich DT: Toxicity of non-nucleoside analogue reverse transcriptase inhibitors. *Semin Liver Dis* 23(2): 173–182, 2003.

14. Sulkowski MS: Drug-induced liver injury associated with antiretroviral therapy that includes HIV-1 protease inhibitors. *Clin Infect Dis* 38(Suppl. 2):S90–S97, 2004.

15. Ena J, Amador C, Benito C, Fenoll V, Pasquau F: Risk and determinants of developing severe liver toxicity during therapy with nevirapine- and efavirenz-containing regimens in HIV-infected patients. *Int J STD AIDS* 14(11):776–781, 2003.

16. Cattelan AM, Erne E, Salatino A, et al.: Severe hepatic failure related to nevirapine treatment. *Clin Inf Dis* 29(2):455–456, 1999.

17. Nunez M, Lana R, Mendoza JL, Martin-Carbonero L, Soriano V: Risk factors for severe hepatic injury after introduction of highly active antiretroviral therapy. *J Acquir Immune Defic Syndr* 27(5):426–431, 2001.

18. Wu CM, Davis F, Fishman EK: Radiologic evaluation of the acute abdomen in the patient with acquired immunodeficiency syndrome (AIDS): The role of CT scanning. *Semin Ultrasound CT MR* 19(2):190–199, 1998.

19. Blanshard C, Francis N, Gazzard BG: Investigation of chronic diarrhea in acquired immunodeficiency syndrome: A prospective study of 155 patients. *Gut* 29:824–832, 1996.

20. Oldfield EC: Evaluation of chronic diarrhea in patients with human immunodeficiency virus infection. *Rev Gastroenterol Disorders* 2(4):176–188, 2002.

21. Wilcox CM: The role of endoscopy in the investigation of upper gastrointestinal symptoms in HIV-infected patients. *Can J Gastroenterol* 13(4):305–310, 1999.

22. Bini EJ, Weinshel EH, Gamagaris Z: Comparison of duodenal with jejunal biopsy and aspirate in chronic human immunodeficiency virus-related diarrhea. *Am J Gastroenterol* 93(10):1837–1840, 1998.

23. Bini EJ, Weinshel EH: Endoscopic evaluation of chronic human immunodeficiency virus-related diarrhea: Is colonoscopy superior to flexible sigmoidoscopy? *Am J Gastroenterol* 93(1):56–60, 1998.

24. Rompalo AM: Diagnosis and treatment of sexually acquired proctitis and proctocolitis: An update. *Clin Infect Dis* 28(Suppl. 1):S84–S90, 1999.

25. Thielman NM, Guerrant RL: Acute infectious diarrhea. *New Engl J Med* 350(1):38–47, 2004.

26. Guerrant RL, Van Gilder T, Steiner TS, et al.: Practice guidelines for the management of infectious diarrhea. *Clin Infect Dis* 32:331–350, 2001.

27. Yusuf TE, Baron TH: AIDS cholangiopathy. *Curr Treat Options Gastroenterol* 7(2):111–117, 2004.

20

Urinary Tract Infections

Jordan C. Foster
Osman Sayan

HIGH YIELD FACTS

1. In a healthy young woman (when there are no symptoms of vaginal discharge), UTI can reliably be diagnosed with just a history of dysuria, frequency, or when symptoms are described by the woman as "similar to prior UTI." When vaginal discharge is present, a physical exam helps to exclude other causes of symptoms.

2. Urine cultures are only recommended in patients with complicated UTIs, upper tract infections (which include any evidence of fever or pyelonephritis), and in recurrent UTIs (RUTIs). Complicated UTIs are defined by the presence of any condition that affects the anatomy, function, or immune responsiveness of the urinary tract.

3. Short course antibiotic therapy (3 days) has been shown to be safe in acute uncomplicated cystitis only when the patient is a healthy nonpregnant woman with no evidence of fever or pyelonephritis.

4. While recurrence of UTI in a healthy woman is common in the months after a UTI, more than two episodes in 6 months or three in a year indicate UTIs will likely continue to recur without specific therapy.

5. Asymptomatic bacteriuria (ASB) needs to be treated in pregnant women to prevent a significant increase in maternal and fetal complications.

6. The rate of incidental asymptomatic bacteriuria in elderly and debilitated patients can be as high as 30–50%. Therefore, bedside testing that indicates the presence of white cells or bacteria (also a possible incidental finding) should not stop testing for other sources of the patient's fever or other acute symptoms.

CASE PRESENTATIONS

1. *Case 1*. A 24-year-old woman with no past medical history presents with dysuria, frequency, and lower abdominal pain. Bedside dipstick urinalysis shows trace leukocyte esterase but no nitrites or blood.

2. *Case 2*. A 75-year-old woman from a nursing home presents with fever and no other symptoms. Her urinalysis shows trace leukocyte esterase and a strong positive result for nitrites.

INTRODUCTION

The goal of the chapter is to describe the important elements in diagnosing and treating the many different groups of adult patients who present to the ED with a urinary tract infection (UTI). The challenge of diagnosing UTI in the ED is that the ED physician rarely is able to confirm the diagnosis with urine culture results before deciding on treatment and disposition. This chapter will focus on the elements that have been shown to have the greatest impact on increasing or decreasing the likelihood that a UTI diagnosis will be confirmed. Once the decision to treat a patient for a UTI is made, the treatment plan is determined by the patient's clinical symptoms and the presence of any other medical conditions.

A urinary tract infection refers to the presence of infectious organisms anywhere along the genitourinary tract. This chapter will concentrate on the two most common sites of infection, the bladder (cystitis) and the kidney (pyelonephritis). Other clinical conditions that will not be covered in this chapter, but that have been classified as UTIs, include urethritis, prostatitis, and perinephric abscess.

Urinary tract infections can be classified as lower or upper tract infections. The clinical diagnosis of upper tract infection is generally made when any of the symptoms of fever, chills, flank, or back pain are present. The diagnosis of lower tract infection is made when these upper tract symptoms are absent and there are symptoms of cystitis such as frequency and dysuria. In addition, there is the category of ASB, which is defined as the presence of significant counts of bacteria in the urine with no signs or symptoms of an upper or lower infection.

After determining the symptoms that indicate the likely site of infection, the next step is to determine if the patient's infection is uncomplicated or complicated (Table 20–1). Uncomplicated UTIs are defined as infections involving a normal urinary tract. Complicated UTIs are present when there are anatomic, metabolic, or functional abnormalities. Most common complicated cases involve diabetic patients and patients using urinary catheters (indwelling, intermittent, condom, or suprapubic). Other complicated cases are defined by the presence of

Table 20–1. Overview of Groups Requiring Treatment for UTIs

Upper tract symptoms Including fever, flank, or back pain	Longer course antibiotics needed. Urine cultures helpful	Longer course antibiotics needed, often requires parental treatment. Urine cultures helpful
Lower tract symptoms Limited to dysuria, frequency, hematuria	Shorter course antibiotics safe. Cultures typically not needed for treatment	Longer course antibiotics needed. Urine cultures helpful
Asymptomatic bacteriuria	No indication for treatment	Treated if pregnant (also if recent kidney transplant or needs GU instrumentation)
	Uncomplicated There are no structural or functional abnormalities to urinary tract	*Complicated* There are structural or functional abnormalities to urinary tract

neurogenic bladder, nephrolithiasis, recent instrumentation, polycystic renal disease, or immunosuppression.

In pregnant women, any UTI including asymptomatic infections are associated with a higher risk of complications in both the mother and the fetus (1). In men, a UTI has a high association with either an anatomic abnormality, such as an enlarged prostate, or functional abnormality (2, 3). Elderly patients who are debilitated or institutionalized who develop UTIs also often have a preexisting anatomic, metabolic, or functional abnormality (4). Therefore, symptomatic infections in these three groups are usually treated as complicated infections. Patients with either an upper UTI or a complicated UTI have a higher risk of treatment failure and progression to more severe infections including abscess formation and septicemia.

One last concept that is important to introduce is that of a RUTI. A recurrent UTI can be either a relapse with the same organism (usually before 2 weeks have passed since treatment) or a reinfection with a different organism (usually after 2 weeks have passed since treatment). A woman is considered to have frequent RUTI if there are two or more episodes in 6 months or three episodes in 1 year. Infections that occur this frequently are likely to continue to recur at an increased rate without intervention (3, 5). While RUTI has not been associated with increased risk for long-term complications, RUTI can still have significant impact on quality of life (6).

The chapter is divided into three sections. Within each section, the elements of epidemiology, microbiology, diagnosis, and treatment will be discussed separately. The first and largest section will focus on uncomplicated UTIs, which mainly involve cystitis and pyelonephritis in young

healthy women. The second section will describe the different concerns pertinent to patients with complicated UTIs. The groups to be discussed in this section include pregnant women, men, elderly, diabetics, catheterized patients, and other immunocompromised patients. The final section will discuss the unique elements regarding treating the incidental finding of an asymptomatic bacteriuria.

UNCOMPLICATED UTI-EPIDEMIOLOGY

Of the over 1 million annual emergency department visits for UTI, young women by far make up the greatest percentage (Fig. 20–1). UTIs occur in about one-third of all women before age 24 and about half of all women in their lifetime (7). In young women, most of the occurrences are in sexually active women who have an average incidence of one infection every $1\frac{1}{2}$ to 2 years (8). Pyelonephritis rates, whether complicated or uncomplicated, are harder to determine, but overall there is estimated to be 250,000 annual cases (9). Recurrence of UTI in 3–4 months can occur in 20–30% of cases. Recurrence in 1 year is as high as 25–50% (3, 10).

In the ED, UTIs diagnosed in males are usually classified as complicated due to disturbances in anatomy or function. However, in males under 50 years of age, certain risk factors for uncomplicated UTI have been identified in outpatient clinic settings. The practice of anal intercourse has been shown to increase the likelihood of an otherwise healthy male developing uncomplicated cystitis. A male with a sexual partner colonized with uropathogenic strains of bacteria is likewise at risk for cystitis. Lack of circumcision may lead to cystitis by allowing colonization of

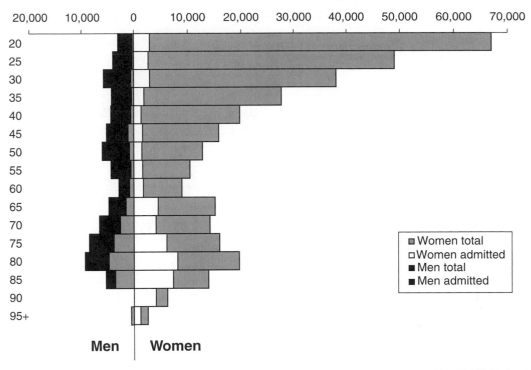

Fig. 20–1. Patients with an emergency department diagnosis of UTI by age and sex (Average Annual NHAMCS National Data 1992–2000).

the glans and prepuce by uropathogenic microorganisms (3). Unless a male patient presents with a prior history of UTIs treated successfully as uncomplicated cases, the ED physician should treat the patient as if he has a complicated UTI.

UNCOMPLICATED UTI–MICROBIOLOGY

Unlike other infectious diseases, the microbiology of UTIs has remained remarkably constant over the last few decades (5). The aerobic gram-negative bacillus, *Escherichia coli*, remains the most common pathogen for all manifestations of UTI and in all groups of patients (3). It is the causative pathogen in approximately 80–90% of patients diagnosed with acute uncomplicated cystitis or acute uncomplicated pyelonephritis. *Staphylococcus saprophyticus*, a coagulase-negative gram-positive coccus, is the second most common pathogen in uncomplicated cystitis, implicated in 10–15% of cases of UTI (11). *Klebsiella*, *Serratia*, *Enterobacter*, and *Proteus* species as well as *Pseudomonas aeruginosa*, *Staphylococcus au-*

reus, group B and group D (enterococcus) *Streptococcus* and fungi are rare causes of UTI in normal hosts (3).

Cases of acute uncomplicated pyelonephritis in women and in otherwise uncomplicated cystitis in males under the age of 50 are almost exclusively caused by *E. coli* with enhanced bacterial virulence factors (known as uropathogenic strains). These virulence factors allow these microbes to evade normal host defenses and infect the urinary system. The uropathogenic *E. coli* belong to a small number of O (lipopolysaccharide), K (capsular polysaccharide), and H (flagellar antigen) subtype groups. They utilize virulence factors such as filamentous surface adhesive organelles known as fimbrae (or pili), flagellae and the production of toxins such as hemolysin and aerobactin to facilitate infection of the urinary tract (12). The presence of multiple virulence factors can increase the likelihood of recurrence, of progression to upper tract infection, and of bacteremic spread even in a normal host (10). Fortunately, the presence of these virulence factors does not influence antibiotic sensitivities (13).

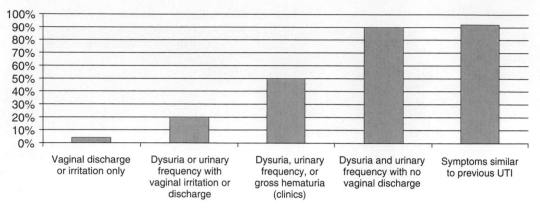

Fig. 20–2. Risk of UTI by chief complaint in young women.

UNCOMPLICATED UTI—CLINICAL PRESENTATION

Uncomplicated Cystitis

In young women, the description of their symptoms is the most powerful predictor of the likelihood that a UTI is present (Fig. 20–2). Most of the symptomatic infections will be uncomplicated cystitis. Therefore, most young women evaluated for UTI will have some combination of dysuria, frequency, or hematuria. When a young woman complains of any one of these symptoms and does not have vaginal irritation or discharge, then the chance of UTI is approximately 50%. If there is both dysuria and frequency (again without vaginal irritation or discharge), then the chance of UTI increases to 90%. Similarly, if a woman complains that she has symptoms similar to a prior UTI, the chance of UTI is approximately 90%. Once a woman also complains of vaginal irritation or discharge, then the chance of UTI decreases to 20%. If a woman complains only of vaginal symptoms, the risk of UTI is only 4% (8, 10, 14).

The duration of these symptoms is usually short. The average duration of symptoms before treatment is sought is 5 days. On average there are 6 days of symptoms with 2 days of restricted activity and less than half a day of bed rest (6). When symptoms extend past 7 days, there is a raised concern that the UTI may not be a simple case of uncomplicated cystitis (10, 14).

From the medical history, the most significant risk factors for acute UTI in this group are previous cystitis and frequent or recent sexual activity. UTIs are rare among healthy, celibate women. Other elements of the past medical history in young women that increase the risk of UTI include use of spermicidal agents, recent antimi-

crobial use, and presence of urinary obstruction. Less significant are the associations with genetic factors of nonsecretor status, ABO blood type, and maternal history of cystitis (6).

Uncomplicated Pyelonephritis

The diagnosis of pyelonephritis or upper tract disease is even more difficult than cystitis to confirm in the ED. Typically, the diagnosis is considered in any person with back or flank pain by history or exam. The presence of costovertebral (CVA) tenderness on exam has been shown to somewhat increase the likelihood that any UTI is present (8). In addition, the presence of fever or chills raises the chance that a UTI has extended beyond simple cystitis. It is important to keep in mind that the presence of back pain or fever often has been used as exclusion criteria for studies on the safety of shorter courses of antibiotics. While pyelonephritis can still be considered uncomplicated when there are no functional or anatomical abnormalities in the patient, the approach to testing (getting cultures) and treatment (longer course of antibiotics) is very similar to the approach recommended for complicated UTIs.

Frequent Recurrent UTIs

Frequent recurring UTIs are a problem for as many as 10–20% of all women, some experiencing infections every few weeks (15). Treatment of the acute infection is similar whether it is an isolated case or one of many UTIs for the patient. When the relapse occurs within 2 weeks, the chance that the same organism is the cause increases and this may prompt a change in antibiotic choice or duration.

Understanding the risk factors associated with recurrent UTIs allows the clinician to further treat the patient by intervening on future UTIs. Healthy, premenopausal women are predisposed to recurrent UTIs by both behavioral and genetic factors. Frequency of sexual intercourse and choice of contraception are the behavioral determinants that most influence the risk for recurrent UTI. Frequent sexual intercourse has long been associated with acute cystitis ("honeymoon cystitis"). Spermicidal contraceptives and barrier methods such as the diaphragm have been associated with a higher rate of recurrent UTIs (10). Spermicides induce colonization of the vagina by *E. coli* (16). When, for example, a pattern of postcoital infection is recognized, a change in behaviors or a plan of self-administered antibiotics can be successfully implemented by the patient. However, many of the behavioral factors once thought to increase the incidence of UTI have not proven to be risk factors. These include wiping patterns, vaginal douching, and pre- and post-coital voiding habits (10).

UNCOMPLICATED UTI—DIAGNOSTIC TESTING

Diagnosing UTIs with Urine Cultures

One of the challenges of treating UTIs in the ED is that confirming a diagnosis requires a result that is not available during ED care: a positive urine culture. Fortunately, in women with no known risk for complicated infections and no symptoms of upper tract infections, the safety of treating without cultures has been established (17). When they have been obtained in studies, the threshold for number of colony forming units per millimeter (CFU/mL) is lower when there are symptoms suggestive of UTI and there is no identifiable reason for incidental bacteriuria. In patients with a normal urinary tract, 100 CFU/mL is predictive of patients who will have progression of disease without treatment (9, 14). Some laboratories find it easier to report a cutoff of 1000 CFU/mL and sensitivity appears not to significantly change (9, 10).

Bedside Urinalysis

The most immediate testing available for UTI is with the bedside dipstick. It is important to remember to test fresh urine ideally within 1–2 h of collection unless refrigerated. Otherwise, organisms such as enterococcus can grow and cause a false positive sample. Also, it is important to wait the recommended time (up to 2 minutes) after dipping the

reagent strip in the urine before interpretation. The three most significant tests for UTI on the dipstick are those that test for leukocyte esterase, nitrite, and blood. Clinicians should bear in mind that the sensitivity and specificity of the urine dipstick decreases with lower CFU/mL bacterial counts (18).

The leukocyte esterase test is a test for the presence of an enzyme produced by WBCs in the urine (pyuria). The limitations of this test are that there are other causes of inflammation besides UTIs and that some causes of UTI cause less inflammation. Other causes of pyuria include urethritis, vaginitis, catheterization, analgesic nephropathy, interstitial nephritis, or any inflammation near the ureters and kidneys (including appendicitis). In the presence of indwelling catheterization, the ability of gram-positive organisms to produce inflammatory response appears to be limited. For the leukocyte esterase test, in patients with 100,000 CFU/mL, the sensitivity has been reported as high as 95% and specificity as high as 98%. In patients with uncomplicated cystitis where a significant infection may be present with only 100 CFU/mL, the sensitivity drops to 71% (14).

The nitrite test is a test for the presence of bacteria that have the enzyme nitrate reductase. Nitrate reductase converts nitrate to nitrite. The limitation of the nitrite test is that it will be falsely negative if either the bacteria present do not produce nitrate reductase or there has not been enough time in the bladder for the conversion (which needs 4-6 h) to take place. The common bacteria that do not produce this enzyme include *S. saprophyticus*, Enterococci spp., and *P. aeruginosa*. Even in microorganisms that do produce this enzyme, if the patient has voided recently before the sample could be collected, or if the patient is taking a diuretic, there may not be enough concentration of nitrite to be detected (9). To achieve the best overall combination of specificity and sensitivity, the leukocyte esterase and nitrite tests are combined. When either one is positive, this improves overall sensitivity to 75–82% and specificity to 82–84%. While adding a positive test for hematuria further increases sensitivity to 99%, there is a great reduction in specificity to just 19% (14, 19).

Microscopic Examination

Microscopic examination of urine can be performed with spun or unspun urine. While bacteria, white cells, and red cells can be detected, the most specific yield is from finding bacteria. If a urine sample has 100,000 CFU/mL of bacteria, the presence of any bacteria per high power field (HPF) in a spun sample (or 10/HPF in unspun sample) has a sensitivity and specificity of 90%, while the presence of

WBCs has a sensitivity only of 60–85%. The limitation of microscopy is that in samples with less than 100,000 CFU/mL, bacteria are found only 10% of the time (9, 20). As stated earlier, in uncomplicated UTIs, the presence of only 100 CFU/mL is still significant.

Some centers only perform microscopy if there is a positive finding on urinalysis, while others always combine the tests. Although there is a small benefit in always using both tests (20), this must be weighed against the high resource cost of microscopy.

UNCOMPLICATED UTI—TREATMENT

While the microbiology of UTIs has remained constant and predictable over the last two decades, selection pressure from the use of antibiotics has produced pathogens with ever-increasing resistance to the traditional antimicrobial agents. Clinicians must be mindful of the resistance patterns that exist within their hospitals and communities. These resistance patterns have increasingly affected the choice of empiric antimicrobial therapy for UTI (21).

Empiric therapy is the standard practice for treatment of UTIs, and management is based on the clinical scenario. In cases of acute uncomplicated cystitis, empiric therapy without culture is usually sufficient. Acute pyelonephritis, complicated UTI, and recurrent UTI warrant the acquisition of cultures prior to the start of empiric therapy with subsequent adjustments based on culture and sensitivity results.

Antibiotics

The selection of an appropriate antimicrobial agent (Table 20–2) must take into account the spectrum of activity of the antimicrobial agent, the prevalence of antibiotic resistance, the incidence and types of adverse effects, the cost, the duration of therapy, and the ease of use (Table 20–3). Most of the ideal antimicrobial agents for the treatment of UTI achieve high drug concentrations in the urine. Lower incidences of recurrent UTI occur with agents that, in addition to high urinary concentrations of drug, also achieve high concentrations in the vaginal secretions, thus eliminating this reservoir for subsequent reinfection (16).

Beta-Lactams

The beta-lactam antibiotics, which include the penicillins and cephalosporins, have long been used for both un-complicated and complicated UTIs. Although still useful for treating enterococci and in combination with beta-lactamase inhibitors, ampicillin and amoxicillin have become less useful due to decreased effectiveness at the standard 3-day dosing schedules, and increasing resistance to these agents among uropathogens. Three-day courses of other antibiotic classes such as the sulfonamides and the quinolones have demonstrated greater effectiveness.

Growing resistance and frequent dosing regimens have limited the utility of first-generation cephalosporins such as cephalexin. Third-generation oral cephalosporins are useful with once daily dosing regimens and low bacterial resistance, but are used sparingly due to cost. Advanced generation parenteral cephalosporins such as ceftriaxone are very effective in treating pyelonephritis that require admission.

Warren et al. postulate that some beta-lactam antibiotics may not perform particularly well in treating UTIs because of very rapid renal excretion resulting in inadequate urinary concentrations and/or ineffectiveness at clearing uropathogens from the vaginal and colonic flora allowing reinfection (22). Nonetheless, beta-lactam antibiotics have excellent safety profiles and can be useful in combination with other agents (e.g., gentamicin or beta-lactamase inhibitors) in treating UTIs.

Trimethoprim/Sulfamethoxazole and Trimethoprim

Trimethoprim/sulfamethoxazole (T/S) is the most studied antibiotic regimen for uncomplicated UTI in women. It is well tolerated and inexpensive with a convenient twice-daily dosing regimen. Care must be taken as the sulfonamide component can potentiate the drug effects of warfarin and oral hypoglycemic agents by displacing these drugs from albumin.

Its spectrum of activity includes the common pathogens for uncomplicated UTI, but there is limited activity against enterococci and *P. aeruginosa*. The greatest concern is the increasing resistance of uropathogens to T/S, which has been increasing over the past decades. Because of these facts, T/S is usually limited to use in uncomplicated UTIs where the known community resistance is low. The host factors independently linked to T/S-resistant *E. coli* include recent hospitalization, current use of any antibiotics, and current or recent use of T/S (21). Some experts prefer to use trimethoprim alone for uncomplicated UTIs and recurrent UTI prophylaxis because of similar efficacy and decreased side effects (9, 16).

Table 20–2. Antibiotic Options for UTIs

Class	Antibiotic	Dosing/Frequency	Route
Beta-lactam	Cephalexin (oral first generation)	250–500 mg QID	Oral
	Cefuroxime axetil (oral second generation)	500 mg BID	Oral
	Amoxicillin	250–500 mg TID	Oral
	Ampicillin po	250–500 mg QID	Oral
	Ampicillin IV	1000 mg QID	IV
	Amoxicillin/clavulanate	500 mg TID or 875 mg BID	Oral
	Ampicillin/sulbactam	3.0 g QID	IV
	Ceftriaxone	1.0–2.0 g QD	IV/IM
	Ceftazadime	1.0–2.0 g Q 8–12 h	IV
	Cefotaxime	1.0–2.0 g Q 4–12 h	IV
	Cefepime	1.0–2.0 g Q 12 h	IV
	Pipercillin	2.0 g BID	IV
	Pipercillin/tazobactam	3.375–4.5 g Q6–8 h	IV
	Ticarcillin	3.0 g Q4–6 h	IV
	Ticarcillin/clavulanate	3.1 g Q4–6 h	IV
Sulfonamide	Trimethoprim	100 mg BID or 200 mg QD	Oral
	Trimethoprim/sulfamethoxazole	One double-strength tablet BID	Oral
Quinolone	Ciprofloxacin po	500–750 mg BID	Oral
	Ciprofloxacin (extended release PO)	500 mg QD	Oral
	Ciprofloxacin IV	400 mg BID	IV
	Ofloxacin	400 mg BID	Oral/IV
	Levofloxacin	250–750 mg QD	Oral/IV
	Gatifloxacin	200–400 mg QD	Oral/IV
Aminoglycoside	Gentamicin (multiple daily dosing)	2 mg/kg load, then 1.7 mg/kg TID	IV
	Gentamicin (once daily dosing)	5–7 mg/kg	IV
	Aztreonam	1.0–2.0 g Q 6–8 h	IV
Other	Nitrofurantoin (macrocrystals)	100 mg QID	Oral
	Nitrofurantoin (monohydrate/macrocrystal)	100 mg BID	Oral
	Fosfomycin	300 mg one dose	Oral
	Imipenum/cilastatin	500 mg Q 6 h	IV

Note: Many of these agents require dosing adjustment for decreased glomerular filtration rate.

Quinolones

Because quinolones are able to maintain high drug concentrations in genitourinary tissue (kidneys, prostate, uterus) and high rates of excretion into urine and vaginal secretions, quinolones are ideal empiric antibiotics for treating genitourinary infections. Within the class, seven drugs are FDA-approved for treating UTI: ciprofloxacin, levofloxacin, gatifloxacin, enoxacin, lomefloxacin, norfloxacin, and ofloxacin. The first three listed are the most commonly used.

Quinolones are well tolerated with mostly once-daily dosing, enhancing patient compliance. Side effects cited include gastrointestinal, dermatologic, and central nervous system effects; these are usually mild and self-limited. Torsades de pointes and QT prolongation has been associated with some of the quinolone agents. Of note, aluminum- and magnesium-containing compounds such as antacids as well as products containing iron, calcium, or zinc can affect quinolone absorption. Like T/S, quinolones can increase warfarin effects. Overall, limitations regarding this class of antibiotic are its cost and its contraindication for use in children under age 18 and pregnant women (23).

The spectrum of activity of quinolones differs based on the generation of the drug. The newer quinolones (levofloxacin and gatifloxacin) have a broader spectrum of activity when compared to the older agents. The

Table 20–3. Empiric Antibiotic Regimens for Uncomplicated UTIs

Scenario	Typical Pathogens	Mitigating Factors	Recommended Empiric Therapy	Route	Duration (days)
Lower tract symptoms: cystitis	E. coli, S. saprophyticus, P. mirabilis, K. pneumoniae	Most cases	T/S, trimethoprim, quinolone	Oral	3
			Fosfomycin	Oral	1
Upper tract symptoms: pyelonephritis	E. coli (particularly uropathogenic), P. mirabilis, K. pneumoniae, S. saprophyticus	Mild-to-moderate illness, no nausea or vomiting— outpatient therapy	Quinolone	Oral	7
			T/S, oral ceph., amoxicillin with clavulanate	Oral	14
			fosfomycin	Oral	3
		Severe illness or possible urosepsis— hospitalization recommended	Quinolone, ceph. (3 or 4 gen), amp/sulbactam, pipercillin- or ticarcillin-containing regimens, gentamicin or aztreonam (with or without ampicillin), imipenem, then	Parenteral	Until afebrile, then
			Quinolone, amp/clavulanate, oral ceph, T/S	Oral	14

newer agents have activity against gram-negative and gram-positive aerobic bacteria (including enterococci) as well as atypical microorganisms such as *Mycobacterium*, *Legionella*, *Mycoplasma*, and *Chlamydia* species. Ciprofloxacin has the best activity against *P. aeruginosa* among quinolones, although recent studies suggest that levofloxacin may be equally efficacious (19, 23).

Cost and concerns about development of resistance with overuse have made quinolones an alternative agent for acute uncomplicated UTI. However, the significant increase in T/S-resistant *E. coli* over the past years has sparked studies to determine when the resistance is high enough to warrant considering quinolones as first line. Le and Miller conducted a decision and cost analysis to determine the resistance rate at which T/S should not be used in favor of a quinolone antibiotic. Their results found that, when the T/S resistance in a community exceeds 22%, the added costs of reinfection and complications from progression of infection when using T/S make quinolones the antibiotic of choice (24).

In patients with allergy to trimethoprim or sulfa compounds, or at high risk for T/S-resistant *E. coli* (recent hospitalization, current use of any antibiotic, current or recent use of T/S, or community with high prevalence of T/S-resistant E. coli), quinolones are the recommended antibiotic. In uncomplicated UTIs, quinolones are usually given as a 3-day course.

Nitrofurantoin

Nitrofurantoin is an effective antibiotic for treating uncomplicated UTIs and has been used for decades as primary therapy for UTI. Gastrointestinal side effects are minimized with the macrocrystalline preparation. Nitrofurantoin has excellent activity against *E. coli* and *S. saprophyticus* and a very favorable resistance pattern that has remained stable and low over the years. Unlike T/S, it also has activity against enterococci. Poor efficacy against *Klebsiella*, *Enterobacter*, and *Pseudomonas* as well as low serum concentrations make nitrofurantoin a poor choice for empiric treatment in uncomplicated pyelonephritis. A clinical trial comparing a 3-day course of nitrofurantoin versus a 3-day course of T/S showed greater efficacy with T/S. Nitrofurantoin is therefore only recommended as a 7-day course (9, 16).

Fosfomycin Tromethamine

Fosfomycin is a phosphonic acid bacteriocidal agent recently introduced to treat UTIs. Fosfomycin is indicated for the treatment of acute uncomplicated cystitis. It has a mild side effect profile of predominantly gastrointestinal symptoms. It is administered as a single 3-g oral dose in uncomplicated lower UTIs. In mild upper or complicated cases, a longer 3 days course is more likely to be needed.

Its spectrum of activity is excellent for the common uropathogens. It includes *E. coli* and enterococci as well as *Klebsiella, Enterobacter, Serratia*, and *Citrobacter* species. Several comparative trials of fosfomycin in acute uncomplicated cystitis have shown it to be equal in efficacy to nitrofurantoin, beta-lactam antibiotics, and trimethoprim alone, but less effective compared to quinolones or trimethoprim-sulfamethoxazole (16). This has relegated fosfomycin to an alternative therapy for cystitis.

Aminoglycosides

Aminoglycosides are only available as parenteral therapy and are reserved for the treatment of acute pyelonephritis that require admission. Aminoglycosides have a spectrum of activity that includes *E. coli, Klebsiella* spp., *Proteus vulgaris, Serratia marcescens, Enterobacter* spp. and *P. aeruginosa* as well as methicillin-sensitive *S. aureus*. Aminoglycosides work in synergy with ampicillin to treat *Enterococcus faecalis*. Aminoglycosides are almost always utilized as combination therapy with a beta-lactam agent. The commonly described but infrequent side effects of nephrotoxicity and ototoxicity are usually not a concern due to the short courses of aminoglycosides therapy (2–3 days) required for UTIs.

Analgesia

Throughout the spectrum of urinary tract infections from uncomplicated cystitis to bacteremia, pain is often present. Clinicians must be mindful of this and seek to provide analgesia with the same interest as they choose antibiotics. Oral agents are often effective. Nonsteroidal antiinflammatory drugs and acetaminophen provide analgesia and antipyresis. Oral opiate narcotics are often combined with the above agents and can provide more potent analgesia. Phenazopyridine (brand name: Pyridium) is a unique therapy for patients with urethritis and/or cystitis. It is a bladder anesthetic that is taken orally and excreted into the urinary system by the kidneys. It provides rapid relief from the discomfort of dysuria. Patients must, however, be advised that phenazopyridine imparts a reddish-orange color to urine and secretions, including tears. Patients should be advised of the risk of contact lens staining.

Other Treatments

A 2004 Cochrane review found two small randomized, controlled trials that demonstrated cranberries may decrease the number of symptomatic UTIs in women over a 12-month period (RR 0.61 95% CI 0.40 to 0.9 compared with placebo-control women) (25). However, with regard to ascorbic acid, a search of the medical literature found no randomized, controlled trials testing the utility of ascorbic acid in treating or preventing UTIs. Some have postulated that the acidification of urine with ascorbic acid would create an unfavorable environment for bacterial growth. Without adequate studies that establish efficacy and safe dosing, it is difficult to recommend the routine use of ascorbic acid.

Summary Treatment of Uncomplicated UTIs

In 1999, the Infectious Diseases Society of America (IDSA) conducted a review of the evidence regarding the treatment of acute symptomatic, uncomplicated cystitis and pyelonephritis in women. Their recommendations were qualified as to the strength of recommendation and quality of evidence. They published their evidence-based guidelines in the journal *Clinical Infectious Diseases* (22). For acute uncomplicated cystitis in women, the evidence presented by the IDSA supports the use of T/S in a 3-day regimen as first-line treatment for acute uncomplicated cystitis in women. The empiric antibiotic regimen is effective and encourages compliance. Trimethoprim alone is equivalent to T/S. Quinolones are noted to likely be of equal efficacy to T/S, but are not the first-line recommendation due to cost (16, 22). Fosfomycin as a single dose therapy is also effective but less so when compared to 3-day quinolone or T/S regimens. Nitrofurantoin requires a 7-day course to achieve equivalent efficacy to 3-day quinolones or T/S treatment.

For most women with acute uncomplicated pyelonephritis, the infection is a progression from bladder to kidney involvement. The microorganisms causing pyelonephritis are thus the same as for cystitis. The antibiotic regimens are similar except that, depending on severity of disease, initial therapy may be parenteral and the duration of therapy longer.

Quinolones are recommended as the first-line antibiotic for acute uncomplicated pyelonephritis in women. T/S, oral cephalosporins and amoxicillin-clavulanate are alternative recommendations for outpatient therapy in the mild to moderately ill patient. In the severely ill patient, parenteral antibiotics should be used until the patient's clinical condition improves. Many advocate that the patient remain afebrile for 24–48 h before converting to an oral regimen. Duration of treatment should be 14 days with one exception. In a mild presentation in which quinolone is chosen, a 7-day course of therapy is equally effective (16, 22).

For frequent RUTIs, antimicrobial treatment options have been developed to limit the morbidity and inconvenience. The options include long-term (6–12 months) low-dose antibiotic prophylaxis, episodic self-treatment, or postcoital prophylaxis. For women with at least two UTIs in 6 months or three in 1 year, long-term low-dose prophylaxis is recommended. This results in 95% reduction in the incidence of recurrent UTIs during the course of therapy. Unfortunately, most patients will have recurrent UTIs within 3 months of discontinuance of the prophylaxis therapy. For patients with less frequent episodes of UTI, self treatment may be the more convenient option. The patient is given a prescription for antibiotics and initiates therapy with the onset of symptoms of UTI. For patients who can relate their UTIs to sexual intercourse, postcoital prophylaxis is a third effective option used when patients take a low-dose of antibiotic immediately after intercourse (16).

The recommended prophylactic antibiotics for RUTIs include trimethoprim, trimethoprim and sulfamethoxazole, nitrofurantoin, cephalexin, and quinolones. The recommendation for self-treatment is the same as that for uncomplicated cystitis (trimethoprim/sulfamethoxazole or quinolone, if resistance to T/S is greater than ~20%) (16). In addition, there may be some utility in encouraging the use of cranberry juice in women with RUTI.

COMPLICATED UTI—EPIDEMIOLOGY

This section will now describe the different concerns pertinent to patients with complicated UTIs. The groups to be discussed in this section include pregnant women, men, elderly, diabetics, catheterized patients, and other immunocompromised patients.

In pregnancy, UTIs are the most common bacterial infection. UTIs affect 4–10% of pregnant women with most having ASB. As many as 1–4% of pregnant women will have their first episode of UTI during the pregnancy. Any prior history of UTI increases risk of developing a new UTI. A history of a childhood UTI further increases the risk to 27% (47% if they had renal scarring). Pyelonephritis is the most common severe infection, affecting 1–2% of pregnant women, usually in the second half of pregnancy (6).

Urinary tract infections in men are a rare condition before age 50 when prostate changes and the development of other medical conditions create conditions that increase the risk of infection (15). In young healthy adults, only about 4% of UTIs occur in men. In elderly nursing home patients, one-third to one-half of UTIs occur in men. In their lifetime, 30% of all men (as compared to 50% of all women) will have experienced a UTI.

Among female patients, diabetes increases the risk of UTI by 2-4 fold. In contrast, the presence of diabetes in men does not appear to significantly increase the risk of UTI. In addition, the progression of infection from lower to upper tract and to bacteremia does appear to be increased in diabetics. This results in more risk for developing complications from even an otherwise simple acute cystitis (5, 26).

Another important group of patients with a unique incidence and prevalence of UTI is those who have urinary catheters. Urinary tract catheter use can be classified as indwelling, intermittent, external (condom-type), or suprapubic. Indwelling catheters can be considered chronic if used for a month or more, with the prevalence of bacteriuria after 1 month approaching 100%. The presence of an indwelling catheter is associated with the highest rates of infection with a daily incidence of bacteriuria of 3–10%. Of these patients, 10–25% will develop symptoms of local infection and 1–4% will develop bacteremia. When using intermittent and condom catheters, the incidence of UTIs drops to 1/10th the infection rate associated with indwelling catheters. When using suprapubic catheterization, the incidence of UTIs is 1/50 times the infection rate associated with indwelling catheters (27–29).

COMPLICATED UTI—MICROBIOLOGY

E. coli remains the most common pathogen for all manifestations of UTI and in all groups of patients (15). However, other bacteria without these virulence factors that are resisted by normal hosts become more successful in establishing infections in patients with abnormal urinary tract anatomy or function. These other bacteria (except for *S. saprophyticus*) become more prevalent in complicated UTIs (9). *Klebsiella, Serratia, Enterobacter,* and *Proteus* species as well as *P. aeruginosa, S. aureus,* group B and group D (enterococcus) *Streptococcus,* and fungi account for a larger percentage of UTIs in complicated cases (5, 6, 9). These latter bacteria are more likely to infect those with structural genitourinary disease, diabetes, spinal syndromes, recent instrumentation, and/or chronic indwelling urinary catheters. These non-*E. coli* microorganisms also account for a larger percentage of nosocomial urinary tract infections (9). The clinical scenario guides the ED clinician in deciding if a microorganism other than *E. coli* is involved.

The influence of age on the incidence of UTIs and the flora that cause them is multifactorial. The elderly are likely to have comorbid diseases that affect the anatomic and immunologic status of their urinary tracts. Males are likely to have urinary stasis secondary to prostatic hypertrophy. Prostatic secretions felt to be protective against the ascent of microorganism via the urethra may be diminished. The elderly are more likely to be on medications that affect bladder tone and result in urinary stasis. There is a greater incidence of type 2 diabetes mellitus as well as a higher likelihood of recent hospitalization, antibiotic use, and urinary tract instrumentation among the elderly. *E. coli, Enterococcus, Staphylococcus epidermidis,* and *S. saprophyticus* are more common in the elderly (29, 30).

Diabetics have a higher incidence of UTIs caused by *Klebsiella* spp., group B streptococci and enterococci. Fungi are a more common cause of UTI in diabetics than in the general patient population (15). Impaired immunity, peripheral and autonomic neuropathy, exposure to antibiotics, and higher rates of urinary tract instrumentation are likely all contributing factors in the incidence and flora of UTIs in diabetics (26).

The introduction of an instrument including a chronic indwelling bladder catheter bypasses many of the defense systems that the host has in place to prevent colonization and subsequent infection by microorganisms. While *E. coli* remains the most common pathogen, a myriad of other microorganisms cause UTIs in these patients. Many of these patients are in hospital or long-term care facilities and many are receiving or have received antibiotics. These patients are more likely to have their periurethral skin or mucous membranes colonized with potent uropathogenic microbes. These pathogens include *Klebsiella* spp., *Proteus mirabilis, Enterobacter* spp., *P. aeruginosa, S. aureus,* enterococci, and fungi (5). The presence of a chronic indwelling bladder catheter usually leads to polymicrobial bacteriuria (15).

Patients with prolonged hospitalizations or residence in long-term care facilities are prone to colonization and infection with nosocomial microorganisms. These pathogens include *Klebsiella* spp., *P. mirabilis, Enterobacter* spp., *P. aeruginosa, S. aureus,* and enterococci (9, 31). Mixed infections are more common in this group. In addition, antibiotic usage places selection pressures on the microorganisms whether these microbes are merely colonizing the patient or causing infection. Some patients will harbor microbes that have unfavorable resistance patterns. Others will experience an overgrowth of nonbacterial microorganisms such as fungi (e.g., *Candida* spp.). While the presence of fungus is more common in diabetics, catheterized, and institutionalized patients, it is still difficult to determine in a given patient when colonization becomes a progressing infection. Fortunately, progression to an upper fungal infection or fungemia from a bladder infection appears to be a rare occurrence (31).

COMPLICATED UTI—CLINICAL PRESENTATION

Pregnant Women

Untreated UTIs (including ASB) in second trimester can progress to pyelonephritis, increased risk premature low-birth-rate infants, anemia, or pregnancy-induced hypertension/preeclampsia. Untreated or treated UTI in third trimester can increase risk for infant complications of mental retardation, developmental delays, cerebral palsy, and death.

Pyelonephritis can present with only lower symptoms, but usually patients have fever, flank pain, costovertebral angle tenderness (usually on the right), and nausea and vomiting. Admission for intravenous hydration and antibiotics is generally warranted. With antibiotics for pyelonephritis, 86% will have contractions during the first hour and 50% after 5 h (6, 7).

Men

Any evidence of a UTI in a man can be considered evidence of a complicated infection. Fortunately, UTI in men is a rare condition until the ages when prostate enlargement creates conditions of obstruction that increase the risk of infection. At times, the prostate itself can become infected. The symptoms of acute prostatitis include all the symptoms mentioned for lower and upper tract infections. Importantly, the absence of perineal pain, painful ejaculation, or a tender prostate is not reliable in excluding the diagnosis of prostatitis in a male patient with a UTI. In males, a UTI that recurs or that does not improve completely with therapy should prompt urology referral for an evaluation of prostate and structural defects of the urinary tract (2, 15).

Elderly Patients

Using the clinical history to diagnose UTI in patients over age 65 becomes more difficult. First, the frequency of atypical presentations increases. Symptoms such as isolated fever, delerium, and decreases in function are more common in the elderly with UTI. Second, common urinary symptoms such as incontinence or frequent urination may be present chronically without infection (30).

There are factors that increase the risk of UTI in elderly. Nonreversible factors include increasing age, dementia, neurologic disease, diabetes requiring medication, urinary incontinence, cystoceles, and previous genitourinary surgery. Factors that are potentially reversible include atrophic vaginitis from estrogen deficiency and even the medications that treat urinary incontinence (6, 29).

The high rate of ASB in the geriatric population living in long-term care facilities can impair the ED physician's ability to accurately make the diagnosis of UTI (Fig. 20–3). In these elderly patients, the prevalence of ASB can be as high as 33% in men and 50% in women. ASB in the elderly rarely requires medical treatment. When investigating elderly patients with fever, there can be the incidental finding of positive urine cultures in one-third to one-half of cases, regardless of the actual etiology of the fever. When a geriatric patient presents with nonurinary symptoms such as fever or delerium, alternative serious causes can be missed if the work-up ends with the finding of a positive urine test. But when no other source is found, symptomatic UTIs in the elderly are usually treated as complicated cases because of the higher risk of progression of symptoms and poor outcomes despite therapy (30).

Diabetic Patients

A UTI in diabetic patients should always be treated as complicated. Severe complications in case reports include emphysematous cystitis/pyelonephritis, abscess formation, and renal papillary necrosis (32). In addition, UTIs in diabetics involve more unusual pathogens including fungi. Markers for functional deficit such as peripheral neuropathy and proteinuria are associated with increased risk of UTI (26). Despite these complications, it is not clear whether incidental ASB, even in women, should be treated. One double-blind study on ASB in diabetic women did not show any benefit with treatment (33).

Catheterized Patients

In elderly nursing home (NH) patients, the symptoms range from those typical for local irritation through to nonspecific abdominal pain, fever, decreased activities of daily living, and altered mental status. About 10–15% of febrile episodes in NH patients are thought to be attributable to UTIs (30, 34). The other challenging group of patients with catheter related infections is those with spinal cord injuries (SCIs). Due to their neurologic dysfunction, SCI patients can experience chills and

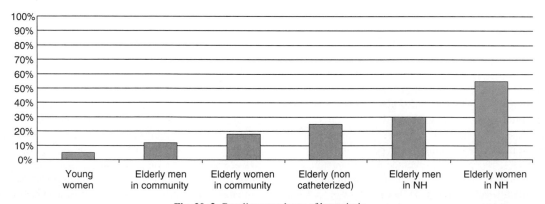

Fig. 20–3. Baseline prevalence of bacteriuria.

sweating without having infection. However, about 45% of febrile episodes in SCI patients are thought to be attributable to UTIs (28).

Other Compromised Hosts

In other groups of immune compromised patients such as those with AIDS (CD4 counts less than 200) (15), ESRD patients (35), or cirrhotic patients with ascites, there do not appear to be any specific differences in presentation of UTIs. There is caution that UTIs may be more prevalent in these groups and so vigilance in getting urine samples in evaluating these patients (including catheterizing ESRD patients without urinary output) who present with febrile illnesses is warranted.

COMPLICATED UTI—DIAGNOSTIC TESTING

Diagnosing Complicated UTIs with Urine Cultures

While in all patients being evaluated for complicated UTIs, cultures are sent from the ED, it is the other tests used in ED (urine dipstick, urinalysis, and urine microscopy) that guide the management. It is important to keep in mind that the cutoff for what constitutes a positive culture varies with the clinical indication for the culture. The threshold for number of CFU/mL is higher when the there are no symptoms suggestive of UTI, especially when there is an identifiable increased risk for incidental bacteriuria. In these patients with an abnormal urinary tract, the cutoff of 100,000 CFU/mL better defines the group of patients who will have progression of disease without treatment. Elderly patients without symptoms, especially those in long-term care facilities, can have rates of 100 CFU/mL approaching 50% (29). In catheterized patients, the prevalence of 100 CFU/mL approaches 100% after a month of indwelling catheterization (27, 34). Therefore, in these patients with either atypical or no symptoms of UTI, the higher the CFU/mL counts, the less likely the infection is an incidental finding and the more likely the patient will benefit from treatment.

Using Microscopic Examination in Complicated UTIs

The added benefit of microscopy in evaluating complicated UTIs is in its ability to predict UTIs with higher CFU/mL counts. The identification of one bacteria/HPF in spun (10/HPF in unspun) urine is 90% specific for predicting urine that will grow 100,000 CFU/mL (9). This cutoff can be helpful in identifying which patients with chronic bacterial colonization have developed a symptomatic infection.

Radiologic Testing in Complicated UTIs

Radiographic testing in evaluating UTIs is rarely indicated. However, CT scanning has the ability to detect structural kidney abnormalities, nephrolithiasis, pyelonephritis, kidney abscesses, and even the rare complication found in diabetics of emphysematous cystitis/pyelonephritis. The most common indication for CT in the ED is the concern for obstructive stone disease which can result in pus collecting above the obstruction. When obstruction is found in the setting of upper tract infection, emergent urologic intervention is required to open up the abscess that has formed above the obstruction. A less common indication would be in evaluating immunosuppressed patients (e.g., diabetics, AIDS patients, post-transplant patients) with evidence of upper tract infection that have not improved after 3 days of treatment. This can detect other abscess complications that may require the services of interventional radiology (36).

COMPLICATED UTI—TREATMENT

While the choices of antibiotics are similar to those used in uncomplicated UTIs, there are some special considerations when choosing an empiric antibiotic regimen for complicated UTIs (Table 20–4). Regimens are generally longer, lasting 10–14 days (up to 21 days for urosepsis). More cases also require parenteral antibiotics and inpatient care. As always, definitive antibiotic therapy is guided by culture results. In complicated UTIs, quinolones are an ideal first-line agent owing to their broad spectrum of activity. The combination of beta-lactam and aminoglycoside is still very effective in the sicker UTI patients (16, 21–23).

Pregnancy and Symptomatic UTI

UTIs are the most common bacterial infections occurring during pregnancy. In pregnant women, asymptomatic bacteriuria and cystitis carry a greater risk of progression to pyelonephritis. Pyelonephritis is associated with an increased risk of premature delivery, low birth weights,

Table 20–4. Empiric Antibiotic Regimens for Complicated UTIs

Scenario	Typical Pathogens	Mitigating Factors	Recommended Empiric Therapy	Route	Duration (days)
Lower tract symptoms: cystitis	E. coli, Klebsiella spp., Proteus spp., Serratia spp., Pseudomonas spp., Staphylococci spp., enterococci	Mild symptoms cystitis	T/S, trimethoprim, quinolone	Oral	7
			Fosfomycin	Oral	3
		Pregnancy	Nitrofurantoin, amoxicillin, oral ceph, (with caution: T/S), trimethoprim	Oral	7
Upper tract symptoms: pyelonephritis		Mild-to-moderate cases, no nausea or vomiting—outpatient therapy	Quinolone	Oral	10–14
		Severe illness or possible urosepsis—hospitalization required	Quinolone, ceph (3 or 4 gen), aminoglycoside or aztreonam (with or without ampicillin), penicillins with beta lactamase inhibitors, imipenem, then	Parenteral	Until afebrile, then
			Quinolone, T/S	Oral	14–21
		Pregnancy – hospitalization recommended	Ceph (3 or 4 gen), amp/sulbactam, pipercillin- or ticarcillin-containing regimens, gentamicin or aztreonam (with or without ampicillin), then	Parenteral	Until afebrile, then
			Amp/clavulanate, oral cephalosporin, T/S	Oral	14

and fetal mortality. Therefore, it is recommended that all forms of UTI including asymptomatic bacteriuria be treated.

While the need for treatment is evident, the choice and duration of antibiotic therapy is less certain. A Cochrane systematic review on studies of antibiotics given for acute cystitis in pregnancy did not find any significant difference in choice or length of treatment among the available antibiotic choices (37). These antibiotics typically available for outpatient therapy include nitrofurantoin and oral cephalosporins. Amoxicillin is also an option but the resistance patterns are often prohibitively high. Any of these choices are usually given as a 7–10 day course. Inpatient treatment can involve third-generation cephalosporins or a combination of ampicillin and aminoglycoside. Treatment is followed by urine culture surveillance (15).

While trimethoprim/sulfamethoxazole is not approved by the Food and Drug Administration (FDA) for use in pregnancy, it has long been used safely in this patient population (9, 22). Some authors recommend caution in using T/S during the first trimester (greater risk of teratogenicity) and the last 2 weeks of gestation (increased risk of kernicterus with sulfonamides). Aminoglycosides, specifically gentamicin, have also long been used safely, although there is some caution in the first trimester over fetal ototoxicity. Nitrofurantoin also requires caution when given near term or in breast-feeding women because of hemolytic anemia in the fetus/newborn. Quinolones are contraindicated during pregnancy and breast feeding (16).

Hospitalization is recommended for all pregnant women with acute pyelonephritis. Parenteral therapy with extended spectrum cephalosporins (e.g., ceftriaxone), ampicillin/sulbactam, pipercillin- or ticarcillin-containing regimens, gentamicin or aztreonam (usually with ampicillin) or T/S (see caution above) is initiated. Twenty-four to 48 h after clinical improvement, the patient can be converted to oral therapy to complete a 14-day course (16).

UTI in Catheterized Patients

Bladder catheterization increases the incidence of UTI as the normal defenses of the genitourinary tract are circumvented. In turn, the catheter can become the very nidus of infection, preventing the complete eradication of the uropathogen. Bacteria have been shown to adhere to the surface of bladder catheters and form biofilms composed of bacteria, bacterial glycocalices, Tamm-Horsfall protein, and urinary salts such as apatite and struvite. These biofilms allow bacteria to adhere and shield them from antibiotics. The treatment regimen should include replacement of the bladder catheter as well as the initiation of systemic antibiotics (15, 27).

Asymptomatic bacteriuria complicates the course of most patients with chronic bladder catheters (more than 30 days). Although systemic antibiotic treatment can reduce bacteriuria and decrease the incidence of UTIs, their routine use has not been recommended. In patients undergoing long-term catheterization, the treatment of episodes of asymptomatic bacteriuria does not reduce the complications of bacteriuria and merely adds cost and risks the development of antibiotic resistance (34). Prophylactic antibiotics are reserved for catheterized patients with bacteriuria at high risk for the development of symptomatic UTIs such as those undergoing invasive urologic procedures or renal transplantation (15). When used, antibiotic treatment of symptomatic UTIs in patients with chronic bladder catheterization is guided by the same recommendations for complicated UTIs. The antibiotic agent chosen must take into account any known resistance patterns.

Patients who undergo intermittent clean bladder catheterization are managed in a different manner. In this group, asymptomatic bacteriuria is treated more aggressively in the hopes of preventing the development of UTI with each successive catheterization (27). Antibiotic regimens include those used for uncomplicated UTI unless cultures warrant different coverage.

Recurrent UTI in Complicated Cases

For postmenopausal women, mechanical and physiologic factors are most strongly associated with the risk of recurrent UTIs. Structural genitourinary disorders associated with recurrent UTIs include bladder and uterine prolapse. Neurologic disorders such as spinal cord injury, multiple sclerosis, and autonomic dysfunction from diabetes can affect bladder tone leading to urinary stasis. Medications with anticholinergic effects also cause urinary stasis and thus predispose to the development of UTIs. Loss of estrogen leads to changes in vaginal mucosa and alteration of vaginal flora. These changes allow uropathogens to colonize the vagina.

Therapy should be aimed at mitigating these risk factors. Structural genitourinary disorders should be addressed, possibly with surgical interventions. Medication which may promote urinary stasis should be eliminated when possible. Estrogen vaginal creams are effective in preventing UTIs in postmenopausal women. The same benefit has not been shown with oral replacement therapy (10, 15, 23).

ASYMPTOMATIC BACTERIURIA—EPIDEMIOLOGY

Asymptomatic bacteriuria is defined as the presence of significant counts of bacteria in the urine with no signs or symptoms of an upper or lower infection, such as dysuria, urinary frequency, urgency, fever, suprapubic, or flank pain. The prevalence of ASB in young women is 3–5%. The prevalence increases with age to over 20% in noninstitutionalized elderly and as high as over 50% in elderly women in nursing homes. The prevalence of asymptomatic bacteriuria is about 10% in men (6% in community and 15–30% in NH) and 20% in women (16%

Table 20–5. Antibiotic Regimens for Treatment of Asymptomatic Bacteriuria

Scenario	Typical Pathogens	Mitigating Factors	Recommended Empiric Therapy	Route	Duration (days)
No symptoms: incidental finding on urine testing	*E. coli*, S. saprophyticus, *P. mirabilis*, *K. pneumoniae*	None	No treatment indicated		
		Pregnancy	Nitrofurantoin, amoxicillin, oral ceph., T/S (with caution), trimethoprim	Oral	7
			Fosfomycin	Oral	3
		Undergoing invasive urologic procedure, immediately postrenal transplant, intermittent sterile bladder catheterization	T/S, quinolone	Oral	7

in community and 17–55% in NH). When patients have indwelling catheters for over 1 month, the prevalence of bacteriuria approaches 100% and is thus common in even asymptomatic catheterized patients (29, 38).

ASB—MICROBIOLOGY

The spectrum of organisms that cause ASB in a given patient population is similar to the organisms that cause symptomatic UTIs. For example, the organisms that cause ASB in pregnant women reflect the microbiology of uncomplicated UTIs in young healthy women. The microbiology discussions of the different groups have already been presented in the uncomplicated and complicated UTI sections.

ASB—CLINICAL PRESENTATIONS REQUIRING TREATMENT

The pertinent question for the clinician is whether treatment is required. The literature seems to overwhelmingly support treatment of ASB in three clinical scenarios: (1) pregnancy, (2) patients prior to undergoing an invasive urologic procedure (e.g., bladder catheterization, cystoscopy), and (3) renal transplant recipients in the early postrenal transplant period (15, 16).

The elderly are another group of special interest for clinicians with regard to ASB. It is a common condi-

tion in the elderly, with females, institutionalized patients, and functionally debilitated patients at particularly highest risk. Early studies had shown an association between bacteriuria and mortality, but these have not been borne out over time. In a large cohort study of elderly ambulatory women conducted over 9 years, there was no association between ASB and mortality (15). Similar results were obtained with institutionalized elderly men and women.

ASB—DIAGNOSTIC TESTING

When a pregnant woman presents to the ED with any complaint, the urine dip is the first line screen. If there is a positive urine dip, urinanalysis, or urine microscopy; then cultures should be sent. If there is a question of adequate follow-up, treatment can be initiated until culture results are available for confirmation.

ASB—TREATMENT

In summary, most cases of ASB do not require antibiotic therapy (Table 20–5). In the nonpregnancy scenarios that require therapy, the treatment regimens include T/S or quinolones for 7 days. The treatment of pregnancy-associated ASB should be guided by the urine culture and sensitivity results with the commonly used antibiotics being nitrofurantoin, amoxicillin, and oral cephalosporins.

T/S and trimethoprim have been used in pregnancy with caution for fetal side effects (16). The needed duration of therapy is not clear with 3–7 day courses typical. What is clear is the need for follow-up on urine cultures before and after therapy (15).

Antibiotic treatment in ASB in the elderly has been shown to produce short-term clearance of the bacteriuria but no reduction in genitourinary symptoms, the rate of future symptomatic UTIs, or overall mortality. In fact, antibiotic use has been associated with higher reinfection rates, greater adverse drug effects, and increased antibiotic resistance (15, 16, 21). Even in the elderly with diabetes, antibiotic treatment for ASB has not been shown to improve clinical outcomes (33).

CASE PRESENTATIONS—OUTCOMES

1. *Case 1.* A healthy young woman presents with possible uncomplicated UTI. It is important to confirm that the patient is not pregnant, that she does not have any upper tract symptoms such as fever or back/flank pain, that she does not have a pattern of recurrent UTI by history, and that she has no history of vaginal discharge. If none of these complicating factors are present, then the patient can be treated empirically with T/S. If community resistance is higher than 20%, the use of a quinolone for 3 days is recommended. Testing does not change this treatment plan, and cultures are not recommended. Of note in this case, the bedside dipstick urinalysis shows trace leukocyte esterase but no nitrites or blood. This could indicate *S. saprophyticus* is more likely, but it is also still consistent with an *E. coli* infection that had not enough nitrite concentration in that particular urine sample to be detected.

   If her symptoms recur before 2 weeks, a relapse with a new infection from the same organism is the likely cause, and a longer course or change in antibiotics is indicated. If her symptoms recur after 2 weeks, then a reinfection from a different organism is now more likely and the same empiric antibiotics can be given. If a third infection occurs, then the patient should be referred to a primary care doctor for possible chronic therapy for RUTI.

2. *Case 2.* An elderly woman from a NH presents with fever and has a urinalysis that shows trace leukocyte esterase and a strong positive result for nitrates. While UTIs are common in NH patients, it is much more common to have incidental urine contamination with bacteria. It is important with this presentation not to limit the

work-up for the patient's symptoms when the presence of bacteria is found in the urine. If no other source is found, it is reasonable to begin antibiotics for UTI that can be modified or stopped in the next days when the culture results are obtained. With nonspecific symptoms such as fever, bacterial counts of 100,000 CFU/mL are more specific for active infection. In the ED, one test that is helpful is when the urine microscopy shows bacteria (1/HPF in spun and 10/HPF in unspun urine). Visualizing bacteria on microscopy indicates the urine culture will likely grow out 100,000 CFU/mL. The choice of antibiotics is similar to that in the uncomplicated case, but the duration of treatment should be longer (usually 1–2 weeks). In addition, there are often parenteral choices in NH patients including IV/IM cephalosporins such as ceftriaxone and IV quinolones. It is also important to remember that if this patient had no symptoms, treatment has no benefit.

REFERENCES

1. Schieve LA, Handler A, Hershow R, et al.: Urinary tract infection during pregnancy: Its association with maternal morbidity and perinatal outcome. *Am J Public Health* 84:405–410, 1994.
2. Lipsky BA: Urinary tract infections in men. Epidemiology, pathophysiology, diagnosis, and treatment. *Ann Intern Med* 110:138–150, 1989.
3. Stamm W, Hooton T: Management of urinary tract infections in adults. *N Engl J Med* 329(18):1328–1334, 1993.
4. Nicolle L: Urinary tract infection in geriatric and institutionalized patients. *Curr Opin Urol* 12(1):51–55, 2002.
5. Ronald A: The etiology of urinary tract infection: Traditional and emerging pathogens. *Am J Med* 113:14S–19S, 2002.
6. Foxman B: Epidemiology of urinary tract infections: Incidence, morbidity, and economic costs. *Am J Med* 113:5S–13S, 2002.
7. Stamm W: Scientific and clinical challenges in the management of urinary tract infections. *Am J Med* 113:1S–4S, 2002.
8. Bent S, Nallamothu B, Simel D, et al.: Does this woman have an acute uncomplicated urinary tract infection? *JAMA* 287:2701–2710, 2002.
9. McBryde C, Redington J: Diagnosis and management of urinary tract infections: Asymptomatic bacteriuria, cystitis, and pyelonephritis. *Prim Care Rev* 4:3–13, 2001.
10. Fihn S: Acute uncomplicated urinary tract infection in women. *N Engl J Med* 349:259–266, 2003.
11. Hooton TM, Stamm WE: Diagnosis and treatment of uncomplicated urinary tract infection.551–81, 1997.
12. Johnson JR: Virulence factors in *Escherichia coli* urinary tract infection. *Clin Microbiol Rev* 4:80–128, 1991.

13. Meyrier A, Zaleznik D: Bacterial adherence and other virulence factors for urinary tract infection, in up to date version 12.2. 2003.

14. Bent S, Saint S: The optimal use of diagnostic testing in women with acute uncomplicated cystitis. *Am J Med* 113:20S–28S, 2002.

15. Stamm W, Hooton T: Management of urinary tract infections in adults. *N Engl J Med* 329:1328–1334, 1993.

16. Nicolle L: Urinary tract infection: Traditional pharmacologic therapies. *Am J Med* 113:35S–44S, 2002.

17. McIsaac W, Low D, Biringer A, et al.: The impact of empirical management of acute cystitis on unnecessary antibiotic use. *Arch Intern Med* 162:600–605, 2002.

18. Lachs M, Nachamkin I, Edelstein P, et al.: Spectrum bias in the evaluation of diagnostic tests: Lessons from the rapid dipstick test for urinary tract infection. *Ann Intern Med* 117:135–140, 1992.

19. Lammers R, Gibson S, Kovacs D, et al.: Comparison of test characteristics of urine dipstick and urinalysis at various test cutoff points. *Ann Emerg Med* 38:505–512, 2001.

20. Leman P: Validity of urinalysis and microscopy for detecting urinary tract infection in the emergency department. *Eur J Emerg Med* 9:141–147, 2002.

21. Gupta K: Addressing antibiotic resistance. *Am J Med* 113:29S–34S, 2002.

22. Warren J, Abrutyn E, Hebel J, et al.: Guidelines for antimicrobial treatment of uncomplicated acute bacterial cystitis and acute pyelonephritis in women. Infectious Diseases Society of America (IDSA). *Clin Infect Dis* 29:745–758, 1999.

23. Schaeffer A: The expanding role of fluoroquinolones. *Am J Med* 113:45S–54S, 2002.

24. Le T, Miller L: Empirical therapy for uncomplicated urinary tract infections in an era of increasing antimicrobial resistance: A decision and cost analysis. *Clin Infect Dis* 33:615–621, 2001.

25. Jepson RG, Mihaljevic L, Craig J: Cranberries for preventing urinary tract infections. *Cochrane Database Syst Rev* 2001, p. CD001321.

26. Stapleton A: Urinary tract infections in patients with diabetes. *Am J Med* 113:80S–84S, 2002.

27. Saint S, Chenoweth CE: Biofilms and catheter-associated urinary tract infections. *Infect Dis Clin N Am* 17:411–432, 2003.

28. Siroky M: Pathogenesis of bacteriuria and infection in the spinal cord injured patient. *Am J Med* 113:67S–79S, 2002.

29. Nicolle L: Urinary tract infection in geriatric and institutionalized patients. *Curr Opin Urol* 12:51–55, 2002.

30. Shortliffe L, McCue J: Urinary tract infection at the age extremes: Pediatrics and geriatrics. *Am J Med* 113:55S–66S, 2002.

31. Sobel JD, Lundstrom T: Management of candiduria. *Curr Urol Rep* 2:321–325, 2001.

32. Calvet HM, Yoshikawa TT: Infections in diabetes. *Infect Dis Clin N Am* 15:407–421, 2001.

33. Harding GK, Zhanel GG, Nicolle LE, et al.: Antimicrobial treatment in diabetic women with asymptomatic bacteriuria. *N Engl J Med* 347:1576–1583, 2002.

34. O'Donnell J, Hofmann M: Urinary tract infections. How to manage nursing home patients with or without chronic catheterization. *Geriatrics* 57:45, 49–52, 55–56, 2002.

35. Minnaganti VR, Cunha BA: Infections associated with uremia and dialysis. *Infect Dis Clin N Am* 15:385–406, 2001.

36. Kawashima A, LeRoy AJ: Radiologic evaluation of patients with renal infections. *Infect Dis Clin N Am* 17:433–456, 2003.

37. Vazquez JC, Villar J: Treatments for symptomatic urinary tract infections during pregnancy. *Cochrane Database Syst Rev* 2003, p. CD002256, 2000.

38. Nicolle L: Asymptomatic bacteriuria: When to screen and when to treat. *Infect Dis Clin N Am* 17:367–394, 2003.

21

Febrile Child

Maureen McCollough
David Talan

HIGH YIELD FACTS

- Vaccines have greatly altered the management of the febrile children over the last two decades.

- Noninfectious disease processes can also be a cause of fever.

- The child's age should be considered when determining the extent of the fever evaluation.

- Careful evaluation of the child's general appearance is mandatory.

- Do not overly rely on laboratory results such WBC or ANC.

- Urinary tract infections in females less than 2 years old and males less than 1 year old should be considered.

CASE PRESENTATION

A 9-month-old female presents with a history of fever for 2 days. The infant was born at term with no significant past medical history. She has had no cough or upper respiratory tract symptoms. She has no vomiting or diarrhea and is eating well. Her pneumococcal and HIB vaccinations are up to date. The infant is very well appearing, is a little girl, simling, and normally interacting on the mother's lap. The pulse rate is 160, respiratory rate 32, and temperature 104.7°F. A blood pressure is not obtained. A pulse oximeter reads 99% on room air. On eximination, the tympanic membranes are normal bilaterally, the oropharynx is moist and clear, and there are no significant lymph nodes on cervical neck examination. The anterior fontanelle is flat. The lings are clear and the heart is tachycardic but without murmurs. The abdomen is soft and nontender. The skin has no rash. The extermities are without swelling and have complete range of motion.

INTRODUCTION/EPIDEMIOLOGY

Fever is a common complaint of children seen in emergency departments, encompassing as much as 25% of all visits. Fever often produces profound parental anxiety that is often reinforced by physicians' and nurses' attitudes. Dehydration and increased metabolic rate may be a result of this increased temperature. Extremely elevated body temperature, above approximately 106.5°F, may potentially be harmful to the central nervous system or other organ systems. Parents should be reassured that generally elevated temperature alone is usually not harmful (1).

The traditional definition of a rectal temperature (for infants and young children) or oral temperature (older children and adolescents) at or above 38°C or 100.4°F has been defined as fever. Temperatures may vary 0.5°C or 1.0°F throughout the day and are typically lowest in the early morning. Therefore, a temperature of 37.0°C (98.6°F) in the early morning hours (e.g., 4 A.M.) may represent a low-grade fever (2, 3). Oral temperatures are generally about 0.3°C to 0.5°F lower than rectal temperatures. Rectal temperatures are not as variable as oral temperatures (4). Axillary temperatures are not generally reliable (5). However, properly used tympanic thermometers may be more reliable than previously thought (6). Bundling of a nonfebrile child should not cause a fever when the temperature is taken rectally (7).

Recent antipyretic use could interfere with identifying a fever in the emergency department. Typically, however, fever is not completely eliminated and the effect of the antipyretic generally dissipates approximately 2 h after the last dose (8). In addition, the response to antipyretic therapy in lowering the temperature does not change the likelihood of bacterial infection, and thus should not be used in determining management (9, 10). At the same time, it is more reassuring when a young child who appears ill when the temperature is very high is playful and smiling when the temperature is lowered.

All children who are evaluated for fever should receive a thorough physical examination. Table 21–1 lists the history and physical findings that are an important part of the emergency evaluation of all febrile children. The initial examination should start with an evaluation of the child's ABCs and identification of life-threatening infections. Obviously, signs of respiratory distress, decreased perfusion, or shock should be treated immediately. The child's mental status and interaction with the environment are especially important to evaluate. A playful, smiling infant with a fever of 40.5°C is less concerning than a lethargic child with no eye contact with a fever of 38.5°C. A thorough history and physical examination also can often identify the source of infection, such as *Varicella* or viral bronchiolitis (i.e., *Respiratory Syncytial virus*). Febrile children should be undressed to look for skin infections and rashes, including petechiae (e.g., meningococcemia)

Table 21–1. Important History and Physical Findings in the Febrile Child

History

Behavior: activity level, consolability, irritability when moved (may be sign of meningitis), lethargy

Hydration: fluid intake, urine output

Respiratory: cough, trouble breathing

Gastrointestinal: vomiting, diarrhea (blood?), travel

Urinary: abdominal pain, dysuria, frequency, urgency, hematuria

Pain: limp, sore throat, earache, abdominal pain, rash

Medical history: chronic medical disease, immunization status, ill contacts

Physical

Appearance: activity, eye contact, muscle tone, color, consolable

Hydration: mucous membranes, fontanelle, capillary refill, skin color, mottling

Respiratory: work of breathing, respiratory rate, grunting, nasal flaring, rales, bronchial breath
   sounds (may be only finding in child with pneumonia), retractions, pulse oximetry

HEENT: adenopathy, meningismus (may not be present in meningitic infants <1 year old),
   pharyngitis, otitis media (bulging, decreased mobility; redness as the only sign is insufficient to
   diagnose otitis)

Cardiovascular: heart rate, murmur, extremity perfusion

Abdomen: tenderness, guarding, organomegaly, costovertebral area (CVA) tenderness

Skin: rash (including viral, Kawasaki disease, measles, Coxsackie virus, scarlet fever, roseola,
   Henoch-Schönlein purpura, varicella)

Musculoskeletal: bone or joint tenderness, swelling, erythema, ability to ambulate

---

and vesicles (e.g., *Coxsackie* or *Varicella* virus infections). Walking an ambulating child will help evaluate for occult joint infections.

The child's age, magnitude of fever, general appearance and behavior, and the presence or absence of a source of infection found during the history and physical examination will determine the need for any further diagnostic tests or empiric antibiotics. The patient's underlying medical conditions, the examiner's experience, the child's behavior and course during a period of observation, and availability of follow-up should also all be considered when deciding the management. Immunocompromised children, such as those with sickle cell anemia or leukemia, are at increased risk for serious infections.

Assessing behavior in very young children can be difficult. Observation of a child's behavior over time, including alertness, consolability, social interactions like playfulness or smiling, and feeding, is perhaps the most sensitive means to discern the presence or absence of a serious infection in a child with an initially equivocal presentation. Signs of serious illness, such as meningitis, can be subtle. Most experts recommend a lumbar puncture in any febrile infant less than 1 month of age. The ability to determine signs of meningitis in older infants will depend on the physician's experience in evaluating and interpreting infant behavior and clinical examination findings. When the examiner's experience is limited, greater reliance on laboratory evaluation may be warranted.

The standard use of empiric antibiotics in young children with fever without a source is rapidly changing. Their use will also depend in part upon the laboratory capability of the hospital. If 2 days are required to identify and report a positive blood culture, then empiric antibiotics may be justified. If faster technology such as radioisotopes is used to identify sources within 12 h, and close follow-up is available, then withholding empiric antibiotics may be a reasonable option.

When follow-up is uncertain, more extensive evaluation and caution with disposition are justified. For example, a 3-year-old well-appearing, toilet-trained girl with reliable follow-up might be discharged to return with a urine specimen for urinalysis and culture in 12 h. But if follow-up is uncertain, it might be more appropriate to catheterize the child during the ED visit. Children at risk for unreliable follow-up include those with parents who are younger, have no access to transportation, or believe their child is not ill (11).

Both infectious and noninfectious causes of fever should be considered when evaluating a child with fever. Tables 21–2 and 21–3 list infectious and other noninfectious causes of fever.

Table 21–2. Infectious Processes Causing Fever in Children

Central nervous system
  Mengingitis
  Encephalitis
Ear, nose, and throat
  Pharyngitis/tonsillitis
  Gingivostomatitis
  Common cold or influenza
  Sinusitis
  Parotitis (viral or suppurative)
  Tonsillar or pharyngeal abscess
  Peritonsillar cellulites or abscess
Respiratory
  Pneumonia
  Croup
  Epiglottitis
  Bronchliolitis
  Bronchitis
Cardiovascular
  Myocarditis
  Endocarditis
Gastroenterology
  Acute gastroenteritis
  Appendicitis
Genitourinary
  Urinary tract infection
  Acute salpingitis (fever generally not the primary
    symptom)
  Epididymitis (fever generally not the primary
    symptom)
Cellulitis and Adenitis
  Periorbital cellulitis
  Facial cellulitis
  Cervical adenitis
  Inguinal adenitis
Musculoskeletal
  Osteomyelitis
  Septic arthritis
Sepsis
  Bacterial sepsis or bacteremia
  Viremia
  Rocky mountain spotted fever
  Toxic shock syndrome

Table 21–3. Noninfectious Causes of Increased Temperature in Children

Environmental
  Overbundling (may raise skin temperature but not rectal
    temperature (17))
  Heat stroke
Collagen-vascular
  Rheumatic fever (prolonged fever, recent sore throat,
    rash, arthralgia)
  Juvenile rheumatoid arthritis (prolonged fever, rash,
    arthritis)
Poisoning
  Atropine or other anticholinergics (dry mucous
    membranes, flushed, decreased, or absent bowel
    sounds)
  Salicylates (tinnitus, hyperventilation)
  Amphetamines (pupillary dilation, agitation, tremor,
    hypertension, tachycardia, hyperreflexia)
  Antidepressants
Other
  Kawasaki disease (prolonged fever, conjunctivitis,
    rash, adenopathy, erythematous mucous
    membranes)
  Drug reaction
  Prolonged seizures
  Hemolysis

certain bacteria from the birth process. Neonates, once infected, are also unable to isolate infections in one organ system, i.e. a neonate who is found to have a urinary tract infection is at higher risk for seeding of the bacteria into other areas, such as the meninges. Up to 25% of febrile neonates will have a bacterial source as a cause of the fever (12). For these reasons, febrile neonates should undergo a thorough evaluation for the source of the fever.

Pathophysiology/Microbiology

Group B *Streptococcus, Listeria monocytogenes,* and *Escherichia coli* are the most common organisms in this age group. A recent study suggested that *Listeria* may not be a continued concern in this age group; however, the study was not of adequate size to make formal recommendations regarding changes in empiric antibiotic coverage (12).

Clinical Presentation

Because of the limitation in examining a neonate, the clinical evaluation cannot be relied upon to reasonably

Fever in the Neonate (0–28 Days)

The evaluation and management of the febrile neonate has remained less controversial than that for older children over the last two decades. Neonates are at unique risk for exclude a serious bacterial infection such as bacteremia or meningitis. A clinical ill appearing neonate e.g. mottled, unresponsive, with labored breathing, should be assumed to be septic until proven otherwise. Other causes of an ill appearing neonate include congenital heart or adrenal problems, or metabolic derangements.

It is the well-appearing neonate with more subtle presentations that can be potentially missed for an infectious process. In this age group, bacterial sepsis and meningitis can present much more subtly (e.g., change in sleep or feeding pattern, apnea, diarrhea, jaundice).

Laboratory, Diagnostic Testing, Management, and Disposition

As was stated earlier, presentations of serious illnesses can be subtle in the very young infant. Therefore, complete septic workup, including lumbar puncture, and hospital admission are generally recommended (13, 14). Most experts recommend neonates be hospitalized and treated with intravenous antibiotics until the culture results are known. Ampicillin (200 mg/kg/day) and gentamicin (7.5 mg/kg/day, or 5 mg/kg/day if less than 1 week post-term age) are recommended as initial empirical therapy. If meningitis is confirmed or highly suspected, cefotaxime (150 mg/kg/day) should be substituted for the gentamicin for better CNS penetration. Other studies suggest that some febrile, well-appearing neonates with negative initial septic workups can be successfully managed with admission and observation without empiric antibiotic treatment, or even discharged (15). Currently, however, this is not considered a standard approach.

Fever in the Young Infant (4–12 weeks)

In the last two decades, the management of febrile young infants, ages 4–12 weeks, has also changed dramatically. Whereas earlier these febrile infants had been admitted to the hospital for intravenous antibiotics, now after a thorough examination, well-appearing febrile infants who are found to be low risk can be discharged home.

Pathophysiology/Microbiology

Group B *Streptococcus, L. monocytogenes,* and *E. coli* continue to be the most common organisms in this age group. The medical history of the mother therefore continues to be important when determining to be more or less conservative with a febrile infant in this age group. As was stated earlier, despite recent literature, *Listeria*

Table 21–4. Rochester Criteria for the Evaluation of Febrile Young Infants (4–12 Weeks Old)

Previously healthy, nontoxic-appearing term infant
No previous past medical history, including maternal birth history
No previous antimicrobial use
No focal infection on examination
WBC count 5,000–15,000/μL
Band count <1500/μL
Stool WBC count $\leq$5 WBC/hpf when diarrhea present
Spun urine $\leq$10 WBCs/hpf

CSF should be evaluated if empiric antibiotics are going to be used in this age group.

should still be considered a potential pathogen in this age group (12).

Clinical Presentation

Infants 4–12 weeks of age also may have subtle manifestations of serious infection, such as decreased oral intake or fussiness. As mentioned earlier, febrile infants as old as 12 weeks had been routinely admitted to the hospital after a complete septic workup. Now several studies support the use of specific guidelines in order to stratify the risk of serious bacterial infection in children 4–12 weeks of age (16, 17). The Rochester criteria (Table 21–4) is a well-validated set of clinical and laboratory criteria that, if met, place a young infant at low risk for a bacterial infection, such that the infant can be managed as an outpatient (16–18). Based on these criteria, the estimated risk of bacteremia and meningitis is 1.1% and 0.5%, respectively.

The transition from a do-everything approach to a selective approach based on risk stratification is now occurring at an earlier age. Traditionally, the Rochester criteria or Philadelphia criteria (Table 21–5) had been recommended for febrile infants 4–12 weeks old. Many experts are now limiting the use of the Rochester criteria and others like it to infants aged 4 weeks to 8 or 10 weeks only, thereby decreasing the number of young infants who require full workups when febrile. For example, the testing and evaluation for occult infections that a well-appearing 9-week-old febrile infant will undergo will today vary greatly depending upon the experience and training of the practitioner. Further studies are needed to support the widespread practice of a less conservative approach to these older yet still vulnerable young infants.

Table 21–5. Philadelphia Criteria for the Evaluation of Febrile Young Infants (4–12 Weeks Old)

Overall clinical appearance
WBC count <15,000/μL
Band-to-neutrophil ratio <0.2
Spun urine <10 WBC/hpf and no bacteria by bright-field microscopy
CSF <8 WBC/microL and negative Gram stain
2-view chest x-ray film with no evidence of discrete infiltrate
Stool for occult blood

Laboratory and Diagnostic Testing

For children meeting the Rochester criteria (i.e., well-appearing term infant with no past medical history), urine and blood cultures are recommended, and routine lumbar puncture and empirical antimicrobials are considered optional (19, 20). Chest x-rays are indicated if the infant has signs of lower respiratory tract disease. Stool evaluation for WBCs and culture are indicated if diarrhea is found in the review of systems. Because of the difficulty in evaluating meningitis in this age group, and the concern for undiagnosed partially treated meningitis, it is recommended that lumbar puncture be performed if antimicrobials are to be administered in this age group. If a source for the fever is found, such as a urinary tract infection, then lumbar puncture should also be considered.

Management and Disposition

If the evaluation of the blood and urine are negative and the child fulfills the other Rochester criteria (or Philadelphia criteria), that infant is considered low risk for a bacterial process and can be discharged home with good follow-up.

For young infants aged 4–12 weeks, if an empiric antibiotic is to be used, intramuscular ceftriaxone (50 mg/kg) is recommended. One should remember that if empiric antibiotics are to be used in this age group, then prior lumbar puncture is recommended. Discharged infants should be followed up in 24 h. Depending upon the timeliness of culture results, a second dose of ceftriaxone may be indicated. Assuring the ability to reach parents at home, i.e. the availability of correct phone numbers, is also imperative.

Fever in Infants and Children Older than 12 Weeks

The evaluation of young children 3 months to 3 years old with fever has changed dramatically in the last two decades. Prior to the advent of the *H. influenza* type b (Hib) and *Streptococcus pneumoniaes* (Prevnar) vaccines, a child with a high fever and no source on examination was of great concern to pediatricians and emergency physicians because of the risk of occult bacteremia and its sequelae. Today, with the widespread use of vaccinations, the routine use of blood tests such as CBC and empiric antibiotics is not recommended.

Pathophysiology/Microbiology

The vast majority of febrile children seen in the emergency department will have a viral process as the underlying cause of fever. Bacterial sources for the fever will depend upon the organ system involved, for example, *E. coli* as a cause of urinary tract infections and *Streptococcus pneumococcus* or *Mycoplasma* as a cause of pneumonia.

More common organisms causing occult bacteremia in this age group have traditionally been *Haemophilus influenzae* type B, *S. pneumoniae,* and *Neisseria meningitidis.* Previously, up to 25% of these bacteremic children would have seeding of other organ systems, causing other serious bacterial infections, such as meningitis or septic arthritis (21).

Prior to the advent of the *H. influenzae* type b (HiB) in 1988 and *S. pneumococcus* (Prevnar) vaccines in 2000, 3–5% of children with no focus of infection and with temperatures above 39.5°C were bacteremic with *S. pneumoniae, H. influenzae,* or *N. meningitidis* (21). With the addition of these vaccines to the pediatric immunization schedule, the rate of invasive disease and bacteremia caused by these organisms has dramatically decreased. Due to the HiB vaccine, this virulent bacterium is now almost nonexistent as a cause of occult bacteremia. Prior to the Prevnar vaccine, *S. pneumoniae* accounted for over 90% of bacteremia cases. The risk of pneumococcal bacteremia causing meningitis compared with *H. influenzae* is much lower, at less than 3% (22). Furthermore, several large multicenter studies have now shown that the overall rate of pneumococcal bacteremia or invasive disease has decreased 66–80% since the advent of the pneumococcal vaccine (23–25). From these studies and others, it can be concluded that the overall bacteremia rate today is probably less than 1%.

Clinical Presentation

Often the source for fever can be found through a thorough history and physical examination. Fever associated with other chief complaints such as a rash or limp should trigger a specific differential diagnosis.

One of the most worrisome causes for fever in children is meningitis. Fortunately, compared to young infants, in this age group, mental status and behavioral changes can be more reliably used to suspect or reasonably exclude this disease process. Young infants with meningitis may have a bulging fontanel. Infants older than 12–18 months usually have meningeal signs such as a stiff neck. Careful and repeated evaluations of the children's general appearance, especially just before discharge from the ED, are the key to reasonably excluding meningitis in children 3–36 months of age. If the febrile child becomes lethargic or is persistently irritable or inconsolable, then a lumbar puncture is recommended, regardless of other physical findings or laboratory parameters.

Fever with a rash can also be a presenting complaint. Ulcers or vesicles isolated to the oropharynx are possibly *Coxsackie* or *Herpes* virus. If vesicles are also present on the hands or feet, then hand-foot-mouth disease (i.e., *Coxsackie*) is likely. Diffuse vesicular lesions on an erythematous base suggest the presence of *Varicella*.

An ill-appearing febrile child with a petechial or purpuric rash should be considered to have meningococcal bacteremia until proven otherwise. Petechiae may develop on the face or neck area, however, due to severe coughing or vomiting. It is recommended, therefore, that any child with fever and petechiae not thought to be due to vomiting or coughing should undergo a complete septic workup. If the child remains well-appearing after a period of observation, no new petechiae have developed, and the child has a negative septic workup, then it may be possible to discharge the child with close follow-up and consideration of empiric administration of ceftriaxone (26). Henoch-Schönlein purpura (HSP), a multisystem vasculitis, results in a petechial or purpuric rash of the lower extremities, associated with painful swollen joints and abdominal pain in a slightly older child. Children with HSP rarely appear acutely ill. If HSP is suspected, stool for occult blood and urine for hematuria should be evaluated.

Roseola infantum is diagnosed by a pink maculopapular after a high fever has defervesced in an otherwise well-appearing infant. Measles will usually present with a maculopapular rash and be associated with an ill-appearing young child with fever, cough, coryza, conjunctivitis, and Koplik spots in the mouth. Kawasaki disease is uncommon but has the potential for serious morbidity. The presentation is usually a several-day history of high fever that progresses to a macular-papular diffuse rash, conjunctivitis, erythematous or fissured lips, strawberry tongue, cervical lymphadenopathy, and edema or desquamation of hands or feet. Kawasaki disease puts the child at risk for developing aneurysms of the coronary arteries. The treatment includes high-dose aspirin, immunoglobulin therapy, and serial echocardiograms. Acute otitis media remains one of the most common discharge diagnoses for young children with fever. Fever or crying alone can result in an erythematous tympanic membrane and therefore this finding alone is not sufficient to diagnose acute otitis media. A bulging membrane or immobility during insufflation is necessary for this diagnosis to be reasonably considered.

Group A beta-hemolytic *Streptococcus* (GABHS) is a cause of pharyngitis and fever in children generally older than 5 years of age. Sequelae of this infection include suppurative infections such as peritonsilar abscess and nonsuppurative complications like rheumatic heart disease and poststreptococcal glomerulonephritis. GABHS is often associated with prominent gastrointestinal symptoms in children. Scarlet fever is likely when a fine, "sandpapery," raised maculopapular rash is also present. A rapid streptococcal antigen test is a relatively specific aid to diagnosis. If it is negative, however, a throat culture is still considered necessary to exclude this diagnosis. Adolescents with exudative pharyngitis accompanied by prominent cervical adenopathy and splenomegaly may have mononucleosis. Atypical lymphocytes on a blood smear or a monospot test will help to confirm this diagnosis.

Respiratory syncytial virus is a cause of fever and upper respiratory symptoms in the winter and early spring. Symptoms can range in severity from mild cough and wheezing to severe respiratory distress with tachypnea, retractions, grunting, and nasal flaring. Hyperinflation and peribronchial cuffing are classic findings on the chest x-ray. A nasal wash for rapid RSV antigen testing can quickly be obtained. If the child clinically appears to have bronchiolitis and the RSV antigen test is positive, the yield from blood cultures and urine cultures looking for other sources of fever is low (27).

Pneumonia in preschool-age children is most often caused by a viral infection; *Mycoplasma* pneumonia is more common in older children and adolescents. Very ill appearing, febrile children of any age may have pneumonia due to pyogenic bacteria such as *S. pneumoniae*. The signs of pneumonia in young children that are indications to consider a chest radiograph include tachypnea, retractions, nasal flaring, grunting, abnormal auscultatory findings, and a pulse oximeter reading of less than 92% (28). Any child without these signs of lower respiratory tract disease does not need to undergo a chest x-ray.

In young children, vomiting, diarrhea, or abdominal pain associated with fever is most likely caused by gastrointestinal causes. Viral or bacterial acute gastroenteritis is a very common cause of fever with vomiting or diarrhea.

The most common in young children is *Rotavirus*. Vomiting frequently precedes diarrhea by 24 h. Rehydration is the cornerstone in treating the vomiting and diarrhea. If oral rehydration appears as an option, the parents should be encouraged to try small amounts of fluids (e.g., 5 cc or 1 teaspoon every 2–3 minutes for young children). The child's diet should be advanced to a regular diet as soon as possible. Intravenous rehydration should be utilized in children who are unable to take oral liquids, have evidence of bowel obstruction, or are moderately to severely dehydrated.

Bacterial sources of diarrhea include *Shigella, Salmonella, Campylobacter,* and enterotoxic and enterohemorrhagic (i.e., Shiga toxin producing) *E. coli.* Stool culture should be considered in children with fever, hematochezia, and abdominal pain, if there are communicability concerns (e.g., a child in a long-term care facility) or if a common source outbreak is suspected. A child found to have a bacterial pathogen as the cause of the diarrhea, with the exception of *Salmonella,* should be treated with the appropriate antibiotic. However, empirical antibiotics are generally discouraged because of the relative likelihood of viral disease and the association of antibiotic treatment with complications from enterohemorrhagic *E. coli* infection. Treating *Salmonella* may lead to a chronic carrier state and is recommended only for infants less than 3 months of age, patients with immunosuppressive illness, and toxic patients. Fluoroquinolones are still relatively contraindicated in young children despite the limited risk to growth.

Appendicitis is one of the more serious causes of fever and abdominal pain in young children. Due in part to the difficulty in making the diagnosis, young children have higher perforation rates compared with older children. Children with appendicitis are often discharged home with diagnoses of gastroenteritis or urinary tract infection (UTI) before the final diagnosis of appendicitis is made. The omentum in young children is less capable of walling off intraperitoneal infections; therefore, peritonitis with diffuse abdominal tenderness is more common. Ultrasound and computed tomography (CT) scan are now used more commonly to diagnose appendicitis in young children. Early antibiotics are recommended in any child with signs of significant peritonitis.

Streptococcal pharyngitis in older children may present with fever, abdominal pain, and associated dysphagia. Lower lobe pneumonia can also be a cause of abdominal pain and fever. Adolescent girls with fever and abdominal pain who are sexually active are at risk for pelvic inflammatory disease. Often, adolescents must be questioned when parents are not present in the room in order to get a more thorough and truthful history. UTIs are also a common cause in girls with fever and abdominal pain. In young children, UTIs may present with fever and vomiting, often without abdominal pain. UTI should be considered in febrile girls less than 2 years old and in uncircumcised boys less than 1 year old.

Fever and vomiting without diarrhea can also be a sign of a neurological process. Meningitis is the most serious cause, particularly bacterial meningitis. Children with a central nervous system (CNS) ventricular shunt should be evaluated for the possibility of shunt obstruction and meningitis. This evaluation would include a head CT scan and lumbar puncture or shunt tap for CSF evaluation. Finally, acute otitis media can also present with fever and diarrhea in young children.

Febrile children who walk with a limp, have local joint symptoms, or refuse to walk should be evaluated for a joint infection. Toxic synovitis is a benign condition related to a recent viral infection; this must be differentiated from septic arthritis which can rapidly be destructive. If the hip joint is suspected, ultrasound appears to be a reliable test to evaluate the presence of an effusion and can then be used to guide joint aspiration. Joint effusions should be analyzed for cell counts, Gram stain, and culture. Discitis is a usually self-limited inflammatory process of the lower thoracic or lumbar disks of the pediatric spine. The patient will often present with a refusal to walk. Careful examination of the back will often show tenderness of the spine and limitation of movement. Disseminated gonococcal infection may also result in arthritis or tenosynovitis in sexually active adolescents.

Laboratory/Diagnostic Testing

After a thorough physical examination, often no identifiable infection source for the fever is found in infants and children 3 months to 3 years old. Studies show that the presence of some defined viral diagnoses can reasonably explain fever, including *Coxsackie* pharyngitis and *Varicella*. Other diagnoses such as otitis media or URI do not necessarily exclude other bacterial causes of fever. If no definitive source for fever can be found after a thorough history and physical examination, then the presence of occult infections must be considered.

In a young child, fever may be the only indication of a UTI. Up to 7% of febrile young children without a source found will have a UTI as a cause of their fever on physical examination (29). In addition, up to 4% of young febrile children less than 2 years old, with either acute otitis media or gastroenteritis as a source for the fever, may also have a UTI (30). A urinalysis and culture are recommended as part of the workup of girls less than 2 years old and of un-circumcised boys less than 12 months old. The urinalysis is insufficiently accurate to be used alone to evaluate the presence of UTI in young children (31). Therefore, a urine culture should be sent in addition to the urinalysis. An enhanced urinalysis, using Gram stain or hemocytometer, has been shown to improve the capabilities of the urinalysis (31). Bag urine specimens are also more likely to produce contaminant flora, compared with catheterized specimens. Pneumonia is rarely present without signs of lower respiratory tract disease and therefore a chest x-ray is generally recommended in the presence of these signs (see previous discussion) (32).

When no source is found on physical examination, and pneumonia and UTI have been ruled out by either physical examination or laboratory tests, the potential for occult bacteremia should also be considered. Prior to the HiB and pneumococcal vaccine era, blood cultures were routinely drawn on highly febrile young children without a source for the fever. The white blood cell count (WBC) or absolute neutrophil count (ANC) was used to determine the need for empiric antibiotics. Today, with the addition of these vaccines, and the declining bacteremia rate, newer recommendations for the management of febrile young children do not advocate the routine use of blood tests or empiric antibiotics. There are little current, postvaccine era data on the risk of occult bacteremia in an unvaccinated young child with a high fever without a source. However, the same approaches as recommended in the prevaccine era should be used.

Management and Disposition

Management and disposition of a child 3 months to 3 years old with fever will depend upon the cause of the fever. Any ill-appearing child should be admitted to the hospital with intravenous antibiotics until the results of cultures are known. If a bacterial source for the fever is known, such as pneumonia or UTI, a well-appearing child with the ability for good follow-up may be discharged home. If the child is to be discharged home, it is recommended that the patient receive the first dose of the appropriate antibiotic prior to discharge. Previous approaches (i.e., prior to HiB and pneumococcal vaccines) to management of the well-appearing febrile child (i.e., rectal temperature greater than or equal to 39.0°C) 3 months to 3 years of age with no source of infection had included (1) blood cultures and empirical antibiotics for all well-appearing febrile children 3–24 months of age without a source; (2) for only those at high risk (e.g., temperature greater than 41.0°C,

under- or nonimmunized, or a combination of temperature greater than 39.0°C and high WBC (>15,000) or absolute neutrophil count (ANC) (>10,000)]; and (3) close follow-up without testing or treatment (33). If empiric antibiotics were to be utilized, intramuscular ceftriaxone (50 mg/kg) was considered appropriate, especially for the child who is not fully immunized against *H. influenzae*. For other children, oral amoxicillin (60–90 mg/kg/d) was considered a reasonable alternative (34).

Today with the advent of the HiB and pneumococcal vaccines, the evaluation and management of febrile young children has changed dramatically. The overall occult bacteremia rate is now estimated to be below 1% in vaccinated (i.e., at least 2 doses of each vaccine) infants and management options using testing to risk-stratify and/or empiric antibiotic treatment are no longer recommended. As stated earlier, in a child who is not adequately immunized, however, the same approaches as recommended in the prevaccine era should be used (35).

When discharging young children with fever, it is important to educate parents that fever alone is not dangerous. Dehydration and increased metabolic demand are the greatest concerns for a child with an elevated temperature. Studies have suggested that fever may be necessary to stimulate the immune system. Fever reduction, however, has not proven to have negative consequences and does improve patient comfort and decrease the metabolic demands and fluid loss. Therefore, fever control with antipyretics is recommended.

Discharge instructions should include the use of acetaminophen (15 mg/kg every 4–6 h) or ibuprofen (10 mg/kg every 4–6 h) for fever control. Cool, clear liquids and light dressing are advised. Sponging may be used but is of questionable value. The hypothalamus regulates body temperature; acetaminophen resets the regulatory center of the hypothalamus, but sponging has no effect on it and a minimal effect on lowering the temperature for any significant period of time. Sponging usually results in an irritated, agitated child (36, 37).

Discharge instructions must also include indications for urgent return for reevaluation. The most important indications for urgent reevaluation are lethargy and persistent irritability. Even with continued fever, if the child's behavior and disposition improve, urgent reevaluation is not necessary. A child who is less than 3 months old, or a child given empiric antibiotics, should be followed up in 12–24 h by a primary care physician or clinic. That follow-up may consist of a telephone call to the caretaker or, if there is reason for additional concern, a repeat examination.

Case Outcome

Because no source for the elevated temperature could be found on physical examination, occult infections were considered. The infant had no evidence of lower respiratory tract disease, so a chest x-ray was not obtained. The infant was fully vaccinated and was therefore at low risk for occult bacteremia. Because of the risk, however, for occult UTI, a catheterized urine specimen was obtained. Urinalysis was positive for blood, leukocytes, and nitrites. Urine was sent to the laboratory for culture. Because the family was considered to be reliable, and because the child was well appearing, the patient was discharged home with a prescription for 10 days of cephalexin. She was given her first dose in the emergency department prior to discharge. Her parents were instructed to follow up with their primary care physician the next day and to return for lethargy, irritability, or inability to take the oral antibiotic.

REFERENCES

1. May A, Bauchner H: Fever phobia: The pediatrician's contribution. *Pediatrics* 90(6):851–854, 1992.
2. Mackowiak PA, Wasserman SS, Levine MM: A critical appraisal of 98.6 degrees F, the upper limit of the normal body temperature, and other legacies of Carl Reinhold August Wunderlich. *JAMA* 268(12):1578–1580, 1992.
3. van der Bogert J: *J Pediatrics* 10:795, 1937.
4. Chamberlain JM, Grandner J, Rubinoff JL: Comparison of a tympanic thermometer to rectal and oral thermometers in a pediatric emergency department. *Clin Pediatr* 30(Suppl. 4): 24–29; discussion, 34–35, 1991.
5. Morley CJ, Hewson PH, Thornton AJ: Axillary and rectal temperature measurements in infants. *Arch Dis Child* 67(1):122–125, 1992.
6. Terndrup TE, Rajk J: Impact of operator technique and device on infrared emission detection tympanic thermometry. *J Emerg Med* 10(6):683–687, 1992.
7. Grover G, Berkowitz CD, Lewis RJ, et al.: The effects of bundling on infant temperature. *Pediatrics* 94(5):669–673, 1994.
8. Vauzelle-Kervroedan F, d'Athis P, Pariente-Khayat A, et al.: Equivalent antipyretic activity of ibuprofen and paracetamol in febrile children. *J Pediatr* 131:683–687, 1997.
9. Baker MD, Fosarelli PD, Carpenter RO: Childhood fever: Correlation of diagnosis with temperature response to acetaminophen. *Pediatrics* 80(3):315–318, 1987.
10. Berkowitz CD, Schiff D, Black JL, et al.: Effect of acetaminophen on clinical assessment of febrile infants. *Am J Dis Child* 142:393(abst), 1988.
11. Scarfone RJ: Compliance with scheduled visits to a pediatric emergency department. *Acad Emerg Med* 1:41(abst), 1994.
12. Sadow KB, Derr R, Teach SJ: Bacterial infections in infants 60 days and younger *Arch Peds Adol Med* 153:611–614, 1999.
13. Bonadio WA: Incidence of serious infections in afebrile neonates with a history of fever. *Pediatr Infect Dis J* 6(10): 911–914, 1987.
14. Roberts KB, Borzy MS: Fever in the first eight weeks of life. *Johns Hopkins Med J* 141(1):9–13, 1977.
15. Baker MD, et al.: The applicability of an established outpatient management protocol for febrile 0–1 month old infants. SAEM 1997 Annual Meeting. *Acad Emerg Med* 427:258(abst), 1997.
16. Baskin MN, O'Rourke EJ, Fleisher GR: Outpatient treatment of febrile infants 28 to 89 days of age with intramuscular administration of ceftriaxone. *J Pediatr* 120(1):22–27, 1992.
17. Jaskiewicz JA, McCarthy CA, Richardson AC et al.: Febrile infants at low risk for serious bacterial infections—an appraisal of the Rochester Criteria and implications for management. *Pediatrics* 94:390–396, 1994.
18. Baskin MN, Fleisher GR, O'Rourke EJ: Outpatient management of febrile infants 28 to 90 days of age with intramuscular ceftriaxone. *Am J Dis Child* 142:391(abst), 1988.
19. Baker MD, Bell LM, Avner JR: Outpatient management without antibiotics of fever in selected infants. *N Engl J Med* 329(20):1437–1441, 1993.
20. Brik R, Hamissah R, Shehada N, et al.: Evaluation of febrile infants under 3 months of age: Is routine lumbar puncture warranted? *Isr J Med Sci* 33(2):93–97, 1997.
21. Baraff LJ, Bass JW, Fleisher GR, et al. (Agency for Health Care Policy and Research): Practice guideline for the management of infants and children 0 to 36 months of age with fever without a source. *Ann Emerg Med* 22(7):1198–1210, 1993.
22. Rothrock SG, Harper MB, Green SM, et al.: Do oral antibiotics prevent meningitis and serious bacterial infections in children with *Streptococcus pneumoniae* occult bacteremia? A meta-analysis. *Pediatrics* 99(3):438–444, 1997.
23. Ling Lin P, Michaels MG, Janosky J et al.: Incidence of invasive pneumococcal disease in children 3–36 months of age at a tertiary care pediatric center 2 years after licensure of the pneumococcal conjugate vaccine *Pediatrics* 111:896–899, 2003.
24. Whitney CG, Farley MM, Hadler J et al.: Decline in invasive pneumococcal disease after the introduction of protein-polysaccharide conjugate vaccine. *N Engl J Med* 348: 1737–1746, 2003.
25. Kaplan SL, Mason EO, Wald ER et al.: Decrease in invasive pneumococcal infections in children among 8 children's hospitals in the United States after the introduction of the 7-valent pneumococcal conjugate vaccine. *Pediatrics* 113:443–449, 2004.
26. Mandl KD, Stack AM, Fleisher GR: Incidence of bacteremia in infants and children with fever and petechiae. *J Pediatr* 131(3):398–404, 1997.

27. Antonow JA, Hansen K, McKinstry CA, et al.: Sepsis evaluations in hospitalized infants with bronchiolitis. *Pediatr Infect Dis J* 17(3):231–236, 1998.

28. Bramson RT, Meyer TL, Silbiger ML, et al.: The futility of the chest radiograph in the febrile infant without respiratory symptoms. *Pediatrics* 92(4):524–526, 1993.

29. Shaw K: Predicting urinary tract infections in febrile young children in the emergency department. SAEM 1997 Annual Meeting. *Acad Emerg Med* 427:257, 1997.

30. Shaw K, Gorelick M, McGowan K, et al.: Prevalence of urinary tract infections in febrile young children in the emergency department. *Pediatrics* 102:E16, 1998.

31. Hoberman A, Wald ER, Penchansky L, et al.: Enhanced urinalysis as a screening test for urinary tract infection. *Pediatrics* 91(6):1196–1199, 1993.

32. Crain EF, Bulas D, Bijur PE, et al.: Is a chest radiograph necessary in the evaluation of every febrile infant less than 8 weeks of age? *Pediatrics* 88(4):821–824, 1991.

33. Green SM, Rothrock SG: Evaluation styles for well-appearing febrile children: Are you a "risk-minimizer" or a "test-minimizer"? *Ann Emerg Med* 33(2):311–214, 1999.

34. American College of Emergency Physicians Pediatric Committee: Clinical policy for children younger than 3 years presenting to the emergency department with fever *Ann Emerg Med* 42(4):530–545, 2003.

35. Baraff LJ: Editorial: Clinical policy for children younger than three years presenting to the emergency department with fever. *Ann Emerg Med* 42(4):546–549, 2003.

36. Friedman AD, Barton LL (Sponging Study Group): Efficacy of sponging vs acetaminophen for reduction of fever. *Pediatr Emerg Care* 6(1):6–7, 1990.

37. Watts R, Robertson J, Thomas G: Nursing management of fever in children: A systematic review. *J Nurs Pract* 9:S1–S8, 2003.

38. Black S, Shinefield H, Ray P, et al.: Efficacy of heptavalent conjugate pneumococcal vaccine in 37,000 infants and children: Results of the Northern California Kaiser Permanente Efficacy Trial (abst LB-9). *Interscience Conference on Antimicrobial Agents and Chemotherapy*, San Diego, California, September 1998.

22

Sepsis

Tonya Jagneaux
David E. Taylor
Stephen P. Kantrow

HIGH YIELD FACTS

Empiric antibiotic therapy should be administered within 1 h with consideration of potential sources and pathogen resistance patterns. Patients with suspected infection should be evaluated for hypoperfusion or organ dysfunction consistent with severe sepsis in order to appropriately administer emerging therapies. Otherwise healthy adults may rapidly develop sepsis due to meningococcus, toxic shock syndrome, pneumococcus, and rickettsial infection. In patients with severe sepsis or septic shock, goal-directed hemodynamic resuscitation should be initiated promptly in the emergency department.

CASE PRESENTATION

A 46-year-old man presents to the emergency department 12 h after onset of fever, chills, nausea, vomiting, and myalgias. He reports eating chicken salad 1 day prior to presentation that tasted "spoiled." Pertinent medical history includes a motor vehicle accident 5 years prior to presentation. He takes no medications and has no allergies.

He is alert but appears acutely ill. Blood pressure is 108/48, pulse 128, respiratory rate 26, and temperature is 39°C. Additional findings on physical exam include sinus tenderness with clear rhinorrhea, a well-healed midline abdominal scar, and cool extremities with palpable pulses. Cardiac, chest, abdominal, and skin examination reveal no further abnormalities. Initial laboratory findings include white blood cell count (WBC) 2600 (70% neutrophils, 20% bands), hematocrit 45%, sodium 146, potassium 3.0, chloride 101, bicarbonate 14, BUN 30, and creatinine 1.6. Arterial lactate level is 6.2. No leukocytes are seen on urinalysis. Chest radiograph demonstrates no focal abnormalities.

INTRODUCTION/EPIDEMIOLOGY

Definitions

Sepsis is systemic inflammation in the setting of infection. Criteria for systemic inflammation have been pro-

posed to aid the clinician in identifying the pathophysiologic response in sepsis (1) and include derangements of temperature, heart rate, respiration, and leukocyte indices (Table 22–1). Severe sepsis is present when organ dysfunction or hypoperfusion supervene. Persistent hypotension despite adequate fluid resuscitation characterizes septic shock. Mortality and the likelihood of bacteremia increase as patients meet criteria for sepsis, severe sepsis and septic shock, and overall mortality for severe sepsis and septic shock remains 25–50% in most studies (2). While febrile and hemodynamically unstable patients are routinely evaluated for sepsis in the emergency department, awareness of more subtle indices of inflammation or organ dysfunction can assist in the identification of this condition (3) (Table 22–2). Recent clinical studies suggest that timely initiation of therapy can improve outcome in this setting.

Epidemiology

In hospitalized patients with sepsis, the frequency and mortality of sepsis increase with age and underlying illness, and competing, noninfectious causes of death are common (4). In one survey of sepsis in academic medical centers, approximately 10% of all cases were identified in the emergency department (5). In a prospective study of patients admitted through the emergency department with suspected infection, investigators derived a prediction rule for stratifying the mortality risk based upon patient demographics (elderly, nursing home resident) and clinical variables (respiratory abnormalities, shock, thrombocytopenia, bandemia, altered mental status, lower respiratory tract infection) (6). Although the prediction

Table 22–1. Definitions (1, 3)

Systemic inflammatory response syndrome (SIRS)	More than one of the following clinical findings: Temperature >38°C or <36°C, heart rate >90 beats/minute, respiratory rate > 20/minute or $PaCO_2$ <32 mmHg, WBC >12,000 cells/uL or <4000 cells/uL or >10% bands
Sepsis	SIRS with infection (proven or strongly suspected)
Severe sepsis	Sepsis with organ dysfunction, hypotension, or hypoperfusion
Septic shock	Sepsis with hypotension despite adequate fluid resuscitation

Table 22–2. Additional Findings Consistent with Sepsis

General
  Altered mental status
  Significant edema or positive fluid balance
  Hyperglycemia in the absence of diabetes
Inflammation
  Elevated plasma C-reactive protein
  Elevated plasma procalcitonin
Hemodynamic alterations
  Arterial hypotension
  High SvO_2
  Increased cardiac index
Organ dysfunction
  Arterial hypoxemia
  Acute oliguria
  Increased creatinine
  Coagulation abnormalities
  Ileus
  Thrombocytopenia
  Hyperbilirubinemia
Tissue perfusion abnormalities
  Hyperlactatemia
  Decreased capillary refill or mottling

rule confirmed the importance of age, comorbidities and organ dysfunction in predicting outcome, use of this MEDS score awaits further validation as a tool for risk stratification of patients with suspected infection in the emergency department setting.

PATHOPHYSIOLOGY/MICROBIOLOGY

Innate Immune Activation

Infections are recognized immediately by highly conserved pattern recognition receptors, and subsequent responses include activation of monocytes, neutrophils, and endothelium (7). If normal host responses fail to contain microbial invasion, spread of infection leads to systemic activation of innate immune pathways. Critical defenses against invading pathogens pose threats to host organ function and survival. Although rapidly effective antibiotics are available for most bacterial pathogens, adequate treatment of infection is frequently accompanied by continued clinical deterioration. Patients with sepsis may die of refractory hypotension or may survive the immediate insult only to develop progressive and prolonged failure of critical organs.

Organ Dysfunction

Mortality in sepsis is strongly correlated to the number of organ failures that occurs during the course of the illness (4). Early identification of organ dysfunction may offer opportunities for interventions to reduce the associated morbidity and mortality.

Upon presentation, *cardiovascular* derangements due to sepsis may include tachycardia, decreased systolic and/or diastolic arterial blood pressure, and cool extremities with mottled skin (8). Patients are typically volume depleted due to decreased oral intake, increased insensible fluid losses, and increased vascular permeability. Additional evidence of organ hypoperfusion may include oliguria, abnormal mental status, and lactic acidosis. Invasive hemodynamic monitoring has demonstrated that venous filling pressures and cardiac output are typically low at the initial presentation of sepsis; appropriate volume resuscitation is followed by development of a high cardiac index and low systemic vascular resistance. Hemodynamic instability can progress to cardiovascular collapse or respond to resuscitation and vasopressor support to resolve in 1 or 2 days.

Early abnormalities of *pulmonary* function include tachypnea in response to metabolic acidosis, fever or increased respiratory drive, and hypoxemia as lung injury progresses. Deteriorating gas exchange, increased ventilation requirements, cardiovascular insufficiency, and abnormal mentation place the septic patient at high risk of respiratory failure. Intubation can avoid complicated cardiopulmonary arrest. Pulmonary dysfunction occurs early in sepsis and commonly lasts for more than a week (9). Sepsis is associated with a risk of developing acute lung injury or the acute respiratory distress syndrome (approximately 40%) (10).

Oliguria at presentation may be a manifestation of *renal* dysfunction caused by volume depletion, hypoperfusion, or local vasoactive mediators, and urine output often responds to management of cardiovascular abnormalities. However, serum creatinine may continue to rise and acute tubular necrosis may occur even in the presence of restored urine output. While mortality is increased if renal injury persists, survival is typically accompanied by eventual return of renal function.

In the setting of systemic endothelial dysfunction in sepsis, abnormal *coagulation* studies are common. Overwhelming activation of the coagulation cascade in its most severe form results in purpura fulminans, characterized by systemic intravascular clot formation, tissue thrombosis, symmetric peripheral gangrene, and organ failure. Despite the dramatic nature of purpura fulminans due to organisms such as *Neisseria meningitidis*, *Staphylococcus aureus*, and *Streptococcus pneumoniae*, the contribution of coagulation to multiorgan dysfunction remains incompletely understood (11). Recent studies suggest that anticoagulant therapy may decrease organ dysfunction during sepsis and may improve survival, even in the absence of overt coagulopathy (12).

Altered mental status should raise suspicion of central nervous system infection, although encephalopathy is also common in elderly patients and with increasing sepsis severity. Intestinal dysfunction (ileus) and hepatic dysfunction (hyperbilirubinemia) are also commonly found in critically ill septic patients.

Microbiology

The most common site of infection in patients hospitalized with sepsis is the *lung* (9). Invasive pyogenic organisms responsible for severe pneumonia from the community include *S. pneumoniae*, *S. aureus*, *Klebsiella pneumoniae*, and *Legionella pneumophila*. Pneumonia is more common and more severe in elderly patients, and mortality is increased when complicated by bacteremia or organ dysfunction (13).

Urinary tract infections are generally mild and caused by *Escherichia coli*. However, cystitis may be complicated by bacteremia, pyelonephritis, and abscess formation (14). In the setting of urinary tract abnormalities such as obstruction, nephrolithiasis, neurogenic bladder, recent instrumentation, and/or indwelling foley catheters, other pathogens to consider include enterococci and *Pseudomonas aeruginosa*. Predisposing conditions and evidence of complicated infection should be sought in patients diagnosed with urosepsis.

Abdominal infection is frequently complicated by sepsis, and causes are similar to those of the acute abdomen: peritonitis, bowel perforation or ischemia, biliary tract infection, complicated pancreatitis, and abscess formation. Infections are frequently polymicrobial and include mixed enteric aerobic and anaerobic pathogens, notably enterococci and *Bacteroides fragilis* (15).

Skin and soft tissue infection is suspected with sepsis and a history or evidence of recent surgery, skin lesions with the potential for superinfection, or minor skin trauma, particularly if there has been additional exposure to salt water (*Vibrio vulnificus*) or fresh water (*Aeromonas hydrophila*). Human and animal bite wounds are also at risk for development of complicating sepsis (*Capnocytophaga canimorsus*, *Pasteurella multocida*). Deep soft tissue infections and toxic shock syndromes, characterized by fever, hypotension, and the rapid development of

multiple organ failure, have been associated with group A streptococci and *S. aureus*. Other important causes of deep tissue infection (necrotizing fasciitis) include *Clostridium perfringens* and *Clostridium septicum*.

Meningitis is most commonly due to *S. pneumoniae* and *N. meningitidis*, organisms that can cause fulminant sepsis in previously healthy individuals. Causes of *bacteremia* in otherwise healthy adults include *S. aureus*, *S. pneumoniae*, *N. meningitidis*, and *Salmonella* species. Underlying immunodeficiency (HIV, hyposplenism), intravascular infection (endocarditis, mycotic aneurysms), and occult foci of infection (abdomen, pelvis) should be considered.

CLINICAL PRESENTATION

Rapidly Progressive Infections

Meningococcemia

Infection with *N. meningitidis* occurs most commonly in children and young adults, with highest attack rates in February and March (16). Acute manifestations include sudden onset of fever, nausea, vomiting, headache, and myalgia. Alternative diagnoses such as streptococcal infection or influenza should be considered. However, when decreased blood pressure, tachycardia, and diaphoresis are prominent, a complete skin examination for petechial rash is essential. Since meningococcemia can present without meningeal signs, the presence of a rash may be critical to consideration of the diagnosis. This infection can progress over hours to shock and disseminated intravascular coagulation. Early administration of antibiotics should be followed promptly by lumbar puncture. Progression of organ dysfunction and development of limb ischemia are common, and transfer of the stabilized patient to a tertiary care facility should be considered. Familial predisposition to overwhelming meningococcemia has been described.

Toxic shock syndrome

Invasive group A streptococcal infection can develop in previously healthy adults, often with a viral prodrome or a history of recent trauma, surgery or varicella infection (17). Fever, confusion, and abrupt onset of pain are frequently noted at presentation and can progress to hypotension within a few hours. Painful soft tissue infection progresses to myositis or necrotizing fasciitis in the majority of patients and often requires aggressive management by fasciotomy, debridement, and/or amputation. Shock and multiple organ failure without focal findings may have a worse prognosis, as definitive source control is delayed. Bacteremia occurs in the majority of patients, and streptococcus is typically recovered from samples of involved tissue. The characteristic diffuse erythema, initially described with toxigenic *S. aureus* infection, may develop after recognition of septic shock and organ dysfunction.

Postsplenectomy sepsis

In splenectomized or hyposplenic individuals, invasive infection with *S. pneumoniae* or *H. influenzae* can progress over a few hours from fever with nonspecific symptoms to hypotension and multiple organ failure, often leading to death in less than 48 h (18). Patients at highest risk for sepsis have undergone splenectomy for a hematologic condition within the previous 2 years, but increased risk persists for decades after surgery. Febrile patients with a history of splenectomy should be treated rapidly with broad-spectrum antibiotics. Asplenia also increases the risk of overwhelming infection by several less common organisms, including *C. canimorsus* (after a dog bite) and malaria or babesiosis in endemic areas.

Rocky Mountain spotted fever

Most patients with infection due to *Rickettsia rickettsii* have a history of tick bite or travel to a tick-infested area during the previous 2 weeks and present between April and September in endemic areas (most commonly in the eastern United States) (19). Typical symptoms include fever and headache, with appearance of a peripheral macular rash within 3 or 4 days of fever onset and then development of petechiae on palms, soles, and axillae. As the infection progresses, direct infection of endothelial cells is accompanied by thrombocytopenia, diffuse capillary leak, confusion, respiratory failure, and limb ischemia. Careful inspection of the head and groin may reveal an engorged tick.

Mimics of Sepsis

Pancreatitis is a cause of systemic inflammation without infection that can be clinically indistinguishable from sepsis (20). Fever, hemodynamic instability, tachypnea, and leukocytosis are common, and progressive organ dysfunction can develop. Severe pancreatitis is often complicated by pancreatic necrosis or infection, both indications for broad-spectrum antibiotics. Other causes of *tissue injury* (trauma, burns, ischemia, surgery) can also trigger a systemic inflammatory response and raise the suspicion of infection.

Acute adrenal insufficiency may present with fever, abdominal pain, and refractory hypotension (21). The initial hemodynamic profile is consistent with cardiogenic shock; however, cardiac output increases and systemic vascular resistance decreases during volume resuscitation. Hypoglycemia, hyponatremia, eosinophilia, hyperpigmentation, or vitiligo may suggest the diagnosis. A plasma cortisol level greater than 25 ug/dL makes this diagnosis unlikely, and ACTH stimulation testing can definitively assess adrenal insufficiency.

The clinical presentation of *thyrotoxicosis* may also suggest the possibility of sepsis. Manifestations of thyroid storm can include tachycardia (often atrial arrhythmias), altered mental status, fevers, and even high output congestive heart failure. Although thyrotoxicosis is typically associated with hypertension, the findings are consistent with the systemic changes in severe sepsis and SIRS. The diagnosis of thyroid storm is confirmed by thyroid function tests including serum thyroid-stimulating hormone and thyroxine levels.

Hyperthermia complicated by organ dysfunction can develop in normal individuals subjected to extreme heat stress and can occur more readily in the setting of underlying illness or medications, particularly drugs with anticholinergic effects. Neuroleptics, including newer atypical antipsychotics, can cause hyperthermia, confusion, and muscular rigidity that require specific therapy for neuroleptic malignant syndrome.

LABORATORY/DIAGNOSTIC TESTING

In the emergency department, *blood cultures* are frequently obtained early in the diagnostic evaluation and can contribute useful, albeit delayed diagnostic information. Blood cultures are positive in 10–20% of critically ill patients with sepsis and in greater than 60% of patients with septic shock (2). Of patients hospitalized with pneumonia, 10% have positive blood cultures, and approximately half of these are caused by pneumococcus. Among patients with pneumococcal pneumonia, clinical findings do not allow accurate prediction of bacteremia (22). The contribution of blood cultures to management of patients hospitalized with community-acquired pneumonia is controversial; however, practice guidelines continue to recommend cultures to allow revision of antibiotic therapy, surveillance for drug resistance, and to support quality improvement efforts (13). The decision to send blood culture may also serve as a marker of clinically suspected infection, and should prompt a review of criteria for SIRS and organ dysfunction to assess for sepsis, even in the absence of hypotension.

Blood smears are rarely revealing in sepsis, as the circulating bacterial load is relatively low in most patients (fewer than 10^3 organisms/mL). However, in splenectomized patients suspected to have overwhelming sepsis, organism burden can be 1000-fold higher and can be identified in peripheral smears (18). Diagnostic evaluation should not delay empiric antibiotic therapy, which is emergent in these cases.

Circulating markers of inflammation or tissue injury offer the potential to identify patients with sepsis well in advance of microbial culture results. Elevated lactate levels may indicate tissue hypoperfusion and can be found when vital signs are deceptively normal. Evidence of intravascular coagulation (markedly increased D-dimer, prolongation of prothrombin and partial thromboplastin times, and consumption of fibrinogen) is another important clue to the diagnosis of sepsis. While cytokines with prominent roles in innate immune activation (tumor necrosis factor, interleukin-8) and markers of systemic inflammation (C-reactive protein) have been the subject of numerous clinical studies, results have generally been disappointing. Procalcitonin, a product of thyroid tissue, is found in very low levels in the serum of normal individuals. Recent investigations have suggested that procalcitonin levels can identify sepsis in patients admitted to the critical care unit and that levels correlate with severity of illness (23). However, other studies suggest a relatively low sensitivity for systemic infection, and the role of procalcitonin as a marker is uncertain in the diagnostic evaluation of the emergency department patient.

MANAGEMENT

Rapid identification of sepsis in the emergency department creates the opportunity for early administration of established and emerging therapies for this condition. In this section we focus on management issues that are important in the emergency setting, and which are critical to the implementation of new sepsis treatments (Table 22–3) (24).

Table 22–3. Management of Severe Sepsis and Septic Shock

Diagnosis	Appropriate cultures should be obtained before antimicrobial therapy is initiated
	Diagnostic studies should be performed promptly to identify the source of infection
Antibiotic therapy	Intravenous antibiotic therapy should be started within 1 h of recognition of severe sepsis
	Empiric antibiotic therapy should include at least one drug effective against the likely pathogens and which penetrates the presumed source of infection
Source control	Every patient presenting with severe sepsis should be assessed for a source of infection amenable to drainage, debridement, or removal
Initial resuscitation	Volume resuscitation of a patient with severe sepsis or sepsis-induced hypoperfusion should begin immediately (Fig. 22–1)[a]
Fluid therapy	Initial volume repletion may be undertaken with crystalloids and/or colloids
Vasopressors	Either norepinephrine or dopamine is appropriate as initial vasopressor therapy of septic shock
	Low-dose dopamine is contraindicated[a]
	All patients should have arterial catheter placed for blood pressure monitoring as soon as is practical
	Vasopressin may be considered for refractory shock
Inotropic therapy	May be used to treat low cardiac output despite fluid resuscitation. Should not be used to reach a goal of elevated cardiac output
Mechanical ventilation	High tidal volumes with high plateau pressures should be avoided for sepsis-induced acute lung injury[a]
	Hypercapnia can be tolerated if required
Recombinant human activated protein C	Recommended for patients at high risk of death with severe sepsis or septic shock[a]
Steroids	Intravenous corticosteroids (<300 mg hydrocortisone/day) are recommended for vasopressor-dependent septic shock

[a]Supported by at least one large randomized trial.
Source: Adapted from (24).

Antibiotics and Source Control

Identifying and addressing the inciting agent for the development of sepsis is critical for therapeutic success. Patients with sepsis should undergo a thorough evaluation for a focus of infection that may require additional intervention to achieve adequate source control. Potential source control measures include abscess drainage, debridement and removal of devitalized and/or infected tissue, removal of potentially infected indwelling catheters, and relief of any obstruction (bowel, hydronephrosis).

Timely initiation of appropriate antibiotic therapy is also necessary in sepsis management (25). Antimicrobial selection is based upon identified sources of infections, and the spectrum of pathogens likely involved based upon epidemiologic risk factors and the immune status of the host. While the appropriate selection of an antibiotic regimen for specific organ systems involved is covered in other chapters, several recommendations for acutely ill septic patients deserve emphasis (Table 22–4) (26).

Recent guidelines for the management of severe sepsis and septic shock recommend administration of antibiotics within 1 h of presentation (24).

Appropriate cultures of blood, urine, sputum, and cerebrospinal fluid, as well as sampling of fluid from normally sterile sites such as the pleural space or the peritoneum, should be obtained expeditiously. Antimicrobial therapy, however, should not be delayed for extensive diagnostic testing. The institution of appropriate empiric antimicrobial therapy can significantly improve survival for patients diagnosed with community-acquired bloodstream infections (27).

Antimicrobial regimens should be selected to cover suspected pathogens based upon the clinical presentation with consideration for local resistance patterns. Pneumonia, soft tissue infection, and bacteremia due to methicillin-resistant *S. aureus* (MRSA) are increasingly presenting from the community, although most patients have had recent contact with a health care facility. Inclusion of vancomycin in the initial therapeutic regimen is

Table 22–4. Common Pathogens and Antibiotic Regimens in Sepsis

Source	Organism	Antibiotic Regimen
Respiratory tract	*S. pneumoniae* *S. aureus* *K. pneumoniae* *L. pneumophila*	Third-generation cephalosporin or β-lactam/β-lactamase inhibitor + macrolide or quinolone
Urinary tract	*E. coli* Enterococcus *P. aeruginosa*	β-lactam + aminoglycoside or β-lactam/β-lactamase inhibitor (with activity against pseudomonas and enterococcus)
Gastrointestinal tract	Polymicrobial Gram-negative enteric Anaerobes Enterococcus *B. fragilis*	Carbapenem or β-lactam/β-lactamase inhibitor + aminoglycoside
Skin/soft tissues	*S. aureus* Group A streptococcus *Clostridium* species *V. vulnificus* *A. hydrophila* *Pasteurella multocida*	Carbapenem or β-lactam/β-lactamase inhibitor + vancomycin $\pm$ clindamycin
Meningitis	*S. pneumoniae* *N. meningitidis*	Third-generation cephalosporin + vancomycin

Third-generation cephalosporin = ceftriaxone, cefotaxime.
β-lactam/β-lactamase inhibitor = piperacillin/tazobactam, ticarcillin/clavulanate.
Macrolide = azithromycin, clarithromycin.
Quinolone = levofloxacin, ciprofloxacin.
Aminoglycoside = gentamicin, tobramycin.
Carbapenem = imipenem-cilastatin, meropenem.

appropriate in critically ill patients for whom MRSA infection is a consideration. Patients at risk for presentation to the emergency department with pseudomonas infections include those with structural lung disease (e.g., bronchiectasis), HIV infection, recent antibiotic treatment, intravenous drug use, and malnutrition (13). The use of two effective antibiotics should be considered when infection with pseudomonal species is suspected as a cause of sepsis.

Immunocompromised patients pose a challenge in selecting appropriate empiric therapy, as they are susceptible to a broader spectrum of pathogens and can have atypical presentations. Patients with neutropenia due to cancer or chemotherapy are at risk for common infections in addition to specifically increased risk of infection from the skin, gastrointestinal tract, and indwelling catheters. Broad-spectrum combination drug therapy directed against resistant gram-positive and resistant gram-negative organisms is indicated. These patients should also be considered for *Pneumocystis jiroveci* pneumonia therapy if there is evidence of pneumonia, acyclovir for the presence of *Herpes* simplex-associated mucositis or gingivitis, and antifungal therapy directed against *Candida* and *Aspergillus* species if the patient has deteriorated despite outpatient antimicrobial therapy.

Patients with HIV infection are at increased risk of invasive infection with community-acquired pathogens, particularly *S. pneumoniae*, *S. aureus*, and *H. influenzae*. In advanced disease, infections with *Pseudomonas* and other resistant gram-negative pathogens are increasingly reported. Depending on the degree of immunosuppression, HIV-infected patients are also at risk for opportunistic infections that can present as sepsis, including disseminated mycobacterial and fungal diseases. Empiric therapy for *P. jiroveci* pneumonia is indicated in critically ill HIV infected patients with a respiratory infection, and clinically suspected fungal or mycobacterial pneumonia should prompt respiratory isolation and induced sputum or interventional procedures to obtain adequate respiratory cultures.

Organ transplant recipients are at particularly high risk for infections with resistant bacterial pathogens, including *P. aeruginosa* and MRSA, likely due to antibiotic use, abnormalities of host defense, and frequent hospitalizations. Immunosuppression required for organ transplantation increases the risk of opportunistic invasive infection with fungal or mycobacterial pathogens, and reactivation of fungal and mycobacterial pathogens from both recipient and donor have been described. While infectious etiologies vary depending upon the organ transplanted, degree of immunosuppression, and prophylaxis regimen, broad spectrum antibacterial therapy followed by early consultation with a transplant physician is indicated. Tissue sampling is often necessary to obtain a diagnosis, and careful attention to drug interactions is required.

Volume Resuscitation and Vasoactive Therapy

Equally important in managing patients with sepsis is aggressive fluid resuscitation. Early recognition of tissue hypoperfusion and appropriate goal-directed therapy may positively affect the survival and recovery of the patient with severe sepsis and/or septic shock. Since maintenance of a normal arterial blood pressure does not exclude tissue hypoperfusion, additional findings such as elevated lactate or organ dysfunction should guide resuscitation. One randomized controlled trial in the emergency department setting provides evidence that a prompt goal-directed approach can improve mortality from sepsis (28). Early assessment of the perfusion status in that trial included measures of central venous pressure and central venous oxygen saturation. Interventions to maintain central venous pressure between 8 and 12 mmHg, mean arterial pressure ≥ 65 mmHg, and superior cava venous oxygen saturation $\geq 70\%$ included administration of crystalloid or colloid boluses, vasopressors, transfusion with packed red blood cells to correct hematocrit less than 30 mg/dL, and dobutamine infusion (Fig. 22–1). Patients received early goal-directed therapy in the emergency department for the first 6 h of hospitalization followed by routine ICU care by intensivists. Patients treated with early goal-directed therapy had a reduction in mortality compared to standard care (30.5% vs. 46.5%), required less vasopressor support, and had fewer days of mechanical ventilation and hospitalization.

Volume replacement typically requires bolus infusions of 1 L of fluid such as normal saline or lactated Ringer and should be given as long as the patient demonstrates improvement in organ dysfunction, such as mean arterial pressure, mental status, urinary output, or central venous oxygen saturation (8). Alternative methods to support blood pressure are necessary if the patient is unresponsive to volume challenges or complications are identified that would limit further volume expansion, such as increased oxygen demands due to pulmonary edema. Patients may require many liters of crystalloid fluid during the first 24 h of treatment.

Vasopressor administration requires central venous access, and arterial catheterization is recommended to

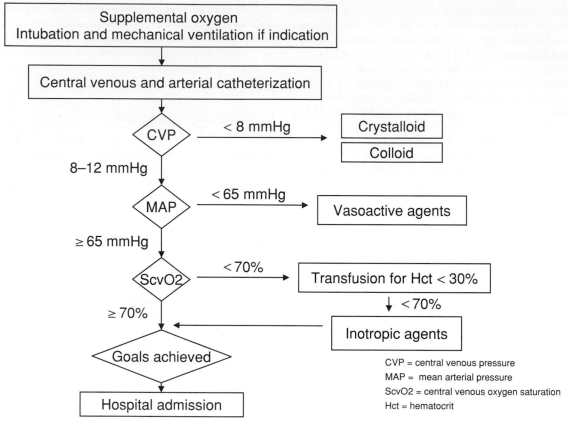

Fig. 22–1. Pathway for resuscitation of severe sepsis or septic shock in the emergency department (adapted from (28)).

follow the arterial pressure response to therapy. A definitive survival advantage of any particular vasopressor usage in septic shock has not been demonstrated, and hemodynamic goals may be met with norepinephrine or dopamine. Inotropic therapy can be used to augment cardiac output in septic shock. While patients with septic shock typically have an elevated cardiac output as part of the hemodynamic profile determined by pulmonary artery catheterization or echocardiography, some patients have a low cardiac output that compromises tissue perfusion despite adequate resuscitation and the addition of vasopressors. In the earlier study of goal-directed therapy in sepsis, dobutamine was implemented when central venous oxygen saturation was persistently low (<70%) after administration of fluid, vasopressors, and, if indicated, blood. Central venous oxygen saturation can be measured continuously using oximetric venous catheters or intermittently by performing blood gas analysis on sampled venous blood.

Airway and Respiratory Support

Patients with sepsis will commonly have multiple etiologies for respiratory failure. Minute ventilation increases due to the hypermetabolic state and lactic acidosis. Acute lung injury and ARDS frequently develop, resulting in profound hypoxemia. Central nervous system dysfunction manifested as septic encephalopathy may result in inability to protect the airway. Also, the combination of increased ventilatory demand and hypoxemia can easily overwhelm the patient who has preexisting cardiopulmonary disease. Therefore, the decision to intubate and mechanically ventilate the septic patient should be considered early in the course of care.

Establishing ventilatory support can be problematic in these patients as they are typically vasodilated, hypotensive, and volume contracted. Administration of sedation to facilitate endotracheal intubation along with initiation of positive pressure ventilation typically reduces preload to the heart and decreases cardiac output, with a potentially precipitous drop in arterial pressure (29). These deleterious cardiovascular effects can be blunted by volume resuscitation prior to intubation.

In delivering ventilatory support, the goal is to reverse or limit physiologic derangement while minimizing iatrogenic injury. To determine the effects of ventilator strategies on outcome in patients with lung injury, subjects enrolled in the ARDS Network trial were randomized to receive assist control mechanical ventilation with traditional tidal volume ventilation (12 mL/kg ideal body weight) versus low tidal volume ventilation (6 mL/kg) (30). Traditional tidal volumes were associated with a higher mortality as compared with low tidal volume ventilation (39.8% vs. 31.0%). Low tidal volume ventilation using 6 mL/kg of predicted body weight is recommended in septic patients with acute lung injury. Patients may require deep sedation, and even neuromuscular blockade, to maintain patient-ventilator synchrony. Since the ongoing risk of developing lung injury throughout the course of sepsis is significant, implementation of low tidal volume ventilation should be considered at the initiation of mechanical ventilation in any patient meeting the criteria for sepsis (24). With low tidal volume ventilation, higher set respiratory rates are often required. However, the hypercapnia and acidemia anticipated as a consequence of low tidal volume ventilation appear to be tolerated by patients with lung injury (24).

Anticoagulation

The use of the anticoagulant agent activated protein C (drotrecogin alfa) is recommended in selected patients with severe sepsis. A phase III trial demonstrated that patients with severe sepsis treated with activated protein C had reduced mortality compared with placebo (24.7% vs. 30.8%) (12). The mechanism of action of activated protein C has not been completely elucidated but is thought to involve both reduction in intravascular coagulation and reduction in the inflammatory response. Patients who meet the criteria for activated protein C include those with evidence of sepsis and organ dysfunction. Bleeding can complicate this therapy and limits its use in patients at high risk of uncontrollable or life-threatening hemorrhage.

Growing evidence suggests that early resuscitation and timely treatment with activated protein C are likely to improve patient mortality and organ dysfunction in sepsis. Although the time frame for initiating drotrecogin alfa in the PROWESS trial was 48 h, the majority of patients were enrolled within a 24-h time period. Once the decision is made to initiate activated protein C, efforts directed to reduce bleeding risk should be undertaken including minimizing arterial punctures, as well as discontinuing drug infusion for 1 h before percutaneous procedures and waiting an hour postprocedure before restarting therapy.

Adrenal Replacement and Glycemic Control

Patient with sepsis and septic shock may have relative adrenal insufficiency or glucocorticoid receptor resistance. Replacement therapy with hydrocortisone and fludrocortisone may reduce mortality in patients with vasopressor-dependent shock in whom relative adrenal insufficiency has been confirmed (31). The use of intensive insulin therapy has also been identified as an adjuvant therapy in critically ill patients. Tight glycemic control in surgical intensive care patients (glucose levels between 80 and 110 mg/dL) resulted in reduced mortality, bloodstream infections, acute renal failure, critical illness neuropathy, and red-cell transfusion (32). This approach has not been evaluated in patients presenting with sepsis, and requires intensive monitoring to prevent hypoglycemic complications. Hyperglycemia should be addressed during the initial period of resuscitation, but at this time, there are no data to support the initiation of intensive insulin therapy for septic patients in the emergency department.

DISPOSITION

The majority of patients meeting the criteria for sepsis upon presentation to the emergency department will require intensive care unit admission to ensure continued resuscitative efforts that often necessitate infusion of vasoactive agents, mechanical ventilation, and close physiologic monitoring. Patients meeting sepsis criteria who do not have organ dysfunction or evidence of hypoperfusion can occasionally be admitted to a monitored medical-surgical bed; however, unrecognized deterioration due to sepsis can substantially increase mortality secondary to delays in appropriate management. Patients should be screened carefully for the presence of preexisting comorbidities, limited cardiopulmonary reserve, and the potential for progressive deterioration even after appropriate treatment has been initiated.

CASE OUTCOME

Additional history obtained from family revealed that the patient had undergone splenectomy secondary to blunt abdominal trauma suffered in the motor vehicle accident

5 years earlier. Blood cultures were drawn and broad-spectrum antibiotic therapy with piperacillin/tazobactam and vancomycin was begun. Two liters of normal saline were administered as central venous access was obtained and central venous pressure measured at 4 mmHg. After two additional liters of saline, the central venous pressure rose to 12 mmHg. However, hypotension progressed and vasopressor therapy with norepinephrine was initiated. Measurement of central venous oxygenation confirmed a hemoglobin saturation of 75%. While awaiting transfer to the intensive care unit, the patient developed hypoxemic respiratory failure and required intubation. He was mechanically ventilated with tidal volumes of 6 mL/kg ideal body weight. No increased risk of bleeding was identified, and infusion of activated protein C was begun.

Upon transfer to the intensive care unit, acute renal failure developed and dialysis was begun. All four blood cultures grew pan-sensitive pneumococcus. The antibiotic regimen was narrowed to a single agent to cover *S. pneumoniae*. Vasopressor support was weaned off on day 2 of hospitalization, and the 96-h drotrecogin alfa infusion was completed without bleeding complications. Mechanical ventilation was discontinued on day 4 after the patient met weaning criteria, and renal function returned to baseline. The patient recovered fully and was discharged home 10 days after presenting to the emergency department.

REFERENCES

1. American College of Chest Physicians/Society of Critical Care Medicine Consensus Conference: Definitions for sepsis and organ failure and guidelines for the use of innovative therapies in sepsis. *Crit Care Med* 20:864–874, 1992.
2. Rangel-Frausto MS, Pittet D, Costigan M et al.: The natural history of the systemic inflammatory response syndrome (SIRS). A prospective study. *JAMA* 273:117–123.
3. Levy MM, Fink MP, Marshall JC et al.: 2001 SCCM/ESICM/ACCP/ATS/SIS international sepsis definitions conference. *Crit Care Med* 31:1250–1256, 2003.
4. Wheeler AP, Bernard GR: Treating patients with severe sepsis. *N Engl J Med* 340:207–214, 1999.
5. Sands KE, Bates DW, Lanken PN et al. (Academic Medical Center Consortium Sepsis Project Working Group.): Epidemiology of sepsis syndrome in 8 academic medical centers. *JAMA* 278:234–240, 1997.
6. Shapiro NI, Wolfe RE, Moore RB et al.: Mortality in emergency department sepsis (MEDS) score: A prospectively derived and validated clinical prediction rule. *Crit Care Med* 31:670–675, 2003.
7. Beutler B, Poltorak A: Sepsis and evolution of the innate immune response. *Crit Care Med* 29:S2–S6, 2001.

8. Dellinger RP: Cardiovascular management of septic shock. *Crit Care Med* 31:946–955, 2003.
9. Bernard GR, Wheeler AP, Russell JA et al. (The Ibuprofen in Sepsis Study Group): The effects of ibuprofen on the physiology and survival of patients with sepsis. *N Engl J Med* 336:912–918, 1997.
10. Ware LB, Matthay MA: The acute respiratory distress syndrome. *N Engl J Med* 342:1334–1349, 2000.
11. Marshall JC: Inflammation, coagulopathy, and the pathogenesis of multiple organ dysfunction syndrome. *Crit Care Med* 29:S99–S106, 2001.
12. Bernard GR, Vincent JL, Laterre PF et al.: Efficacy and safety of recombinant human activated protein C for severe sepsis. *N Engl J Med* 344:699–709, 2001.
13. Niederman MS, Mandell LA, Anzueto A et al.: Guidelines for the management of adults with community-acquired pneumonia. Diagnosis, assessment of severity, antimicrobial therapy, and prevention. *Am J Respir Crit Care Med* 163:1730–1754, 2001.
14. Rubenstein JN, Schaeffer AJ: Managing complicated urinary tract infections: The urologic view. *Infect Dis Clin North Am* 17:333–351, 2003.
15. Solomkin JS, Mazuski JE, Baron EJ et al.: Guidelines for the selection of anti-infective agents for complicated intra-abdominal infections. *Clin Infect Dis* 37:997–1005, 2003.
16. Rosenstein NE, Perkins BA, Stephens DS, Popovic T, Hughes JM: Meningococcal disease. *N Engl J Med* 344:1378–1388, 2001.
17. Stevens DL: The toxic shock syndromes. *Infect Dis Clin North Am* 10:727–746, 1996.
18. Lynch AM, Kapila R: Overwhelming postsplenectomy infection. *Infect Dis Clin North Am* 10:693–707, 1996.
19. Thorner AR, Walker DH, Petri WA, Jr.: Rocky mountain spotted fever. *Clin Infect Dis* 27:1353–1359, 1998.
20. Baron TH, Morgan DE: Acute necrotizing pancreatitis. *N Engl J Med* 340:1412–1417, 1999.
21. Oelkers W: Adrenal insufficiency. *N Engl J Med* 335:1206–1212, 1996.
22. Marrie TJ, Low DE, De Carolis E: A comparison of bacteremic pneumococcal pneumonia with nonbacteremic community-acquired pneumonia of any etiology—results from a Canadian multicentre study. *Can Respir J* 10:368–374, 2003.
23. Harbarth S, Holeckova K, Froidevaux C et al.: Diagnostic value of procalcitonin, interleukin-6, and interleukin-8 in critically ill patients admitted with suspected sepsis. *Am J Respir Crit Care Med* 164:396–402, 2001.
24. Dellinger RP, Carlet JM, Masur H et al.: Surviving sepsis campaign guidelines for management of severe sepsis and septic shock. *Crit Care Med* 32:858–873, 2004.
25. Garnacho-Montero J, Garcia-Garmendia JL, Barrero-Almodovar A et al.: Impact of adequate empirical antibiotic therapy on the outcome of patients admitted to the intensive care unit with sepsis. *Crit Care Med* 31:2742–2751, 2003.
26. Simon D, Trenholme G: Antibiotic selection for patients with septic shock. *Crit Care Clin* 16:215–231, 2000.

27. Valles J, Rello J, Ochagavia A, Garnacho J, Alcala MA: Community-acquired bloodstream infection in critically ill adult patients: Impact of shock and inappropriate antibiotic therapy on survival. *Chest* 123:1615–1624, 2003.
28. Rivers E, Nguyen B, Havstad S et al.: Early goal-directed therapy in the treatment of severe sepsis and septic shock. *N Engl J Med* 345:1368–1377, 2001.
29. Horak J, Weiss S: Emergent management of the airway. New pharmacology and the control of comorbidities in cardiac disease, ischemia, and valvular heart disease. *Crit Care Clin* 16:411–427, 2000.
30. The Acute Respiratory Distress Syndrome Network: Ventilation with lower tidal volumes as compared with traditional tidal volumes for acute lung injury and the acute respiratory distress syndrome. *N Engl J Med* 342:1301–1308, 2000.
31. Annane D, Sebille V, Charpentier C et al.: Effect of treatment with low doses of hydrocortisone and fludrocortisone on mortality in patients with septic shock. *JAMA* 288:862–871, 2002.
32. van den BG, Wouters P, Weekers F et al.: Intensive insulin therapy in the critically ill patients. *N Engl J Med* 345:1359–1367, 2001.

23

Adverse Cutaneous Drug Eruptions

Jeffrey E. Frederic
Lee T. Nesbitt

HIGH YIELD FACTS

1. Most drug eruptions are mild and resolve when the drug is stopped. A morbilliform (measles-like, exanthematous) eruption is the most common morphology.

2. Early in its course, a severe drug eruption may be indistinguishable from a mild one. Some important clinical clues to a severe drug reaction are high fever, eosinophilia, lymphadenopathy, and mucous membrane involvement.

3. Mortality is significant in severe drug eruptions, especially in toxic epidermal necrolysis (TEN), in which secondary sepsis is often the cause of death. The most important intervention is to stop the offending drug, but fluid and electrolyte balance must also be maintained, and secondary infections should be prevented and treated early.

CASE PRESENTATION

A 23-year-old woman presents to the emergency department complaining of an intensely pruritic rash that began 2 days ago on her face and has spread to her upper trunk and extremities. She has been in good health except for a remote diagnosis of epilepsy. One month ago she saw her neurologist because her seizures had begun again. She was started on phenytoin 100 mg three times a day, which is the only medicine she takes aside from oral contraceptives.

The patient is febrile with a temperature of 39°C. Physical exam reveals a widespread eruption of erythematous macules which have produced confluent erythema and scaling on her face and upper trunk. Her face is edematous, and bilateral cervical and axillary lymphadenopathy is noted. She also has tender hepatomegaly. Blood counts are normal except for a significant eosinophilia. Chemistries reveal markedly elevated liver enzymes with the ALT higher than the AST.

INTRODUCTION/EPIDEMIOLOGY

Though not an infectious disease, the subject of adverse cutaneous drug eruptions is important in any discussion of medical emergencies because of its prominent place in the differential diagnosis of fever and a rash. While many drug eruptions result in little more than an annoyance to the patient, about 2% are severe enough to require hospitalization. Without proper treatment these severe reactions may result in disability or death, often because of secondary infectious disease complications. Recognition of a life-threatening drug eruption is of primary concern in the emergency department as prompt intervention can save the patient's life. The focus of this chapter will be on three severe life-threatening drug reactions. The first is the condition with which the aforementioned patient is suffering, drug rash with eosinophilia and systemic symptoms (DRESS), also known as drug hypersensitivity syndrome. Second, we will discuss Stevens-Johnson syndrome (SJS) and TEN, which are now considered to be variations of the same entity. Lastly, we will discuss acute generalized exanthematous pustulosis (AGEP), an eruption that may be confused with infection because of the presence of pustules. These syndromes are summarized in Table 23–1.

Adverse cutaneous reactions to medications are common. Prerelease trials of new medications typically reveal a cutaneous reaction occurring in 0.1–1.0% of patients per course of the drug—a staggering number when one considers how much medication is taken daily throughout the world. Some common drugs such as sulfonamide antibiotics, anticonvulsants, and nonsteroidal antiinflammatory drugs (NSAIDS) show an even higher rate of cutaneous reaction, up to 5% in some estimates (1). Exanthematous, or morbilliform, eruptions account for over 90% of cutaneous drug reactions. The next most common reaction, making up about 6%, is urticaria, followed by drug-induced vasculitis in approximately 1–2% (2). Severe drug reactions are rare. SJS/TEN has an incidence of about 1–2 per million population per year (3). DRESS is more common, occurring in up to one out of every thousand patients taking anticonvulsant medications, with similar numbers estimated for sulfonamides and allopurinol (1). AGEP is a rare condition that has only recently been described. Estimates of its incidence are difficult to provide because it is believed to be underreported.

Several diseases that fall into the category of severe or life-threatening cutaneous drug reactions are not discussed in this chapter. Anaphylaxis, angioedema, drug-induced thrombocytopenia, and warfarin necrosis are all severe drug reactions with prominent skin findings. These

Table 23–1. Comparison of Severe Adverse Cutaneous Drug Reactions

	DRESS	SJS/TEN	AGEP
Time after starting drug	2–6 weeks	1–21 days (mean 14 days)	1–3 days
Distinctive skin findings	Morbilliform eruption, eythroderma	Mucous membrane lesions, skin sloughing	>100 pustules
Site	Face, then upper trunk and upper extremities, then spreads diffusely	Two or more mucous membranes, confluent skin necrosis	Begins face/intertriginous areas
Distinguishing clinical findings	High fever, lymphadenopathy	Prodrome of upper respiratory illness, high fever	High fever
Laboratory findings	Hypereosinophilia, lymphocytosis, ↑LFTs	Electrolyte abnormalities, ↑BUN, ↓CO_2, ↑glucose	Marked leukocytosis, ↑ANC, transient uremia, mild eosinophilia, normal LFTs
Systemic manifestations	Hepatitis (may be fulminant), myocarditis, pneumonitis, nephritis, thyroiditis, cerebritis	Electrolyte imbalance, inflammation of internal epithelia (tracheobronchial tree: respiratory failure, GI: profuse diarrhea)	Transient renal insufficiency
Main differential diagnosis	Morbilliform drug eruption, acute viral infection	Staphylococcal scalded skin syndrome	Pustular psoriasis
Most common drug cause	Anticonvulsants, sulfonamides, allopurinol	Sulfonamides, other antibiotics, anticonvulsants, NSAIDs	Beta-lactam antibiotics, macrolides, calcium channel blockers
Specific treatment	Systemic corticosteroids	ICU/burn unit care, IVIG possibly	Topical steroids, antipyretics
Mortality	Up to 10%	Up to 30%	Up to 2%

Abbreviations: DRESS = Drug rash with eosinophilia and systemic symptoms, SJS/TEN = Stevens-Johnson syndrome/toxic epidermal necrolysis, AGEP = acute generalized exanthematous pustulosis, ↑ = increased, ↓ = decreased, IVIG = intravenous immunoglobulin, ICU = intensive care unit, LFTs = liver function tests, BUN = blood urea nitrogen, CO_2 = bicarbonate, ANC = absolute neutrophil count, GI = gastrointestinal, SSSS = staphylococcal scalded skin syndrome, NSAIDs = nonsteroidal antiinflammatory drugs.

disorders tend to be easily recognized by their distinctive history and physical findings.

PATHOPHYSIOLOGY

The pathogenesis of drug eruptions is poorly understood. Traditionally, most drug eruptions have been considered to be hypersensitivity reactions in which drug molecules or metabolites act as haptens, attaching to cell proteins (4). The drug-protein complex stimulates a delayed-type hypersensitivity reaction causing an attack on skin cells by the patient's own lymphocytes. A type IV hypersensitivity such as this is theorized to play a role in exanthematous eruptions and DRESS. If on the other hand the patient mounted an antibody response to the drug, the result might be a type I IgE-mediated hypersensitivity response such as urticaria, or even a type II cytotoxic hypersensitivity response such as drug-induced thrombocytopenia. This explanation is a gross oversimplification of a process that is far more intricate than originally believed.

Some recent progress has been made in our understanding of SJS/TEN (5). It appears that the massive skin cell death that occurs early in the disease process is caused by apoptosis of keratinocytes. All keratinocytes express on their surface a death-receptor molecule known as Fas. When activated by Fas ligand, Fas causes the programmed death of the cell. In TEN, keratinocytes express an increased amount of Fas ligand on their surface. The interaction with Fas causes widespread cell death, resulting in necrosis of the entire thickness of the epidermis. Use of intravenous immunoglobulin (IVIG) in the treatment of SJS/TEN targets this interaction as an attempt to block apoptosis.

Though most drug reactions are thought to be immunologically mediated, it is clear that other factors play an important role, such as drug metabolism, viral infections, and genetic background of the patient (6). Patients who develop eruptions with sulfonamides are usually slow acetylators, resulting in buildup of the metabolite hydroxylamine which is thought to be the responsible molecule (7). Anticonvulsant hypersensitivity may actually be caused by the metabolite arenae oxide which cannot be detoxified by patients deficient in the enzyme epoxide hydrolase. These alterations in drug metabolism can be inherited producing a genetic tendency for cutaneous drug reactions. Evidence also exists for viral involvement in drug eruptions (8). Recently, titers of HHV-6 and HHV-7 have been shown to rise in patients with DRESS, suggesting that the cytotoxic reaction may be directed against viral antigens in infected keratinocytes. Drug metabolites may bring about the reaction by altering antigens or cytokines. The eruption that occurs in almost all patients with infectious mononucleosis when given amoxicillin is a well-known example of a viral infection working in conjunction with a drug to produce a cutaneous eruption.

Although a clear understanding of the pathogenesis of drug eruptions is still to be reached, several risk factors are known to predispose patients to both mild and severe drug eruptions. Increased age, polypharmacy, and the recent start of a new drug all predispose patients to an adverse cutaneous reaction. A curious risk factor is infection with HIV. The chance of a reaction increases as the CD4 to CD8 ratio decreases (7). This seems paradoxical given that certain drug reactions are thought to be mediated by CD4-positive T cells. However, this may reflect the importance of a patient's own immunoregulation in the mediation of drug reactions. The increased risk for drug eruptions in HIV-infected patients is at least partially explained by the frequent finding of glutathione deficiency, which makes it difficult to detoxify drug metabolites. Although all of the above should be considered in the patient with a suspected drug reaction, the single most important risk factor for developing a drug eruption is the history of a previous drug eruption, even to another medication.

CLINICAL PRESENTATION

Mild Drug Reactions

The most common type of cutaneous drug reaction by far is an *exanthematous eruption*, also know as a morbilliform drug eruption (measles-like) or a maculopapular eruption (Fig. 23–1) (1, 4). Classically, it begins with erythema of the trunk and spreads centrifugally. New lesions appear as macules or papules, which become confluent as the eruption spreads. No vesicles or pustules occur, and pruritus is a common symptom. In the typical time course, the eruption starts about a week after the responsible medication is begun, and resolves 1–2 weeks after the medication is discontinued. Occasionally a slight fever or mild eosinophilia may accompany the skin changes, but no signs of internal organ involvement are appreciated.

The second most common drug eruption, *urticaria*, has a distinctive appearance. Intensely pruritic, erythematous, edematous wheals with a sharp border appear anywhere on the skin surface. Often these lesions will have a pale center as a result of edema in the underlying dermis. The wheals are evanescent, appearing and disappearing rapidly, often within hours. Fever is not an associated finding. There are many causes of urticaria besides drugs, including foods, various infections, insect stings, physical factors such as cold and heat, and idiopathic cases. When drugs are the cause, penicillins and NSAIDS are the most common culprits.

The hallmark of *cutaneous vasculitis* is palpable purpura, typically of the lower extremities. Like urticaria, many factors may result in vasculitis besides medications, including a variety of infections and autoimmune diseases. Although most often confined to the skin, a drug-induced vasculitis may rarely involve other organs, and

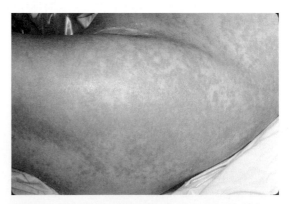

Fig. 23–1. An exanthematous drug eruption (also known as a morbilliform or measles-like eruption).

therefore be classified as a serious drug reaction. Clues to a more serious reaction are fever, arthritis, and signs of internal organ involvement on physical exam and lab testing. Hepatic, renal, and central nervous system involvement are the most dangerous complications.

Severe Drug Eruptions

Drug Rash with Eosinophilia and Systemic Symptoms

The name DRESS replaces the older name of this disease, drug hypersensitivity syndrome, which was confusing because most drug reactions are thought to be immune-related and are therefore technically "hypersensitivity syndromes" (1, 9). The time between starting the drug and the onset of symptoms is typically between 2 and 6 weeks. The long time period may possibly be explained by the time necessary for metabolites of the drug to accumulate. Fever and malaise are often the first symptoms, although the eruption may precede fever. The eruption often begins on the face or upper trunk. It initially has a morbilliform quality and may be indistinguishable from exanthematous drug eruptions and viral exanthems. Although the clinical appearance may be nonspecific early on, the severity of the eruption will increase over the next hours to days, distinguishing it from a mild drug eruption.

The erythema spreads, often covering most of the skin surface. The patient may progress to *erythroderma*, a general term used to describe a severe diffuse eruption from a variety of causes. Pruritus is often intense. Involved skin will become edematous, sometimes so severely that vesicles and bullae erupt. Facial edema is a hallmark of DRESS (Fig. 23–2). The red, edematous skin often begins to scale and exfoliate. Thin sheets of stratum corneum flake off exposing the erythematous epidermis underneath, in contrast to TEN in which the entire epidermis sloughs, leaving a raw, denuded base.

On physical exam generalized lymphadenopathy may be found. The liver may be enlarged and tender. Hepatitis is the most common internal manifestation of DRESS, and a fulminant hepatitis is the most common cause of death (6). Overall mortality is estimated to be between 5% and 10%. Other complications include interstitial nephritis, interstitial pulmonitis, and myocarditis. Thyroiditis may result in a transient hypothyroidism, which typically develops on recovery.

This disease was associated with the anticonvulsants for such a long time that it was sometimes called the "anticonvulsant hypersensitivity syndrome." Phenytoin, carbamazepine, and phenobarbital are the most commonly

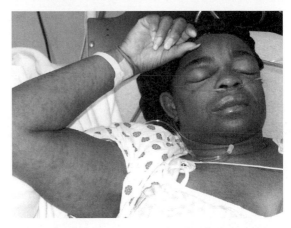

Fig. 23–2. DRESS syndrome due to trimethoprim/sulfamethoxazole. An exanthematous eruption involves the upper extremities and trunk. Edema of the face, most noticeable in the eyelids and lips, is a hallmark of this disease.

involved anticonvulsants, and often cross-react. When a patient has experienced DRESS in the past, administering the responsible drug or one of its cross-reactants a second time results in an accelerated course of the disease. Lamotrigine and valproic acid may also cause DRESS, but do not typically cross-react with the other anticonvulsants, though case reports of this do exist. The antibacterial sulfonamides have probably replaced anticonvulsants as the number one cause of DRESS. Trimethoprim-sulfamethoxazole is a common culprit because of its frequent use. Non-antibacterial sulfa-containing agents such as diuretics and oral hypoglycemics do not generally cause DRESS. Other drugs which can be implicated include allopurinol, NSAIDS, and dapsone.

Stevens-Johnson Syndrome and Toxic Epidermal Necrolysis

The debate over the nomenclature of the erythema multiforme-like spectrum of diseases continues. In the past, erythema multiforme had been considered the mildest variant of the disease entity that includes SJS and TEN. Many experts now feel that SJS and TEN represent the same disease process in differing degrees of severity, but that erythema multiforme is a separate disease. The term erythema multiforme major, which used to be synonymous with the Stevens-Johnson syndrome, is now rarely used. Evidence to support this position comes from recent studies which show that both SJS and TEN are caused by the exact same group of medications (10).

Table 23–2. Medications Most Associated with SJS/TEN

Antimicrobials
  Sulfonamides
  Cephalosporins
  Aminopenicillins
  Tetracyclines
  Macrolides
  Quinolones
  Imidazole antifungals
Antiepileptics
  Carbamazepine
  Barbiturates
  Phenytoin
  Valproic acid
  Lamotrigine
Antiinflammatories
  NSAIDS, in particular:
    Diclofenac
    Indomethacin
    Oxicams
  Acetaminophen
  Aspirin
Allopurinol

Erythema multiforme, in contrast, is uncommonly caused by medications and is most often associated with herpes virus infection. Additional evidence that SJS and TEN are the same illness comes from the numerous cases that cannot be classified as either SJS or TEN, but seem to represent an overlap between the two.

Recent medication use is reported in 97% of patients with TEN (10). Though rare causes include immunizations and infections, a clear relationship between initiation of a new medicine and development of the syndrome is seen in most patients. Typically, skin manifestations begin 1–21 days (mean of 14 days) after initiating the culprit drug, though longer periods have been reported. With reexposure to the drug, the time to onset is usually only 1–3 days. Table 23–2 contains a list of the medications consistently associated with SJS/TEN, but it should be noted that case reports exist for others (11). As with DRESS, antibacterial sulfonamides are the number one cause and are responsible for about one-third of all cases. All other antimicrobials make up another third. The remainder of cases are caused mostly by various antiepileptic drugs, nonsteroidal antiinflammatory drugs, and allopurinol.

SJS and TEN usually begin with a prodrome of fever and flu-like illness that can precede skin manifestations by as little as a day or up to 2 weeks (5, 12, 13). Pain at mucosal sites may begin before the eruption and may cause dysphagia, dysuria, or ocular burning. The eruption presents symmetrically, often starting on the trunk, but occasionally on the head or neck. It appears suddenly and spreads rapidly. It is macular at first and usually erythematous, though lesions may become dusky-colored or purpuric as they evolve. In its early stages SJS/TEN may resemble a common exanthematous eruption. Sometimes the initial erythema is faint and diffuse (scarlatiniform), making early SJS/TEN difficult to distinguish from staphylococcal scalded skin syndrome (SSSS). Atypical target lesions have also been described in which the macules begin to have a dusky-colored center as they spread. The typical target lesions of erythema multiforme in which the dusky center and erythematous ring are separated by a band of pale edema are not seen. The lesions of SJS/TEN are usually painful and tender, sometimes exquisitely so, and patients may complain of a burning sensation. These findings help distinguish SJS/TEN from an exanthematous drug eruption, in which pruritus is the main symptom.

The macules coalesce into wide areas of erythema as the eruption expands. As lesions age, the skin becomes necrotic. Bullae may form underneath the dying epidermis as it separates from the dermis (Fig. 23–3). When fully necrotic, the epidermis may take on a characteristic gray color. Detachment may be detected early when the eruption is still primarily erythematous by placing lateral pressure on the affected skin. The epidermis will detach from the dermis producing what is called a positive

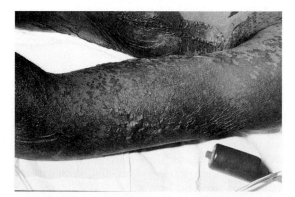

Fig. 23–3. In this patient with TEN, dusky-colored lesions cover over 50% of the body surface area. The lesions are progressing to bullae, and some have already begun to slough, exposing the dermis underneath.

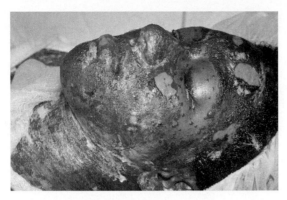

Fig. 23–4. Extensive epidermal necrosis, as well as oral and conjunctival involvement, is seen in this TEN patient.

Table 23–3. The SCORTEN System for Predicting Mortality in SJS/TEN

One point is given for each of the following:
1. Age > 40
2. Presence of a malignancy
3. Tachycardia > 120 beats/minute
4. Initial epidermal detachment > 10% BSA
5. Serum urea > 28 mg/dL (10 mmol/L)
6. Serum glucose > 252 mg/dL (14 mmol/L)
7. Bicarbonate < 20 mEq/L

Number of points	Mortality (%)
0–1	3.2
2	12.1
3	35.3
4	58.3
≥ 5	90

Nikolsky sign. Necrotic epidermis will slough with minor pressure leaving behind a red, oozing or bleeding base.

Mucosal lesions occur in all cases of SJS/TEN (Fig. 23–4). They tend to occur early, either preceding or accompanying the eruption of skin lesions. Any mucous membrane site can be involved. The oral cavity is most common, followed by conjunctival, nasal, and anogenital mucosae. Pain or burning may precede the appearance of erythematous macules. Lesions then mimic the progression of the skin eruption, progressing to erosions with or without a vesicular stage. Erosions may be covered by hemorrhagic crusts or by necrotic tissue that has yet to slough. Involved sites are exquisitely painful. In the mouth, the first lesions are seen on the lips, palate, and buccal surfaces. The eroded surface will expand, possibly covering the entire oral cavity. Sometimes the disease will progress into the oropharynx and larynx, or even as far as the esophagus or tracheobronchial tree.

Maximal skin and mucosal involvement is usually reached within 4–5 days, though progression from the macular stage to sloughing of necrotic epidermis may rarely take less than a day. Recurrent cases tend to progress more rapidly than new ones. It is impossible to predict the extent of the skin disease progression, but the earlier the offending drug is stopped, the better the prognosis. The entire skin surface may necrose and slough. By convention, if less than 10% body surface area (BSA) is involved, the syndrome is given the name Stevens-Johnson syndrome. Toxic epidermal necrolysis is defined as greater than 30% BSA involvement, with cases between 10% and 30% referred to SJS/TEN overlap syndrome. Classification makes a great difference to prognosis: with SJS, mortality is approximately 2%, but mortality in TEN is 30% or higher. A detailed scoring system for predicting

mortality has been developed and independently validated by looking at a large number of TEN cases. The SCORTEN system (see Table 23–3) takes into account clinical and laboratory data to estimate a patient's chance of survival with standard care. Note that HIV infection, while it does increase the risk for developing TEN, does not affect mortality.

The period immediately following maximal skin progression is the most dangerous for the patient. Loss of the barrier function of the skin results in water and electrolyte depletion, and possibly hemodynamic shock. Internal organ involvement is mainly limited to epithelial linings which may undergo a process of necrosis similar to that of the skin. The trachea and bronchi can slough debris into the airway. Small airway involvement may lead to acute respiratory distress syndrome (ARDS). The epithelial lining of the GI tract may also be affected, resulting in diarrhea and bleeding. Renal damage may occur from hypoperfusion due to shock. However, the single most dangerous complication is infection, which accounts for the majority of deaths in SJS/TEN. Bacteria can invade the necrotic epithelia of the skin and internal organs causing sepsis and subsequent multiorgan failure. The patient is at the highest risk for sepsis in the week following maximal progression of skin disease.

If the patient survives this dangerous period, reepithelialization will begin and take about 3 weeks to complete. The skin does not usually scar although pigmentation will be altered, and hair or nails could be permanently lost. Mucosal sites are more likely to scar. Strictures may form at affected mucosal sites such as the trachea, esophagus, anus, vagina, and urethra. If the conjunctiva is involved, synechiae or symblepharon may result. Blindness is possible if corneal scarring occurs. Destruction of salivary and lacrimal glands can cause sicca syndrome. Effective management has the goal of not only minimizing mortality, but avoiding these long-term complications.

Acute Generalized Exanthematous Pustulosis

Acute generalized exanthematous pustulosis, also known as pustular drug eruption or toxic pustuloderma, is not often diagnosed in the United States. It is rare and often mistaken for other diseases such as an acute eruption of pustular psoriasis. The acute eruption of pustules may erroneously suggest infection. Though medications account for the majority of AGEP, a small percentage is attributed to viral infection (14). Ingestion of mercury may also trigger the eruption. Beta-lactam antibiotics are the primary culprit. Other antibiotics, macrolides in particular, are responsible for many of the remaining cases. Many other drugs have been reported, including NSAIDS and calcium channel blockers.

AGEP has an abrupt onset (15, 16). A sudden high fever (average 39°C) begins in close proximity to the skin eruption, usually the same day. The time interval between initiation of the medication and presentation is characteristically short. Symptoms usually begin within 1–3 days of starting the drug, though longer intervals up to 2 weeks have been reported. This short time interval suggests that prior sensitization to the drug may exist. The eruption begins in the intertriginous areas or on the face but disseminates rapidly. Diffuse erythema with underlying edema is seen early, and within a few hours, numerous small pustules appear in the erythematous skin (Fig. 23–5). Usually less than several millimeters each, these superficial pustules may number in the hundreds. The pustules may become confluent and produce a positive Nikolsky sign. Other skin lesions sometimes seen include erythema multiforme-like target lesions, purpura, and mucous membrane erosions, particularly in the mouth (17).

Visceral involvement is rare except for the kidney (18). About a third of patients experience acute renal failure. The finding of red blood cell casts in the urine of several patients with AGEP suggests that this is an acute glomerulonephritis, not an interstitial nephritis as seen in

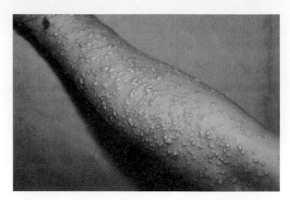

Fig. 23–5. A pustular eruption such as that seen in AGEP.

DRESS. Renal function typically returns to normal in a few days. Pustules and fever persist for approximately 1 week, giving way to superficial desquamation. By 2 weeks the skin typically shows no evidence of the disease. AGEP is usually self-limited; however, it can be dangerous in the elderly and those with preexisting diseases. Mortality is estimated to be about 1–2% and is mainly due to renal complications. Those with previous renal insufficiency may not recover kidney function.

LABORATORY/DIAGNOSTIC TESTING

Standard labs for a patient with a suspected drug eruption should include a complete blood count with platelets and white blood cell differential and a comprehensive metabolic profile that includes measurements of electrolytes, kidney function, and liver function. Laboratory clues that a patient is suffering from more than a simple exanthematous eruption are discussed below.

Drug Rash with Eosinophilia and Systemic Symptoms

Prominent eosinophilia, often as high as 20% or more, is the most common laboratory abnormality as implied by the name of the syndrome (19). However, early in the course it may not be present, and a lymphocytosis will be seen instead. Atypical lymphocytes may be reported, which, when combined with the clinical picture, may cause DRESS to be mistaken for infectious mononucleosis. A history of recently starting one of the "usual suspect" drugs instead of amoxicillin, as well as the severity of the eruption, should alert the clinician to this potentially life-threatening disorder. Additional lab findings are the result of inflammation in the affected internal organs. Most commonly, liver enzymes will be elevated.

Stevens-Johnson Syndrome and Toxic Epidermal Necrolysis

When Lyell first described toxic epidermal necrolysis in 1956, the definition included cases with superficial shedding of the stratum corneum caused by a bacterial exotoxin secreted by *Staphylococcus aureus* (12). This syndrome was later separated out and referred to as SSSS. Although the initial eruption of SSSS is usually scarlatiniform and that of TEN is usually macular, their early lesions may be indistinguishable. Both may have a positive Nikolsky sign. SSSS occurs most commonly in young children, though it may occur in adults, especially in the setting of renal impairment. The most definitive way to distinguish between the two is by skin biopsy, either routine H&E or frozen section. In SJS/TEN the separation will occur at the dermal-epidermal junction, whereas in SSSS the separation is just below the stratum corneum.

Other laboratory tests are important for identifying the complications of SJS/TEN. Serum chemistries may reveal electrolyte imbalances from fluid loss so severe that they can lead to cardiac arythmias. Serum urea will increase from dehydration. Metabolic acidosis may result from volume contraction, hypoperfusion, and sepsis. Blood counts may reveal an eosinophilia. Sepsis may be heralded by either leukocytosis or leukopenia, the latter being associated with poorer prognosis. Blood glucose is often elevated, and severe insulin resistance is another poor prognostic indicator.

Acute Generalized Exanthematous Pustulosis

The most characteristically abnormal lab test in AGEP is the white blood cell count and differential (16). There is often a leukocytosis with an elevated absolute neutrophil count (ANC). The ANC is almost always above 7000 cells per microliter. About 20% of patients will also have an eosinophilia. Liver enzymes are normal. One third of affected patients will have renal function abnormalities. The albumin level may be depressed. Applying the offending medication in solution topically to the skin for 48 h under a small patch will produce a pustular reaction similar to the skin lesions of AGEP in up to 80% of cases.

MANAGEMENT

The first step in management of any drug eruption is to identify the causative agent. This is not always an easy task. Often the temporal relationship between the drug administration and the onset of skin findings does not conform to classically described intervals. Also, the patient may be receiving multiple potential culprit drugs. There is no laboratory test that can reliably identify the offending drug. Sometimes the lesions of an eruption may be reproduced by placing a solution of the medicine against the patient's skin (a patch test), but this finding is rare in all drug eruptions except for AGEP, as described above. However, patch testing takes several days to perform and is of no practical use in emergencies.

The single most important intervention in a life-threatening drug eruption is to stop the causative agent as early as possible (20). When a life-threatening eruption is diagnosed, standard practice is to stop all drugs that are not immediately life-sustaining, as it is often impossible to tell which drug is responsible. In addition to drug cessation, several of the severe cutaneous drug reactions require specific treatments, which are discussed below.

Drug Rash with Eosinophilia and Systemic Symptoms

Systemic corticosteroids are the treatment of choice for DRESS (21). Although controlled-randomized trials are lacking, prednisone at doses of 1 mg/kg or higher is usually given to treat life-threatening complications. The skin eruption responds quickly. Although pulmonary and cardiac manifestations also generally respond rapidly to therapy, liver and kidney disease can be more resistant. Steroids need to be continued for several weeks after clinical resolution and tapered slowly to avoid relapse. Thyroiditis may produce a temporary hypothyroidism 1–2 months later, so thyroid stimulating hormone should be checked and thyroxine given if necessary.

Stevens-Johnson Syndrome and Toxic Epidermal Necrolysis

Again, it should be reiterated that all medicines even remotely suspected of causing SJS/TEN must be stopped as soon as possible. Because SJS/TEN may be confused with staphylococcal scalded skin syndrome, a common treatment dilemma is whether or not to continue an antibiotic. The antibiotics used for treatment of SSSS (penicillins, cephalosporins, and vancomycin) are all potential causes of SJS/TEN. A dermatologist should be consulted early to help with diagnosis. If the distinction is not clear from the clinical presentation, a skin biopsy and frozen section are required.

Treatment for SJS/TEN falls into two main categories: disease-modifying medication and supportive care. Whether treatment can alter the progression of epidermal detachment is still a matter of debate. High-dose corticosteroids were the standard of care until the 1970s, when several retrospective studies showed doubtful benefit of steroid therapy on mortality, complications, or length of hospital stay. Several nonrandomized prospective trials also confirmed this (5). Both oral and intravenous steroid formulations were studied. No large scale randomized study exists. Today, many experts feel that steroid therapy does not help and may even have the deleterious effect of either masking or increasing the risk of infection. If any benefit from steroid therapy exists, it probably occurs only when steroids are given very early in the disease.

More recently, much interest has been generated by case reports suggesting that IVIG can halt progression of the epidermal necrosis if given early in the disease course (22). In vitro studies have demonstrated that many of the commercially available IVIG preparations are able to block the interaction of Fas with Fas ligand. In theory, blocking this interaction should arrest the apoptosis of keratinocytes. However, the benefit has not been as clear as originally hoped (23–25). Several small, nonrandomized studies have shown improved survival over that predicted by SCORTEN; however, others have shown no benefit. Drawing conclusions is difficult because inclusion criteria vary between studies, and the brand of IVIG and dosage vary even within studies. A large, randomized, controlled trial is needed, but will be difficult to perform given the rarity of the disease. If IVIG is to be used, higher doses similar to those used in studies demonstrating benefit are recommended. At least 2 g/kg total dose should be given. Common dosing regimens are 0.75 mg/kg IV for 4 days, or 1 mg/kg for 3 days. Cyclosporine, N-acetylcysteine, and cyclophosphamide have also been touted as beneficial in case reports, but at present, no drug is proven to alter the course of this disease (26).

Good supportive care is arguably more important than any other intervention discussed (5, 6, 12). SJS/TEN is best treated in an ICU or burn unit, and the treatment is similar to the management of severe thermal burns. Patients should be handled gently and with sterile technique in order to prevent further skin loss or introduction of pathogens. Unlike thermal burns, debridement of necrotic skin in SJS/TEN is not recommended. The skin should be left in place, as it forms a biologic dressing. Eroded areas should receive local wound care with a moist, nonadherent dressing. If topical antibiotics are used, silver sulfadiazine

should be avoided as in theory it could cross-react with sulfonamide antibiotics.

Complications must be identified and addressed early to minimize mortality. Electrolyte abnormalities, volume loss, and thermal dysregulation may require correction. The physician should watch for signs of ARDS, renal failure, and above all, sepsis. Pain control is a vital component of care. An ophthalmologist should be consulted early to monitor for signs of severe ocular sequelae. Reepithelialization will usually start within a few days after maximal skin involvement is reached. The patient may require supportive care for several weeks until this process is complete.

Acute Generalized Exanthematous Pustulosis

There is no specific treatment for AGEP. Patients can be treated symptomatically with topical steroids and antipyretics. Renal function should be closely monitored, especially in patients with preexisting renal insufficiency. Hemodialysis may rarely be necessary. Given the short time interval between drug initiation and onset of symptoms, identifying the causative agent is usually not a problem. However, in reported cases when the diagnosis was missed and the drug was not stopped, the eruption became more severe, mimicking SJS/TEN (27).

DISPOSITION

While patients with life-threatening drug eruptions should be admitted to the hospital, common exanthematous drug reactions are easily managed in the outpatient setting. The patient can be sent home with a topical steroid, an oral antihistamine for pruritus, and careful follow-up with a dermatologist. The primary problem is distinguishing a severe drug reaction from a mild one. In their early stages, the eruptions of both DRESS and SJS/TEN can resemble a mild exanthematous eruption. However, as discussed earlier, both of these syndromes have some characteristic clinical findings that would lead the clinician to suspect a more ominous syndrome. Table 23–4 contains a list of some key clinical and laboratory findings that should lead to more cautious treatment of a patient with a suspected drug eruption. Though the presence of one or two of these criteria would not necessarily dictate an admission, it should provoke a higher level of concern, and close follow-up is necessary.

A common question that arises is whether a drug should be stopped if a mild exanthematous eruption is diagnosed.

Table 23–4. Signs of a Severe Drug Eruption

Clinical
  Skin pain or burning
  Blisters, epidermal detachment, or positive
  Nikolsky sign
  Mucous membrane lesions
  Facial edema
  High fever
  Lymphadenopathy
Laboratory
  Eosinophilia
  Lymphocytosis, especially atypical
  Abnormal liver function tests

Typically the drug is discontinued regardless of the severity of the eruption, because there is no way to ensure that life-threatening eruption will not develop. This approach has caused problems in the management of HIV-infected patients, as up to 60% of these patients experience an adverse cutaneous reaction to sulfonamides (7). It has become common practice in HIV clinics to treat through a morbilliform eruption, which often resolves on its own. The decision to continue a drug in the presence of an eruption requires a risk-benefit analysis, and is best made by the patient's primary care physician. In the practice of emergency medicine, it is best to stop any drug suspected of causing an adverse reaction and schedule prompt follow-up with a physician who can decide whether to restart it.

CASE OUTCOME

The phenytoin was immediately stopped, and the patient was given 1 mg/kg of oral prednisone in the emergency department. She was admitted for observation. Her severe pruritus was treated with topical emollients and oral antihistamines. The next day her liver enzymes began to trend downward, though the eosinophilia persisted for several days. On day 2 after admission, the erythema and pruritus decreased, and her skin began to exfoliate. She was discharged on daily prednisone which was tapered over the following 2 weeks. The eruption completely resolved without scarring. Her seizures continued to be a problem, so after a discussion with her neurologist, she was started on valproic acid because of its low cross-reactivity with other anticonvulsants. She was watched closely after starting this new medication but did not develop another eruption.

REFERENCES

1. Revuz J & Valeyrie-Allanore L. Drug Reactions, in Bolognia JL, Jorizzo JL, Rapini RP et al. (eds.). *Dermatology*. London, Mosby, 2003; p333–352.
2. Bigby M. Rates of cutaneous reactions to drugs. *Arch Dermatol.* 137:765–70, 2001.
3. Wolkenstein P & Revus J. Toxic Epidermal Necrolysis. *Dermatology Clinics* 18(3): 485–95, 2000.
4. Shear NH, Knowles SR, Sullivan JR, & Shapiro L. Cutaneous reactions to Drugs, in Freeberg IM, Eisen AZ, Wolff K, et al. (eds.). *Dermatology in General Medicine, 6th ed.* New York, McGraw-Hill, 2003; p1330–7.
5. Prendiville J. Stevens-Johnson syndrome and toxic epidermal necrolysis. *Advances in Dermatology.* 18:151–73, 2002.
6. Revuz J. New advances in severe adverse drug reactions. *Dermatol Clinics.* 19(4): 697–709, 2001.
7. Tilles SA. Practical issues in the management of hypersensitivity reactions: sulfonamides. *Southern Medical Journal.* 94(8): 817–24, 2001.
8. Suzuki Y, Inagi R, Aono T, et al. Human herpesvirus 6 infection as a risk factor for development of severe drug-induced hypersensitivity syndrome. *Arch Dermatol.* 134:1108–22, 1998.
9. Roujeau JC, Stern RS. Severe adverse reactions to drugs. *N Engl J Med* 331(19):1272–85, 1994 Nov 10.
10. Schopf E et al. Toxic epidermal necrolysis and Stevens-Johnson syndrome: An epidemiologic study from West Germany. *Arch Dermatol.* 127:839, 1991.
11. Sane SP & Batt AD. Stevens-Johnson syndrome and toxic epidermal necrolysis – challenges of recognition and management. *J. Assoc Physicians India.* 47(10):999–1003, 2000.
12. French LE & Prins C. Toxic epidermal necrolysis, in Bolognia JL, Jorizzo JL, Rapini RP et al. (eds.). *Dermatology*. London, Mosby, 2003; p323–331.
13. Fritsh PO & Sidoroff A. Drug-induced Stevens-Johnson syndrome/toxic epidermal necrolysis. *Am J Clin Dermatol.* 1(6): 349–60, 2000.
14. Meadows KP, Egan CA, & Vanderfooft SL. Acute generalized exanthematous pustulosis (AGEP), an uncommon condition in children: case report and review of literature. *Pediatric Dermatology.* 17(5):399–402, 2000.
15. Beylot C, Doutre MS, & Beylot-Barry M. Acute generalized exanthematous pustulosis. *Seminars in Cutaneous Medicine & Surgery.* 15(4):244–9, 1996.
16. Roujeau JC, Bioulac-Sage P, Bourseau C, et al. Acute generalized exanthematous pustulosis. Analysis of 63 cases. *Arch Dermatol.* 127(9):1333–8, 1991.
17. Lin JH, Sheu HM, & Lee JY. Acute generalized exanthematous pustulosis with erythema multiforme-like lesions. *European J Dermatol.* 12(5):475–8, 2002.
18. Brandenburg VM, Kurts C, Eitner F, et al. Acute reversible renal failure in acute generalized exanthematous pustulosis. *Nephrol Dial Transplan.* 17(10):1857–8, 2002.

19. Bachot N & Roujeau JC. Differential diagnosis of severe cutaneous drug eruptions. *Am J Clin Dermatol.* 4(3):561–72, 2003.

20. Garcia-Doval I, Le Cleach L, Bocquet H, et al. Toxic epidermal necrolysis and Stevens-Johnson syndrome: does early withdrawal of causative drugs decrease the risk of death? *Arch Dermatol.* 136:323–7, 2000.

21. Ghislain PD & Roujeau JC. Treatment of severe drug reactions: Stevens-Johnson syndrome, toxic epidermal necrolysis and hypersensitivity syndrome. *Dermatology Online Journal.* 8(1):5, 2002.

22. Bachot N & Roujeau JC. Intravenous immunoglobulins in the treatment of severe drug eruptions. *Current Opinion in Allergy & Clinical Immunology.* 3(4):269–74, 2003.

23. Prins C, Kerdel FA, Padilla RS, et al. Treatment of toxic epidermal necrolysis with high-dose intravenous immunoglob-ulins: multicenter retrospective analysis of 48 consecutive cases. *Arch Dermatol.* 139:26–32, 2003.

24. Bachot N, Revuz J, & Roujeau JC. Intravenous immunoglob-ulin treatment for Stevens-Johnson syndrome and toxic epidermal necrolysis: a prospective noncomparative study showing no benefit on mortality or progression. *Arch Dermatol.* 139:33–36, 2003.

25. Trent JT, Kirsner RS, Romanelli P, & Kerdel FA. Analysis of intravenous immunoglobulin for the treatment of toxic epidermal necrolysis using SCORTEN: the University of Miami experience. *Arch Dermatol.* 139:39–43, 2003.

26. Redondo P et al. Drug-induced hypersensitivity syndrome and toxic epidermal necrolysis: Treatment with N-acetylcysteine. *Br J Dermatol.* 136:645, 1997.

27. Cohen AD, Cagnano, & E. Halevy S. Acute generalized exanthematous pustulosis mimicking toxic epidermal necrolysis. *Internat J Dermatol.* 40(7):458–61, 2001.

24

Primary Skin Infections: Impetigo, Erysipelas, Cellulitis, and Necrotizing Fasciitis

Fred A. Lopez
Ellen M. Slaven
Charles V. Sanders

HIGH YIELD FACTS

1. Most skin infections are caused by *Staphylococcus aureus* and/or *Streptococcus* species and may be adequately treated with narrow-spectrum antimicrobial agents such as oral dicloxacillin or cephalexin, or intravenous nafcillin or cefazolin. However, the increasing incidence of community-acquired methicillin-resistant *S. aureus* (MRSA) infections has resulted in the increased utilization of antimicrobials such as vancomycin, quinuprustin/dalfopristin, and linezolid in the treatment of cellulitis.

2. Unusual exposures or host immunodeficiencies can dictate a different microbiologic spectrum of organisms and may require a more broad-spectrum antimicrobial regimen, which includes beta-lactam and beta-lactamase inhibitor combinations such as piperacillin-tazobactam.

3. Necrotizing fasciitis can be polymicrobial (type I) or monomicrobial (type II). Though antibiotics are indicated for both types, the cornerstone of therapy for these infections is prompt surgical debridement.

4. The extent of skin infection may be difficult to assess by physical exam. Computer tomography (CT) and magnetic resonance imaging (MRI) can be helpful in determining the degree of invasiveness.

CASE PRESENTATION

A 45-year-old man with long-standing diabetes mellitus presented to the emergency department with fever and a painful scrotum. He had no trauma to the area but complained of dysuria. He took insulin to control his diabetes and had recently noted that his blood glucose level was elevated. He was febrile and hypotensive. Physical exam showed that he had edema and erythema over the scrotum. Closer inspection revealed a necrotic bullous lesion over the base of the scrotum. Emergent surgical consultation was obtained. A complete blood count revealed a leukocytosis with left shift, and chemistries revealed an anion-gap metabolic ketoacidosis.

INTRODUCTION

Skin infections are typically classified according to the anatomical distribution and resultant clinical syndrome (1). In this chapter we will discuss primary skin infections, including impetigo, erysipelas, cellulitis, and necrotizing fasciitis.

CLINICAL SYNDROMES: EPIDEMIOLOGY AND CLINICAL PRESENTATIONS

Impetigo

Impetigo, most commonly seen in young children, is a superficial cutaneous infection involving the epidermis. Two types of impetigo exist: nonbullous and bullous. Highly communicable, this infection can spread easily over the body of the same individual or to others in closed living situations where crowding and suboptimal hygiene exist. Potential complications include more extensive skin, soft-tissue, or bone infection. Acute glomerulonephritis with hypertension, hematuria, and proteinuria can occur approximately 10–21 days after this skin infection when certain M serotypes of group A streptococcus (*Streptococcus pyogenes*) are implicated.

Nonbullous impetigo is more commonly encountered (i.e., approximately 70% of cases) and usually manifests as a vesiculopustular lesion that eventually develops into a weeping "honey-crusted" sore or plaque (2) (Fig. 24–1). One or more painless pruritic lesions may be present, and despite the usual absence of fever and other systemic signs, localized lymphadenopathy and an elevated white blood cell count are commonly appreciated. Predisposing factors include any disruption of the skin (i.e., wounds, burns, varicella infection, insect bites, ulcers, herpes virus lesions, and preexisting skin disease) as well as immunocompromising conditions including diabetes mellitus, human immunodeficiency virus (HIV) infection, and hypogammaglobulinemia (3). The face and extremities are usually affected, and these infections appear more commonly during hot and humid weather.

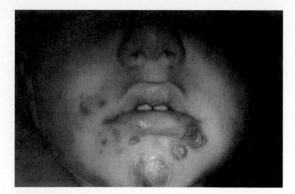

Fig. 24–1. Streptococcal impetigo. Honey-colored crusts of the face. Reproduced with permission from: Lippincott Williams & Wilkins. The Skin and Infection: A Color Atlas and Text, Sanders, CV, Nesbitt LT Jr (Eds), Williams & Wilkins, Baltimore, 1995.

Bullous impetigo manifests as flaccid vesicular and bullous lesions that easily rupture and release a yellow seropurulent fluid (Fig. 24–2). The resultant lesions often layer out in a light-brown crusted pattern that can span a large diameter and intermix with nonruptured bullous lesions. Systemic symptoms are rare. Though lesions can present almost anywhere, including the trunk and perineum, facial lesions are most common.

Erysipelas

Erysipelas is an infection of the epidermis, upper dermis, and superficial lymphatics that typically affects young children and the elderly. This infection is primarily manifest in the lower extremities; however, involvement of the face has also been classically described (4) (Fig. 24–3). Risk factors for erysipelas include disruption of the skin barrier, venous insufficiency, leg edema, lymphedema, obesity, and toe-web intertrigo (5). The characteristic clinical presentation includes well-demarcated erythema that is painful, indurated, and edematous. The borders are elevated and often palpable and can advance quickly. Constitutional symptoms of fever, chills, and malaise are often present; a leukocytosis is frequently noted. Extension of infection can lead to cellulitis, but bacteremia is not common. A bullous form of this disease involving the lower extremities has been described and may portend a more prolonged course of infection (6).

Cellulitis

Cellulitis involves the dermis and subcutaneous tissues, usually resulting from the inoculation of bacteria through tiny breaks in the skin. These disruptions in the skin barrier

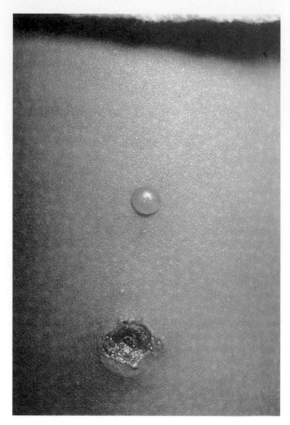

Fig. 24–2. Bullous impetigo, with an early vesicle and later lesion showing a crust formation. Reproduced with permission from: Lippincott Williams & Wilkins. The Skin and Infection: A Color Atlas and Text, Sanders, CV, Nesbitt LT Jr (Eds), Williams & Wilkins, Baltimore, 1995.

can result from tinea pedis, burns, venous insufficiency, lymphedema, traumatic wounds, thrombophlebitis, and ulcers. Host immune defects that result from diabetes mellitus, malnutrition, HIV infection, immunosuppressive medications, and intravenous-drug use may also contribute to the development of infection. Men are more commonly infected, and the extremities (lower more so than upper) are the most commonly involved areas (7) (Fig. 24–4). This infection may be extensive, manifesting as an inflamed, spreading, erythematous, warm, and edematous lesion. The margins of these lesions are not well defined or elevated as they are in erysipelas. Regional lymphadenopathy is usually appreciated, and the clinical presentation can also include fever, chills, malaise, and pain. Some experts have categorized severity of skin and soft-tissue infection into classes ranging from healthy and afebrile patients with cellulitis to those who are septic, with skin and soft-tissue infections that have become

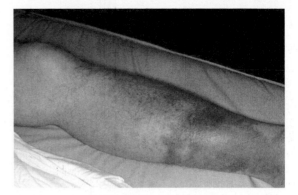

Fig. 24–4. Cellulitis of the leg with hemorrhage and erythematous border. Reproduced with permission from: Lippincott Williams & Wilkins. The Skin and Infection: A Color Atlas and Text, Sanders, CV, Nesbitt LT Jr (Eds), Williams & Wilkins, Baltimore, 1995.

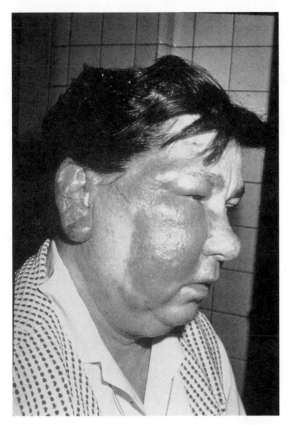

Fig. 24–3. Erysipelas due to group A streptococcus on a female's face. Reproduced with permission from: Lippincott Williams & Wilkins. The Skin and Infection: A Color Atlas and Text, Sanders, CV, Nesbitt LT Jr (Eds), Williams & Wilkins, Baltimore, 1995.

invasive (necrotizing fasciitis, for example) (8). In general, uncomplicated infections refer to immunocompetent patients whose infections are due to *S. aureus* or group A streptococcus. Complicated infections are more likely to include gram-negative or anaerobic organisms and occur in the setting of comorbidities such as diabetes mellitus, burns, chronic pressure ulcers, and postsurgical wounds.

Necrotizing Fasciitis

Necrotizing soft-tissue infections refer to a broad variety of toxic, potentially limb- and life-threatening disorders associated with inflammation, vascular thrombosis, and necrosis of skin, soft-tissue/subcutaneous fat, fascia, and/or muscle. Many confusing terms are used to describe these conditions, and their classifications are usually dictated by the depth of involvement and whether these infections are primarily monomicrobial or polymicrobial. Neither the depth of the infection nor the bacterial

pathogens are known with certainty in the emergency department. A discussion of all of these entities is beyond the scope of this chapter, which will instead concentrate upon the infectious-disease emergency known as necrotizing fasciitis. A proposed microbiologic classification for necrotizing fasciitis includes type I infections, which are mixed anaerobic and aerobic infections, and type II infections, which are due to group A streptococcus either solely (often in the setting of streptococcal toxic-shock-like syndrome) or in combination with *S. aureus* (9). Necrotizing fasciitis can also be due to water-associated organisms including *Vibrio vulnificus*, *Edwardsiella tarda,* and *Aeromonas hydrophila*, and the clinical presentation of these infections is similar to type I and type II infections.

These necrotizing infections of the subcutaneous fat and fascial tissues are abrupt in onset and rapidly progressive, typically sparing the muscle and, early in the process, perhaps even the skin. These devastating infections most commonly affect the extremities though the abdominal wall, head, and neck can often be involved. Fournier's gangrene refers to a necrotizing fasciitis of the skin and subcutaneous fat of the perineum. The testes are generally spared due to an independent vascular supply. Rare in women and children, Fournier gangrene usually affects men greater than 50 years of age and is often associated with genitourinary, anal, or abdominal infections (Fig. 24–5). Risk factors include diabetes mellitus, elderly age, substance abuse, traumatic injury, surgical procedures, renal insufficiency, vascular insufficiency, malignancy, immunosuppression (including secondary to medications such as corticosteroids and chemotherapy), malnutrition, varicella infection, and perineal infection(s) (10, 11).

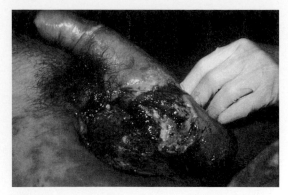

Fig. 24–5. Fournier's gangrene. A mixed aerobic/anaerobic infection. Reproduced with permission from: Lippincott Williams & Wilkins. The Skin and Infection: A Color Atlas and Text, Sanders, CV, Nesbitt LT Jr (Eds), Williams & Wilkins, Baltimore, 1995.

The initial cutaneous presentation in necrotizing fasciitis may be insignificant. When cutaneous findings are present, the skin generally appears erythematous, edematous, and warm, without distinct borders. The patient often experiences pain out of proportion to the cutaneous findings. Fever and systemic signs of toxicity, including hypotension, are common, particularly with the development of hemorrhagic bullous lesions and skin necrosis (Fig. 24–6). Crepitus, a manifestation of subcutaneous emphysema, may be appreciated and can be corroborated by plain radiographs of involved areas. Classic "gas gangrene" is caused by *Clostridium perfringens*; however, not all bacteria capable of producing deep, necrotizing soft-tissue infections produce gas (group A streptococcus, for example). Anesthesia at the site of infection suggests significant subcutaneous necrosis involving destruction of local cutaneous nerves caused by spread of infection in the superficial fascia.

MICROBIOLOGY

Nonbullous impetigo is caused by group A streptococci (*S. pyogenes*) and/or *S. aureus* while bullous impetigo is typically caused by *S. aureus* phage group II type 71 strains that produce exfoliative toxins.

Erysipelas is primarily caused by group A streptococcus (*S. pyogenes*) though other beta-hemolytic streptococci, particularly group G streptococcus, and *S. aureus* can also be causative (12).

Cellulitis is predominantly due to *S. aureus* and *S. pyogenes*. Complicated infections are also due to these organisms but are also more likely to include aerobic Gram-negative or anaerobic organisms and occur in the setting of comorbidities such as diabetes mellitus. In addition, certain host and environmental factors mandate consideration of other etiologic agents (13). For example, patients with liver disease are at increased risk for wound infections and sepsis from *Vibrio vulnificus*, a gram-negative bacterium found primarily in warm coastal waters and undercooked shellfish, especially oysters (14) (Fig. 24–7). *Streptococcus agalactiae* infections are being increasingly reported in nonpregnant adults, including those with diabetes mellitus, cirrhosis, HIV infection, and malignancy (15). Ecthyma gangrenosum is the classic necrotic cutaneous lesion seen in neutropenic patients who develop *Pseudomonas aeruginosa* bacteremia (Fig. 24–8). Patients with pets may also be at risk for skin-associated infections if a bite wound is incurred. Dog bites may result

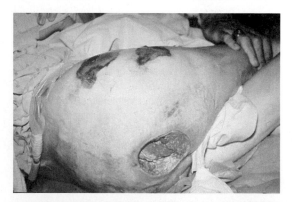

Fig. 24–6. A mixed aerobic and anaerobic infection involving the fascia. Reproduced with permission from: Lippincott Williams & Wilkins. The Skin and Infection: A Color Atlas and Text, Sanders, CV, Nesbitt LT Jr (Eds), Williams & Wilkins, Baltimore, 1995.

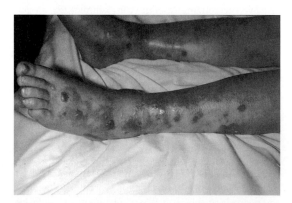

Fig. 24–7. *V. vulnificus.* Hemorrhagic and bullous skin lesions of the feet and lower legs, also showing hemorrhagic necrosis of the dorsum of the left foot. Reproduced with permission from: Lippincott Williams & Wilkins. The Skin and Infection: A Color Atlas and Text, Sanders, CV, Nesbitt LT Jr (Eds), Williams & Wilkins, Baltimore, 1995.

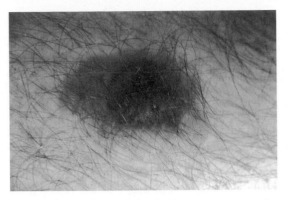

Fig. 24–8. Ecthyma gangrenosum. Ecthyma gangrenosum due to bacteremia from *P. aeruginosa*. Central necrotic eschar with surrounding erythema. Reproduced with permission from: Lippincott Williams & Wilkins. The Skin and Infection: A Color Atlas and Text, Sanders, CV, Nesbitt LT Jr (Eds), Williams & Wilkins, Baltimore, 1995.

in infections with organisms such as *Pasteurella canis, Pasteurella multocida*, anaerobes, *Capnocytophaga canimorsus, S. aureus*, and streptococci, to name a few (16). Cat bites have a similar microbiology to dog bites although *P. multocida* is the most commonly implicated agent (16). Water-associated wound infections deserve special mention. Veterinarians, butchers, and individuals who handle fish are at increased risk for skin infections of the hand (i.e., erysipeloid) caused by *Erysipelothrix rhusiopathiae*. Similarly, cellulitis of the hand secondary to *Streptococcus iniae* has been reported in individuals who have handled the tilapia fish (17). *Mycobacterium marinum* skin infections (i.e., "fish tank granuloma" or "swimming pool granuloma") are primarily seen in individuals who work with fish tanks and can result from contact with salt water, fresh water, and swimming pool water (18).

The polymicrobial infection that characterizes type I necrotizing fasciitis, including Fournier's gangrene, can include facultative non-group A streptococci, *Enterobacteriaceae*, as well as anaerobes such as *Peptostreptococcus, Clostridium*, and *Bacteroides* species. Type II necrotizing fasciitis is primarily due to *S. pyogenes*. Necrotizing fasciitis can be caused by saltwater-associated organisms like *V. vulnificus* (particularly in patients with chronic liver disease) and *E. tarda* (19). *A. hydrophila* is a freshwater-associated Gram-negative bacterium that can also cause necrotizing fasciitis.

DIAGNOSTIC TESTING

The diagnosis of impetigo, erysipelas, or cellulitis is made on clinical grounds. Complete blood count and serum chemistries are rarely useful and never diagnostic. One study demonstrated that the presence of leukocytosis greater than 15.4×10^9/L and serum sodium less than 135 mmol/L may be helpful in identifying necrotizing fasciitis from nonnecrotizing soft-tissue infections (20). In another study, both creatine kinase and C-reactive protein were shown to be significantly higher in patients with necrotizing fasciitis due to group A streptococcus than in those with cellulitis (21). Serum glucose should be measured for patients in whom diabetes is suspected or for diabetic patients with potential abnormalities in glucose control. Streptococcal hyaluronidase and antiDNase B serologic titers can serve as markers for recent group A streptococcal infection although they typically are not available and thus will not impact decision making in the emergency department. A variety of other tests are available to assist the clinician.

Blood Cultures

Blood cultures are often obtained in patients who are being hospitalized for cellulitis. Though bacteremia is uncommon in patients with cellulitis (i.e., blood cultures are positive in only 2–5% of patients), these cultures appear most useful in patients who are immunocompromised, who have underlying lymphedema, or who appear toxic (4, 12, 22–24).

Radiography

Imaging studies, including plain radiographs and CT scans, can be obtained to assess the presence of gas in the soft tissues and underlying bone infection. MRI scans provide a highly sensitive modality for identifying the presence of necrotizing infections (25–27). Imaging studies to evaluate the presence or absence of a necrotizing infection should not delay evaluation by a surgeon. Skin-infection-associated abscesses can be readily identified with the use of ultrasound (28).

Gram Stain and Culture

Gram stain and culture of involved tissue are recommended when the patient with impetigo has failed treatment or when diagnostic uncertainty exists. The crust of the lesion should be removed in a sterile fashion prior to obtaining culture material.

Direct sampling of infected skin lesions can include aspiration and punch biopsy, although these are rarely performed in the emergency department. Aspirates from the leading edge of cellulitis-associated lesions result in a bacteriologic diagnosis in less than one-third of patients (23, 29, 30). The diagnostic yield may be increased slightly by pursuing a skin tissue punch specimen (30). Prompt performance of biopsy and histopathologic evaluation of frozen-section skin biopsy specimens can establish the diagnosis of life-threatening necrotizing fasciitis and precipitate potentially life-saving surgical intervention (31, 32). Microbiologic and histopathologic examination of infected skin or soft tissue can be helpful in not only dictating the need for surgery but also for deciding upon pathogen-directed antimicrobials.

MANAGEMENT

Antibiotic Therapy[33,34]

Impetigo is treated on an outpatient basis in all but the most severe cases or when the patient has severe underlying disease. Topical mupirocin is the drug of choice in mild to moderate infections and for patients whose lesions do not involve the mouth or scalp (see Table 24–1). In patients with more extensive infection, oral dicloxacillin or cephalexin is indicated. Azithromycin is an alternative for those with a penicillin allergy. Impetigo is treated for 10 days.

Erysipelas may also be treated on an outpatient basis unless the patient is toxic appearing or also has severe underlying disease. Oral or intravenous penicillin is the drug of choice for erysipelas. The emergency physician may not be confident in distinguishing erysipelas from cellulitis based on appearance alone, in which case an antimicrobial effective against penicillinase-resistant *S. aureus,* such as dicloxacillin or cephalexin, is indicated. Azithromycin is an alternative for those with a penicillin allergy. Erysipelas is treated for 10 days.

Oral antibiotics are given to patients with cellulitis who are afebrile and without comorbidities. Empiric antibiotic therapy in the emergency department must be active against both group A streptococcus and penicillinase-resistant *S. aureus.* Ideally, the antimicrobial prescribed should be the least expensive, most effective, and the best tolerated. Appropriate oral agents include dicloxacillin or cephalexin. Azithromycin may be used for the penicillin-allergic patient (see Table 24–1.) Cellulitis is usually treated for 10–14 days. Intravenous therapy is typically reserved for patients with high fever; comorbidities (including diabetes mellitus); hypotension; extensive involvement; involvement of face, perineum, or hands; or rapid evolution of infection. Parenteral antibiotics historically recommended in the treatment of cellulitis include nafcillin and cefazolin.

The increasing incidence of MRSA infections has resulted in the increased utilization of antimicrobials such as vancomycin, quinupristin/dalfopristin, and linezolid (35). This emergence of community-acquired MRSA (CA-MRSA) skin and soft-tissue infections has cast doubt over past recommendations for treatment of these infectious-disease syndromes. (For a complete discussion of CA-MRSA, refer to Chapter 25.)

Hemodynamically unstable patients with skin and soft-tissue infections and those with known or suspected necrotizing fasciitis should be evaluated immediately for surgical debridement and possible amputation. Aggressive intravenous fluid administration must be initiated, and vasopressor agents and transfusions should be undertaken as needed to restore normal hemodynamic parameters. Empiric antibiotics must be broad in spectrum to provide adequate coverage for the possible etiologic pathogens. Empiric regimens for necrotizing fasciitis include clindamycin plus imipenem, meropenem, piperacillin/tazobactam, or ticarcillin/clavulanate. The addition of vancomycin to these regimens should be considered when there is suspicion of methicillin-resistant *S. aureus.* Sea-water exposure, particularly in the setting of liver disease, should prompt the inclusion of anti-*V. vulnificus* agents, which include antibiotics such as a tetracycline, cefatzidime, gentamicin, or a fluoroquinolone. The combination of intravenous penicillin and intravenous clindamycin is the regimen of choice for classic necrotizing fasciitis type II due to group A streptococcus. Like penicillin, clindamycin is active against group A streptococcus but has the added advantage of inhibiting streptococcal toxin production (see Table 24–1).

Adjunctive intravenous immunoglobulin (IVIG) may be beneficial in patients with type II necrotizing fasciitis and toxic shock syndrome caused by group A streptococcus. Though definitive controlled, randomized prospective data are lacking, antibodies in IVIG may neutralize the streptococcal toxins responsible for this syndrome (36, 37). Adjunctive hyperbaric oxygen may also be useful although prospective randomized, controlled data are lacking (38, 39). This modality should not delay surgical intervention and the initiation of appropriate empiric antimicrobials.

SURGICAL CONSULTATION

Prior to establishing the diagnosis of necrotizing fasciitis, the emergency physician must consider the possibility. The distinction between cellulitis and more deeply seated necrotizing infections may be exceedingly difficult, particularly in the early stages of necrotizing infection. Suspicion of a potentially deadly underlying soft-tissue

Table 24–1. Antibiotics for Skin and Soft Tissue Infections

Syndrome	Antimicrobial
Impetigo	Topical:
	Mupirocin TID (for limited disease not involving mouth/scalp)
	Oral:
	Dicloxacillin, 250 mg q 6 h
	Cephalexin, 250–500 mg q 6 h
	If Penicillin allergic:
	Erythromycin, 250 mg q 6 h
	Azithromycin, 500 mg on day 1 then 250 mg q day × 4 days
	Clindamycin, 300 mg q 6 h
Erysipelas	Oral:
	Penicillin VK, 500 mg q 6 h
	Dicloxacillin, 500 mg q 6 h
	Cephalexin, 250–500 mg q 6 h
	If penicillin allergic:
	Clindamycin, 300 mg q 6 h
	Erythromycin, 500 mg PO q 6 h
	Azithromycin, 500 mg on day 1 then 250 mg q day × 4 days
	Intravenous:
	Penicillin G, 2 million units q 4 h
	Nafcillin, 1–2 g q 4 hr
	Cefazolin, 1 g q 8 h
	If penicillin-allergic:
	Vancomycin, 1 gm q 12 h
	Clindamycin, 450–900 mg q 8 h
	Erythromycin, 500 mg −1 g 6 h
Cellulitis	*Uncomplicated (S. aureus or S. pyogenes)*
	Oral:
	Dicloxacillin, 500 mg q 6 h
	Cephalexin, 250–500 mg q 6 h
	If Penicillin allergic:
	Clindamycin, 300–450 mg q 6 h
	Azithromycin, 500 mg on day 1 then 250 mg q day × 4 days
	Linezolid, 600 mg q 12 h
	Intravenous:
	Nafcillin, 1–2 g q 4 hr
	Cefazolin, 1 g q 8 h
	If Penicillin allergic or MRSA infection:
	Vancomycin, 1 g q 12 h
	Clindamycin, 900 mg q 8 h
	Linezolid, 600 mg q 12 h
	Quinupristin/dalfopristin, 7.5 mg/kg q 12 h
	Daptomycin, 4 mg/kg q 24 h
	Complicated (also including Gram-negative bacilli, anaerobes):
	Oral:
	Amoxicillin-clavulanic acid, 500 mg q 8 h
	Clindamycin, 300–450 mg q 6 h

(continues)

Table 24–1. Antibiotics for Skin and Soft Tissue Infections (*Continued*)

Syndrome	Antimicrobial
	Levofloxacin, 500 mg q day or
	Ciprofloxacin, 750 mg q 12 h
	Intravenous:
	Imipenem, 500 mg q 6 h
	Piperacillin-tazobactam, 4.5 g q 8 h
	Ticarcillin-clavulanic acid, 3.1 g q 4–6 h
	Ceftriaxone, 2 g q 24 h plus
	Metronidazole, 500 mg q 6 h or
	Clindamycin, 900 mg q 8 h
	Plus/minus
	Vancomycin, 1 g q 12 h (based on suspicion of concomitant MRSA infection)
Necrotizing fasciitis	Intravenous:
	Imipenem, 500 mg q 6 h
	or
	Meropenem, 1 g q 8 h
	or
	Piperacillin-tazobactam, 4.5 g q 6 h
	or
	Ticarcillin-clavulanic acid, 3.1 g q 4–6 h
	Plus
	Clindmaycin 900 mg q 8 h
	Add vancomycin 1g q 12 h if suspicious of MRSA
	If penicillin allergic:
	Ciprofloxacin 400 mg q 12 h (or equivalent fluoroqinolone) plus vancomycin, 1 g q 12 h plus clindamycin, 900 mg q 8 h or metronidazole, 500 mg q 6 h
	If known to be group A streptococcus, then:
	Penicillin G, 4 million u IV q 6 h (or 24 million u over 24 h) plus
	Clindamycin, 900 mg IV q 8 h

infection must begin when a patient with "cellulitis" is experiencing extreme pain, classically "out of proportion" to the observed process. In reality, the pain is not out of proportion to a rapidly spreading infection leading to necrosis of unseen tissue. Cellulitis with associated restricted movement of the involved area due to severe pain must alert the emergency physician to the possibility of deep necrotizing infection. Frank necrosis of the skin is a late but remarkable finding. Ecchymosis or hemorrhagic bullae associated with cellulitis are indicators of underlying necrosis that require emergent surgical debridement. Subcutaneous gas, either detected as crepitus by palpation of the involved area or as seen on radiographs, is another indication of necrotizing infection and the need for immediate surgery (see Table 24–2).

Table 24–2. Indications for Emergency Surgical Consultation for Patients with Skin and Soft-Tissue Infections

Cellulitis associated with "pain out of proportion" to clinical findings
Cellulitis associated with inability to move affected areas due to pain
Cellulitis associated with crepitus
Cellulitis associated with hemorrhagic bullae
Cellulitis associated with ecchymosis
Cellulitis associated with necrotic or black tissue
Cellulitis that is rapidly expanding

Emergent surgical consultation is warranted when the possibility of a necrotizing infection is present. It is prudent to involve the surgeon prior to the results of laboratory tests or radiographs, which may not aid in the diagnosis and, worse, may delay limb- and life-saving surgery.

The diagnosis may still be uncertain even after a surgeon has been consulted. At this point, radiographic imaging studies may be utilized. The patient can be admitted to the surgical service for serial examinations of a potential rapidly spreading infection. Alternatively, a small 2-cm incision may be made in the affected skin at the bedside. Ease of passage of a probe or finger placed within the incision along the deep fascial planes is indicative of necrotizing fasciitis (40–42).

Ultimately, the diagnosis of necrotizing infection is made in the operating room by direct visualization of the involved subcutaneous tissues. Surgical consultation may be considered for skin infections overlying a joint or bursa to eliminate the possibility of an overlooked septic joint (see Chapter 28).

DISPOSITION

There is no "evidence-based medicine" regarding admission criteria for patients with skin and soft-tissue infections. The decision to admit is based upon a subjective impression of the severity of illness. Patients with hypotension, persistent tachycardia, or tachypnea require admission not only for intravenous antibiotics but also for management of possible sepsis and/or septic shock. Host factors, such as age and underlying immune status, are important in decision making regarding admission. Skin infections that are extensive, rapidly spreading, and potentially deep (as suggested by marked induration) also warrant strong consideration for admission. Additionally, when the possibility of deep, necrotizing soft-tissue infection cannot be excluded, admission for intravenous antibiotics and observation is indicated. The location of the infection is also critical; cellulitis involving vital areas, such as the face, hands, or perineum, should dictate admission. Additional considerations include patients' abilities to care for themselves, afford their prescriptions, and tolerate their medications.

CASE OUTCOME

Intravenous saline, an insulin drip, and broad-spectrum antibiotic therapy consisting of piperacillin-tazobactam and clindamycin were initiated. The patient was immediately taken to the operating room, where debridement confirmed the diagnosis of Fournier's gangrene. No muscle involvement was appreciated. Tissue cultures revealed a polymicrobial aerobic and anaerobic infection. The patient required an additional extensive debridement procedure, but the surgeries and antibiotics eventually proved curative. Ultimately, he required a skin-grafting procedure over the involved area.

REFERENCES

1. Chiller K, Selkin BA, Murakawa GJ: Skin microflora and bacterial infections of the skin. *J Invest Dermatol Symp Proc* 6:170–174, 2001.
2. Darmstadt GL, Lane AT: Impetigo: An overview. *Pediatr Dermatol* 11:293–303, 1994.
3. Sadick NS: Current aspects of bacterial infections of the skin. *Dermatol Clin* 15:341–349, 1997.
4. Bishara J, Golan-Cohen A, Robenshtok E, Leibovici L, Pitlik S: Antibiotic use in patients with erysipelas: A retrospective study. *Isr Med Assoc J* 3:722–724, 2001.
5. Dupuy A, Benchikhi H, Roujeau JC, et al.. Risk factors for erysipelas of the leg (cellulitis): Case-control study. *BMJ* 318:1591–1594, 1999.
6. Guberman D, Gilead LT, Zlotogorski A, Schamroth J: Bullous erysipelas: A retrospective study of 26 patients. *J Am Acad Dermatol* 41:733–737, 1999.
7. Dong SL, Kelly KD, Oland RC, Holroyd BR, Rowe BH: ED management of cellulitis: A review of five urban centers. *Am J Emerg Med* 19:535–540, 2001.
8. Eron LJ: Infections of skin and soft tissue: Outcomes of a classification scheme. *Clin Infect Dis* 31:287, 2000.
9. Giuliano A, Lewis F, Hadley K, et al.: Bacteriology of necrotizing fasciitis. *Am J Surg* 134:52–57, 1977.
10. Aronoff DM, Bloch KC: Assessing the relationship between the use of nonsteroidal antiinflammatory drugs and necrotizing fasciitis caused by group A streptococcus. *Medicine* 82:225–235, 2003.
11. Callahan EF, Adal KA, Tomecki KJ: Cutaneous (non-HIV) infections. *Dermatol Clin* 18:497–508, 2000.
12. Eriksson B, Jorup-Ronstrom C, Karkkonen K, Sjoblom AC, Holm SE: Erysipelas: Clinical and bacteriologic spectrum and serologic aspects. *Clin Infect Dis* 23:1091–1098, 1996.
13. Lopez FA, Sanders CV: Dermatologic infections in the immunocompromised (nonHIV) host. *Infect Dis Clin North Am* 15:1–32, 2001.
14. Slaven E, Lopez F: *Vibrio vulnificus. Infect Dis Pract Clin* 24:77–80, 2000.
15. Farley MM: Group B streptococcal disease in nonpregnant adults. *Clin Infect Dis* 33:556–561, 2001.
16. Talan DA, Citron DM, Abrahamian FM, et al.: Bacteriologic analysis of infected dog and cat bites. *N Engl J Med* 340:85–92, 1999.

17. Weinstein MR, Litt M, Kertesz DA, et al.:. Invasive infections due to a fish pathogen, *Streptococcus iniae*. *N Engl J Med* 337:589–594, 1997.

18. Aubry A, Chosidow O, Caumes E, Robert J, Cambau E: Sixty-three cases of *Mycobacterium marinum* infection: Clinical features, treatment, and antibiotic susceptibility of causative isolates. *Arch Intern Med* 162:1746–1752, 2002.

19. Slaven EM, Lopez FA, Hart SM, Sanders CV: Myonecrosis caused by *Edwardsiella tarda*: A case report and case series of extraintestinal *E. tarda* infections. *Clin Infect Dis* 32:1430–1433, 2001.

20. Wall DB, Klein SR, Black S, de Virgilio C: A simple model to help distinguish necrotizing fasciitis from nonnecrotizing soft tissue infection. *J Am Coll Surg* 191:227–231, 2000.

21. Simonart T, Simonart J-M, Derdelinckx I, et al.: Value of standard laboratory tests for the early recognition of group A β-hemolytic streptococcal necrotizing fasciitis. *Clin Infect Dis* 32:e9–e12, 2001.

22. Perl B, Gottehrer NP, Raveh D, Schlesinger Y, Rudensky B, Yinnon AM: Cost-effectiveness of blood cultures for adult patients with cellulitis. *Clin Infect Dis* 29:1483–1488, 1999.

23. Swartz MN: Cellulitis. *N Engl J Med* 350:904–912, 2004.

24. Eriksson B, Jorup-Ronstrom C, Karkkonen K, Sjoblom AC, Holm SE: Erysipelas: Clinical and bacteriologic spectrum and serological aspects. *Clin Infect Dis* 23:1091–1098, 1996.

25. Schmid MR, Kossmann T, Duewell S: Differentiation of necrotizing fasciitis and cellulitis using MR imaging. *AJR Am J Roentgenol* 170:615–620, 1998.

26. Brothers TE, Tagge DU, Stutley JE, et al.: Magnetic resonance imaging differentiates between necrotizing and non-necrotizing fasciitis of the lower extremity. *J Am Coll Surg* 187:416–421, 1998.

27. Rahmouni A, Chosidow O, Mathieu D, et al.: MR imaging in acute infectious cellulitis. *Radiology* 192:493–496, 1994.

28. Bureau NJ, Chhem RK, Cardinal E: Musculoskeletal infections: US manifestations. *Radiographics* 19:1585–1592, 1999.

29. Sachs MK: The optimum use of needle aspiration in the bacteriologic diagnosis of cellulitis in adults. *Arch Intern Med* 150:1907–1912, 1990.

30. Hook EW III, Hooton TM, Horton CA, Coyle MB, Ramsey PG, Turck M: Microbiologic evaluation of cutaneous cellulitis in adults. *Arch Intern Med* 146:295–297, 1986.

31. Stamenkovic I, Lew PD: Early recognition of potentially fatal necrotizing fasciitis: The use of frozen-section biopsy. *N Engl J Med* 310:1689–1693, 1984.

32. Majeski J, Majeski E: Necrotizing fasciitis: Improved survival with early recognition by tissue biopsy and aggressive surgical treatment. *South Med J* 90:1065–1068, 1997.

33. Eron LJ: The admission, discharge, and oral-switch decision processes in patients with skin and soft tissue infections. *Curr Treat Options Infect Dis* 5:245–250, 2003.

34. Fung HB, Chang JY, Kuczynski S: A practical guide to the treatment of complicated skin and soft tissue infections. *Drugs* 63:1459–1480, 2003.

35. Eron LJ, Lipsky BA, Low DE, Nathwani D, Tice AD, Volturo GA: Managing skin and soft tisuue infections: Expert panel recommendations on key decision points. *J Antimicrob Chemother* 52(Suppl. S1):i3–i17, 2003.

36. Perez CM, Kubak PM, Cryer HG, et al. : Adjunctive treatment of streptococcal shock syndrome using intravenous immunoglobulin: Case report and review. *Am J Med* 102:111–113, 1997.

37. Kaul R, McGeer A, Norrby-Teglund A, et al. (The Canadian Streptococcal Study Group): Intravenous immunoglobulin therapy for streptococcal toxic shock syndrome: A comparative observational study. *Clin Infect Dis* 28:800–807, 1999.

38. Riseman JA, Zamboni WA, Curtis A, et al.: Hyperbaric oxygen therapy for necrotizing fasciitis reduces mortality and the need for debridements. *Surgery* 108:847–850, 1990.

39. Monestersky JH, Myers RA: Hyperbaric oxygen treatment of necrotizing fasciitis. *Am J Surg* 169:187–188, 1995.

40. Wilson B: Necrotizing fasciitis. *Am J Surg* 18:416–431, 1970.

41. Andreasen TJ, Green SD, Childers BJ: Massive infectious soft tissue injury: Diagnosis and management of necrotizing fasciitis and purpura fulminans. *Plast Reconstr Surg* 107:1025–1035, 2001.

42. Childers BJ, Potyondy LD, Nachreiner R, et al.: Necrotizing fasciitis: A fourteen-year retrospective study of 163 consecutive patients. *Am Surg* 68:109–116, 2002.

25

Pyogenic Skin and Soft Tissue Infections

Ellen M. Slaven
Fred A. Lopez

1. Uncomplicated subcutaneous abscesses in otherwise healthy hosts do not require culture or antibiotic therapy following incision and drainage.

2. Fluctuance may not be noted on physical examination of a subcutaneous abscess. Aspiration should be performed to identify pus within the lesion and dictate the need for incision and drainage.

3. A single incision the length of the abscess cavity, and not simply a stab-like incision, should be made during incision and drainage to allow for proper drainage.

4. Perianal abscesses must be distinguished from deeper perirectal abscesses because perianal abscess should be incised and drained in the emergency department while deeper perirectal abscesses should be drained in the operating room.

CASE PRESENTATION

A 27-year-old man presents with a painful swelling on his left thigh. He claims to have been bitten by an insect several days earlier. He reports no drainage from the site. He denies having fever. He has no significant past medical history. He takes no medications and has no medication allergies.

He is moderately obese but does not appear acutely ill. His blood pressure is 145/90, his pulse 88, his respiratory rate is 16, and his temperature is 99.0°F. Further physical examination reveals a 6 cm × 8 cm indurated and tender soft tissue swelling on his posterior left thigh. There is no fluctuance. The overlying skin is intact, warm, mildly erythematous, and without evidence of a recent insect bite. There are no signs of drainage, lymphangitis, or localized lymphadenopathy.

INTRODUCTION/EPIDEMIOLOGY

Localized pyogenic skin and soft tissue infections make up a spectrum of diseases that may be as simple and uncomplicated as folliculitis or as painful and dangerous as an extensive perirectal abscess. In between these extremes are several discrete skin and soft tissue conditions, including furuncles, carbuncles, and subcutaneous abscesses, that are commonly encountered in the emergency department. One report noted that approximately 2% of all adult patients visiting the emergency department did so for evaluation of cutaneous abscesses (1). Pyogenic skin infections can occur in any area of the body, but have a predilection for skin containing hair and glandular tissue such as face, neck, axilla, and buttock. In the vast majority of patients the microbiology of cutaneous abscess is not important due to the impressive resolution attained after incision and drainage alone.

PATHOPHYSIOLOGY/MICROBIOLOGY

Folliculitis describes a small pustular infection of the hair follicle that is usually caused by *Staphylococcus aureus*. The pustules are typically erythematous, pruritic, and range in size from 2 to 5 mm in diameter.

Furunculosis is a form of folliculitis albeit with a greater degree of inflammation due to the extension of the infection spreading outward from the hair follicle to include the surrounding dermis. A furuncle is often referred to as a deep-seated subcutaneous nodule or boil. Furuncles are located on hairy skin with a predilection for the face, neck, axillae, and buttock. A carbuncle is a collection of contiguous furuncles which have enlarged to produce a deep subcutaneous mass of inflammation. Pus may drain freely from a number of follicular orifices. Carbuncles are commonly found on the nape of the neck where the infection extends laterally in the subcutaneous tissue due to overlying thick skin. Patients with carbuncles tend to exhibit signs and symptoms of systemic illness, such as fever and malaise.

A subcutaneous abscess is a painful localized collection of purulent materials that can occur anywhere on the body. These abscesses are typically spherical and contain semiliquid whitish-yellow material composed of dead and dying neutrophils, fibrin, necrotic tissue, and bacteria. The surrounding tissue is indurated and of variable thickness. Often peripheral to the induration is a rim of hyperemic tissue that is warm and tender. The microbiology consists of bacteria that normally colonize the affected

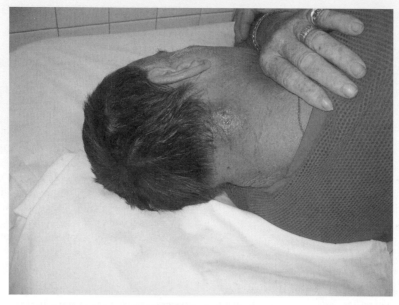

Fig. 25–1. Carbuncle.

host. *S. aureus* is the most common single pathogen iso-lated from subcutaneous abscesses (2). Most abscesses, however, yield a mixed culture of bacteria, including *S. aureus*, *Streptococcus* species, gram-negative bacilli, and anaerobes. Anaerobes, such as *Bacteroides fragilis*, tend to be isolated more frequently from abscesses in the perineal area. Minor abrasions or other trauma may allow for the entry of bacteria into the skin where an abscess may form. Obstruction of skin-associated apocrine and sebaceous glands can predispose to the development ab-scesses. Occasionally, abscesses develop following inoc-ulation of unusual bacteria such as *Pseudomonas aerug-inosa* in plantar puncture wounds and *Pasturella* species in mammalian bite wounds. Abscesses may also form fol-lowing the systemic spread of bacteria or they may arise spontaneously.

Patients who inject illicit drugs are certainly at risk for infectious complications, including infective endocardi-tis, but skin and soft tissue infections are the most com-mon reason for hospital admission in this patient pop-ulation (3). One report described greater than one-third insert of injection drug users with soft tissue infections had abscesses located deep in the soft tissue, muscle, or fascia that were not obvious at initial presentation (4). Ul-trasound, computer tomography, or magnetic resonance imaging can be useful in making the diagnosis. In the ma-

jority of cases these abscesses are found to be polymicro-bial in origin with a mixture of both anaerobic and aerobic bacteria, although *S. aureus* is the most common pathogen isolated by culture (5). Patients with a history of injection drug use should also be carefully evaluated for evidence of infective endocarditis and/or underlying HIV infection.

An abscess on the buttock may be a simple and uncom-plicated subcutaneous abscess or it may reflect an under-lying perirectal abscess that has tracked to the subcuta-neous tissue. A thorough understanding of the perineal anatomy is important to be able to recognize these po-tentially dangerous and often occult abscesses. Perirectal abscesses are thought to develop from the anal crypts. Any abscess that tracks deep to the perineum or ish-iorectal space requires drainage in the operating room so that adequate exposure can be ensured while pro-viding definitive drainage and delivering adequate anal-gesia. Patients with these extensive abscesses are often febrile and appear clinically ill. The physician may ap-preciate a tender mass in the intersphincteric space on digital rectal exam. Perirectal abscesses must be recog-nized and managed appropriately because these serious infections are associated with a mortality rate greater than 6% (6). The pathogens identified in perirectal abscesses are frequently a combination of aerobic and anaerobic bacteria, including a preponderance of anaerobes, such

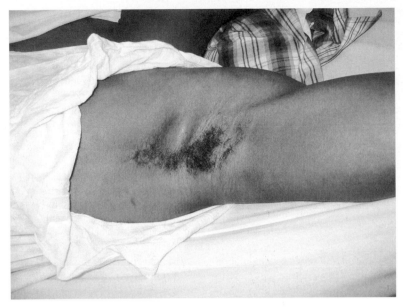

Fig. 25–2. Subcutaneous abscess.

as *B. fragilis* and *Peptococcus* species (1, 6). Abscesses located in the genital area, particularly in men, must also be evaluated for the possibility of a deeper spreading infection such as Fournier gangrene. Fournier gangrene is a life-threatening necrotizing soft tissue infection in the perineum and genital region. Early presentation of these infections may appear innocuous and patients may not appear toxic. A surgeon should be consulted when suspected.

CLINICAL PRESENTATION

Folliculitis classically presents with small tender pustules at the base of the hair. The surrounding skin may be erythematous and warm. Furuncles appear as larger deep seated nodules or pustules which are tender and may be spontaneously draining. Patients with carbuncles present with an enlarged and painful subcutaneous swelling, generally at the base of the neck, with overlying orifices that often are draining pus (see Fig. 25–1). These patients are usually systemically ill and have fever.

A painful and swollen subcutaneous mass is generally the presenting symptom of a subcutaneous abscess (see Fig. 25–2). Patients frequently attempt to treat themselves by pinching or squeezing the site and may present with incomplete drainage of the abscess. Fever is unusual and,

if present, suggests illness beyond a localized subcutaneous abscess. Abscesses may be complicated by cellulitis and the cellulitis may even mask the presence of an abscess. Clues to occult abscesses include marked swelling, painful range of motion of the affected extremity, and poor response to antibiotic therapy.

Perianal abscesses produce tender swollen areas around the anal region. Deeper perirectal abscesses may present similarly yet they extend deeper into the perineum. Patients with perirectal abscesses may also present with complaints of pain while sitting or with defecation. Systemic signs of infection such as fever and tachycardia may occur with perirectal abscesses.

LABORATORY/DIAGNOSTIC TESTING

Pyogenic skin infections are usually diagnosed by their clinical appearance: folliculitis—small pustules, 2–5 mm, at the base of the hair; furuncles—tender nodules associated with hair follicles that are larger in size than folliculitis; carbuncles—indurated and tender skin with multiple orifices draining purulent material; and subcutaneous abscess—tender and fluctuant soft tissue mass. With subcutaneous abscesses there may be erythema of the overlying skin and a surrounding area of induration. Frequently

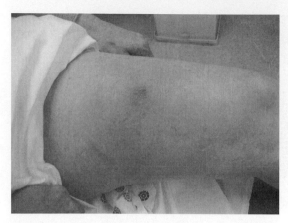

Fig. 25–3. Subcutaneous abscess with surrounding cellulitis.

Table 25–1. Management of Folliculitis, Furuncles, and Carbuncles

Folliculitis
Warm moist compresses
Topical antibiotic ointment
Mupirocin, apply TID
If associated with cellulitis add an antibiotic
Cephalexin, 500 mg po QID × 7–10 days
Dicloxacillin, 500 mg po QID × 7–10 days
Azithromycin, 500 mg po × 1 then 250 mg po q day × 4
Clindamycin, 300 mg po QID × 7–10 days
Furuncles
Incision and drainage in ED
If associated with cellulitis add an antibiotic:
Cephalexin, 500 mg po QID × 7–10 days
Dicloxacillin, 500 mg po QID × 7–10 days
Azithromycin, 500 mg po × 1 then 250 mg po q day × 4
Clindamycin, 300 mg po QID × 7–10 days
Carbuncles
Incision and drainage in operating room
Parenteral antibiotic:
Cefazolin, 1 g iv q 6–8 h
Oxacillin/nafcillin, 1–2 g iv q 4 h
Azithromycin, 500 mg iv q day
Clindamycin 600 mg iv q 8 h

the abscesses are not fluctuant and only tense induration can be palpated. Aspiration with a needle may help to identify the abscess cavity by confirming the presence of pus and the need for complete incision and drainage.

Routine laboratory testing is generally not indicated. Blood glucose measurements may be useful in known or suspected diabetic patients.

Microbiological testing, such as Gram stain and culture of aspirated purulent material from an abscess, may be useful in patients who are immunocompromised, acutely ill, or who have complicated abscesses, such as those associated with cellulitis (see Fig. 25–3). These patients will require empiric antibiotic therapy, in addition to incision and drainage, and knowledge of offending bacteria and their antimicrobial susceptibilities may alter the initial selection of antibiotics.

Aspiration of purulent material from the abscess cavity prior to incision and drainage is the best method to obtain material for culture in order to prevent possible contamination with bacteria from the overlying skin.

Radiographs are of limited utility in the diagnosis and management of subcutaneous abscesses. If there is suspicion of a foreign body (e.g., tooth or needle) or gas in the soft tissue then radiographs should be obtained. If there is suspicion of an abscess deep in the subcutaneous space, or even muscle, ultrasound, computed tomography (CT), or magnetic resonance imaging (MRI) may be utilized.

MANAGEMENT

Folliciulits. It is generally treated with moist warm compresses and topical antibiotic ointment such as mupirocin (7, 8). Oral first-generation cephalosporins, such as

cephalexin, or oral antistaphylococcal penicillins, such as dicloxacillin, are first line agents if systemic therapy is desired. Azithromycin or clindamycin are alternatives for penicillin-allergic patients (see Table 25–1).

Furuncles. These are collections of pus and require incision and drainage (see section Procedure: incision and drainage). Local wound care is all that is required if the furuncle is spontaneously draining. Antibiotics are reserved for signs of systemic illness such as fever or associated cellulitis (see Table 25–1).

Carbuncles. They almost always require surgical drainage. Because carbuncles can become quite large, simple incision in the emergency department is usually not adequate. Antibiotic therapy is indicated for carbuncles due to the greater extent of infection (see Table 25–1).

If a soft tissue swelling is not fluctuant and/or no pus is found by needle aspiration, there is no benefit of incision and drainage. The patient should be instructed to apply warm moist heat and return in 24–48 h to reassess the need for incision and drainage. There is no clinical data

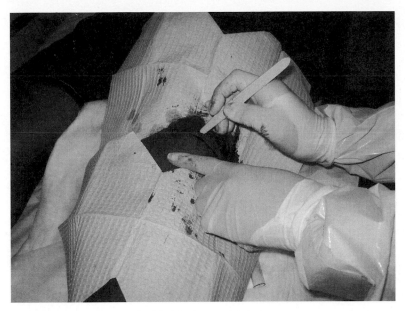

Fig. 25–4. Incision and drainage.

Subcutaneous Abscesses

There is no indication for antibiotic therapy in the healthy host with a cutaneous abscess who is not systemically ill. Treatment consists entirely of surgical incision and drainage (9, 2).

Procedure: incision and drainage

Consider the use of narcotics such as intravenous morphine or oral hydrocodone for analgesia (and possibly benzodiazepines if patients are particularly anxious) in patients with all but the smallest abscesses.

The incision and drainage of an abscess is not a sterile procedure. Though there is no data to support the utility of iodine surgical scrub and the use of sterile drapes, many physicians, including the authors, choose to do so (see Fig. 25–4).

Infiltrating local anesthesia, such as 1% lidocaine, may be difficult due to the thinning of the skin overlying an abscess. Careful attention must be paid to the total dose of lidocaine injected into a large abscess due to the highly vascular nature of abscesses and the potential for lidocaine toxicity (i.e., maximum dose is 3–5 mg/kg for lidocaine

and 5–7 mg/kg for lidocaine with epinephrine). A small gauge (i.e., 25-gauge) needle should be used to inject the dome of the abscess. A single linear incision should be made with an 11-blade scalpel to continue along the entire length of the abscess cavity. Skin incisions should be made in the direction of natural skin lines to minimize scarring. Cruciate incisions and elliptical excisions are to be avoided to prevent unnecessary scarring. A small stab-like incision should also be avoided because it may inhibit adequate drainage and prevent thorough disruption of loculations within the abscess.

It is important to disrupt loculations within the abscess cavity with a blunt probe or closed hemostats. Beware of probing abscesses with a gloved finger due to unanticipated potentially sharp foreign bodies that may be retained in the abscess, including broken needles (10).

There is no evidence to support irrigation of the abscess cavity with saline, or any other irrigants, although some authors recommend it to aid in the removal of necrotic tissue and pus (2).

Loose packing is then placed within the abscess cavity to prevent premature closure of the wound edges and to aid in drainage. While iodoform gauze is frequently used, there is no data to suggest that it provides any benefit over plain gauze strips (see Fig. 25–5).

Most small and uncomplicated abscesses can be drained in the emergency department. Some abscesses

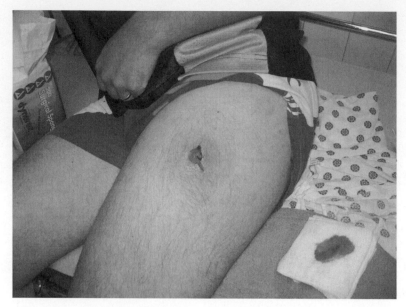

Fig. 25–5. Packing following incision and drainage.

are better managed in the operating room where the surgeon can provide for adequate anesthesia and allow for more extensive exposure. These may include large abscesses, those located near neurovascular structures (such as the anticubital fossa, neck, groin, axilla, and popliteal fossa), potentially deep abscesses (such as those involving the deep perirectal areas), and abscesses where there is suspicion for associated necrotizing infection. Necrotizing infections should be suspected when the patient is experiencing severe pain that restricts movement of the involved extremity, where ecchymotic or necrotic skin is observed, and in the presence of hemorrhagic bulla. Abscesses located on the breast and hand may complicate incision and drainage due to delicate underlying structures and all but the most superficial should be drained in the operating room (see Table 25–2).

INDICATIONS FOR ABSCESS CULTURE AND INITIATION OF ANTIBIOTIC THERAPY

Antibiotic therapy, in addition to surgical incision and drainage, has not been demonstrated to improve outcomes of subcutaneous abscesses in randomized double-blind placebo controlled clinical trials in healthy adults (9, 11). Although no evidence supports the practice, most authorities agree it is prudent to administer antibiotics, in addition to incision and drainage, to patients with subcutaneous abscesses who also have underlying immune suppression. These patients include those with advanced HIV infection, diabetes, liver disease, those taking chronic steroids or chemotherapy, and transplant patients (see Table 25–3).

Antibiotics should also be provided to patients who are systemically ill with fever, cellulitis, lymphangitis,

Table 25–2. Pyogenic Skin Infections Requiring Surgical Consultation

Carbuncles
Perirectal abscesses (other than perianal abscesses)
Large and extensive abscesses
Abscesses overlying neurovascular structures
Suspicion of necrotizing infection
Breast or hand involvement

Table 25–3. Immune Suppressing Conditions Warranting Antibiotics for Patients with Subcutaneous Abscesses

Advanced HIV infection
Diabetics
Patients on chronic steroids
Chemotherapy patients
Patients with liver disease/alcoholics
Transplant patients

Table 25–4. Indications for Antibiotics for Patients with Subcutaneous Abscesses

Immunocompromised host
Concomitant cellulitis, lymphangitis, fever, or sepsis
Abscesses located on the central face

Table 25–5. Antibiotics: Outpatient Treatment of Cutaneous Abscesses

Healthy host with signs of mild systemic illness[a]
Host with immune compromise but no signs of systemic
   illness
 Abscess on extremities, head, trunk, not perineal
  Cephalexin, 500 mg po QID × 7–10 days
  Dicloxacillin, 500 mg po QID × 7–10 days
  Azithromycin, 500 mg po first day then 250 mg po
   q day × 4 days
  Clindamycin, 300 mg po QID × 7–10 days
 Perirectal abscess
  Amoxicillin/clavulanate, 500/125 po TID × 7–10
   days
  Trimethoprim/sulfamethoxazole, DS 1 tab po BID
   × 7–10 days
   and
  Metronidazole 500 mg po QID × 7–10 days
  Ciprofloxacin 500 mg po BID × 7–10 days
   and
  Metronidazole 500 mg po QID × 7–10 days

[a]Fever, cellulitis, or lymphangitis.

or hypotension. Many abscesses manifest changes in the overlying skin consistent with cellulitis, that is, erythema, warmth, and tenderness. Some authors suggest that patients with subcutaneous abscesses associated with a "large area of cellulitis" or a "significant amount of cellulitis" should receive antibiotic therapy although these terms are not well-defined (12, 13). Additionally, some authorities recommend antibiotic therapy for abscesses located in the midface due to theoretical concerns of venous cavernous sinus thrombosis (2) (see Table 25–4 for indications for antibiotic therapy).

Culture of the abscess should be obtained when an antibiotic regimen is initiated. Knowledge of the bacteria and local antibiotic susceptibilities may aid in adjusting the initial antibiotic selection.

No studies have assessed the timing of administration of antibiotics. It appears logical to give antibiotics prior to, and within 1 h, of the incision and drainage (2, 13). One report in 1985 reviewed 10 patients with blood cultures obtained before and 1, 5, and 20 minutes after incision and drainage (14). None of the cultures preceding incision and drainage were positive, but 11 out of 30 drawn after the procedure were positive. A more recent study examined 50 patients with separate aseptic venipuncture-obtained blood cultures prior to incision and drainage and at 2 and 10 minutes following the procedure (15). Interestingly, no blood cultures were positive. However, none of the patients in this study were febrile.

Recommendations for the selection of empiric antibiotics are based on likely pathogens. Following incision and drainage, a patient with an uncomplicated abscess on the trunk or extremities can be treated as an outpatient with an antibiotic that provides coverage for grampositive bacteria (*S. aureus* and *Streptococcus* sp.). Examples include cephalexin or dicloxacillin. Alternatives include azithromycin or clindamycin for the penicillin-allergic patient (see Table 25–5). In contrast, outpatient antibiotic therapy for patients with uncomplicated abscesses located in the perineum or in injection drug users should include antibiotics that are active against *S. aureus*, *Streptococcus* sp., gram-negative bacilli, and anaerobes. Examples include ampicillin/sulbactam, a combination of trimethoprim/sulfamethoxazole and metronidazole, or

a combination of ciprofloxacin and metronidazole (see Table 25–5). Patients who are acutely ill and those with deep perirectal abscesses should be treated with a parenteral antibiotic regimen that is active against anaerobic organisms and gram-negative bacilli, in addition to *S. aureus* and *Streptococcus* sp. Examples include ampicillin/sulbactam, ticarcillin/clavulanate, and piperacillin/tazobactam (see Table 25–6). Alternatives include second-generation cephalosporins with anaerobic activity such as cefoxitin or cefotetan. For patients allergic to penicillin, ciprofloxacin with metronidazole is appropriate. When there is a suspicion of methicillin-resistant *S. aureus* (MRSA), vancomycin should be added. For life threatening infections imipenem or meropenem with vancomycin is recommended (16).

The duration of antibiotic therapy depends upon the patient's clinical course. Recommendations range from 3 to 14 days, though in most cases 7–10 days are sufficient.

SPECIAL CIRCUMSTANCES
Methicillin-Resistant S. aureus

Patients with skin and soft tissue infections caused by community-associated methicillin-resistant *S. aureus* CA-MRSA are increasingly reported in the medical

Table 25–6. Antibiotics: Inpatient Treatment of Subcutaneous Abscesses

---

Abscess located on face, extremities or trunk—not perineal—not septic
    Nafcillin, 1–2 g iv q 4–6 h
    Oxacillin, 1–2 g iv q 4–6 h
    Cefazolin, 1 g iv q 6–8 h
    Azithromycin, 500 mg iv q day
    Clindamycin, 600 mg iv q 8 h
Abscesses located on the perineum or patient septic
    Beta-lactam/beta-lactamase inhibitors
        Ampicillin/sulbactam, 1.5 g iv q 6 h
        Ticarcillin/clavulanate, 3.1 g iv q 4–6 h
        Piperacillin/tazobactam, 3.375 g iv q 4–6 h
    Second-generation cephalosporins
        Cefotetan, 1–2 g iv q 12 h
        Cefoxitin, 1 g iv q 8 h
    Carbapenems
        Imipenem + cilastin, 0.5 g iv q 6 h
        Meropenem, 0.5–1 g iv q 8 h

---

literature and the lay press. Many such patients were previously healthy without any traditional risk factors for MRSA infection, such as recent hospitalization, dialysis, injection drug use, immunocompromise, prior antibiotic administration, and residence in long-term care facilities (17,19). Outbreaks of CA-MRSA skin and soft tissue infections have been reported in prisons, in children in day care centers, and in athletes, including professional football players (20–24). No systematic population based surveillance of CA-MRSA exists so the true prevalence remains unknown. Based on the experience of penicillin-resistant strains of *S. aureus* that first spread within hospitalized patients and then moved into the community, one expert speculates that the prevalence of CA-MRSA may be as high as 25% within the next 5–10 years (25).

CA-MRSA differs from hospital-acquired MRSA (HA-MRSA) in more ways than the locale of acquisition. They are differentiated by antimicrobial susceptibilities, the types of infections they cause, their genetics, and perhaps their virulence. CA-MRSA strains are resistant to methicillin and other β-lactams, but generally are susceptible to a broader array of antibiotics than are HA-MRSA strains. Many of the CA-MRSA strains remain susceptible to trimethoprim/sulfamethoxazole, clindamycin, aminoglycosides, and tetracycline. One report found skin and soft tissue infections were more common among CA-MRSA than among HA-MRSA infections (75% vs. 37%, respectively) (26). It is the *mec*A gene (that encodes a

penicillin binding protein with a low affinity for beta-lactam antibiotics) in staphylococci that confers resistance to beta-lactams. In CA-MRSA isolates the *mec*A gene is carried within a genetic element known as the staphylococcal cassette chromosome *mec* (SCC*mec*) type IV whereas HA-MRSA predominantly contain SCC*mec* types I, II, and III. CA-MRSA strains may also be more virulent than HA-MRSA strains. In 1998 four pediatric fatalities were attributed to fulminant infection with CA-MRSA (27). Another report found 31 out of 32 CA-MRSA strains isolated in the United States produced enterotoxin B and C, toxins which are associated with non-menstrual toxic shock syndrome (28). And a report from France describes strains of CA-MRSA that carry the gene for Panton-Valentine leukocidin caused more severe and rapidly progressive pneumonia than strains that did not carry the gene (29). The Panton-Valentine leukocin gene is rarely found in HA-MRSA or methicillin-susceptible community-associated isolates (30).

There are no clinical data that support abandoning beta-lactam antibiotics, such as cephalexin or oxacillin, that have traditionally been the first choice for empiric therapy of skin and soft tissue infections. Although the incidence of CA-MRSA is apparently on the rise many experts agree that β-lactam antibiotics remain the drug of choice for empiric therapy (31–33). In the setting where CA-MRSA is likely (e.g., in areas of high prevalence or in patients with prior CA-MRSA infection or colonization), it seems reasonable to select an antibiotic that is not a beta-lactam, such as trimethoprim/sulfamethoxazole. It is important to note, however, that a common cause of cellulitis is group A streptococcus, an organism that is not adequately sensitive to trimethoprim/sulfamethoxazole. This dilemma has led some clinicians to prescribe both cephalexin and trimethoprim/sulfamethoxazole, or more expensive agents such as linezolid, for empiric therapy of skin and soft tissue infections.

Once MRSA is isolated from a clinical specimen the selection of antibiotics is dictated by the pathogen's antibiotic susceptibility pattern. Typically, CA-MRSA strains are sensitive to clindamycin, trimethoprim/sulfamethoxazole, rifampin, and tetracycline. Fluoro-quinolones, such as ciprofloxacin and levofloxacin, and macrolides, such as erythromycin or azithromycin, are not recommended for CA-MRSA skin and soft tissue infections due to the high rates of resistance to these antibiotics (see Tables 25–7 and 25–8). Two new agents have recently been approved for use in proven drug resistant gram-positive cocci infections (including MRSA): quinupristin-dalfopristin and linezolid. Quinupristin-dalfopristin is available for intravenous use only and requires infusion

Table 25–7. Oral Antimicrobial Agents for Mild Community-Associated MRSA Skin Infections

Clindamycin, 150–450 mg po QID
Trimethoprim/sulfamethoxazole (double strength), 1 tab po BID
Doxycycline 100 mg po BID

through a large bore central venous line due to the high incidence of thrombophlebitis. Linezolid is available in oral and intravenous forms. Side effects of linezolid include diarrhea and thrombocytopenia. Both of these newer agents are expensive and are not routinely recommended for empiric therapy. Vancomycin is the drug of choice for serious MRSA infections. These alternative antibiotics should be reserved for patients who cannot tolerate vancomycin.

Empiric treatment of moderate to severe subcutaneous abscesses requiring hospitalization and intravenous antibiotics should include a broad spectrum agent, or agents, in addition to vancomycin.

The Food and Drug Administration (FDA) recently approved a new intravenous antibiotic, daptomycin, for the treatment of complicated skin and soft tissue infections. Daptomycin is the first of a new class of antibiotics called cyclic lipopeptides that target gram-positive bacteria. Early reports describe the safety and efficacy of daptomycin in skin and soft tissue infections (34).

There are no reports on the efficacy of decolonization procedures for CA-MRSA in the outpatient setting; they are not routinely recommended. For patients with recurrent CA-MRSA skin abscesses, some suggested decolonization regimens include: (1) systemic therapy with rifampin and trimethoprim/sulfamethoxazole or rifampin and doxycycline, (2) topical intranasal mupirocin ointment, and (3) chlorhexidine body wash (see Table 25–9). Consultation with an infectious disease specialist is recommended prior to initiation of therapy to eradicate CA-MRSA colonization.

Table 25–8. Intravenous Antimicrobial Agents for Moderate to Severe Community-Associated MRSA Skin Infections

Vancomycin, 1 g iv q 12 h
Alternatives
    Clindamycin, 600–900 mg iv q 8 h
    Quinupristin-dalfopristin, 7.5 mg/kg iv q 8–12 h
    Linezolid, 400–600 mg iv q 12 h
    Trimethoprim/sulfamethoxazole, 15–20 mg/kg (based on TMP) iv q 6–8 h
    Daptomycin, 4 mg/kg iv q 24 h

Table 25–9. Possible Regimens to Eradicate Community-Associated MRSA Colonization

1. Systemic therapy
    Rifampin
    Adult dose: 300 mg po BID × 5 days
    Pediatric dose: 10–20 mg/kg/day in two divided
        doses—not to exceed 600 mg/day × 5 days
        AND
    Trimethoprim/sulfamethoxazole
    Adult dose: 1 tablet (160 mg TMP/800 mg SMX)
        double strength po BID × 5 days
    Pediatric dose: 8 mg/kg TMP/40 mg SMX po divided
        BID × 5 days
    OR
    Rifampin × 5 days
        AND
    Doxycyline
        100 mg po BID × 5 days
        (not recommended for use in pediatric patients)
2. Topical intranasal mupirocin ointment BID × 5 days
    with or without systemic therapy
3. Chlorhexadine body wash daily × 5 days
    with or without systemic therapy

Endocarditis Prophylaxis

The American Heart Association has published recommendations for the prevention of bacterial endocarditis in patients with cardiac disease (35). Those at risk include patients with prosthetic cardiac valves, prior history of endocarditis, congenital heart disease, surgically constructed shunts or conduits, hypertrophic cardiomyopathy, acquired valvular disease (e.g., rheumatic heart disease), and mitral valve prolapse with regurgitation (see Table 25–10). These patients should receive a single dose of antibiotics 1 h prior to incision and drainage of an abscess. An oral antistaphylococcal penicillin (dicloxacillin), first-generation cephalosporin (cephalexin),

Table 25–10. Indications for Infective Endocarditis Prophylaxis

Prosthetic cardiac valves
History of previous endocarditis
Congenital heart disease
Surgically constructed shunts or conduits
Hypertrophic cardiomyopathy
Acquired valvular disease (e.g., rheumatic heart disease)
Mitral valve prolapse with regurgitation

Table 25–11. Antibiotic Regimens for Infective
Endocarditis Prophylaxis[a]

Dicloxacillin, 2 g po × one
Cephalexin, 2 g po × one
Clindamycin, 600 mg po × one
If unable to tolerate oral medications or if MRSA is
    involved
Vancomycin, 1 g iv × one

[a] All antibiotics should be administered 1 h prior to incision and
drainage.

or clindamycin for penicillin allergic patients is recommended (see Table 25–11). For patients who cannot take oral medications, or those in whom methicillin-resistant *S. aureus* are suspected, intravenous vancomycin may be given.

DISPOSITION

The vast majority of patients with pyogenic skin infections may be treated as outpatients. Admission should be considered for patients with large and extensive abscesses, concomitant cellulitis, involvement of deep perirectal spaces, immunocompromised states, and signs of systemic illness.

All patients who have undergone surgical incision and drainage must be reevaluated within 24–72 h. Most authors suggest 48 h as an appropriate interval for reassessment. Some recommend reexamination within 24 h for central facial abscesses due to concerns of potential complications such as cavernous sinus thrombosis. Packing material should be removed and the wound reexamined since further incision and drainage may be required. Large abscesses and perirectal abscesses should be referred for surgical follow-up within 3–5 days.

If the patient was treated with antibiotics and cultures were obtained at the time of the incision and drainage, the results of those cultures should direct further antibiotic therapy accordingly.

CASE OUTCOME

The patient was administered hydrocodone/acetaminophen 10/650. Lidocaine 1% was infiltrated over the suspected abscess. An 18-gauge needle was used to aspirate purulent material. A 4-cm incision was made along the entire length of the abscess cavity. The cavity was probed with a blunt surgical probe disrupting loculations

and enhancing drainage of pus. The abscess was then loosely packed with gauze and a bandage placed. He was sent home with his wife with a prescription for hydrocodone/acetaminophen and told to return for reexamination in 48 h.

The patient was seen in a surgical clinic 2 days later at which time the packing was removed and the abscess was reexamined. There were no signs of cellulitis and the abscess cavity was healing well without evidence of purulent drainage. The patient reported subjective improvement and no fever.

REFERENCES

 1. Meislin HW, Lerner SA, Graves MH, et al.: Cutaneous abscesses: Anaerobic and aerobic bacteriology and outpatient management. *Ann Intern Med* 87:145–149, 1977.
 2. Meislin HW, McGehee MD, Rosen P: Management and microbiology of cutaneous abscesses. *JACEP* 7:186–191, 1978.
 3. Orangio GR, Pitlick SD, Della Latta, et al.: Soft tissue infection in parenteral drug abusers. *Ann Surg* 199:97–100, 1984.
 4. Henriksen BM, Alberktsen SB, Simper LB, et al.: Soft tissue infections from drug abuse, a clinical and microbiological review of 145 cases. *Acta Orthop Scand* 65:625–628, 1994.
 5. Summanen PH, Talan DA, Strong C, et al.: Bacteriology of skin and soft-tissue infections: Comparison of infections in intravenous drug users and individuals with no history of intravenous drug use. *Clin Infect Dis* 20(Suppl. 2):S279–S282, 1995.
 6. Beavens DW, Westbrook KC, Thompson BW, et al.: Perirectal abscess: A potentially fatal illness. *Am J Surg* 126:765–768, 1973.
 7. Rhody C: Bacterial infections of the skin. *Prim Care* 27:459–473, 2000.
 8. Feingold DS: Staphylococcal and streptococcal pyodermas. *Semin Dermatol* 12:331–335, 1993.
 9. Llera JL, Levy RC: Treatment of cutaneous abscess: A double-blind clinical study. *Ann Intern Med* 14:15–19, 1985.
10. Blumstein H, Roberts JR: Retained needle fragments and digital dissection. *N Engl J Med* 19:1426, 1993.
11. Macfie J, Harvey J: The treatment of acute superficial abscesses: A prospective clinical trial. *Br J Surg* 64:264–266, 1977.
12. Powers RD, Meislin HW, Talan DA: Diagnosis and management of skin and soft tissue infections. *Emerg Med Rep* 11:229–236, 1990.
13. Blumstein H: Incision and drainage, in Roberts JR, Hedges JR (eds.): *Clinical Procedures in Emergency Medicine.* Philadelphia: W. B. Saunders, 1998; pp 634–659.
14. Fine BE: Incision and drainage of soft-tissue abscesses and bacteremia. *Ann Intern Med* 102:645, 1985.

15. Bobrow BJ, Pollack CV, Gamble S, et al.: Incision and drainage of cutaneous abscess is not associated with bacteremia in afebrile adults. *Ann Emerg Med* 29:404-408, 1997.

16. Gilbert DN, Moellering RC Jr., Sande MA: *The Sanford Guide to Antimicrobial Therapy, 33rd ed.* Hyde Park, VT, Antimicrobial Therapy Inc.

17. Gorak EJ, Yamada SM, Brown JD: Community-acquired methicillin-resistant *Staphylococcus aureus* in hospitalized adults and children without known risk factors. *Clin Infect Dis* 29:797–800, 1999.

18. Gosbel IB, Mercer JL, Neville SA, et al.: Non-multiresistant and multi-resistant methicillin-resistant *Staphylococcus aureus* in community-acquired infections. *MJA* 174:627–630, 2001.

19. Frank AL, Marcinak JF, Mangat PD, et al.: Community-acquired and clindamycin-susceptible methicillin-resistant *Staphylococcus aureus* in children. *Peditr Infect Dis J* 18:993–1000, 1999.

20. MMWR: Methicillin-resistant *Staphylococcus aureus* skin or soft tissue infections in a state prison—Mississippi, 2000. *Morb Mortal Wkly Rep* 42:919–922, 2001.

21. Shahin R, Johnson I, Jamieson F, et al.: Methicillin-resistant *Staphylococcus aureus* carriage in a children day care center following a case of disease. *Arch Pediatr Adolesc Med* 153:864–868, 1999.

22. MMWR: Methicillin-resistant *Staphylococcus aureus* infections among competitive sports participants—Colorado, Indiana, Pennsylvania, and Los Angeles County, 2000–2003. *Morb Mortal Wkly Rep* 52:793–795, 2003.

23. Fang YH, Hsueh PR, Hu JJ, et al.: Community-acquired methicillin-resistant *Staphylococcus aureus* in children in northern Taiwan. *J Microbiol Immunol Infect* 37:29–34, 2004.

24. Kazakova SV, Hageman JC, Matava M, et al.: A clone of methicillin-resistant *Staphylococcus aureus* among professional football players. *N Engl J Med* 352:468–475, 2005.

25. Chambers HF: The changing epidemiology of *Staphylococcus aureus*? *Emerg Infect Dis* 7:178–182, 2001.

26. Naimi TS, LeDell KH, Como-Sabetti K, et al.: Comparison of community- and health care-associated methicillin-resistant *Staphylococcus aureus* infection. *JAMA* 290:2976–2984, 2003.

27. Center for Disease Control and Prevention: Four pediatric deaths from community-acquired methicillin-resistant *Staphylococcus aureus*—Minnesota and North Dakota, 1997–1999. *Morb Mortal Wkly Rep* 48:707–710, 1999.

28. Fey PD, Said-Salim B, Rupp ME, et al.: Comparative molecular analysis of community- or hospital-acquired methicillin-resistant *Staphylococcus aureus*. *Antimicrob Agents Chemother* 47:196–203, 2003.

29. Gillet Y, Issartel B, Vanhems P, et al.: Association between *Staphylococcus aureus* strains carrying genes for Panton-Valentine leukocidin and highly lethal necrotizing pneumonia in young immunocompetent patients. *Lancet* 359:753–759, 2002.

30. Chambers HF: Community-associated MRSA—resistance and virulence converge. *N Engl J Med* 352:1485–1487, 2005.

31. Ferraro MJ: Methicillin-resistant *Staphylococcus aureus*: History and genetics of resistance. *Inform Decis Clin Strategies Gram positive Infect* 1:15–24, 2003.

32. The Medical Letter. *Treat Guidelines Med Lett* 2:13–26, 2004.

33. Swartz MN: Cellulitis. *N Engl J Med* 350:904–912, 2004.

34. Lipsky BA, Stoutenbugh U: Daptomycin for treating infected diabetic foot ulcers: Evidence from a randomized, controlled trial comparing daptomycin with vancomycin or semi-synthetic penicillins for complicated skin and skin-structure infections. *J Antimicrob Chemother* 55:240–245, 2005.

35. Dajani AS, Taubert KA, Wilson W, et al.: Prevention of bacterial endocarditis. Recommendations by the American Heart Association. *JAMA* 277:1794–1801, 1997.

26

Viral-Associated Exanthems

Jeffrey C. Poole

VIRAL-ASSOCIATED EXANTHEMS

Viruses are noncellular, obligatory intracellular parasites that require host machinery for their replication. Viral particles (virions) contain a central nucleic acid core, surrounded by a protective protein coat (capsid). Some viral groups, such as the Herpesvirus group, also contain an outermost membrane (envelope) that surrounds the capsid, making them susceptible to drying. The life cycle of a virus consists of two phases: (1) the virion or extracellular stage and (2) the intracellular parasitic stage in which the viral genome is incorporated into its host's. This second, or infectious, phase may last from hours to many years, depending on the virus involved.

Three general patterns of viral infection occur: (1) acute infection followed by clearance, classically demonstrated with measles virus, (2) acute infection followed by latency and possible reactivation as seen with Herpes Simplex virus (HSV) and varicella-zoster virus (VZV), and (3) chronic infection, as with HIV. As it is primarily acute viral infections, and their associated exanthems, that may prompt an emergency department evaluation, we will focus on a few of the most significant viral exanthems and their broad differentials in this chapter.

VARICELLA

High Yield Facts

1. Varicella infection presents as a febrile, pruritic eruption, occurring in crops, consisting of multiple "dew drops on a rose petal" in multiple stages of healing.

2. Persistence or recrudescence of fever, or worsening pain and redness around a vesicle, may herald secondary bacterial infection with *Staphylococcus aureus* or *Streptococcus pyogenes*.

3. Varicella vaccination has markedly reduced the incidence of varicella and its sequelae.

4. Patients are infectious until crusting of all lesions occurs.

Case Presentation

A mother, 7 months pregnant, presents late one evening with her 3-year-old son who has had fever for 3 days, and an itchy rash that was first noted that morning. He is a previously healthy young boy with no allergies, but his mother is unsure about his immunization history and they have no regular pediatrician. He has been given ibuprofen for his fever, and his skin is smeared with calamine lotion. His mom reports that his activity and appetite are somewhat decreased, but he is still playing and drinking well.

On physical exam the child is somewhat apprehensive and miserable, but does not appear toxic. He has multiple lesions consisting of erythematous macules, papules, vesicles, pustules and crusts, many of which have excoriations. There is a predominately truncal distribution and a few vesicular lesions on the palate. The rest of his exam is otherwise normal. Of note, the child plays frequently with his 3-year-old cousin, who is on maintenance chemotherapy for acute lymphocytic leukemia which is in remission.

Introduction/Epidemiology

Varicella, or chicken pox, is the result of primary infection with the VZV. Humans are the only source of the infection (1). Ninety percent of cases occur in children less than 10 years of age (2), with the highest incidence in children 1–4 year old (154 cases/1000 individuals). Though fewer than 5% of cases occur in persons over 15 years old (3), increasing age portends increasing severity of illness. Death rates in children are 1.4/100,000, compared to adults at 30.9/100,000 (2), and increasing to 535/100,000 in those over 65 years of age. Patients at increased risk from varicella infection include infants, the elderly, the immunosuppressed, patients with chronic cutaneous or pulmonary disease, and patients on long term salicylate therapy (1). Until 1995, 4 million cases, 11,000 hospitalizations, and 100 deaths per year were attributable to varicella. These numbers are in dramatic decline, by as much as 84%, since the introduction of the varicella vaccine in 1995 (5). Importantly, secondary family cases tend to have more severe disease than the index case.

Varicella is seasonal in temperate climates, with most cases occurring in children during the late winter and early spring. Tropical climates show no seasonal variation, and adults comprise a higher proportion of cases (1).

Pathophysiology/Microbiology

Varicella is a highly infectious agent that is spread primarily via respiratory droplets. Direct contact with infectious

Table 26–1. Pertinent Features of VZV, HSV, and Measles

	Varicella	**Zoster**	**Herpes Simplex**	**Measles**
Pseudonyms	Chicken pox	Shingles, Herpes Zoster	Cold sores, genital herpes	Morbilli
Virus	VZV (primary)	VZV (recurrent)	HSV-1, HSV-2	Rubeola
Age	<10 y/o	Increases with age	Any; HSV-2 primarily in the sexually active	6–15 months; early school age
Season	Late winter and early spring	None	None	Winter and spring
Spread	Respiratory droplets > direct contact	Direct contact of lesions	Direct contact of mucosal surfaces or secretions	Respiratory droplet
Incubation	10–21 days	Reactivation of dormant disease	1–2 weeks	8–12 days
Infectivity	Until last lesion has crusted (6–7 days)	Up to 7 days	Primary: 7 days Recurrent: 3–4 days Asymptomatic shedding occurs	3–5 days before until 4 days after rash
Prodrome	Fever; chills; malaise; anorexia	Pain; dysesthesia; allodynia in dermatome involved	Cutaneous sensory changes; fever; malaise	Fever; malaise; irritability; "3 Cs"; Koplik spots
Rash	Diffuse pruritic vesicles with an erythematous base; multiple stages of evolution	Unilateral; dermatomal; grouped papulo-vesicles on an erythematous base	Grouped vesicles on an erythematous base in a localized distribution	Erythematous macules and papules start on head/neck spreading centrifugally
Complications	Secondary bacterial infection; necrotizing fasciitis; pneumonia	PHN; scarring; dissemination; ophthalmic disease; motor neuropathy; secondary infection	Eczema herpeticum, keratoconjunctivitis, disseminated dz, meningitis, encephalitis, recurrent EM	Pneumonia; encephalitis; ITP; fetal death with pregnancy; SSPE
Immunization	VZV at 1 year	VZV at 1 year	None	MMR at 15 months and 4–6 year

VZV = varicella zoster virus; HSV = herpes simplex virus; PHN = postherpetic neuralgia; MMR = measles, mumps, and rubella immunization; ITP = idiopathic thrombocytopenic purpura; SSPE = subacute sclerosing panencephalitis.

lesions is also another mechanism for infection. The incubation period is approximately 2 weeks, with a range of 10–21 days. Initial viremia occurs on days 4–6 with seeding of the liver, spleen, lungs, and perhaps other organs. A secondary viremia occurs on days 11–20, and it is during this stage that skin lesions appear (2). Patients are infectious up to 4 days before, and as long as 6 days after the appearance of the exanthem (2, 3), with immunosuppressed patients potentially having a much longer contagious period. A more clinically relevant guide to infectivity is to consider the patient contagious until crusting of all lesions (1), and patients should be excluded from school or day care until that time.

Immunity from varicella infection is generally life long and primarily mediated by cellular immunity. As such, patients with decreased cellular immunity may present with reinfection (recurrent varicella) and are at increased risk for reactivation of latent virus (herpes zoster). Most cases of "recurrent varicella" actually represent incorrect diagnosis of the patient's initial episode, or possibly a case of disseminated zoster (3).

Clinical Presentation
(see Table 26–1, Fig. 26–1)

Chicken pox is one of the classic exanthems of childhood and is characterized by a febrile patient with an extremely pruritic rash consisting of vesicles on an erythematous base ("dewdrop on a rose petal") in multiple stages of healing/evolution. There is often a prodrome in older children and adults, but it may not be apparent in younger children. This may consist of fever, chills, malaise, headache, anorexia, sore throat, or dry cough (3). The rash often begins as faint erythematous macules that rapidly progress to papules, vesicles, pustules, and then crusts. Lesional count typically numbers 250–500 lesions (1) which occur in successive crops most concentrated on the trunk, face, and oral mucosa, with relative sparing of the extremities. Cutaneous lesions tend not to scar except when excoriated or secondarily infected.

Of importance is the fact that secondary household cases are often more severely affected than the index patient. Aggressive treatment, or prophylactic measures, should be considered in these patients. Complications and severe disease are generally more common in adults than children.

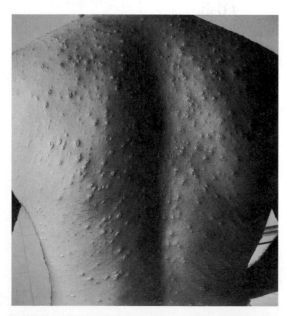

Fig. 26–1. Varicella (Sugathan Paramoo, MD, Dermatlas; http://www.dermatlas.org).

Secondary infection with *S. aureus* and *S. pyogenes* is the most common complication of varicella (2) and may be manifest as prolonged fever or fever recrudescence. While severe infection is rare in normal patients, up to one-third of invasive group A streptococcal diseases (i.e., "flesh eating bacteria") are associated with varicella (3). NSAID use has been postulated to increase the risk of bacterial complications (1), but more recent evidence does not support this theory (8).

Other complications of varicella may include pneumonia, acute otitis media, secondary bacterial osteomyelitis, cerebellar ataxia, encephalitis, thrombocytopenia, and purpura fulminans/disseminated intravascular coagulation. Primary varicella pneumonia is a frequent complication in adults (i.e., 1/400), but is quite rare in children (2). Mortality is less than 10% in the immunocompetent patient (3). Other associated findings may include an asymptomatic myocarditis or hepatitis, both of which resolve spontaneously and are rarely of significance.

Reye syndrome (i.e., acute hepatic encephalopathy) has been associated with varicella and aspirin use, though this association has been disputed (7). Nevertheless, aspirin should be avoided in children, especially those with varicella infection. Reye syndrome should be considered in a child with varicella and severe vomiting.

Congenital varicella syndrome refers to infection of the nonimmune mother during the first 20 weeks of gestation, with resultant fetal injury. Limb atrophy, cutaneous scarring, CNS abnormalities, and ocular abnormalities may occur. Fortunately, the incidence is quite low, occurring in 0.4–2% of infected mothers (1, 2).

Neonatal varicella occurs in a newborn whose mother develops varicella 5 days before to 2 days after delivery. The neonate is exposed to the initial viremia stage, but does not acquire the protective maternal VZV IgG antibodies. Disease is very severe and may be fatal (1).

Immunocompromised patients are at increased risk for severe disease and death from varicella infection, and prior infection is not necessarily protective. Pneumonia, hepatitis, and encephalitis are quite frequent, and hemorrhagic varicella may be seen. Lesions tend to be more necrotic, ulcerative, and chronic, especially in patients with HIV coinfection.

Laboratory/Diagnostic Testing
(see Table 26–2)

The diagnosis of varicella infection is classically a clinical one. Morphology and evolution of the rash, as well as exposure history, have been the primary evaluation

Table 26–2. Diagnostic Options for VZV, HSV, and Measles

Test/Disease	VZV	HSV-1, HSV-2	Measles
Tzanck smear	Scraping base of fresh vesicle; cannot differentiate VZV from HSV; may help to rule out other blistering disorders	Scraping base of fresh vesicle; cannot differentiate VZV from HSV; may help to rule out other blistering disorders	N/A
Viral culture	Vesicular fluid; less sensitive and rapid than DFA; differentiates VZV from HSV	Vesicular fluid; slightly more sensitive than DFA; differentiates HSV serotypes and from VZV	From blood, urine, and nasopharynx- state public health labs or CDC to process
DFA	Scraping base of fresh vesicle; more rapid and sensitive than culture; differentiates VZV from HSV	Scraping base of fresh vesicle; rapid; slightly less sensitive than culture; differentiates HSV serotypes and from VZV	N/A
PCR	Vesicular fluid or tissue; most sensitive, not readily available	Vesicular fluid or tissue; most sensitive, not readily available	N/A
Serology	Acute and convalescent IgG; not useful in the acute setting	Acute and convalescent IgG; not useful in the acute setting	Acute IgM; acute and convalescent IgG
Histopathology	Differentiate VZV from other blistering disorders; does not differentiate VZV from HSV	Differentiate HSV from other blistering disorders; does not differentiate VZV from HSV	
Single best test	DFA	DFA and culture; PCR for CSF	Serology

VZV = varicella zoster virus; CSF = cerebrospinal fluid; HSV = herpes simplex virus; DFA = direct fluorescent antibody test; CDC = centers for disease control; PCR = polymerase chain reaction.

methods. Interestingly, a negative past history of varicella is associated with a seronegativity rate of only 20% in adults (2). Since universal immunization of all children has been recommended since 1995, it may be helpful to seek other confirmatory tests, especially in severe or confusing cases. Confirmatory measures typically include a Tzanck smear, direct fluorescent antibody (DFA) test, viral culture, or biopsy.

Tzanck smear scrapings are best obtained from the base of a fresh vesicle. A positive result reveals typical multinucleated giant cells and can help to confirm a herpes virus etiology versus other blistering disorders. However, it cannot differentiate between VZV or HSV. Even in experienced hands the test is not very sensitive or accurate (1).

Viral culture, best obtained as an aspirate from a clear vesicle, can differentiate VZV from HSV, and results may be obtained within 24–72 h (3). It is less sensitive and less rapid than DFA, and often is a "send-out" for many labs.

Direct fluorescent antibody is the most rapid, sensitive, and readily available test in most centers (1). It can distinguish between VZV and HSV, the turnaround time can be as rapid as a few hours, and virus can be detected in situations where culture is negative (3). Fresh vesicles or prevesicular lesions are the optimal test sites.

Biopsy for histopathology is helpful to differentiate VZV from other blistering disorders, but will not differentiate VZV from HSV.

Other confirmatory tests may include PCR and serologic testing. While PCR is very sensitive and specific, it is not readily available. Serologic testing, most commonly with enzyme linked immunoassay (EIA) (1), is not very helpful in the acute setting, as acute and convalescent titers must be obtained for comparison.

The differential diagnosis of VZV (Table 26–3) includes disseminated HSV, impetigo, vesicular enteroviral infections (Coxsackie, Echovirus), rickettsialpox,

Table 26–3. Differential Diagnosis VZV, HSV, and Measles

Varicella	Disseminated HSV, impetigo, vesicular enteroviral infections, rickettsialpox, insect bites, papular urticaria, scabies, contact dermatitis, dermatitis herpetiformis, pityriasis lichenoides et varioliformis acuta, drug eruption, secondary syphilis, erythema multiforme
Zoster	Prodrome: Angina pectoris, duodenal ulcer, biliary colic, renal colic, appendicitis, pleurodynia, glaucoma
	Eruption: impetigo/bullous impetigo, allergic contact dermatitis, chemical burns, zosterifrom HSV, varicella (for disseminated disease)
HSV (cutaneous)	Impetigo, zoster, hand-foot-mouth disease, EM, apthosis, pemphigus, allergic contact dermatitis, varicella, diphtheria, BehÇets
HSV (genital)	Syphilis, chancroid, zoster, trauma, impetigo, molluscum contagiosum
Measles	Rubella, scarlet fever, secondary syphilis, enteroviral infections, drug eruptions

VZV = varicella zoster virus; HSV = herpes simplex virus; EM = erythema multiforme.

insect bites, papular urticaria, scabies, contact dermatitis, dermatitis herpetiformis, pityriasis lichenoides et varioliformis acuta, drug eruption, secondary syphilis, and erythema multiforme (2).

MANAGEMENT (SEE TABLE 26–4)

Symptomatic therapy for uncomplicated varicella is still considered by many to be the standard of care. Antipyretics and analgesics, cool compresses, calamine, oral antihistamines, and colloidal oatmeal baths are frequently utilized. Aspirin, due to its possible association with the Reye syndrome, and possibly NSAIDs, due to concern for increased incidence of severe infection (1), should be avoided. Nails should be clipped to prevent excoriations, occlusive ointments or corticosteroids avoided, and patients monitored for signs of secondary bacterial infection.

While some sources do not recommend the routine use of antivirals in otherwise healthy children (1), therapy does shorten illness period, decrease disease severity, allows parents and the patient to return to work sooner, and does not inhibit the immune response (3, 9). If therapy is decided upon, initiation should be as soon as possible and ideally within 24 h. As most viral replication has stopped by 72 h following the onset of the rash (1), treatment beyond this period is probably not beneficial.

Therapy should be considered in the following at risk cases: secondary household cases, adolescents and adults, patients with chronic cardiopulmonary disease, immunodeficiency, diabetes, severe disease, and pregnant women.

For the immunocompetent, dosing typically is with acyclovir 20 mg/kg qid (up to 800 mg per dose) for 5–7 days (6). Valacyclovir, a prodrug of acyclovir with higher oral bioavailability, and famciclovir, a penciclovir prodrug which has a much longer intracellular half-life (6), require less frequent dosing and may be considered as alternatives. Dosing for valacyclovir is 1000 mg orally tid for 5 days and that for famciclovir is 500 mg orally tid for 5 days.

For the severely infected, pregnant, or immunosuppressed individual, IV therapy is recommended. Dosing is typically 10 mg/kg every 8 h for 10 days. When patients are improved and new vesicles are no longer developing, switching to oral valacyclovir or famciclovir may be considered (2). Some immunosuppressed patients, especially with HIV coinfection, may develop acyclovir-resistant disease. In these cases, foscarnet is the treatment of choice (6).

At risk patients exposed to VZV should be considered for both active (VZV vaccine) and passive (VZIG) immunization. Varicella-zoster immunoglobulin (VZIG), if warranted, should be given within 72–96 h of a significant exposure (1, 2). Active immunization with VZV vaccine is also effective if given within 3 days to *immunocompetent* individuals (3). The value of prophylactic antivirals is unknown (1). It is critical to isolate potentially infectious patients with VZV infection from immunosuppressed patients in the hospital.

Disposition

Since the introduction of the *Oka* strain varicella vaccine in 1995, there has been a dramatic decline in the incidence of varicella infection. This live, attenuated vaccine, is recommended for children at 12–18 months, with a 95% antibody seroconversion after one dose. It has proven 90% effective in preventing varicella during outbreaks,

Table 26–4. Antiviral Management of VZV and HSV Infections (1, 6, 24)

	Acyclovir	Valacyclovir	Famciclovir
Varicella—children	20 mg/kg/dose po qid up to 800 mg/dose for 5–7 days	Insufficient data	Insufficient data
Immunocompromised	10–12 mg/kg IV q8 h for 7–10 days		
Varicella—adult	800 mg po qid for 5–7 days	1000 mg po tid for 5 days (not FDA approved)	500 mg po tid for 5 days (not FDA approved)
Immunocompromised	10–12 mg/kg IV q8 h for 7–10 days	Insufficient data	Insufficient data
Zoster—children	Nonsevere: as varicella	Insufficient data	Insufficient data
Immunocompromised	Severe: as varicella (immunocompromised) $\geq$ 12year/o: treat as adult Consider as adult		
Zoster—adult	800 mg po 5×/day × 7 days	1000 mg po TID × 7 days	500 mg po TID × 7 days
Immunocompromised	Not severe: as normal Severe: 10–12 mg/kg IV q8 h for 7–14 days	Insufficient data	Insufficient data
HSV—primary	200 mg po 5×/day × 10 days	1000 mg po bid × 10 days	250 mg po tid × 10 days
Children	40–80 mg/kg po divided qid × 10 days	Insufficient data	Insufficient data
Immunocompromised	200–400 po5×/day or 5–10 mg/kg IV q8 h × 7–14 days	Insufficient data	Insufficient data
HSV—recurrent	400 mg po tid × 5 days	500 mg po bid × 5 days	125 mg po bid × 5 days
Children	400 mg po tid × 5 days	Insufficient data	Insufficient data
Immunocompromised	Insufficient data	Insufficient data	500 mg po bid × 7 days
HSV—suppression	400 mg po bid	500–1000 mg po qd	250 mg po bid
Immunocompromised	At least 400 mg po bid	Insufficient data	500 mg po bid
HSV—neonatal	20 mg/kg IV q8 h × 14–21 days	Insufficient data	Insufficient data

and 100% effective at preventing severe disease (1, 3). Varicella infection in the immunized individual is milder (15–32 median lesion count), is associated with a lower fever, and results in a more rapid recovery. Current studies show lasting immunity up to 20 years (10), though it is quite possible booster immunizations will be required as the reservoir or wild virus exposure declines. In the future we can expect fewer cases, and less complications, from this "routine" childhood illness.

Case Outcome

Though the child had no significant risk factors, the physician and parent decided to initiate a course of oral acyclovir suspension, 20 mg/kg qid for 5 days. The mother had a positive history for chicken pox as a child, so no therapy was necessary for her. Varicella serology was drawn

for confirmation and revealed an immune status. The cousin's oncologist was contacted, who recommended that the patient receive VZIG and be closely monitored for signs of varicella.

ZOSTER (HERPES ZOSTER, SHINGLES)
High Yield Facts

1. Zoster is the reactivation of latent varicella infection.

2. The eruption consists of grouped vesicles on an erythematous base in a dermatomal distribution, usually associated with pain or other sensory abnormalities.

3. Oral antiviral therapy should be instituted within 72 h to be effective. Oral corticosteroids are also helpful for the acute pain of zoster.

Case Presentation

A 69-year-old man presents with complaints of severe pain and a very tender, red rash on his scalp that has now progressed onto his face over the last 36 h. The patient is concerned that he came in contact with poison ivy while hiking over the weekend. Most recently, he reports his vision being somewhat blurry in the right eye. He otherwise is in good health and is taking no medications.

On physical exam the patient appears well and his vital signs are normal. The right side of his forehead, scalp, upper eyelid, and nose are markedly erythematous with multiple small papulo-vesicles. The eruption is very tender, sensitive to the touch, and does not cross the midline. He has injection of his right eye, with tearing and photophobia.

Introduction/Epidemiology

Herpes zoster, or shingles, represents a reactivation of the latent VZV virus. Patients must have had prior exposure and infection with chicken pox or have received the varicella vaccine. The eruption is sporadic, there is no seasonal prevalence, and an increasing incidence of disease is seen with increasing age. The lifetime incidence of zoster in the United States is 10–20%, equating to nearly 850,000 cases per year (3). African-Americans are four times less likely to develop zoster (2).

Immunosuppression, especially associated with hematologic malignancies and HIV, also dramatically increases the incidence of zoster by up to 50–100 fold (11). While the incidence of herpes zoster is markedly increased in the immunosuppressed, it should not be used as a marker for malignancy. Instead, appropriate history, risk factors, and physical exam should be undertaken to assess this risk (2). "Recurrent zoster," in fact, most likely represents a recurrent form of zosteriform HSV.

Zoster is less contagious than its primary infection, varicella. Unlike varicella, it is spread mainly by direct contact, and vesicles remain infectious for up to 7 days. Exposure of a nonimmune individual to the lesions of zoster will result in chicken pox, not shingles.

Pathophysiology/Microbiology

After primary infection with VZV, the virus becomes dormant in the sensory dorsal root ganglion cells where it persists indefinitely. At some future date, often for factors not fully understood, the virus may become reactivated and spread distally from the sensory ganglion along its given dermatome. This dermatome is often the one where varicella achieved its highest density during the primary

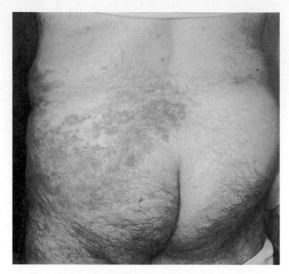

Fig. 26–2. Herpes zoster.

infection. V1, and T1 to L2 are the dermatomes most commonly involved. Factors that are known to play a contributing role in reactivation often involve waning cellular immunity and may include increasing age, immunosuppression, frontal sinusitis, and irradiation, trauma, tumor or manipulation of the spinal column (3).

Clinical Presentation (see Table 26–1, Fig. 26–2)

Zoster is frequently heralded by several days of pain, itching, and paraesthesia or dysethesia in the affected area, though the sensory complaints may begin with or follow the eruption. Less commonly, the eruption may be relatively asymptomatic, or pain may develop in dermatomes with no rash. Descriptions used to describe the pain often include "itching," "tingling," "burning," or "lancinating." It may be constant or intermittent, with significant tenderness or hyperesthesia (11). Allodynia, pain, and/or unpleasant sensations elicited by stimuli that are not normally painful is a characteristic finding.

The typical rash of zoster is unilateral and dermatomal in distribution, manifesting grouped papular and vesicular lesions on an erythematous base, with its most frequent areas of involvement being along cranial or spinal sensory nerves. Involvement of surrounding dermatomes may occur. The trigeminal nerve is the most common single nerve involved (20% of cases), but the vast majority of eruptions occur in thoraco-lumbar-sacral areas (75% of cases). Occurrence distal to the elbows or knees is rare. Lesions may become hemorrhagic, bullous, with necrotic lesions often resulting in significant scarring. Evolution is slower than seen with varicella infections. New lesions continue to develop for 5–7 days, but the illness may persist for 2–6 weeks or more, with prolonged illness more common in the elderly (2).

Pain, the most common complaint of zoster, is often divided into zoster-associated pain (ZAP) and postherpetic neuralgia (PHN). PHN refers to pain persisting after all skin lesions have healed (2). Nearly all patients with zoster will experience ZAP, while 10–70% will develop PHN (11). The elderly typically have more severe and chronic pain problems as the incidence of PHN increases with age.

Various complications of zoster may include disseminated zoster, ophthalmic zoster, motor nerve neuropathy, secondary bacterial infections, scarring, and the Ramsay-Hunt syndrome. Disseminated zoster is a varicelliform eruption defined as more than 20 lesions outside the affected dermatome and most commonly is seen in patients with lymphoreticular malignancies or AIDS. Ophthalmic zoster involves the V1 distribution of the trigeminal nerve and should be suspected in patients with tearing, visual complaints, diplopia, or photophobia. Hutchinson sign, described as vesicles on the nasal tip and sidewall, and vesicular lesions occurring on the lid margin are both strong indicators of eye involvement. Acute retinal necrosis is the most severe form of ocular disease, representing a fulminant, sight threatening event. Ocular lesions of zoster and their complications tend to recur (2, 3).

The Ramsay-Hunt syndrome, another complication of zoster, represents inflammation of the facial and auditory nerves. The resulting clinical findings include ipsilateral facial paralysis and auditory symptoms of tinnitus, deafness, vertigo, nauseua, vomiting, or nystagmus. Zoster is often evident on the external ear or tympanic membrane.

Immunosuppressed patients often have a more severe, protracted course, with a significantly higher incidence of complications and recurrences. Lesions often appear the same, but may be more ulcerative or necrotic, and may scar more easily. Disseminated, ophthalmic, or neurologic disease complications are more common. Patients with bone marrow transplants represent the highest risk group, with an associated mortality rate of 5% (2), while HIV patients tend to represent a large proportion of recurrent disease (3).

Laboratory/Diagnostic Testing (see Table 26–2)

As with varicella, the diagnosis of herpes zoster is normally made solely on clinical criteria. An accurate history revealing the appropriate prodrome, evolution, and morphology of the rash will generally be all the evaluation that is necessary. Disseminated disease may be easily mistaken for varicella and should be considered in the immunosuppressed. Recurrent disease, especially near the gluteal cleft, mouth, and genitals, should be suspect for zosteriform HSV. Clinically, this may be impossible to distinguish, but multiple recurrences in the same site are more consistent with HSV infection.

Other differential diagnoses (see Table 26–3) to consider, especially relating to prodromal pain, include angina pectoris, duodenal ulcer, biliary or renal colic, appendicitis, pleurodynia, or glaucoma (2). When considering lesional disease, other conditions could include impetigo/bullous impetigo, allergic contact (rhus) dermatitis, and chemical or thermal burns.

In those situations where additional information may be necessary, the same testing strategy outlined for varicella infections would apply. DFA is the preferred test as it is more rapid and has a higher yield than culture, and it can differentiate between HSV types and VZV (2). The Tzanck smear and histopathology help to differentiate herpes zoster from other blistering disorders. PCR, while not readily available, may some day become an important diagnostic tool.

Management (see Table 26–4)

Management issues for zoster focus upon treatment during the acute phase of illness and pain as well as the treatment of PHN.

In the acute phase, and for zoster-associated pain, pharmacologic and nonpharmacologic measures may be helpful. Activity restriction and bed rest, especially in the elderly, may help to reduce the incidence of postherpetic neuralgia (2). Local application of heat or topical anesthetics may be beneficial. Acetaminophen, NSAIDs, and opiates have all been used to alleviate the acute pain, with the minimum goal of allowing a restful sleep.

Corticosteroids have been proven to improve the acute neuritis more rapidly and shorten the period of analgesia needed, but are unproven at preventing PHN (11). Treating with 40–60 mg of prednisone per day and tapering over a 2–4-week course, providing the patient has no contraindications, may be considered.

Antiviral therapy should be instituted in all patients, provided there are no contraindications. Topical antivirals are ineffective, and treatment should be via the oral or IV route. Therapy should be started within 72 h of onset of rash, but may be considered beyond that time in patients with ophthalmic zoster (3). Antivirals have been proven to reduce ZAP, lead to more rapid resolution of lesions, and reduce the duration of infectivity. Their efficacy in preventing PHN is controversial (2, 11).

The efficacy of oral therapy with acyclovir, valacyclovir, and famciclovir is roughly equivalent. The advantages of the latter two oral preparations include increased oral bioavailability and prolonged intracellular half-life, respectively, allowing for less frequent dosing. Treatment for 7 days is as good as 21 days of therapy (3). Dosing for acyclovir is 800 mg po five times daily. Valacyclovir dosing is 1 g po tid, and famciclovir dosing is 500 mg po tid. For immunosuppressed patients, ophthalmic zoster, disseminated disease, severe pain, or the Ramsay-Hunt syndrome, IV therapy is generally warranted. Ophthalmology should be consulted in all cases of ophthalmic zoster.

Treatment of PHN should ideally involve consultation with a dermatologist, neurologist, or pain clinic. Therapies include capsaicin, topical lidocaine preparations, opiates, nerve blocks, tricyclic antidepressants, and anticonvulsants. The anticonvulsant gabapentin has become a first line agent for many cases of PHN.

Appropriate control measures include contact precautions, strict hand washing for anyone having contact with lesions, and airborne and contact precautions for the immunosuppressed.

Disposition

With the advent of the VZV vaccine in 1995, there has been a reduction in the natural pool of varicella infections. There is some concern that those individuals with a past history of chicken pox may see a higher incidence of zoster, as their opportunity for wild virus rechallenge, and resultant immunologic boosting, is decreased. Vaccination boosters may help to decrease the incidence of zoster and PHN (3). What has been witnessed is a marked reduction in zoster in those who have received immunization compared to those with natural infection, i.e., 2.6/100,000 person years versus 68/100,000 person years, respectively.

Zoster will remain a pertinent clinical entity in the future. With more patients receiving immunosuppressive drugs, the increase in HIV infections, and the universal vaccination of all children for varicella, patient demographics and the epidemiology of infection will continue to evolve.

Case Outcome

The distribution of the patient's lesions, including the nasal tip and upper eyelid, along with the ocular symptoms supported a diagnosis of ophthalmic zoster. Due to the high risk of complications and the advanced age of the patient, he was admitted for IV acyclovir at a dose of 10 mg/kg every 8 h. Ophthalmology was consulted and additional therapy instituted. After a discussion of the benefits of oral corticosteroids, therapy with prednisone was begun for the severe nature of the pain.

HERPES SIMPLEX

High Yield Facts

1. HSV infections typically manifest as painful, grouped vesicles on an erythematous base in a localized distribution.

2. HSV-1 infections typically occur "above the waist" and HSV-2 "below the waist," but both infections may occur in either location.

3. Viral shedding may occur despite an absence of signs or symptoms of reactivation.

4. While generally a localized infection is observed, more severe disease with extensive cutaneous, visceral, or neurological manifestations may be seen.

Case Presentation

A 4-year-old, irritable boy presents with a 4-day history of a suddenly worsening skin eruption. The mother reports a high fever with rash and an inability to tolerate anything by mouth. The rash began with marked vesiculation and erosions to the perioral, gingival, and buccal mucosa, including the tongue, and has made oral intake very difficult. In the last 24 h, the grouped erythematous vesicles, pustules, and erosions have spread to the rest of the skin, with somewhat more marked concentration on the flexural arms, legs, and neck region. The eyes are uninvolved, as are the soft palate and posterior oropharynx.

The patient, although arouseable and interactive, is somewhat listless, with dry, slightly sunken eyes. Vitals reveal a 101.5°F temperature and a mild tachycardia. The mother feels that the child's urine output has been decreased. When compared to a weight obtained at his pediatrician's office 3 weeks ago, his current weight documents an approximately 5% weight loss. The child has a history of severe atopic dermatitis that is partially controlled with daily tacrolimus and triamcinalone ointment. He has no prior history of cold sores and has received no recent oral medications.

Introduction/Epidemiology

Herpes simplex virus is one of the most prevalent infectious agents worldwide. Up to 60% of the U.S. population is infected during childhood with HSV-1, and over 90% is seropositive after the age of 50 years (3). HSV-2 seropositivity approaches 23% in the U.S. population, correlates with sexual activity, and has been increasing. Compounding this problem is the high rate of asymptomatic infection, often approaching 80%, or asymptomatic reactivation that contributes to further viral spread (2).

Typically, diseases caused by these two serotypes have been divided into "above the waist" (HSV-1) and "below the waist"(HSV-2), but infection is not limited to these areas. In fact, HSV-1 disease has become increasingly prevalent in genital lesions (1). Prior infection with HSV-1 offers some cross immunity and will reduce the likelihood of experiencing symptomatic HSV-2 infection, and vice versa. In some cases this may offer a protective benefit, as in maternal transmission of HSV-2 to a newborn, while in others it may mask the initial HSV-2 symptoms perhaps leading to asymptomatic spread of virus to future sexual contacts. In general, the frequency and severity of both disease types decrease with time (2).

Pathophysiology/Microbiology

Herpes simplex is an enveloped double-stranded DNA virus which infects humans primarily through mucosal surfaces by way of direct contact or secretions. Incubation period is from as few as 2 days to as long as 4 weeks (1), but generally is 1–2 weeks. Three stages of infection are recognized: acute infection, latency, and reactivation.

Acute infection is primarily epidermal, resulting in cytolytic activity that involves the host cells. The virus spreads centrally via sensory nerves where it eventually establishes latency in the dorsal root ganglion. Intermittent reactivation is the rule, with many known and unknown triggers. UV light, hyperthermia, trauma, and physiologic stressors are all known triggers for HSV reactivation. Most common sites of reactivation include the trigeminal ganglion (HSV-1) and sacral ganglion (HSV-2) (3). Primary infections often shed virus for 1 week or more, while reactivated disease may be infectious for 3–4 days. Viral shedding during times of no signs or symptoms of disease also occurs.

Clinical Presentation
(see Table 26–1, Fig. 26–3)

Clinical manifestations of HSV infection will depend on the site of infection and the immune status of the host. Most commonly grouped vesicles on an erythematous base are found in a localized distribution, as is classically seen in herpes labialis. Less common, but more significant, findings can include eczema herpeticum resembling

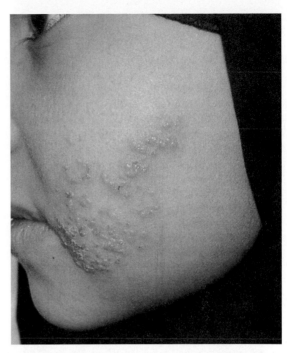

Fig. 26–3. Herpes simplex virus (Yahia Albaili, MD, Dermatlas; http://www.dermatlas.org).

varicella, herpes meningitis, and disseminated herpes. Primary infection is typically more severe than recurrent disease, but prior infection with either HSV-1 or HSV-2 will result in less severe infection when exposed to the alternate viral serotype.

Orolabial Herpes can present as herpes labialis ("cold sore, fever blister"), herpetic gingivostomatitis, or herpetic pharyngitis. HSV-1 is the most prevalent serotype for infection, and most primary infections are asymptomatic. Infection caused by HSV-2 is much less commonly seen, and recurrent disease is 120 times less likely with this serotype (3). Symptomatic gingivostomatitis occurs in less than 1% of infected persons, with the highest prevalence rate in the 10-month- to 5 year-old age group (13). Vesicles and ulcerative lesions on the hard palate, tongue, buccal mucosa, and perioral area are most common. Associated symptoms include fever, lymphadenopathy, malaise, poor oral intake, and decreased appetite leading to possible dehydration and the need for hospitalization. A prodrome consisting of burning or tingling commonly precedes the eruption by up to 24 h. Untreated, lesions persist for 1–2 weeks (15). Recurrent disease presentation is variable, but typically briefer and less severe. Recurrent disease may represent a complication following surgical, dental, or cosmetic procedures to the orofacial

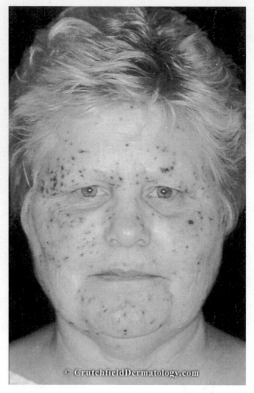

Fig. 26–4. Eczema herpeticum (contributor Charles Crutchfield, MD).

region, as well as following physiologic stressors or after a sunburn (14). Differential diagnosis includes impetigo, zoster, hand-foot-mouth disease, erythema multiforme, apthosis, pemphigus, and allergic contact dermatitis.

Eczema Herpeticum (i.e., Kaposi varicelliform eruption) is a severe cutaneous manifestation of HSV most commonly seen in patients with atopic dermatitis (Fig. 26–4). Disease may also be seen in any disorder of epidermal barrier function including seborrheic dermatitis, ichthyosis, Darier disease, pemphigus, and burns. The eruption resembles varicella, with fever, hundreds of vesicles, malaise, irritability, and generalized lymphadenopathy. Lesions tend to be more monomorphous and concentrated in areas of eczema (12), which helps to differentiate the eruption from chicken pox. Infected eczema may also be considered in the differential. While the disease is often self-limited, prior to antiviral therapy deaths occurred from diffuse disease, rhabdomylosis with renal failure, or sepsis from secondary bacterial infections (12). Therefore, it is recommended that all cases be treated with oral or systemic antiviral therapy.

Herpetic Keratoconjunctivitis, another potentially severe form of localized cutaneous disease, is the most common cause of blindness in the United States (2). Disease should be suspected when vesicles involve the lid margin and there is associated tender preauricular lymphadenopathy. Other signs and symptoms of keratitis or dendritic corneal ulcers include severe purulent conjunctivitis, edema, erythema, pain, photophobia, and increased lacrimation. Ophthalmology consultation should be obtained on an emergent basis and systemic therapy begun.

Other cutaneous manifestations of HSV include *herpetic whitlow* (infection of the fingertip pulp typically in young children with orolabial herpes or in adults via HSV-2 direct contact), *herpetic sycosis* (infectious spread of shaved areas), and *herpes gladiatorum* and *herpes rugbiaform* (spread via skin to skin contact in these sports). *Recurrent erythema multiforme (EM) minor* is usually associated with orolabial HSV-1 flares. Signs of EM include symmetrical targetoid lesions on the hands, feet, elbows, knees and face, minor mucosal signs, and a duration of 2–3 weeks (3).

Genital Herpes (herpes progenitalis) infections are the most common manifestations of HSV in adolescents and adults (1). Severity of genital herpes, like other forms of cutaneous herpes simplex, is often of reflection of initial versus recurrent disease. Primary infection can present as a severe, systemic illness with fever, tender bilateral lymphadenopathy, and flu-like symptoms that may last 3 or more weeks. In contrast, recurrent disease may by asymptomatic and go unnoticed by the patient. Viral shedding may even occur asymptomatically between outbreaks.

Typically disease, especially recurrent disease, is heralded by a prodrome. Within 24 h a vesicular-erosive, nonindurated (in contrast to syphilis) eruption will occur that lasts about 1 week and heals without scarring. The gluteal cleft is a common site of zosteriform recurrence as is the distribution of the trigeminal nerve.

Intrauterine and Neonatal HSV represent some of the most potentially severe HSV infections. Intrauterine infections are fortunately quite rare and are the result of primary infections occurring during pregnancy. This infection represents one of the *TORCH* infections, and may result in microcephaly, microophthalmia, chorioretinitis, encephalitis, intracerebral calcifications, diffuse cutaneous scarring, and other skin findings. Neonates may suffer severe CNS damage and may die from its complications.

Neonatal HSV, occurring in approximately 1/3000–20,000 live births (1), most commonly results via passage through an infected birth canal. Primary infection in the mother has up to a 50% risk of neonatal transmission, while recurrent maternal infection results in neonatal disease in less than 3% of cases (3). Infection may also occur via direct contact of the neonate with lesions on an infected caregiver. The manifestations of disease are divided into SEM (skin, eye, mouth disease), disseminated, CNS, and asymptomatic disease. Skin vesicles are often the presenting sign, though they may be absent, may appear late, or may be difficult to appreciate. Culture or PCR of vesicles, mouth or nasopharynx, eye, urine, blood, stool or rectum, and CSF should be obtained in all cases of suspected neonatal disease for evidence of active viral replication (1).

SEM disease represents classic, localized HSV cutaneous disease, and all patients should be evaluated for more severe systemic disease. Disseminated disease results in high mortality rates even with treatment (up to 55%) due to causes such as meningitis, hepatitis, pneumonia, adrenal hemorrhage, and coagulopathy. CNS disease is manifested by encephalitis with a predilection for the temporal lobes often resulting in hemorrhagic necrosis. With treatment, mortality still approaches 15% and approximately 50% of all patients develop neurologic sequelae.

HSV in the immunocompromised may often present with more severe, more persistent, more recurrent, or atypical disease patterns. Any erosive mucocutaneous lesion should be considered as possible HSV in these patients (2).

Laboratory/Diagnostic Testing (see Table 26–2)

The variety of tests available for HSV detection are the same as for VZV. Tzanck smears are rapid but nonspecific determinants of herpes family virus infections and have a low positivity rate even in experienced hands. They will not differentiate between HSV-1, HSV-2, or VZV, but the finding of multinucleated epidermal giant cells will differentiate herpes-associated disease from other blistering disorders. Tissue biopsy is generally not necessary, though characteristic epidermal changes will be seen. Histopathological differentiation between HSV and VZV is not possible, and other tests generally yield more useful information. If other blistering disorders are high on the differential, then tissue biopsy may be helpful.

Viral cultures, best obtained from fresh vesicular lesional fluid, have a positive yield of only 60–70% (3) with results available in 2–3 days. DFA and EIA are rapid tests, with specificity and sensitivity approximating that of culture. Material is best obtained by scraping a fresh lesional base, and results may be available within 1–4 h (12). PCR is the most sensitive test, though not readily available in all labs. It is the recommended test for CSF in the evaluation of both neonates and for HSV encephalitis, as culture is often negative (1). Temporal lobe biopsy and culture remains a means for definitive diagnosis in these cases. A bloody spinal tap should raise the suspicion of HSV encephalitis. Serologies are not useful in the acute setting.

Differential diagnosis (see Table 26–3) will depend on the site and clinical patterns involved, but may include aphthous stomatitis, impetigo, hand-foot-mouth disease, streptococcal disease, EM, diphtheria, Behcet syndrome, varicella, zoster, syphilis, and chancroid.

Management (see Table 26–4)

Effective treatment of herpes simplex virus infections first and foremost relies upon accurate diagnosis and classification of disease risk and treatment benefit. In general, the use of antivirals has become more accepted for even routine cases of HSV infection, such as orolabial herpes, though some would still advocate that many infections require no treatment. Treatment is considered primarily for protracted, severe, or complicated HSV disease.

Therapy for HSV infection typically includes the antivirals acyclovir, valacyclovir, and famciclovir. All three agents offer comparable efficacy at appropriate dosing, with acyclovir having the longest history of usage and the most clinical data to support its use. Valacyclovir and famciclovir offer the primary advantage of increased oral bioavailability, allowing for less frequent dosing and the possibility of blood levels equivalent to IV therapy with acyclovir (6). Of note, famciclovir and valacyclovir are not FDA approved for use in children. Topical agents, such as penciclovir and docosanol cream, play only a limited role in therapy for recurrent orolabial HSV infections. Topical acyclovir cream is also relatively ineffective (3). Foscarnet is selectively used for resistant HSV disease which is primarily seen in patients with HIV coinfection (2).

Orolabial herpes is often not treated in otherwise healthy individuals, although treatment should be instituted in severe primary infections such as acute herpetic gingivostomatitis (15), and in the immunocompromised patient. Symptomatic therapy in acute gingivostomatitis, with topical anesthetics and mucosal protectants, is a mainstay of therapy in helping to maintain oral intake and prevent the need for IV rehydration. Exclusion of children from school with acute gingivostomatitis is necessary only in those children who cannot control their oral secretions. The regular use of sunblock to prevent recurrent disease, often triggered by ultraviolet light, or suppressive doses of antivirals in patients with frequent recurrences are useful measures (2). The benefit of oral therapy in recurrent disease is minimal (1).

Other cases of cutaneous herpes simplex, such as herpetic whitlow and herpes gladiatorum, can also be considered for oral therapy. Recurrent EM minor can be treated with suppressive doses of antivirals (2).

Severe HSV disease should always be treated with oral or IV antivirals, depending upon the severity (2), and possibly hospitalization. These conditions would include eczema herpeticum, herpetic keratoconjunctivitis, disseminated disease, neonatal disease, and disease in the immunocompromised. Contact precautions are necessary for all hospitalized patients. Topical corticosteroids may induce corneal perforation in ocular disease, and therapy should be guided by ophthalmology consultation. In cases of suspected acyclovir resistance in the immunosuppressed, treatment should be with foscarnet (2).

Primary *genital HSV* is treated with oral or IV antivirals and should be instituted within 6 days of infection. For recurrent disease, therapy should begin by day 2 (1). Long-term suppressive therapy is safe, and lab monitoring is not required. One should consider discontinuing the therapy once a year to reassess disease status (2) (see Chapter 36 for more details regarding sexually transmitted infections).

Disposition/Future Trends

Antiviral therapies have drawn increased interest in recent years, particularly with the advent of the AIDS epidemic. Therapies on the horizon include helicase primer inhibitors, the first nonnucleoside antiviral compounds, which promise superior clinical activity when compared to current therapy (16). Other measures, aimed primarily at control of the genital HSV epidemic, include HSV-DNA (3) and disabled infectious single cycle HSV (6) vaccines.

Case Outcome

This dehydrated child is diagnosed with primary acute herpetic gingivostomatitis and eczema herpeticum. He is admitted for IV rehydration and IV acyclovir at a dose of 10 mg/kg/dose every 8 h. Culture for HSV and VZV is obtained from an aspirate of fresh vesicles, and material for DFA testing is obtained by scraping the base of these vesicles. A liquid diet is started and advanced as tolerated. Topical therapy for his eczema is switched to heavy emollients only, until the HSV is under control, and he is monitored closely for signs of secondary bacterial infection.

MEASLES

High Yield Facts

1. Measles is a reportable communicable disease. If the clinical picture is sufficiently suspect, appropriate laboratory evaluation and reporting are necessary.

2. Fever, myalgias, irritability, the 3 Cs (cough, coryza, and conjunctivitis), and Koplik spots form the classic prodrome of measles.

3. Rash progresses outwards from the head and neck, completing its whole body progression by day 3.

4. High dose vitamin A is the recommended therapy for the very ill or malnourished.

Case Presentation

An 8-year-old boy presents with a 3-day history of worsening rash, high fever, and irritability. The rash began on his face and now has spread to the trunk and extremities. On questioning, he reports frequent coughing, a profuse rhinitis, and decreased physical activity, but no nausea or vomiting. He is a recent immigrant from southeast Asia, and he has no prior history of immunization. He denies any recent medication use.

On physical exam, the patient is alert but very thin and moderately ill-appearing. He is tachypneic, febrile with a temperature of 104°F, and coughing frequently. His rash consists of macules and papules which blanch and are present on the head, neck, trunk, and extremities. He has conjunctival injection, but no discharge or photophobia. Mild cervical lymphadenopathy is present, but there is no evidence of hepatosplenomegaly. Fine blue-white papules are present on the buccal mucosa.

Introduction/Epidemiology

Measles, also known as *Rubeola* or *Morbilli*, is considered one of the classic childhood exanthems, with the first reported description dating back to the 10th century (17). Derived from the Latin *miser* (meaning miserable) and a diminutive of *morbus*, *morbilli* referred to measles and other minor rashes, while *morbus* applied to the bubonic plague. *Morbilliform* is a synonym for measles-like rashes (3).

Measles is a worldwide disease, most commonly affecting children less than 15 months of age (2) with another peak in the early school age years (3). Disease peaks in March and April, but may occur throughout the winter and spring. Mandatory immunization strategies in the United States since the 1960s have resulted in a more than 99%

reduction in measles, with a record low of 86 confirmed cases in 2000 (17). Most U.S. cases are now generally acquired outside this country and imported due to the ease of international travel. Measles still infects approximately 30 million people in Africa and Asia each year, resulting in 900,000 fatalities annually (3). Because of its public health impact and due to its many imitators, it is important to be familiar with the differentiation of measles from other morbilliform exanthems.

Pathophysiology/Microbiology

The measles virus is a highly contagious RNA paramyxovirus that is spread via respiratory droplet(s). Human beings are the only natural host of infection. Incubation period is 8–12 days, with patients becoming contagious 1–2 days before symptoms and 3–5 days before onset of the rash. Viremia with nasopharyngeal shedding continues up to 4 days after the appearance of the rash (1, 3, 17). The cause for the rash is unclear and is possibly a result of direct viral cytopathic effects on the skin or a result of virus-antibody complex deposition (3).

Clinical Presentation
(see Table 26–1, Fig. 26–5)

Clinical disease first begins with a prodrome of symptoms lasting 1–7 days prior to the onset of the eruption. Fever, malaise, irritability, and the 3 Cs of measles—cough, coryza, and conjunctivitis—are classically seen. Symptoms of infection may increase until the rash has peaked. Fever can reach 105°F, often peaking with the appearance of the rash and then promptly resolving. Patients are often quite tired and irritable, as opposed to the milder rubella infection and other nonspecific viral morbilliform exanthems. Cough, often barking in nature (from source 17) can be quite severe, may persist longer than other symptoms, and may be complicated by pneumonia. Coryza refers to a heavy nasal discharge, as seen with a severe common cold. Lacrimation, photophobia, and lid edema may accompany conjunctivitis; generalized adenopathy may also be seen (2, 3, 17).

The enanthem of measles, the Koplik spots, is pathognomonic for the disease. These typically appear 2 days prior to rash onset and persist for approximately 3 days. Often referred to as "grains of sand on a red background," these 1-mm blue-white papules generally occur on the buccal mucosa opposite the second molars. Similar lesions are occasionally seen on the conjunctiva at the medial canthus and in the large intestine (17). Herman spots

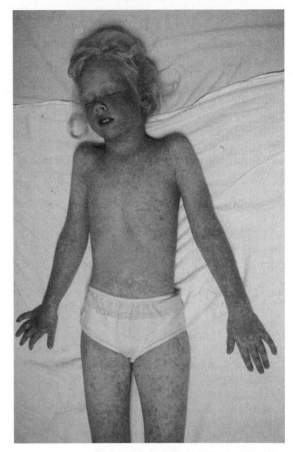

Fig. 26–5. Measles (Peter Rowe, MD, Dermatlas; http://www.dermatlas.org).

are bluish-gray areas on the tonsils which are another, less common, enanthem typical of measles.

The rash of measles consists of erythematous macules and papules initially presenting along the scalp margin and behind the ears. Lesions coalesce quickly, spreading distally and centrifugally, with the eruption involving the entire body by 3 days. The evolution is not unlike someone "pouring" the rash on the scalp with it slowly dripping down the trunk and extremities. Lesions remain most prominent and confluent in the areas initially involved, becoming more discrete and sparse on the extremities. The rash fades in similar fashion to its appearance, generally clearing by 7 days. Fine desquamation and brownish hemosiderin staining may accompany the clearance of the rash.

Complications of measles are varied, including acute otitis media, pneumonia, croup, diarrhea, encephalitis,

ITP, and fetal death with pregnancy. Death may occur in 1–3/1000 childhood cases, predominately from respiratory or neurological complications (1). Secondary bacterial infections should be suspected in patients with prolonged fever or a secondary fever spike (3). Complications are most common in the very young, malnourished, and those with underlying disease such as HIV and tuberculosis. Interestingly, the rash of measles may not appear in the immunocompromised. Subacute sclerosing panencephalitis (SSPE) is a late developing complication characterized by mental and motor deterioration, often with seizures, years after the initial, frequently uneventful, infection. Disease is caused by persistent, defective measles virus, resulting in gradual deterioration over 1–3 years. With immunization, this commonly fatal disease has virtually disappeared; the incidence is approximately 0.1/million in vaccinated children (1, 3).

Two other measles variants of interest include *atypical measles* and *modified measles*. Atypical measles, now of historic interest, was an atypical presentation of rash similar to Rocky Mountain Spotted Fever in patients who received the killed measles vaccine in the 1960s and were subsequently infected with natural measles. Modified measles is a clinically milder form of disease as a result of partial immunity obtained by prior infection, persistence of maternal antibodies, or immunization. This disease may be indistinguishable from other, nonspecific viral exanthems.

Laboratory/Diagnostic Testing (see Table 26–2)

The actual incidence of measles, and its close relative *rubella* (i.e., *German measles* or *3 day measles*), approaches near insignificance in general primary care practice. While the frequency of morbilliform eruptions are quite common, the vast majority of these infections are relatively innocuous, self-limited diseases (19). Since rubeola and rubella are both reportable communicable diseases, it becomes necessary, then, to definitely diagnose any case of suspected measles.

In the evaluation of most morbilliform eruptions, measles can be excluded by a thorough history and physical. The lack of significant prodromal signs or symptoms, a positive measles, mumps and rubella (MMR) immunization history, recent drug exposures, and a careful evaluation of rash progression, distribution and morphology will often quickly rule out measles. A decreased peripheral white blood cell count and lymphopenia that is typically seen in measles may also be helpful (2).

In those situations where the diagnosis is still suspect, acute measles IgM and acute and convalescent IgG titers should be obtained, with follow-up titers obtained in 2–3 weeks. Serum IgM titers, most reliable by enzyme immunoassay (EIA) method, may be negative in the first 72 h and should be repeated if measles is still being considered (1, 20). In suspected cases, definitive diagnosis should also be made by viral isolation. This requires special viral laboratory facilities, which either state public health or CDC labs will process. Viral isolates should be obtained from blood, urine and, nasopharyngeal secretions (1). Immediate notification of state public health agencies is important, and one should not wait for laboratory confirmation in suspected cases.

In cases concerning SSPE, characteristic EEG changes and raised measles antibody in the plasma and CSF will be appreciated (18).

The differential diagnosis for measles (see Table 26–3) includes rubella, scarlet fever, secondary syphilis, enteroviral infections, and drug eruptions. Rubella is a much milder, more rapidly clearing disease. Scarlet fever has its own classic signs and symptoms, and rapid strep testing is generally confirmatory. Many morbilliform eruptions involve the enteroviruses, including echovirus and coxsackie viruses, and are often nonspecific in presentation.

Management

No specific therapy for measles is generally effective, and supportive care is the mainstay in most cases. Rest, hydration, proper nutrition, antipyretics, analgesics, and respiratory isolation are basic aspects of care. Prophylactic antibiotics are not indicated and may predispose the individual to superinfection. Antibiotics should be reserved for those with clinical signs of pneumonia or sepsis (22).

For the very ill or for those at risk of malnutrition, high dose vitamin A (100–200,000 IU/day for 2 days) is recommended (1, 17, 21). These groups may include children 6–24 months old, immunodeficient patients, malnutrition-associated disorders such as cystic fibrosis or inflammatory bowel disease, or recent immigrants from high risk areas. In high risk areas, studies have shown a 36% reduction in mortality with the use of vitamin A (21). Ribavirin, though not clinically proven or FDA approved, has shown in vitro activity against measles and may be considered in severe cases (17).

In exposure or outbreak control, immediate reporting of disease is necessary. Vaccine given 3–5 days after exposure (1) may prevent infection in susceptible persons. For the immunosuppressed and in children less than 1 year of age, serum immune globulin should be given within 6 days of exposure (2, 3).

For SSPE, no treatment has been determined. Oral isoprinosine along with intraventricular interferon alpha appears to be the most effective treatment, with lifelong therapy necessary (18).

Disposition

Routine measles vaccination in the United States has resulted in the near elimination of disease. The two dose immunization schedule will afford greater than 99% of the population life-long immunity (3). While morbilliform exanthems are quite common, the actual incidence of measles is exceedingly rare, and any case truly suspected of measles should be confirmed by laboratory methods and reported to the local public health department. Appropriate knowledge of measles prodrome, enanthem, and exanthem will generally allow a practitioner to disregard, or further pursue, the diagnosis. Recent immigrants without a measles vaccination history should be most suspect. If the infected individual is at risk for malnutrition, high dose vitamin A should be given for therapy.

Some recent reports in the lay press have expressed concern about a possible association between autism and the MMR vaccination. This has resulted in unnecessary fear and rejection of vaccination by some parents. Current scientific evidence does not support the hypothesis of a link between MMR vaccine and autism. No evidence from a number of epidemiologic studies suggest an association, while the evidence against such an association is compelling (23).

Case Outcome

Our patient is diagnosed with probable measles and possible pneumonia. A chest x-ray is ordered, revealing a mild interstitial pattern with no focal infiltrates. Routine labs as well as measles serum IgM and IgG are obtained. The case is reported to the public health department, and an inquiry to verify immune status of all staff members who have had contact with the patient is made. Infectious disease and dermatology are consulted and the patient is admitted into the hospital and placed in respiratory isolation. He is given vitamin A, 200,000 IU in a single oral dose, to be repeated the next day.

REFERENCES

1. Pickering LK (ed.): *Red Book: 2003 Report of the Committee on Infectious Diseases, 26th ed.* Elk Grove Village, IL, American Academy of Pediatrics.
2. Odom RB, James WD, Berger TG, et al.: *Andrew's Diseases of the Skin, 9th ed.* Philadelphia, W.B. Saunders, 2000.
3. Freedberg IM, Eisen AZ, Wolff K, et al.: *Fitzpatrick's Dermatology in General Medicine, 6th ed.* New York, McGraw-Hill, 2003.
4. Boelle PY, Hanslik T: Varicella in non-immune persons: Incidence, hospitalization and mortality rates. *Epidemiol Infect* 129(3):599–606, 2002.
5. Seward JF, Watson BM, Peterson CL, et al.: Varicella disease after introduction of varicella vaccine in the United States, 1995–2000. *JAMA* 287(5):606–611, 2002.
6. Wolverton SE: *Comprehensive Dermatologic Drug Therapy.* Philadelphia, WB Saunders Company, 2001.
7. Orlowski JP, Hanhan UA, Fiallos MR: Is aspirin a cause of Reye's syndrome? A case against. *Drug Saf* 25(4):225–231, 2002.
8. Lesko SM, O'Brien KL, Schwartz B, et al.: Invasive group A streptococcal infection and nonsteroidal anti-inflammatory drug use among children with primary varicella. *Pediatrics* 107(5): 1108–1115, 2001.
9. Klassen T, Belseck E, Wiebe N, et al.: Acyclovir for treating varicella in otherwise healthy children and adolescents. *Cochrane Database Syst Rev* 2:CD002980, 2004.
10. Ampofo K, Saiman L, LaRussa P, et al.: Persistence of immunity to live attenuated varicella vaccine in healthy adults. *Clin Infect Dis* 34(6):774–779, 2002.
11. Kost RG, Straus SE: Postherpetic neuralgia—pathogenesis, treatment, and prevention. *N Engl J Med* 335(1):32–42, 1996.
12. Kramer SC, Chadwick JT, William BT, et al.: Kaposi's varicelliform eruption: A case report and review of the literature. *Cutis* 73:115–122, 2004.
13. Hurwitz S: *Clinical Pediatric Dermatology, 2nd ed.* Philadelphia, W.B. Saunders Company, 1993.
14. Nikkels AF, Pierard GE: Treatment of mucocutaneous presentations of herpes simplex virus infections. *Am J Clin Dermatol* 3(7):475–487, 2002.
15. Amir J: Clinical aspects and antiviral therapy in primary herpetic gingivostomatitis. *Paediatr Drugs* 3(8):593–597, 2001.
16. Kleymann G: New antiviral drugs that target herpesvirus helicase primase enzymes. *Herpes* 10(2):46–52, 2003.
17. Scott LA, Stone MS: Viral exanthems. *Dermatol Online J* 9(3):4, 2004.
18. Garg RK: Subacute sclerosing panencephalitis. *Postgrad Med J* 78(916):63–70, 2002.
19. Vega AT, Gil Costa M, Rodriguez Recio MJ, et al.: Incidence and clinical characteristics of maculopapular exanthems of viral aetiology. *Aten Primaria* 32(9):517–523, 2003.
20. Bellini, WJ, Helfand RF: The challenges and strategies for laboratory diagnosis of measles in an international setting. *J Infect Dis* 187(Suppl. 1): S283–S90, 2003.
21. D'Souza RM, D'Souza R: Vitamin A for the treatment of children with measles—a systematic review. *J Trop Pediatr* 48(6):323–327, 2002.
22. Shann F, D'Souza RM, D'Souza R: Antibiotics for preventing pneumonia in children with measles. *Cochrane Database Syst Rev* (4):CD001477, 2000.
23. Miller E: Measles-mumps-rubella vaccine and the development of autism. *Semin Pediatr Infect Dis* 14(3):199–206, 2003.

Osteomyelitis/infected Prosthetic Devices

Cedric J. Tankson

Peter C. Krause

HIGH YIELD FACTS

1. The principal associated etiologies for osteomyelitis are infection after open fractures, infection after surgery, hematogenous spread, vascular insufficiency, and diabetes mellitus.

2. Bone infections may be acute or chronic. Chronic infections are distinguished by the presence of necrotic bone (sequestrum) which cannot be penetrated by antibiotics.

3. Early osteomyelitis can present without radiographic changes and can sometimes be treated with antibiotics alone.

4. Chronic osteomyelitis can be relapsing and remitting over many years, can be suppressed by antibiotics, and requires surgical resection of the sequestrum to achieve cure.

5. Septic arthritis can occur secondary to osteomyelitis of the metaphysis of bone where the metaphysis is intraarticular, i.e., the proximal humerus, proximal femur, distal tibia, and proximal radius.

CASE PRESENTATION

Case 1

A 7-year-old boy presents with a limp and knee pain of one day duration. There is a history of minor trauma to the knee and a recent upper respiratory tract infection. Past medical history is otherwise negative. On physical exam he is lying on a stretcher and appears comfortable; however, he is unable to bear weight, complaining of pain in the proximal tibia. His temperature is 37.5°C. There is minimal swelling in the extremity. There is no knee joint effusion and the knee joint is nontender. Range of motion is full although he is reluctant to move. There is a small area on the proximal tibia which is exquisitely tender and slightly erythematous. There is no palpable fluctuance. Radiographs are negative. His white blood cell count (WBC) is 8700/mm³ (normal: 4000–10,000/mm³), his erythrocyte sedimentation rate (ESR) is 60 mm/h (normal: 0–15 mm/h), and his C-reactive protein (CRP) is 6.8 (normal: <0.80 mg/dL).

Case 2

A 50-year-old man underwent total knee arthroplasty 6 months earlier. He has had minor discomfort in the knee since the time of surgery. He now presents with delirium and pain and swelling in the knee of 1 day duration. Past medical history is significant for diabetes mellitus and obesity. On physical exam he appears ill and is confused. His temperature is 38.5°C, his pulse is 110, and his BP is 100/70. The knee is swollen and there is a tense effusion. The surgical wound appears well healed but there is mild erythema present. The knee is held at about 10° of flexion and he is unable to flex or extend the knee. There is diffuse tenderness of the knee to palpation. Radiographs reveal a well-positioned knee replacement and an effusion but are otherwise negative. His WBC is 16,000/mm³, his ESR 90 mm/h, and his C-reactive protein is 15 mg/dL.

INTRODUCTION/EPIDEMIOLOGY

Osteomyelitis has been reported since ancient Egypt, but before the modern medical era both bone infections and open fractures were frequently fatal conditions (1). During World War I, gunshot wounds to the femur had a mortality rate of 80%. Similarly, before the introduction of penicillin in 1944, acute hematogenous osteomyelitis had a mortality rate as high as 45%. Today the mortality rate is dramatically less, i.e., probably less than 1% (2, 3). With the development of antibiotics and refinement of surgical and anesthetic techniques, the treatment of deep infections of the bone has become much more sophisticated and successful. Conversely, a greater number of invasive surgical techniques, such as total joint arthroplasty, have resulted in many more serious infections, and an increased incidence of high-speed motor vehicle accidents has led to more traumatic infections. In addition, osteomyelitis has also become a frequent late complication of diabetes mellitus and peripheral vascular disease. The spectrum of osteomyelitis and prosthetic-related infections encompasses an enormous range of conditions complicated and difficult to treat, which are defined by their mode of spread (hematogenous, traumatic, surgical, or contiguous extension), by their chronicity, by the patient's age (pediatric versus adult), and by the local and systematic characteristics of the host.

PATHOPHYSIOLOGY/MICROBIOLOGY

Osteomyelitis is a consequence of a bacterial inoculum (direct or hematogenous) in the setting of traumatized, ischemic, or devitalized tissues. The condition of the local soft tissue environment is the critical factor. Bacteria are always present in contaminated wounds and often in surgical wounds, but infection does not invariably follow. This combination of circumstances (i.e., devitalized tissue and a bacterial inoculum) can occur in open fractures and in clean surgical procedures especially when a large quantity of material is implanted, such as a total joint. The local soft tissue environment also predisposes patients with vascular insufficiency and diabetes mellitus to infection. The diabetic patient often has poor circulation, poor host immune defenses, and a sensory neuropathy. Minor neglected foot wounds with consequent deep infection can frequently ensue.

After initial contamination occurs, infection can only develop if bacteria successfully adhere to either bone or implanted material. This occurs via weak attractive forces that depend on the type of surface as well as the kind of material; for example, smooth surfaces are more resistant than porous ones and titanium is more resistant than stainless steel (4). Adhesion also occurs via special proteins called adhesins, which are specific for the different components of bone (e.g., fibronectin, laminin, and collagen) and expressed by many bacteria. After initial adhesion, bacteria create a glycocalyx biofilm on the surface of implants (also known as a "slime" layer) which encases bacteria, promotes bacterial nutrition, and interferes with the host immune response. Once the slime layer develops, eradication of the bacteria becomes more difficult (5). The bacterial infection and the host inflammatory response disrupt the periosteal vascular supply producing local tissue and bone necrosis. The dysvascular environment subsequently makes the host inflammatory response ineffective and provides a conducive environment for persistent bacterial growth.

Acute pediatric hematogenous osteomyelitis occurs by a somewhat different mechanism. The ends of the long bones are areas of rapid growth and increased vascularity. As the vessels make sharp angles near the growth plate (the physis), there is sludging of blood which predisposes to thrombosis and bacterial seeding. This thrombosis is accompanied by a suppression of the recruit-

ment of macrophages to fight infection (6). The infection starts in the metaphyseal venous sinusoids, where there is a change from high flow arterioles to low flow venous sinusoids. If the infection is left untreated, it will eventually track through the porous metaphyseal cortical surface and elevate surrounding periosteum. If the metaphysis is intraarticular (proximal humerus, proximal femur, proximal radius), infection may result in a concurrent septic arthritis. The elevated periosteum produces new bone known as involucrum and the original cortex, stripped of its blood supply, becomes a sequestrum.

The microbiology of osteomyelitis varies. Chronic osteomyelitis is frequently polymicrobial, but the most commonly involved organism in both chronic and acute disease is *Staphylococcus aureus*. *Staphylococcus epidermidis*, which was once thought of as commensal skin organism, is also a common pathogen (7). Other specific organisms are thought to be more common in specific hosts, such as *Pseudomonas aeruginosa* in IV drug users and anaerobes in diabetics. Infections that occur after open fractures contaminated by soil are at risk for *Clostridium* species. Aeromonas and Pseudomonas infections can occur after fresh water wounds. Acute infection after total joint arthroplasty is most often due to *S. aureus*, but late infection is commonly due to *S. epidermidis*. Gram-negative and mixed bacterial infections are less common, but may be more difficult to treat (8, 9).

The most common organisms in cases of hematogenous osteomyelitis are *S. aureus*, *Streptococcus pneumoniae*, and *Haemophilus influenzae* type B. However, *Haemophilus influenza* type B has become less common since the widespread implementation of specific immunization against this organism (10). Both group B streptococcus and *Escherichia coli* are common causative organisms in neonatal osteomyelitis. Children with sickle cell disease are at increased risk of bacterial infections, especially *Salmonella* species. Other common pathogens in sickle cell patients are *S. aureus*, *Serratia* species, and *Proteus mirabilis* (11).

Infections by gram-negative bacteria such as *P. aeruginosa* or *E. coli* occur after puncture wounds to the feet or open injuries involving bone. Anaerobes can also lead to infection especially after human or animal bites. Rarer causes of osteomyelitis include fungal organisms, such as *Candida* species, *Aspergillus* species, and *Coccidioides immitis*, all seen more often in immunocompromised hosts. Lastly, infections secondary to *Brucella* species, *Mycobacterium tuberculosis*, and *Bartonella henselae* are seen more frequently in patients with AIDS.

CLINICAL PRESENTATION

The history and physical exam are the most important factors in determining the diagnosis of osteomyelitis. Initial symptoms can range from malaise and low grade fever to severe constitutional symptoms and high grade fever. Not all patients with osteomyelitis present with an acute severe illness. Many of the signs and symptoms are the same as in cellulitis, thus creating a source of confusion (for a differential diagnosis see Tables 27-1 and 27-2).

In acute hematogenous osteomyelitis there is a history of another recent or current infection elsewhere in one-third to one-half of the patients. Neonates tend to have a very nonspecific exam and pseudoparalysis of the limb may be the only initial finding. Children may present with a limp or refuse to bear weight on the affected extremity. Some young patients appear restless secondary to futile attempts to relieve their pain by changing positions. In their series of children with acute hematogenous osteomyelitis, Scott et al. (12) demonstrated that 36% of the children had an admission temperature less than 37.5°C and 47% had a WBC less than 10,500/mm^3 (12). Physical examination often reveals restriction of motion and swelling of the extremity. Usually there is point tenderness at the nidus of the infection, but there is no true joint irritability unless there is a concurrent septic arthritis. The adult presentation of hematogenous osteomyelitis is rare, but most commonly occurs in the spine, and typically appears in intravenous drug users, immunocompromised patients, or patients who have had recent urinary tract manipulation.

Table 27–1. Differential Diagnosis for Pediatric Osteomyelitis

Cellulitis

Soft tissue abscess
Septic arthritis
Inflammatory arthritis
Fracture
Benign tumor of bone (especially eosinophilic granuloma)
Malignant tumor of bone (especially Ewing sarcoma)
Leukemia
Diskitis
Aseptic bone necrosis
Slipped capital femoral epiphysis
Legg-Perthes disease
Rheumatic fever

Table 27–2. Differential Diagnosis for Adult Osteomyelitis

Cellulitis
Soft tissue abscess
Septic arthritis
Inflammatory arthritis
Fracture
Charcot arthropathy (neuropathic arthropathy)
  • Diabetes mellitus
  • Syringomelia (shoulder arthropathy is classic)
  • Syphilis
Benign or Malignant tumor of bone
Skin cancer
Metastatic cancer
Soft tissue sarcoma

In chronic osteomyelitis there may be a history of chronic intermittent drainage or a history of a previous infection at the site which appeared to resolve with antibiotics. A draining sinus should definitely arouse suspicion of a deep infection when associated with previous internal fixation (Fig. 27-1). Diabetics most often present with chronic foot wounds associated with drainage. These patients usually have sensory neuropathies and these wounds can be related to poorly fitting shoe wear. Confusion sometimes arises because these patients are also at risk for developing neuropathic arthropathies of the foot (known as Charcot arthropathy). Patients with acute Charcot changes can have feet that appear infected, radiographs that show destructive changes, and other studies (nuclear, CT, and MRI) that can be equivocally interpreted. Sometimes only a bone biopsy can verify the diagnosis.

Another potential pitfall when evaluating a chronic wound is the possibility of missing a scar carcinoma, also known as a Marjolin ulcer. A Marjolin ulcer is an aggressive neoplasm that occurs when a chronic wound, such as a sinus, burn, fistula, or pressure sore, undergoes malignant transformation, most often becoming a squamous cell carcinoma. This underscores the importance of the surgical pathology specimen whenever treating a patient with chronic osteomyelitis.

Infections involving orthopedic hardware, including total joint replacements, can have an extremely variable presentation, ranging from fulminant sepsis to chronic indolent infections (Figs. 27-2 and 27-3). Chronic infections are sometimes difficult to differentiate from hardware failure for other reasons, such as aseptic loosening. In the case of joint arthroplasty, septic failure is said to be associated with constant pain while aseptic

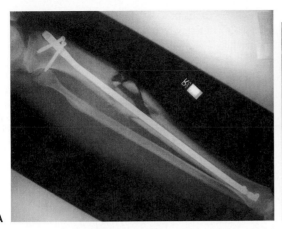

A

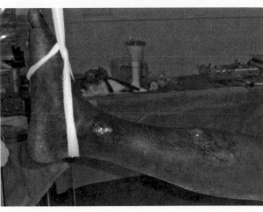

B

Fig. 27–1. Open tibia fracture treated with intramedullary nail now with chronic osteomyelitis. The bony fragments seen anteriorly on the lateral radiograph (*A*) were likely devitalized at the time of injury and now may be a source of persistent infection.

Clinical photographs (*B*) of the leg show multiple draining sinuses. Treatment consisted of multiple debridements, placement of antibiotic beads, intravenous antibiotics, and stabilization with an external fixator.

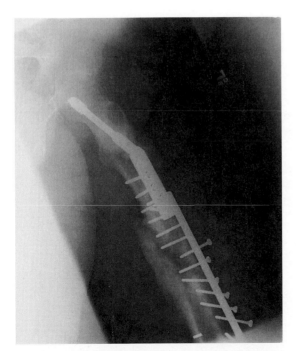

Fig. 27–2. Infected total hip replacement with loose acetabular component. This patient had an acetabular fracture that resulted in arthritis and was treated by arthroplasty. Loosening of components, especially early loosening, raises the possibility of infection.

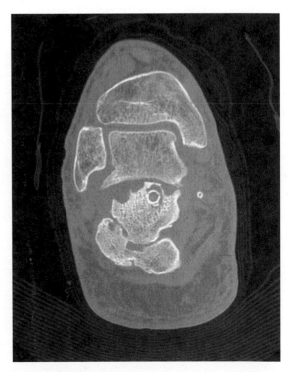

Fig. 27–3. Infected total knee arthroplasty with loose tibial component. Note erosion of proximal tibial bone, again suggestive of infection.

loosening is worse with load bearing. Total joint infections can also occur via late hematogenous seeding, and therefore routine antibiotic prophylaxis is recommended for high-risk patients (patient during the first 2 years after total joint replacement, immunocompromised patients, and patients with significant other comorbidities) before dental and genitourinary procedures that produce bacteremia (13, 14).

LABORATORY/DIAGNOSTIC TESTING

Diagnostic tests for osteomyelitis include laboratory data, diagnostic imaging studies, and tissue specimens. Laboratory tests alone cannot establish the diagnosis. A normal peripheral white blood cell count has been reported in as many as 75% of patients and a normal polymorphonuclear cell count in 35% of patients. The ESR is elevated in the majority of patients. However, it is a less reliable indicator of infection in neonates with osteomyelitis, patients with sickle cell anemia, and patients taking steroids. Of note, an elevated ESR is also only about 60% sensi-

tive in the evaluation of infected total joints. Typically, the ESR rises slowly and peaks at 3–5 days and begins to decline 1–2 weeks after initiation of therapy. The C-reactive protein level rises rapidly and peaks in 2 days, and then begins to decline within 6 h after therapy has been started. The CRP is therefore, theoretically, a better indicator of the effectiveness of therapy and predicting recovery from osteomyelitis than either the WBC or ESR (15). Blood cultures in the setting of acute hematogenous osteomyelitis are positive in approximately 40–50% of cases (16).

Plain radiographs may demonstrate displacement of muscle planes within 3 to 5 days of infection onset. Bony changes on plain films—usually not evident until 7 to 14 days—consist of periosteal reaction or new bone formation at the outer cortex (Fig. 27-4). When plain radiographs are negative, the nuclear bone scan is a useful modality. A bone scan may detect bone involvement as early as 2 to 3 days after infection has begun. These studies are especially helpful in identifying sites of involvement in the pelvis or spine, and are also useful in looking for multiple sites of involvement, such as in hematogenously

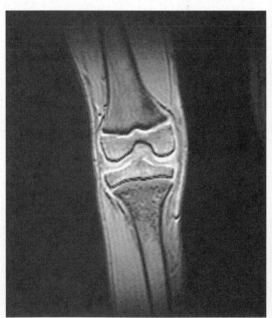
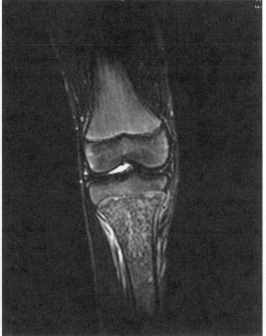

A **B**

Fig. 27–4. Chronic infection and nonunion after plating of an open femur fracture. Hardware is loose and there is abundant periosteal new bone formation, both typical of infection. Treatment consisted of debridements until the wound was clean and then repeat plating with an autologous bone graft.

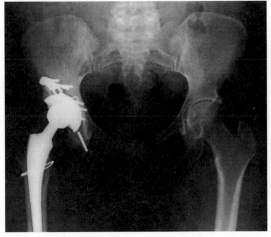

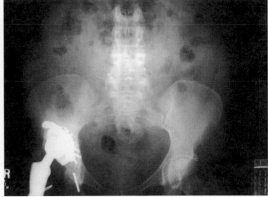

A

B

Fig. 27–5. Calcaneal osteomyelitis after percutaneous fixation of a closed fracture with a large pin left out of the skin. Thermal necrosis of bone from drilling has resulted in a ring sequestrum around the path of the pin, best shown on the CT scan. This sequestrum needed to be removed in order to control the infection.

derived infections. Technetium-labeled bone scans may, however, be misleading in the early stage of infection or after recent bony surgery or trauma. In the setting of total joint replacements, bone scans may not be able to differentiate loosening from infection. Adding the indium-111 white blood cell scan can increase the sensitivity and specificity for infection in both chronic osteomyelitis and the infected total joint arthroplasty (17, 18).

Computed tomography is not very helpful in the early stages of osteomyelitis. As the disease progresses, CT scans can help delineate the extent of cortical destruction, extraarticular abscesses, and bony sequestration (Fig. 27-5). MRI is very sensitive, but not specific for osteomyelitis. Changes associated with osteomyelitis can be detected as early as 3 to 5 days, although abnormal MRI signal changes can be difficult to distinguish from a fracture or bone infarct. Typically, on MRI there is an area of abnormal marrow with decreased signal intensity on T1 weighted images and increased signal intensity on T2 weighted images (Fig. 27-6). The addition of gadolinium intravenous contrast can help define areas of necrosis. Ultrasonography is also being used more often to detect subperiosteal abscesses in symptomatic children, although caution is recommended since this modality is operator-dependent. Characteristic findings include thickening of periosteum with both superficial and deep hypoechogenic zones. When the periosteum is elevated by 2 mm, a purulent fluid collection is usually visible (19).

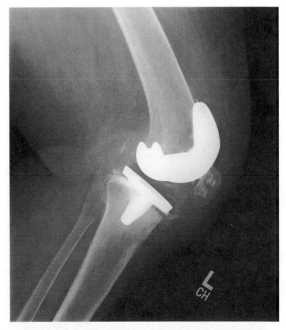

Fig. 27–6. MRI of proximal tibial osteomyelitis in a child. This study shows bone edema in the metaphysis, which is dark on T1 and bright on T2, a finding that is suggestive but not specific for the diagnosis of osteomyelitis.

Sampling of infected tissue is considered the gold standard for diagnosis. Aspiration in acute osteomyelitis is important in determining the causative organism and guiding therapy. Diagnostic aspiration of a possibly infected total joint arthroplasty is commonly done, but remains very low-yield unless infection is strongly suspected. Needle biopsy in the setting of chronic osteomyelitis has a high false-negative rate. Sinus and wound cultures will routinely miss organisms in what are usually polymicrobial infections and thus operative cultures are considered the gold standard (20, 21).

MANAGEMENT

Acute Hematogenous Osteomyelitis

Aspiration with either a core biopsy needle or a spinal trocar needle is an important diagnostic tool in the initial evaluation of a patient with suspected osteomyelitis. The needle is usually directed to the area of maximal tenderness. In inaccessible locations, CT-guided aspiration is recommended. Empiric antibiotics are begun and then adjusted according to culture results. Historically, the most common organism is methicillin-sensitive *S. aureus* and oxacillin is the preferred treatment. Clindamycin or vancomycin may be used when patients are allergic to penicillin. Vancomycin is used for infections caused by methicillin-resistant *S. aureus*. Antibiotics are initially administered parenterally. The duration and route of antibiotic administration is still controversial. Although animal studies and retrospective studies support current practice, randomized studies are lacking. Adults are usually treated with 4–6 weeks of intravenous antibiotics. Children are usually treated with 3 weeks of intravenous pathogen-directed antibiotics followed by 3 weeks of oral antibiotics. Patients are not switched to oral antibiotics until a clinical response to treatment has been seen and appropriate organism sensitivities are known. The patient's temperature, clinical picture, and CRP can be used to follow the response to antibiotics and determine the duration of therapy (for antibiotic therapy see Table 27-3).

Surgery is indicated in children with subperiosteal or soft tissue abscesses, intramedullary purulence, sequestra, pyogenic arthritis, or avascular bone. At the time of surgery, the abscess should be drained, the periosteum incised, and all devascularized bone removed. Primary bone cultures should be taken during the procedure. Persistent fever and pain after surgical drainage may indicate inadequate drainage and repeat drainage should be considered.

The adult patient with hematogenous osteomyelitis of the spine is usually managed with bacteria-specific antibiotics. A CT scan is used to obtain a diagnostic percutaneous biopsy. Surgery is indicated for patients with spinal instability, neurologic deficits requiring decompression, and abscess formation. Nonoperative treatment is more likely to be successful in immunocompetent patients younger than 60 years with decreasing erythrocyte sedimentation rates during the first month of treatment (22).

Chronic Osteomyelitis

The management of chronic osteomyelitis is dictated by both local disease and host factors. If the host is significantly compromised to the point where the treatment would be more debilitating or dangerous than the disease, chronic suppressive antibiotic therapy or amputation is chosen. If cure is planned, a thorough debridement is performed based on the location of the infection, which may be cortical, intramedullary, or involving a segment of bone or a bony nonunion. In addition, any associated hardware is usually removed. If the bone is unstable or destabilized by the debridement, then external fixation is usually applied. The wound may be managed with delayed primary closure, but frequently a muscle flap is required. Dead space can be filled with beads made from bone cement and antibiotics. When the soft tissue envelope has healed, the beads are then exchanged for autologous bone graft. Organism-specific antibiotics are given intravenously for 4–6 weeks. Using this method, Cierny and others have reported success rates between 80 and 100 percent (23, 24). Two other techniques for managing the soft tissue are used. One is the technique of Ilizarov which may be used to transport both bone and soft tissue to close down an open wound as well as an underlying bone deficit (25). The other technique was described by Papineau and consists of open wound care to allow granulation and then repeated open autologous bone grafting on top of the granulation tissue. Both of these two techniques are less well tolerated by patients than muscle flap coverage; in addition, the Papineau technique appears to produce inferior results (26, 27).

Infected Orthopedic Hardware/Total Joint Replacement

Infected total joint replacements and infected fracture fixation are usually best managed surgically if the patient can tolerate surgery. If a total joint infection occurs in the early postoperative period (i.e., less than 1 month),

Table 27–3. Antibiotic Therapy for Osteomyelitis in Adults

Organism Cultured	Treatment (Based on Antibiotic Susceptibility)	Alternative (Based on Antibiotic Susceptibility)
Methicillin-sensitive *S. aureus*	Nafcillin, 2 g IV q4	Cefazolin, vancomycin, clindamycin
Methicillin-resistant *S. aureus*	Vancomycin, 1 g IV q12 h	Infectious diseases consultation; linezolid, minocycline with or without rifampin, quinupristin/dalfopristin, daptomycin, trimethoprim/sulfamethoxazole
Coagulase-negative *Staphylococcus* species	Vancomycin, 1 g IV q12 h	Infectious diseases consultation; trimethoprim-sulfamethoxazole or minocycline with or without rifampin, clindamycin, linezolid
Streptococcus pyogenes	Penicillin G, 3–4 million U IV q4 h (20 million U total daily)	Clindamycin, cefazolin, vancomycin, erythromycin
Streptococcus agalactiae	Penicillin G, 3–4 million U IV q4 h (20 million U total daily)	Cefazolin, ceftriaxone, vancomycin, clindamycin
S. pneumoniae	Penicillin G, 3–4 million U IV q4 (20 million U total daily); ceftriaxone, 2 g IV q24 h; vancomycin, 1 g IV q12 h; levofloxacin, 750 mg IV/po q24 h	Clindamycin, erythromycin
Enterococcus species	Ampicillin, 2 g IV q4 h or vancomycin 1 g IV q12 h and consider initial addition of gentamicin for up to 2 weeks	Infectious diseases consultation; ampicillin-sulbactam, linezolid
Vancomycin-resistant *Enterococcus faecium*	Infectious diseases consultation; quinupristin/dalfopristin, 7.5 mg/kg IV q8 h or linezolid, 600 mg IV/po q12 h	Infectious diseases consultation
Enterobacteriaceae (gram-negative enteric rods)	Ceftriaxone, 2 g IV q 24 h or ciprofloxacin, 750 mg po/IV q 24 h	Cefepime
P. aeruginosa	Cefepime, 2 g IV q12 h or piperacillin, 3 g IV q4 h or ceftazidime, 2 g IV q8 h plus an aminoglycoside for at least 2 weeks	Ciprofloxacin or imipenem plus an aminoglycoside for at least 2 weeks
Anaerobes	Clindamycin, 900 mg IV q8 h	Ampicillin-sulbactam, metronidazole, ticarcillin-clavulanic acid, piperacillin-tazobactam, cefotetan, penicillin G

Sources: Lew DP, Waldvogel: Osteomyelitis. *Lancet* 364:369–379, 2004. Mader JT, Wang J, Calhoun JH: Antibiotic therapy for musculoskeletal infections. *J Bone Joint Surg Am* 83:1878–1890, 2001. Gilbert DN, Moellering RC, Eliopoulos GM, Sande MA: *The Sanford Guide to Antimicrobial Therapy, 34th ed.* Hyde Park, VT, Antimicrobial Therapy, Inc., 2004. Osmon DR, Steckelberg JM: Osteomyelitis, infectious arthritis, and prosthetic joint infection, in Wilson WR, Sande MA (eds.): *Current Diagnosis and Treatment in Infectious Diseases.* Stamford, CT, Appleton and Lange 2001; pp 669–679.

some evidence exists that debridement, retention of the components, and intravenous antibiotic therapy may be successful. If the total joint infection is chronic, however, a two-stage revision is usually recommended. First, the old components and cement are removed, and the joint is thoroughly debrided. Then appropriate intravenous antibiotic therapy is given for 6 weeks and a reimplantation procedure is performed when the wound has healed and laboratory indices of infection have decreased. Successful outcomes are reported using this approach in about 80% of hip and knee infections. One-stage revision—in which the old components are removed, a debridement is performed, and new components are placed all at once—has a success rate that is somewhat less although the data appear somewhat variable. Older reports suggested that gram-negative infections may be more difficult to treat, although this is now disputed. Other options for treatment include chronic suppressive antibiotics, resection arthroplasty, fusion, and amputation (28,29,30). Retention of components versus removal in the case of fracture fixation is controversial and depends on the status of fracture healing, the fracture location, and the virulence of the infection.

DISPOSITION

Acute orthopedic infections should be managed aggressively to avoid chronic deep infections. Although acute hematogenous osteomyelitis can often be managed with antibiotics alone, acute hardware-associated infections usually require surgical debridement. Orthopedic consultation should be obtained when these patients are initially evaluated in the emergency department.

Chronic orthopedic infections, in the absence of systemic illness such as sepsis, should be managed on a more elective basis. Prior to surgery, all appropriate preoperative studies should be performed to delineate the extent of the infection. If systemic illness occurs, the patient should be resuscitated and the initial surgery should be designed to decompress the infection.

CASE OUTCOME

Case 1

Acute osteomyelitis was initially suspected in the case of the child with tender metaphysis. The negative radiographs suggested an early infection. Aspiration at the area of maximal tenderness produced scant purulent fluid that represented a subperiosteal abscess. Gram stain showed gram-positive cocci in clusters. Empiric clindamycin was started to cover *S. aureus*, which was confirmed by subsequent culture. An MRI demonstrated tibial metaphyseal edema consistent with osteomyelitis. Symptoms in this child failed to resolve although the organism was sensitive to clindamycin and repeat radiographs showed a lucent area in the metaphysis. Surgical debridement of cortical and medullary bone guided by the radiographs was performed and purulent material was drained. Symptoms resolved over several days and the CRP began to decrease. Oral antibiotics were initiated after 3 weeks of intravenous antibiotics and the child was discharged home.

Case 2

The patient's high temperature, tachycardia, and hypotension suggested sepsis. Knee joint aspiration revealed purulent fluid with gram-positive cocci in clusters. Blood cultures also revealed gram-positive cocci. Empiric intravenous vancomycin therapy was started for presumptive methicillin-resistant *S. aureus*. Surgical debridement of the knee was performed after hemodynamic stabilization. Consideration was given to acute amputation, but the patient responded to treatment. The total knee was removed and replaced with an antibiotic impregnated cement spacer. Intravenous antibiotics were continued for 6 weeks and the ESR returned to near normal. Options at this point included placing a new total knee or knee fusion. The patient elected to have a knee fusion which was performed successfully.

REFERENCES

1. Holtom PD, Smith AM: Introduction to adult posttraumatic osteomyelitis of the tibia. *Clin Orthop* 360:6–13, 1999.
2. Gilmour WN: Acute haematogenous osteomyelitis. *J Bone Joint Surg Br* 44:841–853, 1962.
3. McHenry MC, Alfidi RJ, Wilde AH, et al.: Hematogenous osteomyelitis: A changing disease. *Cleve Clin Q* 42:125–153, 1975.
4. Schmidt AH, Swiontkowski MF: Pathophysiology of infections after internal fixation of fractures. *J Am Acad Orthop Surg* 8:285–291, 2000.
5. Gristina AG, Costertom JW, Webb LX: Microbial adhesion, biofilms, and the pathophysiology of osteomyelitis, in D'Ambrosia RD, Marier RL (eds.): *Orthopaedic Infections.* Thorofare NJ, SLACK, 1989; pp 49–69.
6. Green NE, Edwards K: Bone and joint infections in children. *Orthop Clin North Am* 18(4):555–576, 1987.
7. Cierny G, Mader T: Adult chronic osteomyelitis: An overview, in D'Ambrosia RD, Marier RL (eds.):

Orthopaedic Infections. Thorofare NJ, SLACK, 1989; pp 31–47.

8. Gustilo RB, Leagogo LAC: Management of infected total hip replacement, in Gustilo RB, Gruninger RP, Tsukayama DT (eds.): *Orthopaedic Infections: Diagnosis and Treatment*. Philadelphia, W. B. Saunders, 1989; pp 224–233.

9. Gustilo RB: Management of infected total knee replacement, in Gustilo RB, Gruninger RP, Tsukayama DT (eds.): *Orthopaedic Infections: Diagnosis and Treatment*. Philadelphia, W. B. Saunders, 1989; pp 234–242.

10. Howard AW, Viskontas D, Sabbagh C: Reduction in osteomyelitis and septic arthritis related to *Haemophilus influenzae* type B vaccination. *J Pediatr Orthop* 19:705–709, 1999.

11. Epps CH Jr., Bryant DD III, Coles MJ, et al.: Chronic osteomyelitis in patients who have sickle-cell disease: Diagnosis and management. *J Bone Joint Surg* 73-A:1281–1294, 1991.

12. Scott RJ, Christofersen MR, Robertson WW Jr., et al.: Acute osteomyelitis in children: A review of 116 cases. *J Pediatr Orthop* 10:649–652, 1990.

13. American Academy of Orthopaedic Surgeons. Advisory Statement: Antibiotic prophylaxis for urological patients with total joint replacements. December 2002.

14. American Academy of Orthopaedic Surgeons. Advisory Statement: Antibiotic prophylaxis for dental patients with total joint replacements. September 2003.

15. Unkila-Kallio L, Kallio MJT, Eskola J, et al.: Serum C-reactive protein, erythrocyte sedimentation rate, and white blood cell count in acute hematogenous osteomyelitis of children. *Pediatrics* 93:59–62, 1994.

16. Fink CW, Nelson JD: Septic arthritis and osteomyelitis in children. *Clin Rheum Dis* 12:423–435, 1986.

17. Hanssen AD, Rand JA: Evaluation and treatment of infection at the site of a total hip or knee arthroplasty. *J Bone Joint Surg Am* 80:910–922, 1998.

18. Nepola JV, Seabold JE, Marsh JL, et al.: Diagnosis of infection in ununited fractures. Combined imaging with indium-111-labeled leukocytes and technetium-99m methylene diphosphonate. *J Bone Joint Surg Am* 75:1816–1822, 1993.

19. Kaiser S, Jorulf H, Hirsch G: Clinical value of imaging techniques in childhood osteomyelitis. *Acta Radiol* 39:523–531, 1998.

20. Perry CR, Pearson RL, Miller GA.: Accuracy of cultures of material from swabbing of the superficial aspect of the wound and needle biopsy in the preoperative assessment of osteomyelitis. *J Bone Joint Surg Am* 73:745–749, 1991.

21. Patzakis MJ, Wilkins J, Kumar J, et al.: Comparison of the results of bacterial cultures from multiple sites in chronic osteomyelitis of long bones. A prospective study. *J Bone Joint Surg Am* 76:664–666, 1994.

22. Carragee EJ: Pyogenic vertebral osteomyelitis. *J Bone Joint Surg Am* 79:874–880, 1997.

23. Kelly PJ, Fitzgerald RH Jr., Cabanela ME, et al.: Results of treatment of tibial and femoral osteomyelitis in adults. *Clin Orthop* 259:295–303, 1990.

24. Patzakis MJ, Mazur K, Wilkins J, Sherman R, Holtom P: Septopal beads and autogenous bone grafting for bone defects in patients with chronic osteomyelitis. *Clin Orthop* 295:112–118, 1993.

25. Paley D, Maar DC: Ilizarov bone transport treatment for tibial defects. *J Orthop Trauma* 14:76–85, 2000.

26. Koval KJ, Meadows SE, Rosen H, Silver L, Zuckerman JD: Posttraumatic tibial osteomyelitis: A comparison of three treatment approaches. *Orthopedics* 15:455–460, 1992.

27. Esterhai JL Jr., Sennett B, Gelb H et al.: Treatment of chronic osteomyelitis complicating nonunion and segmental defects of the tibia with open cancellous bone graft, posterolateral bone graft, and soft-tissue transfer. *J Trauma* 30:49–54, 1990.

28. Masterson, EL, Masri, BA, Duncan, CP: Treatment of infection at the site of total hip replacement. *J Bone Joint Surg Am* 79:1740–1749, 1997.

29. Haleem AA, Berry DJ, Hanssen AD: Mid-term to long-term followup of two-stage reimplantation for infected total knee arthroplasty. *Clin Orthop* 428:35–39, 2004.

30. Tsukayama DT, Goldberg VM, Kyle R: Diagnosis and management of infection after total knee arthroplasty. *J Bone Joint Surg Am* 85-A(Suppl. 1):S75–S80, 2003.

28

Septic Arthritis

Javier Marquez
Liliana Candia
Luis R. Espinoza

SEPTIC ARTHRITIS

High Yield Facts

- When a joint effusion is present, arthrocentesis of the affected joint is mandatory especially in children.

- Both blood and synovial cultures should be obtained before initiation of antibiotics.

- Coexistence of septic arthritis and crystal-induced arthritis is relatively common; therefore, a search for crystals in synovial fluid should always be done.

- One should always try to identify risk factors for septic arthritis, that is, diabetes, trauma, previous arthritis.

- Septic arthritis, especially in children, constitutes a medical emergency which requires prompt recognition and institution of appropriate antibiotic therapy.

Representative Case History

A 38-year-old woman with diabetes mellitus presents with severe pain in her right knee that awakened her from sleep that morning. She had been in her usual state of health until 2 days earlier when she accidentally fell down the stairs and excoriated both knees. Malaise, low grade fever, and chills developed the evening before. Past medical history included insulin-dependent diabetes mellitus since age 16, and her most recent glycosylated hemoglobin had been markedly elevated.

She had difficulty ambulating because of knee pain. Her vital signs included temperature 101°F, pulse 98 beats per minute, and blood pressure 145/94 mmHg. She was diaphoretic, and two small abrasions were noted over each knee. Examination of chest, eyes, cardiovascular, abdomen, genitourinary, and central nervous systems was unremarkable. Her right knee, however, was swollen, erythematous, warm, and diffusely tender to palpation. Both active and passive flexion and extension were limited by pain.

Introduction

Musculoskeletal disorders including septic arthritis have a significant impact on health care. Musculoskeletal disorders account for 30% of all physician visits in the United States and its direct and indirect costs related to treatment and complications, including loss of resources and productivity, represent 2.5% of the gross national product (1). Septic arthritis represents a medical emergency and the clinician dealing with an afflicted individual should try to establish an early diagnosis based on a focused history and physical exam, joint aspiration in the presence of joint effusion, and pertinent laboratory tests including radiographs of involved joint(s), complete blood count with differential, and Gram stain and culture of both peripheral blood and synovial fluid.

The term septic arthritis refers to all joint infections caused by pyogenic bacteria and encompasses the terms pyogenic arthritis, suppurative arthritis, purulent arthritis, pyarthrosis, or infectious arthritis. The inflammatory response is seen in the synovium and the destructive effects are manifested on articular cartilage. Septic arthritis can lead to rapid joint destruction and irreversible loss of function. *Neisseria gonorrhoeae* infection is the most common cause of septic arthritis in the United States and is identified in approximately one half of human sexually acquired infections. In addition the gram-positive cocci of the Micrococcaceae and Streptococcaceae families cause most cases (50–90%) of nongonococcal bacterial arthritis. Septic arthritis remains a relevant issue in clinical medicine, and despite significant advances in diagnostic approaches and the development of newer and more powerful antibiotics over the past 20 years, its impact in terms of human morbidity and mortality remains unchanged (2).

EPIDEMIOLOGY

Incidence

The overall incidence of septic arthritis is about 6–10 cases per 100,000 population per year. Interestingly, in one study Gupta et al (3) found an annual incidence of culture-proven septic arthritis of 1 in 62,500 people. Their findings were part of a multicenter study incorporating 11 teaching and district general hospitals serving a combined population of 2.3 million people in the central belt of Scotland. The incidence is higher in warm and humid geographic areas and is probably also related to socioeconomic conditions (4). The incidence is age dependent, with the highest incidence observed under 15 and over 55 years of age. About one-third of the patients are under the age of 2 years, and half are under 3 years. Under the age of 3 months, however, the incidence is low. Men are affected more often than women. Patients with rheumatoid arthritis and patients with joint prostheses have a higher incidence of septic arthritis. Actually it has been reported to be 30–70 cases per 100,000 persons per year. Improvement in surgical procedures and antibiotic prophylaxis has led to a reduction in the infection rate to less than 0.5% in hip surgery and 1% in knee prosthetic surgery (5, 6).

Pathogenesis

Bacteria or other infectious agents may reach the joint from a remote focus via the hematogenous route. These foci are usually abscesses or infected wounds in the skin, infections in the teeth, upper or lower respiratory tract infections, or endocarditis. In small children, a second potential route is dissemination of bacteria from an acute osteomyelitic focus in the bone metaphysis or epiphysis. A third potential pathway of septic arthritis is from an infection in the vicinity of the joint with progression or spread via the lymphatic route.

The synovium is an extremely vascular tissue and contains no limiting basement membrane, thus promoting easy access of blood contents to the synovial space. Certain bacteria, such as *N. gonorrhoeae, Staphylococcus aureus,* and *Streptococcus pneumoniae,* are particularly prone to infecting a joint during a bacteremic episode. In addition, pneumonia, urinary tract infection, or skin infection are common extraarticular foci of infection causing seeding of a joint. Within hours of entering the closed joint space, bacteria trigger an acute inflammatory synovitis. Every hour that an acute suppurative process continues within a joint portends a potentially poorer prognosis. Ultimately, an influx of acute and chronic inflammatory cells as well as release of proinflammatory cytokines such as tumor necrosis factor-alpha (TNF-α) and proteases such as elastases, collagenases, and metalloproteinases lead to cartilage degradation. Within a few days, irreversible subchondral bone loss can be demonstrated (7). Recently published work suggests a role for Toll-like receptors in the pathogenesis of septic arthritis. Proost et al. (8) have shown that Toll-like receptor ligands differentially regulate chemokine expression (CXCL10/IP-10) in fibroblasts and monocytes in synergy with interferon-alfa (IFN-α) and provide a mechanism for enhanced synovial chemokine levels in septic joints.

Other mechanisms which may allow bacteria to enter the joint space include a deep penetrating wound presenting as chronic synovitis caused by a foreign body reaction or acute pseudoarthritis. Orthopedic surgeons may encounter patients with joint infections as a result of prosthetic joint procedures. Lastly, infection resulting from the introduction of bacteria into the joint during an intraarticular steroid injection is a very uncommon event occurring at a rate of one per 10,000 procedures (9).

Risk Factors

Normal joints are very resistant to infection compared to diseased joints or prosthetic joints. Identification of predisposing factors is very important for prevention and treatment of septic arthritis (Table 28–1). Host factors that predispose to bacterial arthritis include the patient's age, decreased immunocompetence, and preexisting joint diseases. Age greater than 80 years, diabetes mellitus, and rheumatoid arthritis were found to be important independent risk factors in a large-scale prospective study from the Netherlands (10). In addition, liver disease, chronic renal failure, pregnancy, menses, malignancy, hemodialysis, alcoholism, HIV infection, hemophilia, organ transplantation, and hypogammaglobulinemia have been recognized as risks factors (11). Local factors, such as previous joint damage, recent articular trauma, surgery or arthroscopy, occupational exposure (e.g., brucellosis in

Table 28–1. Risk Factors for Septic Arthritis: Gonococcal and Nongonococcal

Gonococcal	Nongonococcal
Menses	Diabetes mellitus
Pregnancy	Rheumatoid arthritis
Complement deficiency	Prosthetic joint
HIV infection	Hemophilia
Systemic lupus	Immunosuppression
erythematosus	Hypogammaglobulinemia
IV drug use	Malignancy
	Hemodialysis
	Alcoholism
	Liver disease
	Age: greater than 80 years
	Skin ulceration and/or
	infection
	Steroid therapy
	TNF-α antagonists

shepherds, farmers, and/or livestock producers), and low socioeconomic status, are additional predisposing factors.

Recently, anti-TNF-α therapy has been associated with a variety of undesirable effects, among them being infections including septic arthritis. Anti-TNF-α treatment for rheumatoid arthritis, Crohn disease, and other autoimmune and non-autoimmune conditions is rapidly becoming well established and high level of clinical suspicion is necessary in patients receiving this treatment because the nature and course of infectious diseases may be altered by TNF blockade (12).

In summary, well-known host risk factors described in nongonococcal septic arthritis include age greater than 80 years, cancer, cirrhosis, diabetes mellitus, rheumatoid arthritis, previous damage to a joint, indwelling catheters, and intravenous drug addiction (11, 23). Repeated intraarticular corticosteroid injection can also slightly increase the risk of bacterial arthritis.

Microbiology

Theoretically, any infectious agent can cause septic arthritis (Table 28–2). However, the most common nongonococcal causes of acute septic arthritis are grampositive cocci particularly *S. aureus* in native septic joint infections; *Staphylococcus epidermidis* has been reported slightly more often than *S. aureus* in prosthetic joint infections.

Staphylococcus aureus is responsible for 30–50% of nongonococcal septic arthritis. Methicillin-resistant *Staphylococcus aureus* (MRSA) has emerged as an important pathogen among hospitalized patients. According to recent estimates from the National Nosocomial

Infection Surveillance System of the Centers for Disease Control and Prevention (CDC), the rate of MRSA causing nosocomial infections in intensive care unit patients has approached 50% in U.S. health care facilities, while community-acquired MRSA has reached a prevalence of 30.2–37.3% (13). After *S. aureus*, pneumococcus is the most common gram-positive aerobe responsible for nearly 10% of native joint bacterial arthritis. Gram-negative bacilli and *Haemophilus influenzae* are more common in elderly people, children younger than 5 years of age and newborn, immunocompromised hosts, and patients with systemic lupus erythematosus. Overall, the incidence of infection caused by *H. influenzae* among children younger than 5 years of age has fallen by 70–80% since the introduction of the *H. influenzae* type b conjugate vaccine. Anaerobic infections are more common in prosthetic joint infections and in diabetics who develop septic arthritis. Ten to twenty percent of clinically diagnosed septic arthritis cannot be confirmed with synovial fluid or blood cultures (14). *Neisseria gonorrhoeae* remains the most common causative agent in bacterial arthritis among young and sexually active adults in the United States. Up to 3% of patients infected with *N. gonorrhoeae* develop disseminated gonococcal infection (DGI) and septic arthritis.

Gonococcal Arthritis

Gonococcal arthritis results from blood dissemination of *N. gonorrhoeae* from its mucosal portal of entry (Table 28–3). The term "gonorrhea" was first used by Galen in AD 130 and comes from the Greek *gonos* (seed) and *rhoea* (flow) because urethral discharge was mistaken for semen.

Table 28–2. Septic Arthritis: Frequency of Causative Microorganisms

Agent	Adults	Children < 5 Years Old	Prosthetic Joint
S. aureus	30–50%	30–50%	15–30%
S. epidermidis	15–30%	15–30%	30–50%
Streptococci	30–50%	5–15%	5–15%
N. gonorrhoeae	30–50%	Very rare	Very rare
H. influenzae	5–15%	15–30%	5–15%
Pseudomonas	1–5%	5–15%	15–30%
Salmonella	1–5%	5–15%	15–30%
Mycobacteria	1–5%	Rare	Rare
Fungal	Rare	Very rare	Very rare
Viral	5–15%	15–30%	Very rare
Protozoal	Very rare	Very rare	Very rare

Table 28–3. Clinical Characteristics of Gonococcal and Nongonococcal Septic Arthritis

Findings	Gonococcal	Nongonococcal
Patients	F > M; 18–40 years; sexually active	F = M; children and elderly
Arthritis	Polyarthralgia; monoarthritis; Tenosynovitis; rash	Monoarthritis or oligoarthritis
Predisponent conditions	Pregnancy; menses; HIV; complement deficiency	RA; SLE; crystals, prosthetic joints
Microorganism	*N. gonorrhoeae*	*S. aureus; S. pneumoniae, H. influenzae; E. coli; Pseudomonas* sp.
Blood culture	<10%	50%
Synovial fluid	<50%	90%
Outcome	Excellent	Often poor

F: female; M: male; RA: rheumatoid arthritis; SLE: systemic lupus erythematosus.

Disseminated gonococcal infection develops in 0.5–3% of patients with mucosal infection. It has long been proposed that some manifestations of gonococcal arthritis, such as the migratory arthralgia, are immunologically driven, and not strictly septic, as defined by the presence of viable organisms in the involved joints.

The biological characteristics of gonococcal strains influence their virulence, resistance to complement-mediated bactericidal activity of human serum, and the risk of dissemination. The ability of gonococci to disseminate has been associated with certain protein serotypes in the gonococcal outer membrane, certain nutritional requirements for specific aminoacids, and antibiotic susceptibility profiles (15). Pregnancy and menses increase the risk for DGI as a result of associated changes in gonococcal phenotype and endometrial exposure of submucosal vessels to the infecting organism. Inherited complement deficiency (mainly C5–C8), systemic lupus erythematosus, intravenous drug use, and human immunodeficiency virus infection have also been reported as risk factors for gonococcal arthritis.

Migratory or additive polyarthralgia is the most common initial presentation of gonococcal arthritis. Tenosynovitis, dermatitis, and fever occur in 30–70% of cases. Multiple tendons of the wrist, ankles, and small joints may be inflamed and exquisitely tender. The skin lesions are typically multiple, painless macules and papules, most often found on the arms or legs or on the trunk. True arthritis is observed in less than 50% of cases, and, when present, monoarticular involvement is most commonly seen. Any joint can be affected; however, knees, wrists, ankles, and finger joints are the most often involved (16). Unusual

manifestations of DGI can be life threatening and include gonococcal endocarditis, myocarditis and conduction defects, pericarditis, osteomyelitis, pyomyositis, hepatitis (Fitz-Hugh-Curtis syndrome), meningitis, Waterhouse-Friderichsen syndrome, and adult respiratory syndrome. These complications have become rare since the introduction of antibiotics (17).

Diagnosis

The definite diagnosis of septic arthritis requires identification of bacteria in the synovial fluid by Gram stain or by culture. Clinical suspicion of joint sepsis should prompt immediate synovial fluid aspiration (arthrocentesis). If synovial fluid cannot be obtained with closed needle aspiration, the joint should be aspirated again with imaging guidance. This approach may be necessary for joints that are not easily accessible, such as hips, shoulders, or sacroiliac joints. Such joints may even require surgical arthrotomy to obtain synovial fluid. When infected, the synovial fluid is generally inflammatory consisting of leukocyte counts in the range of 50,000–100,000 cells/mm^3, with a polymorphonuclear predominance greater than 70%.

Leukocytosis and elevated erythrocyte sedimentation rate (ESR) and C-reactive protein (CRP) levels are present in most patients with DGI. However, these abnormalities are not consistent and are frequently of only mild intensity. *Neisseria gonorrhoeae* is a fastidious aerobic organism, with various nutritional requirements, whose growth can be inhibited by drying or planting on a cold and dehydrated medium. Chocolate agar media supplemented with glucose can be used to grow gonococci from otherwise sterile sites. Isolation of gonococci from mucosa or skin lesions requires the use of selective media supplemented with antibiotics (such as modified Thayer-Martin medium) to eliminate saprophytic organisms (18). Synovial fluid Gram stain is positive in less than 25% of patients with gonococcal arthritis. In contrast blood or synovial fluid cultures are positive in approximately 50% of cases. Approximately 80% of patients have a positive culture from a mucosal site. The genitourinary tract has the best yield for a positive culture. It is also important to look for concomitant HIV or chlamydial infections which are frequently associated with gonorrhoea (*Chlamydia* has been reported as high as 30%) and require specific treatment.

Ligase chain reaction (LCR) or polymerase chain reaction (PCR) techniques can be used to detect nucleic acid sequences specific for *N. gonorrhoeae* in urogenital samples or synovial fluid even when culture is negative. Specificity and sensitivity of nucleic acid diagnostic testing has been estimated at 96–98% and 78–89%, respectively. However PCR cannot test for antibiotic resistance and therefore should not replace culture (19).

In the acute stages of septic arthritis, radiographs initially show evidence of soft tissue swelling and effusion. Cartilage destruction or evidence of osteomyelitis at the time of diagnosis suggests infection with nongonococcal agents or prior ineffective antibiotic(s) treatment. Characteristic juxtaarticular osteoporosis and bone erosions take weeks to develop. Scintigraphy, computed tomography (CT), or magnetic resonance imaging (MRI) are far more sensitive than plain films in early septic arthritis. CT is most useful to detect effusions and to guide the joint aspiration of the hip, sternoclavicular, and sacroiliac joints. MRI demonstrates adjacent soft-tissue edema and may be especially helpful in detecting septic sacroiliitis (20).

Treatment and Prognosis

The treatment of acute gonococcal arthritis requires antibiotics and joint drainage. The initial choice of antibiotic(s) should be based on the Gram stain and the age and risk factors of the patient. If the Gram stain is negative, empirical therapy with ceftriaxone 1 g/day parenterally or ceftizoxime or cefotaxime, 1 g parenterally every 8 h, for 24–48 h are the initial antibiotics of choice for suspected DGI. Patients can then be switched to oral cefixime, 400 mg twice daily, or oral ciprofloxacin, 500 mg twice daily, to complete 7–10 days of treatment. If the patient is allergic to beta-lactam drugs, ciprofloxacin, 500 mg IV every 12 h, or spectinomycin, 2 g IM every 12 h, may be initially used. If the infecting strain proves to be peni-

cillin sensitive, treatment can be changed to penicillin G (2–4 million U IV every 4–6 h daily), ampicillin 1 g IV every 6 h or amoxicillin 500 mg po every 8 h with probenecid 1 g/day (21, 22). Surgical drainage or arthroscopy is rarely needed. Lack of response to treatment suggests incorrect diagnosis or infection with an antibiotic-resistant organism. In general the response to treatment and outcome are excellent within a few days of antibiotic therapy (2).

Nongonococcal Septic Arthritis

Nongonococcal septic arthritis usually involves one joint, most commonly the knee, but the shoulder, hip, wrist, interphalangeal, and elbow joints may be affected. *Staphylococcus aureus* or *S. pneumoniae* are the common causative organisms. However, gram-negative bacteria such as *H. influenzae*, *Escherichia coli*, *Proteus* sp., and *Pseudomonas* sp. have been reported.

Clinical Features

Nongonococcal bacterial arthritis usually presents with the abrupt onset of a single hot, swollen, and very painful joint (Table 28–3). The knee is the site of infection in about 50% of the cases, but any joint may be involved. Mild fever is common but rigors are rare. Oligoarticular infection (less than four joints involved) usually involving two or three joints occurs in 10–20% of cases and is more often seen in patients with rheumatoid arthritis, systemic connective tissue diseases, or in patients with overwhelming sepsis. Hips are infected more often in children (24). The hip is often held in a flexed and externally rotated position and there is extreme pain on motion, and in 50% of cases a source of infection, from the skin, lungs, or bladder, will be found. Sometimes, it is very difficult to detect an effusion of the hip or shoulder although the joint is frequently warm and very tender. The sacroiliac joints are involved in 10% of infections and are very difficult to assess with physical examination; imaging studies can be very helpful in this setting.

Diagnosis

A high index of suspicion for septic arthritis should be maintained in the setting of a patient with acute monoarthritis, fever, toxic appearance, and extraarticular sites of infection. The synovial fluid culture is positive in 90% of cases of nongonococcal bacterial arthritis, but Gram stains are positive in only 50% and clumps of stain or cellular debris may be mistaken for bacteria. Fluid from septic joints contains on average 100,000 white cells/mL with a range of 25,000–250,000 cells/mL. If there are more than 50,000 white cells/mL and more than 90% are polymorphonuclear leukocytes, infection is highly likely even when organisms are not isolated. In addition, plain radiographs are necessary to provide a baseline assessment of the affected joint and to rule out a possible contiguous osteomyelitis. The earliest findings include joint effusion with displacement of the fat pads. Periarticular osteoporosis is evident during the first week of bacterial arthritis. Joint space narrowing and erosions may be detectable within 7–14 days, but the rapidity of appearance depends on the virulence of the microorganism. Gas formation within the joints suggests *E. coli* or anaerobic infection (26).

The radiological findings in a suspected infected prosthetic joint are difficult to distinguish from mechanical loosening of the prosthesis since both may cause zones of radiolucency at the bone-cement interface. In such a situation, arthrography, particularly with hip aspiration, may be helpful to document pathologic bone and cement separation as well as to demonstrate synovial hypertrophy and abscess formation. In joints that are particularly difficult to evaluate clinically or that have a complex anatomic structure, CT scanning, radionuclide imaging, or magnetic resonance imaging may be of diagnostic value (27).

Differential Diagnosis

A wide range of rheumatic diseases can mimic septic arthritis. Even more challenging is that these can occur simultaneously, such as with rheumatoid arthritis and gouty arthritis. The crystal-induced arthritides including gout and pseudogout are very difficult to differentiate, but a history of recurrent monoarthritis, typical podagra, the presence of tophi, radiological evidence of chondrocalcinosis, identification of crystals in the synovial fluid, negative Gram stain and cultures are indicative of crystal-induced arthritis (28).

Several forms of chronic inflammatory joint diseases such as rheumatoid arthritis, reactive arthritis (formerly Reiter syndrome), ankylosing spondylitis, and psoriatic arthritis should be considered in the appropriate clinical and radiological setting. For these reasons, routine synovial fluid examination from any joint with acute effusion of unknown etiology is mandatory (29) (Table 28–4).

Treatment and Prognosis

The treatment of acute bacterial arthritis requires broad-spectrum parenteral antibiotics and joint drainage. Early and aggressive therapy is very important to prevent joint

Table 28–4. Differential Diagnosis between Septic and Reactive Arthritis

Characteristics	Reactive Arthritis	Septic Arthritis
Patients	Commonly young; M = F	All ages; F > M in gonococcal septic arthritis
Genetics	Family clustering; HLA-B27	None
Infectious agents	*Salmonella; Shigella; Yersinia; Campylobacter; Chlamydia; N. gonorrhoeae*	*N. gonorrhoeae; S. aureus;* streptococci
Triggers	Enteric or urogenital infections	Skin infection; bacteremia
Clinical	Conjunctivitis; acute uveitis; pustulosis palmoplantaris and nail lesions	Skin rash
Laboratory	Normal or mild leukocytosis; microhematuria; proteinuria	Moderate or severe leukocytosis; normal urine
Synovial fluid	"Sterile" leukocytosis	Leukocytosis; Gram stain and culture can be positive
Treatment	NSAIDs, sometimes antibiotics, DMARDs and TNF-α inhibitors	Antibiotics
Prognosis	In general good spontaneous recovery is common. Some patients develop ankylosing spondylitis (15–30% in 10–20 years)	Generally good Mortality: 10–30%

F: female; M: male; DMARDs: disease modifying antirheumatic drugs.

destruction especially in childhood. The initial choice of antibiotics should be based on patient risk factors, Gram stain, and clinical setting.

When gonococcal infection is not suspected, empirical treatment should usually include antimicrobial activity against *S. aureus,* streptococci, and gram-negative bacilli. Therapy is modified according to Gram-stain, culture, and sensitivity results of the synovial fluid or blood culture isolates. Most antibiotics penetrate well into inflamed joints.

The combination of semisynthetic penicillins and a third-generation cephalosporin such as ceftriaxone or cefotaxime are often administered empirically in many cases. Combinations of semisynthetic penicillins and ciprofloxacin have also been used. Intravenous vancomycin, 1 g every 12 h, is indicated in lieu of nafcillin or oxacillin when MRSA infection is suspected (30).

The appropriate duration of therapy has been the subject of much discussion in the past several years. New effective oral antibiotics are leading to changes in clinical practice, particularly regarding the duration of therapy. Treatment should last until the infected joint has been sterilized and the infection eradicated from intraarticular sites. A 3-week treatment period (1 week of parenteral therapy followed by 2 weeks of oral antibiotics) is appropriate for most patients with septic arthritis. The duration of treatment should be extended in immunocompromised patients and those with nonremovable prosthetic material (31).

The drainage of purulent synovial effusions is essential in order to facilitate an environment that facilitates antibiotic activity and to remove bacteria, inflammatory mediators, and degradative enzymes. Two methods of drainage exist: (1) closed drainage with repeated aspirations of the infected joint (in general, not necessary to drain small joints) which has the advantage of preserving the integrity of the joint and (2) open drainage that allows for a better joint lavage but adds to potential morbidity. Open drainage is most indicated in deep-seated joints (including hip and shoulders), joints with preexisting damage, joints not responding to appropriate medical management, or joints with loculated effusion or contiguous osteomyelitis. Joint drainage by arthroscopy is gaining popularity and is associated with less morbidity when compared to open drainage.

Nongonococcal arthritis is a serious condition with a 5–15% mortality rate and a 25–60% rate of chronic joint damage and disability. A raised peripheral white blood cell count at presentation and the development of abnormal renal function have been reported as predictors of poor prognosis. Hip and polyarticular infection are also negative prognostic factors. The mortality of polyarticular septic arthritis in all patients is 23%, but in RA patients it may reach 56% (25, 32).

Viral Arthritis

An increasing number of viruses are being identified as causes of arthritis including hepatitis B, hepatitis C, HIV, parvovirus, and rubella among others (Table 28–5). Small and large joint involvement is frequent, and acute

Table 28–5. Viral Arthritis

Virus	% Arthritis	Findings	Duration	Additional Features
Parvovirus	Children 10% Adults 50–70%	Polyarticular Symmetric	2–8 wks or chronic	Pancytopenia
Rubeola	10–30%	Polyarticular	5–10 days	Autoantibodies
VZV	<1%	Monoarticular	1–7 days	Latency
EBV	1–5%	Poly or monoarticular	1–12 weeks	Autoantibodies
HBC	10–25%	Migratory	1–3 weeks	Vasculitis
HCV	10–50%	Polyarticular	Chronic	Vasculitis
HIV	10–50%	Mono or oligoarticular	Chronic	>viral load (higher than 10,000 copies of HIV RNA) <CD4 count (less than 500 cells/mL)
Alphavirus	>50%	Oligoarticular	1–4 weeks	Fever; myalgias
Adenovirus	Rare	Polyarticular	1–2 weeks	Pharyngitis
Coxsackie	Rare	Oligoarticular	Acute or chronic	Serositis

VZV: Varicella Zoster virus; EBV: Epstein-Barr virus; HBV & HCV: Hepatitis B and C viruses.

polyarthritis, fever, and sometimes rash are characteristic features (33, 34).

HIV infection is associated with a variety of musculoskeletal manifestations including septic arthritis. The natural course including etiologic agents and response to therapy of HIV-associated septic arthritis is similar to the non-HIV-associated form (35).

Case Outcome

Laboratory investigation of this patient with monoarthritis revealed a peripheral white blood cell count of 18,000/mm^3 with a differential of 95% neutrophils. The differential diagnosis included traumatic synovitis, crystal-induced arthritis, prepatellar bursitis, and septic arthritis. Prepatellar bursitis was ruled out in this case because it produces pain, swelling, and erythema but does not limit the mobility of the affected joint, in this case the right knee. The next step in the management of this patient included joint aspiration and synovial fluid analysis in order to differentiate between infection and crystal-induced arthritis. Synovial fluid findings included 95,000 white blood cells/mm^3 with a differential of 98% neutrophils, a negative Gram stain, and no crystals. Blood and synovial cultures eventually grew out *S. aureus*. Vancomycin was initiated until sensitivity test results became available. In addition, the affected joint was aspirated daily or until the infectious process was under control. Arthroscopic aspiration with or without lavage was not needed since needle drainage was adequate.

REFERENCES

1. Yelin E, Collahan LF: (National Arthritis Data Work Groups): The economic cost and social and psychological impact of musculoskeletal conditions. *Arthritis Rheum* 38:1351–1362, 1995.
2. Espinoza LR: Infectious arthritis, in Goldman L, Ausiello D. (eds.): *Cecil Textbook Of Medicine, 22nd ed*. Philadelphia, W. B. Saunders, 2004; Chapter 286, pp 1696–1698.
3. Gupta MN, Sturrock RD, Field M: A prospective 2-year study of 75 patients with adult onset septic arthritis. *Rheumatology* 40:24–30, 2001.
4. Cucurull E, Espinoza LR: Gonococcal arthritis. *Rheum Dis Clin North Am* 24:305–322, 1998.
5. Lidgren L: Joint prosthetic infections: A success story. Guest editorial. *Acta Orthop Scand* 72:553–556, 2001.
6. Lidgren L: Infection of prosthetic joints. *Best Pract Res Clin Rheumatol* 17(2):209–218, 2003.
7. Goldenberg DL: Septic arthritis. *Lancet* 351:197–202, 1998.
8. Proost P, Vynckier AK, Mahieu F, et al.: Microbial Toll-like receptor ligands differentially regulate CXCL10/IP-10 expression in fibroblasts and mononuclear leukocytes in synergy with IFN-γ and provide a mechanism for enhanced synovial chemokine levels in septic arthritis. *Eur J Immunol* 33:3146–3153, 2003.
9. Gray RG, Tenenbaum J, Gottlieb NL: Local corticosteroid injection treatment in rheumatic disorders. *Semin Arthritis Rheum* 10:231–254, 1981.
10. Kaandorp CJE, van Schaardemburg D, Krijnen P, Habbeme JDF, van de Laae MAFJ: Risk factors for septic arthritis in patients with joint disease: A prospective study. *Arthritis Rheum* 38:1819–1825, 1995.
11. Barzilai A, Varon D, Martinowitz U, Heim M, Schulman S: Characteristics of septic arthritis in human immunodeficiency virus-infected haemophiliacs versus other risk groups. *Rheumatology* 38:139–142, 1999.
12. Kroesen S, Widmer AF, Tyndall A, Hasler P: Serious bacterial infections in patients with rheumatoid arthritis under anti-TNF-α therapy. *Rheumatology* 42:617–621, 2003.
13. Salgado CD, Farr BM, Calfee DP: Community-acquired methicillin-resistant *Staphylococcus aureus*: A meta-analysis of prevalence and risk factors. *Clin Infect Dis* 36(15):131–139, 2003.
14. Dubost JJ, Soubrier M, De Champs C, et al.: No changes in the distribution of organisms responsible for septic arthritis over a 20 years period. *Ann Rheum Dis* 61:267–269, 2002.
15. Bardin T: Gonococcal arthritis. *Best Pract Res Clin Rheumatol* 17(2):201–208, 2003.
16. Angulo JM, Espinoza LR: Gonococcal arthritis. *Compr Ther* 25(3):155–162, 1999.
17. Mahowald ML: Gonococcal arthritis, in Hochberg MC, Silman AJ, Smolen JS, Weinblatt ME, Weisman MH (eds.): *Rheumatology, 3d ed*. London, Mosby, 2003; pp 1067–1075.
18. Beverly A, Bailey-Griffin JR, Schwebke JR: InTray GC medium versus modified Thayer-Martin agar plates for diagnosis of gonorrhea from endocervical specimens. *J Clin Microbiol* 38(10):3825–3826, 2000.
19. Liebling M, Arkfeld D, Michelini G, et al.: Identification of *N. gonorrhoeae* in synovial fluid using the polymerase chain reaction. *Arthritis Rheum* 37:702–709, 1994.
20. Nade S: Septic Arthritis. *Best Pract Res Clin Rheumatol* 17(2):183–200, 2003.
21. Garcia-De La Torre I: Advances in the management of septic arthritis. *Rheum Dis Clin North Am* 29(1):61–75, 2003.
22. Van Oosterhout M, Sont JK, Van Laar JM: Superior effect of arthroscopic lavage compared with needle aspiration in the treatment of inflammatory arthritis of the knee. *Rheumatology* 42:102–107, 2003.
23. Fleisch F, Zbinden R, Vanoli C, Ruef C: Epidemic spread of a single clone of methicillin-resistant *Staphylococcus aureus* among injection drug users in Switzerland, Zurich. *Clin Infect Dis* 32(4):581–586.
24. Shaw BA, Kasser JR: Acute septic arthritis in infancy and childhood. *Clin Orthop* 257:212–225, 1990.
25. Carreno-Perez L: Septic arthritis. *Ball Best Clin Pract* 13(1):36–58, 1999.

26. Shirtliff ME, Mader JT: Acute septic arthritis. *Clin Microbiol Rev* 15(4):527–544, 2002.

27. Goldenberg DL: Bacterial arthritis, in Kelley WH, Harris ED, Ruddy Jr., S, and Sledge CB (eds.): *Textbook of Rheumatology, 5th ed.* Philadelphia, W. B. Saunders, 1997; Chapter 90, pp 1435–1449.

28. Lo TS, Buettner AM, Ingebretson MC: Concurrent acute gouty and gonococcal arthritis. *Lancet Infect Dis* 2(5):313, 2002.

29. Colmegna I, Cuchacovich R, Espinoza LR: HLA-27-associated reactive arthritis: Pathogenetic and clinical considerations. *Clin Microbiol Rev* 17(2):348–369, 2004.

30. Khare M, Keady D: Antimicrobial therapy of methicillin resistant *Staphylococcus aureus* infection. *Expert Opin Pharmacother* 4(2):165–177, 2003.

31. Stengel D, Bauwens K, Sehouli J, Ekkernkamp A, Porzsolt F: Systematic review and meta-analysis of antibiotic therapy for bone and joint infections. *Lancet Infect Dis* 1:175–188, 2001.

32. Lidgren L: Septic arthritis and osteomyelitis, in Hochberg MC, Silman AJ, Smolen JS, and Weisman MH (eds.): *Rheumatology, 3d ed.* Spain, Mosby-Elsevier, 2003; Chapter 93, pp 1055–1065.

33. Scroggie DA, Carpenter MT, Cooper RI, Higgs JB: Parvovirus arthropathy outbreak in Southern United States. *J Rheumatol* 27(10):2444–2448, 2000.

34. Cuellar ML, Espinoza LR: Viral arthritis, in Koopman WJ, Boulware DW, and Hexdebert GR (eds.), *Viral arthritis in Clinical Primer of Rheumatology.* Baltimore, Williams and Wilkins, 2003; pp 350–354.

35. Marquez J, Restrepo C, Candia L, Berman A, Espinoza LR: Human immunodeficiency virus-associated rheumatic disorders in the HAART era. *J Rheumatol* 31:741–746, 2004.

29

Plantar Puncture Wounds

Kathleen C. Hubbell

HIGH YIELD FACTS

1. The interventions most likely to prevent complications after a plantar puncture wound are unknown.

2. Cellulitis and superficial, localized abscesses caused by *Staphylococcus* and *Streptococcus* are the most common infections after plantar puncture. They present within the first week after the puncture.

3. Retained foreign bodies, often pieces of rubber from the shoe sole, will cause infection, continued or worsening symptoms, and failure to resolve symptoms despite antibiotic therapy.

4. Osteomyelitis is an uncommon complication but should be suspected in any patient who has continued or worsening symptoms 1 week or more after the puncture, regardless of previous antibiotic therapy.

5. Three-phase bone scan, ultrasound, CT, and MRI are effective imaging methods to diagnose osteomyelitis.

6. Erythrocyte sedimentation rate (ESR) is the laboratory test most likely to be abnormal in a patient with osteomyelitis following a plantar puncture wound.

7. *Pseudomonas aeruginosa* is the most common cause of osteomyelitis after a plantar puncture wound. *Staphylococcus* may be seen as a copathogen.

8. Surgical treatment followed by a short course of antibiotic therapy appears to be the best treatment for plantar-puncture-associated osteomyelitis.

Case Presentation

The patient was a 49-year-old man who had stepped on a nail in a board 17 days previously while wearing sandals. He had gone to the emergency department (ED) that day and received wound care and a prescription for ciprofloxacin that he did not fill. He returned to the ED 1 or 2 days later complaining of continued foot pain and received a prescription for cephalexin, which he took for 7 days. Despite this treatment, his foot became swollen and he was unable to bear weight on it. He denied fever or wound drainage.

Examination revealed a patient ambulating only with the aid of a crutch. He was afebrile. There was a pinhead-sized sealed wound on the sole of the midfoot without surrounding redness or drainage. The dorsum was minimally red and warm but moderately tender and swollen with loss of all landmarks. X-ray of the foot was normal except for generalized soft tissue swelling. White blood cell count was 5700.

Introduction/Epidemiology

The puncture of the sole of the foot is known to progress to a spectrum of endpoints, including rapid, complete healing; cellulitis or localized abscess; and development of the most dreaded complications, osteochondritis, osteomyelitis, and septic arthritis. The literature offers little guidance in identifying those patients at risk for the more serious infections. Similarly, there are no randomized trials studying the effects of various treatments such as wound cleaning, probing, debriding, or antibiotic use when applied at the initial ED visit after the puncture. In fact, there is only one prospective study on initial treatment of these wounds and it involved only 63 patients (2).

Despite these limitations, the statistics and case descriptions available do illustrate the natural history of the infectious complications and highlight "red flags" in the patient's course that can suggest the need for more aggressive diagnostic and management steps.

The true incidence of plantar punctures has not been determined, as most do not come to medical attention. A 4-year review of pediatric emergency department visits in one study revealed that 0.8% of visits were due to plantar punctures (1). Nails are the most common cause of puncture (1), but sewing needles, wire, glass, plastic spikes, toothpicks, branches, cactus thorns, and catfish spines are also involved.

Although many of the patients who develop complications are wearing tennis shoes at the time of the puncture, it is not clear whether this predisposes to infection or if this simply reflects current footwear fashion. Socks, pieces of rubber sole, and foam inner lining from shoes have been found as foreign bodies when exploring plantar punctures. Conversely, infectious complications have also developed in patients who were barefoot at the time of puncture.

The incidence of infection after a plantar puncture is similarly difficult to define because not all punctures present to medical attention. Fitzgerald and Cowan (1) found that of the 774 patients who presented within the first 24 h after puncture, 8.4% either had cellulitis or returned within 4 days with cellulitis. In 113 patients who presented 1–7 days after the injury, 57% developed cellulitis or abscess. The only prospective study in the literature found a 12% complication rate (cellulitis, abscess, foreign body) among its 63 patients (2). All complications were evident 1–8 days postpuncture.

The incidence of osteomyelitis is very low, 0.04–1.8%, yet rightly feared due to the medical morbidity for the patient and legal liability issues for the physician (3, 1, 4).

Pathophysiology/Microbiology

The inoculation of bacteria from the puncturing object and any materials it passes through on its path into the soft tissues of the foot provides the basis for infection. The depth of penetration is the most important determining factor in the likelihood of infection. Most infections are found in the forefoot and heel, the weight-bearing areas of the foot (5). Also important are the immune and vascular status of the patient. Diabetics are almost three times more likely to develop osteomyelitis after plantar puncture than healthy patients (6).

Because of the relatively small amount of soft tissue under the bones of the foot, a nail can easily penetrate the deep tissues to the depth of the joints and cartilaginous areas of joints or growth plates. The avascular nature of the cartilage renders it particularly susceptible to infection. There can also be direct penetration to the bones of the foot by the impaling object or osteomyelitis may develop as a result of extension from adjacent soft tissue or cartilage infection.

The soft tissue infections, usually cellulitis and localized abscesses, that manifest early, within the first week postpuncture, are generally caused by *Staphylococcus* and *Streptococcus*. Infections manifesting later are more likely to be osteochondritis, septic arthritis, and osteomyelitis. *Pseudomonas* is the responsible organism in about 93% of these bone-joint infections. *Staphylococcus* and *Streptococcus* are frequent copathogens with *Pseudomonas* (1). *Klebsiella, Escherichia coli, Serratia, Bacteroides*, various *Mycobacteria*, and other bacteria are sometimes cultured (1, 7–9). In diabetics, *Staphylococcus* is the most common pathogen in both osteomyelitis and soft tissue infections. Polymicrobial infections are also common in these patients (6).

The source of the *Pseudomonas* in most cases is probably the tennis shoes through which the nail penetrated before entering the foot. In a study of cultures from the skin of the heel and the inside surface of the corresponding shoes of 100 healthy pediatric patients, only three yielded *Pseudomonas*, one from the skin and two from the shoe inner surface (10). However, when the soles of tennis shoes of patients with puncture wound osteomyelitis were cut open and the inner foam layers were cultured, *Pseudomonas* was recovered from 11 shoes of the eight studied patients. Enzyme typing of isolates from the sneaker and the infected foot was done in four of the eight patients, revealing an exact match in one case and minor variation in the other three (11). In the same study *Pseudomonas* was cultured from the inner foam layers of 4 of 66 pairs of discarded sneakers from healthy teenagers. No *Pseudomonas* was obtained from the culture of foam from 47 pairs of new, never-worn sneakers.

Pseudomonas and other organisms have also been cultured from patients with osteomyelitis who were wearing rubber-soled work boots and sandals when they suffered a plantar puncture. Rubber foreign bodies were almost always found at surgery (8).

The source of *Pseudomonas* in patients who developed osteomyelitis while walking barefoot is unclear. Some have suggested that it is water used for soaking the foot, but this has never been studied.

Clinical Presentation

Many patients present to the ED within hours of a plantar puncture wound. Their main concern is often tetanus prophylaxis or evaluation of an as yet asymptomatic wound.

Patients presenting after 24 h usually have swelling or pain that is increasing rather than resolving, raising the possibility of infection or foreign body. Most of these patients will receive antibiotic therapy and their symptoms will completely resolve. A small percentage will experience transient or incomplete improvement from antibiotic treatment. These patients almost always have an undiscovered foreign body, an abscess, or are manifesting early symptoms of osteochondritis, osteomyelitis, or septic arthritis.

It is essential to recognize the significance of these phases in the presentation of patients with plantar punctures and to perform the appropriate investigation.

A thorough and well-documented history will aid the physician in determining an appropriate course of action. The following may be helpful:

1. Description of the puncturing object—material, length, size, intactness post removal, contaminated or clean

2. Depth of penetration

3. Footwear at time of penetration

4. Time of injury

5. Foreign body sensation

6. Tetanus immunization status

7. Health status—diabetes, vascular disease, etc.

8. Previous diagnostic measures and treatment—antibiotics, radiographs, scans

Physical examination should be performed in such a way as to maximize the physician's view of the wound, preferably with the patient prone on a stretcher, using bright light, and magnification (12). The puncture site should be inspected for foreign body and signs of infection. A neurovascular exam of the limbs should be documented. It is wise to use a drawing to illustrate the puncture site and to measure the size of the wound. The ability to bear weight should be noted.

The dorsum of the foot should be examined for swelling, tenderness, erythema, and warmth. Many patients with abscesses or osteomyelitis will have no residual tenderness around the puncture, but will have diffuse soft tissue swelling of the dorsum of the foot with loss of dorsal landmarks and minimal to moderate dorsal erythema and tenderness. Fever is rare, even with osteomyelitis.

Pain caused by the movement of a specific joint or by axial compression of the involved toe may suggest septic arthritis in the later stages of presentation (13).

Management and Diagnostic Testing

Patients who present to the emergency department after sustaining a plantar puncture wound are hoping to receive treatment that will prevent all complications of this injury. Unfortunately, due to the lack of any randomized, prospective trials comparing the effectiveness of initial interventions, management must be based on general principles of wound care and an appreciation for the natural history of the development of the infectious complications of this injury as well illustrated in the literature. It must be emphasized that it is currently not known whether any intervention applied at the initial patient visit can prevent the development of cellulitis, abscess, or osteomyelitis.

Presentation within 24 h

The priorities of management for the ED visit that occurs within 24 h of the puncture include tetanus prophylaxis, assessment of the possibility of foreign body, and wound care. Most puncture wounds would be considered tetanus-prone wounds and prophylaxed accordingly with Td and, when appropriate, Tetanus Immune Globulin.

A foreign body can be suspected on the basis of history and searched for on exam. An x-ray to assess for foreign body need not be routine at the first visit, but should be done in the case of foreign body sensation, stepping on glass, removal of a nonintact foreign body by patient or physician, or a thin, brittle foreign body such as wire. Metal, bone, teeth, pencil graphite, glass, gravel, and some plastics are easily seen on plain radiography. Small strands of sock fiber or pieces of rubber or foam will not appear on x-ray, but can be sought on exam. Aluminum, fishbones, some plastics, most wood, splinters, thorns, and spines are also not seen well on x-ray and require another imaging modality (14, 15).

Ultrasound can detect non-radiopaque foreign bodies of 1 × 2 mm with a 95–98% sensitivity and an 89–98% specificity (14). Air, sutures, fresh blood, small bones such as sesamoids, and scar tissue can cause false positives.

Computerized tomography also has great sensitivity for detection of non-radiopaque foreign bodies. After 48 h, however, wooden foreign bodies will have absorbed enough water from surrounding tissues to become isodense and difficult to identify (14, 15).

The nature and aggressiveness of the wound care that should be provided on the initial visit is the area of greatest controversy (7). The proposed benefits of more aggressive intervention, that is, greater access to the depths of the wound for inspection and cleaning, have never been proven to decrease infection and must be contrasted against the increased pain, need for regional anesthesia or procedural sedation, and possible development of plantar scars from more aggressive debridement.

Cleaning the sole of the foot with soap and water will facilitate the exam and application of betadine to the skin surface may decrease bacterial contamination. Removal of jagged, insensate epidermal skin edges from larger wounds will expose the outer aspect of the puncture tract and any superficial foreign bodies.

Coring, which usually involves using a scalpel or punch biopsy to remove the margins of the puncture down to dermal or even subdermal depth, has been advocated by some as providing improved drainage and visualization. Sedation or regional anesthesia is required and some patients develop painful scars.

Probing of wounds also requires anesthesia and while it may reveal the presence of metal or glass foreign bodies, it may fail to detect softer foreign bodies like rubber, foam, or cloth and push them deeper into the tissues.

Irrigation of the superficial areas of the wound tract is possibly helpful and probably harmless. Injecting deeper into a closed tract may push contamination deeper or out along tissue planes.

The benefit of antibiotic therapy at the initial presentation of plantar puncture is as theoretical as all other interventions. It has not been studied either alone or as an adjunct to specific wound management (16). Seventy-five percent of the 77 children who developed osteomyelitis after plantar puncture in a 10-year study received antibiotics as initial treatment for the puncture (13).

A 24–48-h period of non-weight bearing may be beneficial.

Presentation between 2 and 7 Days

Those patients who present between 2 and 7 days after the puncture generally have worsening symptoms and most have an infection. In the Fitzgerald and Cowan study, 57% of 113 children presenting to the ED within that interval had cellulitis or localized abscess. Forty-one were cultured and 87% of the cultures yielded *Staphylococcus* or *Streptococcus*. Most patients were treated with antibiotics and experienced prompt improvement. Nine patients, who were treated with appropriate antibiotics based on their culture results, failed to improve and all nine required incision and drainage of an abscess. Five of those procedures also revealed a foreign body, which was removed. These patients then did well without further intervention (1).

Schwab and Powers studied the course of 63 patients with plantar punctures who presented within 24 h of the puncture and received minimal wound care. Twelve percent of their patients returned within 7 days and were found to have cellulitis, abscess, or foreign body and responded fully and quickly to antibiotic therapy or removal of the foreign body (2).

Since patients presenting on days 2–7 commonly have cellulitis or abscess, the evaluation should concentrate on identifying those conditions. If signs of infection are present and the patient has not previously had an x-ray, one should be ordered to search for a foreign body. Individual circumstances will dictate whether other imaging is needed to detect a non-radiopaque foreign body.

Although of unproven benefit, it would seem prudent in the face of established infection to debride and possibly to core the puncture wound under regional anesthesia or procedural sedation to search for a foreign body.

Anti-*staphylococcal* antibiotics such as cephalexin, dicloxacillin, or one effective against community-acquired methicillin-resistant *Staphylococcus aureus* (MRSA), if dictated by local resistance patterns, should be prescribed orally and rapid improvement expected. A scheduled, not "as needed," 48-h follow-up appointment with the patient's primary care physician should be arranged. The patient should remain non-weight-bearing and elevate the foot. Failure to resolve signs of infection should prompt an evaluation for deep abscess, occult foreign body, or osteomyelitis.

Presentation More than 7 Days after Puncture

When a patient presents after the first week, his symptoms usually have failed to resolve despite earlier treatment or he may be seeking medical attention for the first time due to progressive worsening since the puncture. This must prompt suspicion of osteomyelitis, septic arthritis, or abscess, with or without a foreign body. The physician must remember that fever, localized fluctuance, tenderness around the wound, and drainage from the puncture wound are rare. Diffuse dorsal foot swelling, tenderness, and pain with weight bearing are often the only signs and symptoms (17, 18).

Although most such patients seek attention within 2–3 weeks of the initial visit, some may present months or years later. It is essential to elicit the history of the perhaps forgotten puncture and pursue the search for osteomyelitis. All of these patients have retained foreign bodies, many despite previous surgical management (8, 19).

When symptoms persist beyond the first week, labs should be drawn and imaging ordered to look for signs of osteomyelitis. Suspicion of osteomyelitis should not diminish because of a normal peripheral white blood cell count; the mean value in puncture-associated osteomyelitis is 10,000/mm^3 (1). Blood cultures are usually negative. The ESR is the most valuable test to support suspicion of osteomyelitis. Crosby and Powell (20) noted an elevated ESR in 12 of 12 cases of plantar-puncture-associated osteomyelitis with a range of 22–54 and a mean of 41 mm/h. Jacobs et al. (13) found an abnormal ESR in 70 of 77 children (90%) with osteomyelitis with a median value of 38 mm/h. However, a normal ESR does not rule out osteomyelitis.

Fewer than one-third of patients with osteomyelitis will have any plain film abnormality in the first 7–10 days of symptoms. Ninety percent will have typical radiographic changes by 28 days (21). In the Jacobs series of children with osteomyelitis in which the mean time from puncture to hospitalization was 12 days, only 14% had a diagnostic plain x-ray (13).

The earliest, although nonspecific, sign of osteomyelitis on plain film is deep soft tissue swelling. Periosteal elevation is the first bony abnormality to appear. It is much more common in children because the periosteum of adults is tightly adherent to the bone. Signs of cortical destruction will follow, but 30–50% of bone mineral must be destroyed before lucency can be appreciated (21).

Ultrasound can demonstrate soft tissue swelling most pronounced near the bone and periosteal thickening and elevation.

The three-phase technetium 99m bone scan, contrast- and non-contrast-enhanced spiral CT, and MRI are positive as early as the second or third day of bone infection. The bone scan has a sensitivity of 90% and is the imaging method of choice for diagnosis. CT and MRI also have 90% sensitivity. They can be used to delineate the extent of bony involvement and the location of soft tissue or joint capsule pus collections in planning for surgery (21).

MRI cannot be used if metal foreign bodies are present. Choice of imaging modality often depends on institutional availability.

The patient who presents to the ED in the second week after the puncture with unresolved signs and symptoms should be admitted to the hospital with a presumed diagnosis of osteomyelitis to receive IV antibiotics which are active against *Pseudomonas* and *Staphylococcus* and to undergo imaging as described above and orthopedic consultation.

If osteomyelitis is confirmed, surgical management is required, not only to debride the infected bone and cartilage, but to find and drain infected joints and to explore for foreign bodies (17, 22, 23). Jacobs et al. (13) found 14 foreign bodies during surgical exploration in their 77 patients. One foreign body was a 2.5 cm piece of rubber from a tennis shoe sole. Cultures taken at surgery grew *Pseudomonas* alone or in combination with *Staphylococcus* and/or *Streptococcus* in 91 patients in two studies (13, 22).

Antibiotics are continued after surgery; the appropriate duration is unknown. In most studies, 1–2 weeks of parenteral anti-*Pseudomonal* antibiotics are given with good result. In one study in adults, oral ciprofloxacin was given for 2 weeks after surgical debridement with complete clinical resolution of symptoms (23). The 4–6-week regimen of IV antibiotics used to treat hematogenous osteomyelitis does not appear to be necessary in patients with disease caused by plantar puncture when managed with surgical debridement. However, there are no studies comparing various antibiotic treatment regimens.

Patients who do not demonstrate rapid resolution while on antibiotics after surgical treatment often require a second surgical intervention at which a previously undetected septic arthritis, soft tissue abscess, foreign body, or area of bone necrosis is found (13, 20, 22).

Crosby and Powell (20) have suggested that the ESR may be used to further monitor improvement after treatment and possibly to help determine the duration of antibiotic treatment. In their study of 14 cases of *Pseudomonas* osteomyelitis, the ESR decreased at a mean rate of 1.1 mm per day in all but 5 patients after treatment was started. In four of the five, ESR decreased when the antibiotic regimen was changed or surgery was done. The fifth patient's ESR declined but remained elevated despite 26 days of antibiotic therapy after surgery. He was readmitted a year later with foot pain and a still elevated ESR. He underwent incision and drainage. Culture grew the same *Pseudomonas*.

Disposition

The medical literature demonstrates that, among patients with plantar puncture wounds who come to medical attention, it can be anticipated that about 8–12% will develop an early cellulitis or superficial abscess and 0.04–1.8% will go on to develop the limb-threatening complication of osteomyelitis. Unfortunately, the lack of prospective studies comparing the efficacy of various wound care measures and antibiotic regimens leaves the physician without evidence-based recommendations to predict which patients will develop complications or to decrease their incidence.

However, physicians should not be misled by the relatively subtle physical examination findings and normal results of routine laboratory tests associated with these infectious complications. A "wait-and-see" approach applied to the patient with continued pain and swelling would reflect a lack of appreciation of the natural history of plantar-puncture-wound-associated infections and would allow progression of bone and joint destruction, possibly increasing the need for amputation.

The author offers the following suggestions for care of patients with plantar puncture wounds at the various stages at which they may present to the emergency department. These recommendations emphasize close follow-up and aggressive pursuit of a diagnosis of significant infection should the patient fail to improve rapidly on the treatment given at each stage (Tables 29–1 and 29–2).

The patient should be educated regarding the lack of certainty about the best way to treat plantar puncture wounds to prevent complications and this should be documented on the medical record. The possible complications of plantar punctures and the importance of follow-up must be emphasized. Written discharge instructions should include arrangements for definite, not "as needed," follow-up at 48 h.

Table 29–1. Treatment Recommendations

Patient presents on day of puncture
  Well-documented history
  Physical exam with light and magnification
  Tetanus immunization, as appropriate
  Surface wound cleaning
  Minor debridement, if needed, possibly with irrigation of superficial portion of puncture track
  X-ray for foreign body, if history and exam suggest
  No antibiotics
  Crutches for non-weight-bearing for 24–48 h
  Elevate limb
  Mandatory follow-up at 48-h

Patient presents on day 2–7 with signs of infection
  History and exam
  X-ray for foreign body
  Coring and exploration for foreign body
  Treat for cellulitis with anti-*Staph/Strep* antibiotics, usually as outpatient
  Crutches for non-weight-bearing for 48 h
  Elevate limb
  48-h scheduled follow-up with admission for IV antibiotics and imaging if not significantly improved

Patient presents >7 days after puncture with signs of infection
  History and exam
  Labs
  Admit for anti-*Pseudomonal* IV antibiotics and imaging for osteomyelitis
  Orthopedic consultation

Table 29–2. Recommendations for Antibiotic Therapy

Patient presents on day of puncture
  No antibiotics

Patient presents on day 2–7 with signs of infection (outpatient)
  Treat for *Staphylococcal/Streptococcal* infection
    First-generation cephalosporin, e.g., cephalexin
    Penicillinase-resistant penicillin, e.g., dicloxacillin
      Penicillin-allergic patient-first-generation cephalosporin, macrolide, clindamycin, TMP/SMX
    Endemic community-acquired MRSA—TMP/SMX or as suggested by local susceptibility patterns

Patient presents > 7 days after puncture with signs of infection (inpatient)
  Treat for *Pseudomonas* infection±possible *Staph/Strep* coinfection
    Anti-*Pseudomonal* cephalosporin, e.g., cefepime
    Anti-*Pseudomonal* penicillin, e.g., ticarcillin/clavulanate
    Anti-*Pseudomonal* aminoglycoside, e.g., gentamicin, tobramycin
    Meropenem, imipenem
    Ciprofloxacin
    Add vancomycin if CA-MRSA endemic

Case Outcome

The emergency physician placed a consult for admission for further evaluation. The consultant noted that the foot was not red, warm, fluctuant, or indurated and that there was no fever or drainage. The consultant's diagnosis was resolving cellulitis and he discharged the patient with instructions to elevate the foot and a follow-up in clinic in 2 weeks.

Three days later the patient returned to the ED with continued inability to bear weight due to foot pain. A bone scan showed osteomyelitis of the third, fourth, and fifth metatarsals. White blood count was 6600/mm^3. ESR was 35 mm/h. The patient was admitted to the orthopedic service and received 2 days of intravenous fluoroquinolone therapy. A PICC line was placed for planned 6 weeks of IV antibiotic therapy.

At the end of 6 weeks of IV antibiotic therapy, the patient was symptomfree. His ESR was 8 mm/h.

Author's Comment

This patient's initial care typified the widespread lack of knowledge about the signs, symptoms, and natural history of complications of plantar puncture wounds. After several visits, the correct diagnosis was made and the patient received treatment that was apparently effective. He did not, however, have surgical exploration of his wound, which is a necessary component of treatment to ensure that foreign bodies are removed, infected bone and cartilage debrided, and septic joints drained. He underwent a prolonged course of antibiotics that may not have been necessary had he undergone the surgical procedure.

REFERENCES

1. Fitzgerald RH Jr., Cowan JDE: Puncture wounds of the foot. *Orthop Clin North Am* 6:965–972, 1975.
2. Schwab RA, Powers RD: Conservative therapy of plantar puncture wounds. *J Emerg Med* 13:291–295, 1995.
3. Houston AN, Roy WA, Faust RA, et al.: Tetanus prophylaxis in the treatment of puncture wounds of patients in the deep South. *J Trauma* 2:439–446, 1962.
4. Gonzalez SM, Hamilton FN, Lydon DR, et al.: Watch your step: Avoiding lawsuits for management of plantar puncture wounds. *Emerg Legal Brief* 4:89–95, 1993.
5. Patzakis MJ, Wilkins J, Brien WW, et al.: Wound site as a predictor of complications following deep nail punctures to the foot. *West J Med* 150:545–547, 1989.
6. Lavery LA, Walker SC, Harkless LB, et al.: Infected puncture wounds in diabetic and nondiabetic adults. *Diabetes Care* 18:1588–1591, 1995.
7. Chisholm CD, Schlesser JF: Plantar puncture wounds: Controversies and treatment recommendations. *Ann Emerg Med* 18:1352–1357, 1989.
8. Chong CH, Verhoeven W, Mun CW: Rubber foreign bodies in puncture wounds of the foot in patients wearing rubber-soled shoes. *Foot Ankle Int* 22:409–414, 2001.
9. Wilson S, Casio B, Neitzschman HR: Nail puncture wound to the foot. *J La State Med Soc* 151:251–252, 1999.
10. Goldstein EJC, Ahonkhai VI, Cristofaro RL, et al.: Source of *Pseudomonas* in osteomyelitis of heels. *J Clin Microbiol* 12:711–713, 1980.
11. Fisher MC, Goldsmith JF, Gilligan PH: Sneakers as a source of *Pseudomonas aeruginosa* in children with osteomyelitis following puncture wounds. *J Pediatr* 106:607–609, 1985.
12. Roberts JR: Stepping on a nail: Some rational clinical guidelines. EMN 12:9–13, 1998.
13. Jacobs RF, McCarthy RE, Elser JM: *Pseudomonas* osteochondritis complicating puncture wounds of the foot in children: A 10-year evaluation. *J Inf Dis* 160:657–661, 1989.
14. Lammers RL, Magill T: Detection and management of foreign bodies in soft tissue. *Emerg Med Clin North Am* 10:767–781, 1992.
15. Ginsburg MJ, Ellis GL, Flom L: Detection of soft tissue foreign bodies by plain radiography, xerography, computed tomography, and ultrasonography. *Ann Emerg Med* 19:701–703, 1990.
16. Harrison M, Thomas M: Towards evidence based emergency medicine: Best BETs from Manchester Royal Infirmary. Antibiotics after puncture wounds to the foot. *Emerg Med J* 19:49, 2002.
17. Inaba AS, Zukin DD, Perro M: An update on the evaluation and management of plantar puncture wounds and *Pseudomonas* osteomyelitis. *Pediatr Emerg Care* 8:38–44, 1992.
18. Saha P, Parrish CA, McMillan J: *Pseudomonas* osteomyelitis after a plantar puncture wound through a rubber sandal. *Pediatr Infect Dis J* 15:710–711, 1996.
19. Markiewitz AD, Karns DJ, Brooks PJ: Late infections of the foot due to incomplete removal of foreign bodies: A report of two cases. *Foot Ankle* 15:52–55, 1994.
20. Crosby LA, Powell DA: The potential value of the sedimentation rate in monitoring treatment outcome in puncture-wound-related *Pseudomonas* osteomyelitis. *Clin Orthop* 188:168–172, 1984.
21. Perron AD, Brady WJ, Miller M: Orthopedic pitfalls in the ED: Osteomyelitis. *Am J Emerg Med* 21:61–67, 2003.
22. Jacobs RF, Adelman L, Sack CM, et al.: Management of *Pseudomonas* osteochondritis complicating puncture wounds of the foot. *Pediatrics* 69:432–435, 1982.
23. Raz R, Miron D: Oral ciprofloxacin for treatment of infection following nail puncture wounds of the foot. *Clin Infect Dis* 21:194–195, 1995.

30

Diabetic Foot Ulcers

Heather Murphy-Lavoie
Keith Van Meter

HIGH YIELD FACTS

- Diabetic foot ulcers are precursors to lower extremity amputation and should be treated aggressively to reduce the likelihood of amputation.
- *Staphylococcus aureus* is the most important pathogen in diabetic foot infections; however, as severity increases infections become polymicrobial.
- Antibiotic coverage should include Staphylococcus and Streptococcus species at a minimum; increasing severity of disease warrants broader antimicrobial coverage.
- Hyperbaric oxygen therapy (HBOT) reduces amputation rates in selected cases of diabetic foot ulceration.

CASE PRESENTATION

A 67-year-old insulin-dependent diabetic male presents with a 2-year history of a nonhealing ulcer of his left foot. He has been appropriately off-loaded in a custom orthotic and has had a vascular evaluation to rule out operable peripheral vascular disease. Over the last month he has received wound care through home health; however, the foot has begun to swell and become more painful.

His vital signs on presentation were: blood pressure 149/84, heart rate 105, respiratory rate 12, temperature 100.4°F, and pulse oximetry revealed 99% hemoglobin oxygen saturation. Physical examination revealed a tender fluctuant plantar foot with a dusky 1.5 cm ulcer over the first metatarsal-phalangeal joint (Fig. 30–1) and 1+ peripheral pulses at points of palpation of both dorsalis pedis and posterior tibial arteries. He has Achilles tendon contracture and decreased ability to dorsiflex his foot, leading to increased pressure on the plantar surface of his foot at the ulcer. He has erythema and edema of the entire foot but not extending to the calf. There is purulent drainage and tenderness to deep palpation, although a significant peripheral sensory neuropathy is present.

INTRODUCTION/EPIDEMIOLOGY

Diabetes is an increasingly prevalent and costly illness. There are approximately 16 million diabetics in the United States with more than 18% of persons over 65 having diabetes. The 3-year incidence of ulceration among all diabetics is 6%. The 3-year mortality of diabetics with foot ulceration is 28%. Of those with ulcers 15% will require amputation and 15% will develop osteomyelitis (1, 2). Infection is a significant predisposing risk factor for amputation in 68% of diabetics who undergo lower extremity amputation (3). The estimated cost of a single ulcer episode is $5000 and this increases to between $40,000 and $70,000 if amputation, hospitalization, and rehabilitation are required (2, 4). The impressive morbidity, mortality, and cost of diabetic foot ulcers demand diligence to minimize impact.

PATHOPHYSIOLOGY/MICROBIOLOGY

Diabetics are more susceptible to foot ulceration than patients without diabetes for a variety of reasons. The quatrad of ischemia, neuropathy, infection, and nutritional dysfunction predisposes diabetics to ulcer formation (5). A poorly perfused foot is more resistant to healing than a well-perfused foot. Also, autonomic neuropathy in diabetics leads to less recruitment of capillaries and a diminished effectiveness of perfusion. In addition, the loss of sensation impedes the natural response to pressure or injury and a loss of sweat and oil gland activity causes dry cracking skin that fissures easily (5). For these reasons diabetics are more likely to develop an ulcer and have a more difficult time healing an ulcer once it forms. And it is from these ulcers that infection typically begins.

Staphylococcus aureus and *Streptococcus* species predominate in early infections; however, more chronic and severe infections tend to be polymicrobial. Lipsky et al. (6) reported a prospective evaluation of diabetic patients with non-limb-threatening lower extremity infections and who were not yet treated with antibiotics, and cultures revealed aerobic gram-positive cocci as pathogens in 89% of patients and were sole pathogens in almost one half of those patients (6). *Enterococcus* species follows *S. aureus* as the most commonly cultured organism, especially in patients previously treated with cephalosporins (3). As infection and necrosis deepens and becomes more severe, gram-negative and anaerobic pathogens are also likely to be isolated. Many of these are resistant organisms, specifically methicillin-resistant *S. aureus*, and they are becoming increasingly common (3).

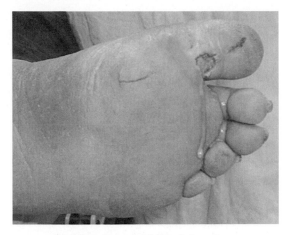

Fig. 30–1. Example of diabetic foot ulcer.

CLINICAL PRESENTATION

Diabetic patients may not always be aware of pressure points or early ulcer formation on their feet since they are often insensate. Additionally their visual acuity may be impaired by ophthalmologic diabetic end organ damage. Muscle, tendon, and joint flexibility are also impaired by structural protein glycolization. This lack of flexibility makes it difficult for diabetics to inspect the bottoms of their feet without a mirror even when they can see clearly. They may not recognize a problem area until malodorous discharge or extensive infection develops. Therefore, the goal in these patients is to identify and treat patients at risk prior to the ulcer formation.

Risk factors for ulcer formation are listed in Table 30–1. Patients with these risk factors should be referred for protective footwear, screened for reversible peripheral vascular disease, and have screening foot exams at least every 6 months.

Once an ulcer forms, staging of the ulcer can facilitate multidisciplinary care and aid in monitoring progress and predicting outcome. Patients with stage-3 ulcers or higher, for example, are candidates for hyperbaric oxygen

Table 30–1. Risk Factors for Ulcer Formation

History of previous ulcer or amputation
Sensory neuropathy
Peripheral vascular disease
Foot deformity
Age over 65
Poor glycemic control
Renal disease

Table 30–2. Wagner Ulcer Classification System (7)

Grade	Lesion
0	No open lesion; may have deformity or cellulitis
1	Superficial ulcer (partial or full thickness)
2	Ulcer extends to ligament, tendon or joint without abscess or osteomyelitis
3	Deep ulcer with abscess, osteomyelitis, tendonitis, or joint sepsis
4	Gangrene of a portion of the forefoot or heel
5	Extensive gangrene of the entire foot

therapy. Several classification systems have been described, but the Wagner system is the most widely used (7) (Table 30–2).

Infections of the lower extremities in diabetic patients commonly occur on the plantar surface of the forefoot, in particular the toes and metatarsal heads. The diagnosis of infection in the diabetic ulcer is a clinical one based upon the presence of fever, purulent secretions, and two or more of the following classic signs or infection: erythema, warmth, swelling, pain or tenderness, foul odor, lymphangitis, or gas formation (8). Interestingly, many patients do not report pain and fewer than 50% have fever (9). Severe pain and tenderness in the foot, especially in a previously insensate foot, suggests the presence of a deep space infection.

Limb- and/or life-threatening infections may present with signs of necrotizing infection, such as hemorrhagic bullae, crepitus, necrosis, and gangrene. These patients will also demonstrate systemic signs of infection, including fever, chills, leukocytosis, altered mental status, hypotension, and dehydration. Laboratory abnormalities include hyperglycemia, leukocytosis, azotemia, and electrolyte abnormalities (8).

LABORATORY/DIAGNOSTIC TESTING

Diabetic foot ulcers are usually diagnosed by their clinical appearance; however, it is important to screen for reversible pathology and underlying infection. Blood glucose measurement and control is essential. Uremia impairs healing by interfering with collagen deposition and by decreasing the amount of granulation tissue in the wound. Screening for and control of uremia is therefore important (10). Other blood tests are commonly performed to aid in the diagnosis of an infected diabetic foot, including WBC count and erythrocyte sedimentation rate (ESR). However, these tests are not sensitive nor specific. Two reports suggest that up to 50% of diabetic patients with deep foot infections do not demonstrate a leukocytosis (11, 12).

Obtaining samples for microbiological testing is worthwhile, particularly for patients with more severe infection. However, samples may be easily contaminated by surface bacteria and reveal little information on the true pathogen. Simply swabbing the surface of an infected ulcer and sending purulent material for culture or debris will not yield useful data. Aspiration of deep purulent secretions and obtaining tissue by curettage or biopsy are superior methods. Tissue scrapings and biopsy are more reliable than superficial swabs.

Since 15% of patients with diabetic foot ulcers develop osteomyelitis, patients with ulcers should have radiography to screen for osteomyelitis. Additional information obtained by radiographs may include evidence of subcutaneous emphysema (suggesting infection with gas forming bacteria, such as *Clostridium perfringens*), abscesses, or foreign bodies (2). Advanced osteomyelitis on radiograph shows periosteal reaction and destructive osteolytic lesions; however, early in the course of the disease the radiograph may appear normal. Probing the ulcer with a sterile blunt probe and palpating bone has a 66% sensitivity and a 85% specificity to detect osteomyelitis (13). If the foot appears infected, an erythrocyte sedimentation rate (ESR >40) is associated with a 12-fold increased likelihood of osteomyelitis and may help identify those patients who should undergo In-labeled leukocyte scan or magnetic resonance imaging (MRI) to identify early osteomyelitis not yet evident on plain radiography (14). False positive results can occur with each of these radiographic studies in diabetic osteolysis (boney destruction or neuropathic osteopathy that occurs in diabetics) and/or charcot foot. The clinician should be mindful of the radiographic mime of osteomyelitis in the diabetic patient, which presents itself as diabetic osteolysis. Early charcot foot presents itself as soft tissue sterile inflammation with diabetic osteolysis with signs and symptoms not unlike diabetic osteomyelitis. The gold standard for diagnosis of osteomyelitis is bone biopsy and culture (2).

Optimization of blood flow and oxygen delivery significantly improves chances of healing; therefore, these patients should undergo screening for peripheral vascular disease and local tissue hypoxia. Transcutaneous oxygen measurements can identify local tissue hypoxia and are useful in predicting peripheral vascular disease and those patients who may benefit from hyperbaric oxygen therapy (15). Arterial Doppler studies are less expensive and less invasive than angiography; however, patients with peripheral vascular disease often have to ultimately undergo angiography to determine if the patient is a candidate for stenting, angioplasty, or bypass surgery. These studies are traditionally not done as part of the emergency department evaluation although they play a critical role in determining the treatment course.

MANAGEMENT

The presence and severity of infection in diabetic foot ulcers dictates management; therefore, careful assessment is mandatory. Ulcers and their surrounding tissues must be assessed for depth of soft tissue involvement, presence of foreign bodies, and necrotic tissue.

Mild infections generally only involve the local skin with less than 2 cm of surrounding cellulitis. These infections tend to be slowly progressive. The patient will not show any systemic signs of infection. Laboratory abnormalities are generally limited to hyperglycemia.

Severe infections of diabetic ulcers tend to be acute and/or rapidly progressive. The infection extends deep into the dermis, and possibly into the subcutaneous tissues, even deep enough to involve the fascia, muscle, and bone. It may also spread to tissues distant to the ulcer.

Mild to moderate infection of diabetic foot ulcers are primarily infected with *S. aureus*, or other aerobic grampositive cocci, and therefore antibiotic selection must target these pathogens initially. These patients may be managed as outpatients with an oral antibiotic such as cephalexin, amoxicillin/clavulanate, or clindamycin (8) (Table 30–3).

Polymicrobial involvement (gram-positive cocci predominantly plus gram-negative bacilli and anaerobes) is the rule in severe diabetic foot infections (3). Increasing severity of infection leads to decreased margin of error for coverage and more broad spectrum antibiotics are recommended pending culture results. For example, for patients with infected diabetic ulcers and moderate to severe cellulitis, intravenous ampicillin/sulbactam or clindamycin is recommended (8). Those with limb- or life-threatening infections should be treated with imipenem or meropenem plus vancomycin. Depending on local incidence of methicillin-resistant *S. aureus*, vancomycin should be considered in all but the most superficial ulcers. All infected ulcers treated with systemic antibiotics should have cultures obtained so that the antibiotic regime can be tailored to the specific infection.

Emergency physicians should maintain a low threshold for surgical consultation for patients with infected

Table 30–3. Antibiotic Regimens for Infected Diabetic Foot Ulcers (7–9)

Depth/Severity of Infection	First Line	Alternatives
Mild to moderate localized cellulitis	Cephalexin 500 mg po qid	Amoxicillin/clavulanate 875/ 125 mg po bid OR Clindamycin 450 mg po qid
Moderate to severe cellulitis	Ampicillin/sulbactam 3 g iv qid	Ticarcillin/clavulanate 3.1 g iv qid OR Pipericillin/tazobactam 3.3 g iv qid OR Vancomycin 1g iv Q D OR Clindamycin 600 mg iv tid PLUS Ceftazidime 2g iv TID
Life or limb threatening infection	Imipenem/cilastin 500 mg iv qid OR Meropenem 1 g iv tid PLUS Vancomycin 1.0 g in bid	Aztreonam 2 g iv tid PLUS Metronidazole 7.5 mg/kg in tid PLUS Vancomycin 1 g iv bid

diabetic foot ulcers. Any suspicion of abscess formation, deep space infection, necrotizing infection, or foreign body mandates a prompt surgical evaluation.

Grade 1 or 2 ulcers without infection can be managed with local moist wound care and outpatient follow-up. Moist wound healing improves epidermal migration, promotes angiogenesis and connective tissue synthesis, and also aids in autodebridement of necrotic tissue. Moist dressings must have the precaution of not overextending wound margins to prevent the common problem of maceration of intact wound margin dermis. Sharp debridement is indicated for grossly necrotic tissue except in cases of dry gangrene and peripheral vascular disease in which case autoamputation may be physiologically preferable to surgical amputation (2). Emergency physicians should feel comfortable with local superficial debridements in patients not requiring abscess drainage or extensive resections. In diabetic patients these procedures can usually be done without local anesthesia or sedation since the patients are often insensate. Topical antibiotic ointments (e.g., Mupirocin) can be used in conjunction with systemic antibiotics when wound beds appear infected; however, usage should be limited to not more than 2 weeks to avoid the development of resistant organisms. Occlusive or semiocclusive dressings retain moisture better than topical antibiotics. In cases of copious drainage and mac-

eration of surrounding tissue an absorptive dressing (e.g., Calcium alginate) would be preferred.

In a fresh wound a platelet plug forms and platelets are stimulated to release their growth factors into the wound. These growth factors attract macrophages into the area, stimulate the proliferation of macrophages and fibroblasts, cause fibroblasts to lay down the collagen matrix, and stimulate angiogenesis. In a chronic wound these processes are often stalled. The addition of platelet derived growth factors through autologous graft or becaplermin can "jump-start" a stalled wound (2, 18). Several skin substitutes have been developed to aid in healing of diabetic ulcers theoretically by providing growth factors and chemotatic agents to the wound bed (19–21). Use of these agents is reserved for wounds that are not infected and is probably beyond the prevue of most emergency physicians.

Altered foot mechanics in diabetics from stiffening and shortening of tendons has been blamed for contributing to ulcer formation. In a case series of 16 patients, Laborde (22) showed 87.5% healing rate of diabetic foot ulcers following Achilles tendon lengthening. In a prospective controlled trial, Mueller et al. (23) found patients with Achilles tendon lengthening were 75% less likely to have ulcer recurrence than controls. Patients with diabetic foot ulcers presenting to the emergency department should be screened for the presence of Achilles tendon contracture and referred for repair as necessary.

Hyperbaric oxygen therapy has been shown in multiple trials to reduce amputation rates and improve healing in patients with diabetic foot ulcers (2426). The largest, best-designed trial was published in 1996 by Faglia. This study included 68 patients with severe infected or gangrenous diabetic foot ulcers randomized to a hyperbaric oxygen treatment or standard moist wound care. Of the patients treated with hyperbaric oxygen therapy, 8.6% underwent lower extremity amputation compared to a 33.3% amputation rate in the control group (26). HBOT works on a variety of pathways. It increases the efficiency of leukocyte activity by oxidative killing, thereby diminishing infection. It reduces tissue edema through hyperoxic vasoconstriction while still augmenting tissue oxygenation. It stimulates fibroblast growth, collagen synthesis, and angiogenesis. In addition, HBOT upregulates the expression of platelet derived growth factor receptor sites in the wound bed. For these reasons, patients with refractory ulcers or extensive infection (Wagner grade III or higher) should be considered for hyperbaric oxygen therapy.

DISPOSITION

Deep space infections (involvement of fascia, muscle, join, or bone), abscesses, necrotizing infections (crepitus, bullae, or ecchymosis), and/or rapidly progressing, extensive cellulitis in association with an infected diabetic foot ulcer all require acute surgical intervention and warrant emergent surgical consult and hospital admission. Additional considerations for hospitalization include severe hyperglycemia, sepsis, acidosis, azotemia, dehydration and electrolyte abnormalities. Social considerations affecting admission decisions include the ability of the patients to care for themselves (e.g. , off-load the affected area and to perform wound care) and the ability to afford and tolerate antimicrobial therapy.

CASE OUTCOME

The patient was admitted to the hospital for intravenous ampicillin/sulbactam, surgical debridement, Achilles tendon lengthening, and hyperbaric oxygen therapy. His transcutaneous oxygen measurements increased from TcPO2 of 30 on his dorsal foot on room air to 250 under hyperbaric oxygen conditions, which was a positive predictor of his chances of healing with hyperbaric oxygen support. Pre- and postoperatively he underwent a course of 40 hyperbaric oxygen treatments. During hyperbaric

oxygen therapy the wound was followed closely and a moist wound healing environment was maintained. His wound healed within 6 weeks and remained healed at 3-year follow-up.

REFERENCES

1. CDC: History of Foot Ulcer Among Persons with Diabetes—United States, 2000–2002. *Morb Mortal Wkly Rep* 2002.
2. Peterson KA, et al.: Advances in managing the diabetic foot. *J Fam Pract* 49:11, 2000, S1–S49.
3. Frykberg R: An evidence-based approach to diabetic foot infections. *Am J Surg 186(5A)*, 2003.
4. Green M, et al.: Diabetic foot: Evaluation and management. *South Med J* 95:1, 95–101, 2002.
5. LoGerfo FW, Gibbons GW: Chronic complications of diabetes: Vascular disease of the lower extremities in diabetes mellitus. *Endocrinol Metab Clin* 25:2, 439–445, 1996.
6. Lipsky BA, Pecoraro RE, Larson SA, Hanley ME, Ahroni JH: Outpatients management of uncomplicated lower-extremity infections in diabetic patients. *Arch Intern Med* 150(4):790–797, 1990.
7. Wagner FW, et al.: The Diabetic Foot. *Orthopedics* 10:163–167, 1987.
8. van Baal JG: Surgical treatment of the infected diabetic foot. *Clin Infect Dis* 39:S123–S128, 2004.
9. Lipsky B: Medical treatment of diabetic foot infections. *Clin Infect Dis* 39:S104–S114, 2004.
10. Deery H, et al.: Infections in patients with chronic renal failure: Saving the diabetic foot with special reference to the patient with chronic renal failure. *Infect Dis Clin North Am* 15:3, 2001.
11. Armstrong DG: Leucocytosis is a poor indicator of acute osteomyelitis of the foot in diabetes mellitus. *J Foot Ankle Surg* 35:280–283, 1996.
12. Eneroth M: Clinical characteristics and outcome in 223 diabetic patients with deep foot infections. *Foot Ankle Int* 18:716–722, 1997.
13. Grayson ML, Gibbons GW, Balogh K, Levin E, Karchmer AW: Probing to bone in infected pedal ulcers. A clinical sign of underlying osteomyelitis in diabetic patients. *JAMA* 273(9):721–723, 1995.
14. Lipsky B: Osteomyelitis of the foot in diabetic patients. *Clin Infect Dis* 25:1318–1326, 1997.
15. Strauss MB, Bryant BJ, Hart GB: Transcutaneous oxygen measurements under hyperbaric oxygen conditions as a predictor for healing of problem wounds. *Foot Ankle Int* 23(10):933–937, 2002.
16. Lipsky B, et al.: Treating foot infections in diabetic patients: A randomized, multicenter, open-label trial of linezolid versus ampicillin-sulbactam/amoxicillin-clavulanate. *Clin Inect Dis* 38:17–24, 2004.
17. The Sanford Guide to Antimicrobial Therapy
18. Wieman TJ, et al.: Efficacy and safety of a topical gel formulation of recombinant human platelet-derived growth factor-BB (becaplermin) in patients with chronic neuropathic

diabetic foot ulcers: A phase III randomized, placebo-controlled, double blind study. *Diabetes Care* 21:822–827, 1998.

19. Veves A: Graftskin, a human skin equivalent, is effective in the management of noninfected neuropathic diabetic foot ulcers: A prospective randomized multicentered clinical trial. *Diabetes Care* 24:290–295, 2001.

20. Gentzkow GD: Use of dermagraft, a cultured human dermis, to treat diabetic foot ulcers. *Diabetes Care* 19:350–354, 1996.

21. Redekop WK: The cost effectiveness of Apligraf treatment of diabetic foot ulcers. *Pharmacoeconomics* 21:1171–1183, 2003.

22. Laborde JM: Treatment of forefoot ulcers with tendon lengthenings. *J South Orthop Assoc* 12(2):60–65, 2003.

23. Mueller MJ, Sinacore DR, Hastings MK, Strube MJ, Johnson JE: Effect of Achilles tendon lengthening on neuropathic plantar ulcers. *J Bone Joint Surg* 2003.

24. Hunt D, et al.: Foot ulcers in diabetes. *Clin Evidence* 5: 397–402, 2001.

25. Baroni G, Porro T, et al.: Hyperbaric oxygen in diabetic gangrene treatment. *Diabetes Care* 10:1, 81–86, 1987.

26. Faglia F, et al.: Adjunctive systemic hyperbaric oxygen in treatment of severe prevalently ischemic diabetic foot ulcers—a randomized trial. *Diabetes Care* 19(12):1338–1343, 1996.

31

Paronychias, Felons, and Tenosynovitis

Fiona E. Gallahue
Rafael E. Torres

HIGH YIELD FACTS

1. Paronychias are caused by mixed flora involving both aerobic and anaerobic bacteria.

2. Chronic paronychias are indolent and cyclical, best treated by avoidance of inciting factors.

3. Immobilization of the involved hand is critical in the management of tenosynovitis and felons.

4. Disseminated gonorrhea should be considered as the underlying etiology of acute flexor tenosynovitis in all sexually active persons especially if there is no apparent traumatic etiology.

CASE PRESENTATION

A 23-year-old woman presents with a swollen, painful left index finger for 3 days. She notes that the finger has progressively become more swollen, warm, and tender over the 3 days and notes erythema, which began yesterday. She denies any history of trauma to the site or prior swelling of any fingers or joints. She has no past medical history, takes oral contraceptives, and has no allergies. She is sexually active with a few partners and does not always remember to use barrier protection. Her family history is noncontributory. She has a negative review of systems except for a mild sore throat for 1 week.

On physical exam, her vital signs are within normal limits including a temperature of 98.9°F. Pharyngeal examination reveals erythema of the tonsils with no hypertrophy or exudates. She has no cervical lymphadenopathy. Her left index finger is erythematous with fusiform swelling. The digit at rest is held in slight flexion; there is no evidence of trauma to the digit. When the examiner passively extends the left index finger, the patient winces and notes increased pain. There is tenderness over the flexor tendon of the left index finger. The rest of the exam is unremarkable.

PARONYCHIA

Introduction

Paronychia is the most common hand infection (Table 31–1), representing approximately one-third of all hand infections. It is found along the nails of the hand (most commonly) and foot. The infection is categorized as either acute or chronic depending on time to development, duration of symptoms, and etiology. Each condition has a unique pathophysiology, clinical presentation, and management, therefore proper recognition is essential. Care must be taken to differentiate it from other diseases (e.g., felons, psoriasis, malignant melanoma, herpetic whitlow) that involve the area adjacent to the nail plate.

Acute and chronic paronychias can occur concomitantly and should be treated appropriately. Repeat exacerbations do occur for both acute and chronic paronychias; in these cases, other potentially life-threatening etiologies (e.g., primary and metastatic carcinoma) should be considered.

ACUTE PARONYCHIA

Epidemiology/Pathophysiology

Acute paronychias develop from repeated local trauma (e.g., nail biting, hangnail, poor hygiene, manicuring, foreign body) that disrupts the junction of the nail plate and nail fold (1). Bacterial invasion easily follows the loss of this natural barrier. Although common skin bacteria predominate, paronychias have come to be recognized as infections of mixed flora, including both aerobic and anaerobic organisms. The most common aerobic pathogens isolated are *Staphylococcus aureus* (21%), group A beta-hemolytic streptococcus (6%), and eikenella corrodens (7%). The most common anaerobic pathogens isolated are gram-positive anaerobic cocci (42%), bacteroides species (19%), and fusobacterium species (19%) (2).

Clinical Presentation

Acute paronychias present with the classic signs of infection: erythema, edema, tenderness, and warmth. Early on, these characteristics are primarily localized to the dorsolateral aspect of the nail plate and along the eponychial fold. Cellulitis encompassing a greater portion of the distal tip may be present as well. Because a suppurative collection has yet to form during this early stage, most patients do not present to the E.D. during this time. However, most patients affected seek medical attention later, when extension to the contralateral nail plate margin develops

Table 31–1. Hand Infections, Common Etiology, and Appropriate Therapy

	Organism Most Commonly Involved	**Recommended Treatment**
Acute paronychia	Mixed flora	Outpatient Amoxicillin/clavulanic Acid Tetracycline Inpatient Cefoxitin Ticaricillin/clavulanic Acid
Chronic paronychia	Fungal (*Candida* spp. sp.) versus Contact dermatitis	1. Avoidance of moist environments 2. Topical antifungal agents or Nystatin Miconizole Ketoconazole Ciclopirox Systemic antifungal agents Fluconazole Itraconazole
Felon	*S. aureus*	Dicloxicillin Cephalexin
Tenosynovitis	*S. aureus*, Streptococcal sp. consider *Neisseria gonococcus*	Routine: No unusual organisms suspected I.V. antibiotics directed against *S. aureus* and streptococcal sp., multiple regimens acceptable If *N. gonococcus* suspected Ceftriaxone or Cefotaxime or Ciprofloxin or Ofloxin or Levofloxin PLUS Rx for concomitant *Chlamydia trachomatis* with Doxycycline or Azithromycin

along with a purulent collection. This stage is known as a "run around" infection. Finally, when left untreated, perionchial spread develops, which involves the potential space between the nail plate and nail bed. By this time, a defined area of fluctuance will be universally present or actively draining.

Management

In most cases of acute paronychia, a clinical diagnosis is sufficient. When a defined collection of pus is present, the mixed flora limits the utility of a Gram stain and culture; therefore, this testing is not routinely advised. Only complicated cases where healing is delayed or patient characteristics exist that may promote growth of an unusual organism (e.g., nursing home, diabetic patients, etc.) should have microbiologic testing. Similarly, radiographs of the digit are rarely useful. Radiographs are only advised if a foreign body, osteomyelitis, or subcutaneous gas is a clinical possibility.

Management of an acute paronychia is dependent on the stage of infection. Early signs of infection without a defined collection for drainage should be managed with warm water soaks 3–4 times daily, elevation, and if evidence of bacteria is present (i.e., cellulitis, signs of systemic involvement), an antistaphylococcal antibiotic, preferably amoxicillin and clavulanic acid (Augmentin). Due to the resistance demonstrated by anaerobic bacteria such as Bacteroides species, oxacillin and first-generation cephalosporins are poor antibiotic choices. Tetracycline is a cheaper alternative but cannot be used in pregnant or pediatric patients (2). Patients who are systemically ill or who have extensive cellulitis should be admitted for parenteral antibiotics, preferably cefoxitin or the combination of ticaricillin and clavulanic acid.

For a more advanced paronychia there are three stages to treatment in the emergency department: (1) incision and drainage, (2) irrigation, and (3) packing and dressing. If a collection is present, surgical drainage is the standard of care.

Adequate pain is paramount for this painful condition. Using analgesics and a complete digital block, using no more than 5 mL of 2% lidocaine without epinephrine is sufficient. There are several acceptable techniques for performing nerve blocks; however, the conventional method is as follows. After prepping the area with povidone-iodine and applying sterile drapes, 25-gauge needle is introduced dorsally or ventrally to infiltrate 1.0–2.5 cc of lidocaine to the ulnar aspect of the base of the involved digit, and one should repeat this on the radial side (3). If there is a need for prolonged anesthesia, there is evidence that 1% lidocaine with epinephrine is safe to use in selected patients with no vasospastic, thrombotic, or extreme medical conditions (4, 5).

Treatment consists of an incision with # 11 scalpel or a single puncture with an 18-gauge needle. It should be noted that these methods of drainage have never been compared for outcomes in a prospective randomized fashion. If the collection is extensive, a # 11 scalpel should only be employed. The incision or puncture should be from the medial direction into the nail fold, being careful to avoid the nail plate. The preferred approach is medial, as it reduces the likelihood of a visual and/or painful scar (see Fig. 31–1). If perionchial spread has occurred, removal of a 2–3-mm longitudinal section of the nail plate may be required to achieve adequate drainage. In a "run around" infection the proximal eponychial fold should be drained. This can be accomplished by sliding the # 11 scalpel into the sulcus, followed by gentle lifting of the fold. For more severe cases, bilateral dorsolateral incisions should be made. If this still fails to provide adequate drainage, removal of the proximal third of the nail plate should follow (see Fig. 31–2). Caution must be advised with such an extensive dissection due to the scar-

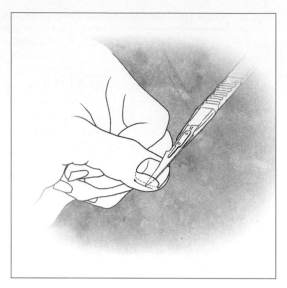

Fig. 31–1. Courtesy of Retsu Takahashi.

ring that may result (6). Following surgical treatment, the wound should be copiously irrigated. When feasible, a dry gauze packing is placed to prevent reaccumulation. Petroleum gauze should always replace any nail removed from the eponychial sulcus, in order to prevent fold adherence and scar formation. As with the management of an earlier-stage paronychia, the surgically treated hand or foot should be kept elevated, clean, and dry, and an antistaphylococcal antibiotic prescribed. Because of the

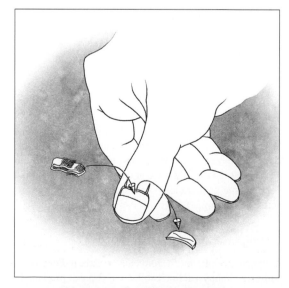

Fig. 31–2. Courtesy of Retsu Takahashi.

mixed flora comprising the infection, antibiotic coverage must be carefully tailored for those predisposed to uncommon, more virulent pathogens (e.g., diabetic, immunosuppressed, etc.).

Prior to discharge, one shoul check tetanus immunization status and administer when appropriate. The original dressing should be removed after 24–48 h. If the paronychia has not reaccumulated or spread, twice-daily 15-minute warm water soaks for the next 5–7 days should be recommended followed by dressing changes. Patients should be reevaluated within 48–72 h to assess clinical response to therapy.

CHRONIC PARONYCHIA

Introduction/Epidemiology

Chronic paronychias are caused most commonly by recurrent acute paronychias or chronic exposure to a moist environment or chemical irritant (e.g., alkali) (7). Those at risk include bartenders, dishwashers, or housecleaners. Although a bacterial super-infection with mixed flora can occur, the organisms most often isolated are *Candida* spp. (95%) and atypical mycobacterium.

Chronic paronychias are easily differentiated from an acute infection by the patient history and physical. First, chronic paronychias have an indolent cyclical course and often do not improve with repeated treatments (8). Second, they often occur in individuals with occupational exposures that promote their development. Third, the infection is most commonly isolated to the proximal eponychial nail fold without lateralization and is frequently not suppurative but rather indurated and protruding in appearance. Finally, chronic paronychias are more common in those who are immunosuppressed. As with acute paronychias, Gram stain, culture, and radiographs have a limited role in diagnosis.

Management

The management of chronic paronychias begins with recognizing inciting factors and educating patients on modifying activity to reduce exposure. Initial treatment usually involves topical (e.g., nystatin, amphotericin B, ketoconazole, ciclopirox, miconazole applied BID-QID for 3 weeks) or if topical fails, systemic (e.g., fluconazole 100 mg or itraconazole 200 mg daily for 3 weeks) antifungal therapy (8). Patients who are started on oral antifungal therapy in the emergency department should have baseline liver function tests drawn and checked before starting therapy since the most worrisome complication of these medications is hepatotoxicity.

The predominant theory is that *Candida* spp. sp. are the causative etiology of chronic paronychias. However, Tosti et al. theorize that a chronic paronychia is actually a contact dermatitis and should be responsive to steroid therapy. In a prospective randomized double-blind study, they were able to demonstrate an improved outcome with a 3-week topical application of 1% methylprednisolone aceponate compared to systemic antifungal therapy (9). These findings make an argument for the use of steroid therapy along with antifungal agents. Patients started on medication in the emergency department should be followed within a week by a physician to ensure appropriate response to therapy and for surveillance of side effects of these medications.

Surgical treatment is definitive and is known as eponychial marsupialization. Given the indolent nature of chronic paronychias, this is rarely, if ever, required in the emergency setting. A 3×7 mm window is removed proximal to, but with subsequent conservation of, the eponychial fold. All subcutaneous layers up to the germinal matrix should be removed (6). Extensive involvement may require partial or complete nail plate removal. These procedures should be performed only in consultation with a hand surgeon due to the propensity for germinal matrix damage, subsequent nail disruption, and to ensure proper care following emergency department management.

Antibiotic coverage has no role in the treatment of chronic paronychia and should not be prescribed. After the initial 24–48 h with the original dressing, twice-daily dressing changes should be preceded by 15-minute full-strength hydrogen peroxide soaks for the next 5–7 days.

Reevaluation in 2–3 days is needed to ensure appropriate response to therapy.

FELONS

Introduction/Epidemiology

A felon is the infection or abscess of the fat pad volar to the terminal phalanx and less commonly involves the foot. The organisms involved are predominantly gram positives such as *S. aureus*; however gram-negative organisms have been reported (10).

Pathophysiology

These infections are closed space infections with the crease of the DIP joint bordering proximally, the thick skin bordering volarly and distally, and the bone of the distal phalanx bordering dorsally. Approximately 15–20 vertical fibrous fascial strands attach the periosteum of the distal phalanx to the thick fibrous skin and are needed to provide structural support to the digit. Purulent material in the fat pad can cause increased pressure within the limited space, leading to soft tissue necrosis. Ischemic necrosis can extend to the surrounding skin, tendon, and bone.

Usually the organisms are introduced by a minor penetrating trauma to the fingertip such as an abrasion or small cut. Another mechanism is the iatrogenic inoculation from a fingerstick to check blood glucose levels leading to the phrase "fingerstick felon." Foreign bodies such as toothpicks or slivers of glass, as well as untreated paronychias can also lead to the development of felons (11–13).

Clinical Presentation

Felons initially present with erythema and gradually progressive inflammation and tenderness. Untreated, the felon progresses to form an abscess in the pulp space. Severe throbbing pain with tension and swelling of the entire fat pad of the finger with erythema are hallmark signs and symptoms. Complications of untreated felons include skin necrosis, tenosynovitis, osteomyelitis of the distal phalanx, septic arthritis of the DIP joint, lymphangitis, or extension of the infection into the palm or other digits.

Management

In the very early stages of a felon, the patient can be treated with warm soaks, antistaphylococcal oral antibiotics, and elevation of the extremity with follow-up within 24 h. Once an abscess cavity has formed, incision and drainage are necessary to treat a felon and prevent the development of ischemia to the distal digit.

Prior literature allowed for various types of incisions to be made to drain felons (fish-mouth and hockey-stick). Current literature discourages incisions that disrupt the anatomical boundaries of the distal finger. These aggressive incisions can cause poor cosmetic outcome leading to an unstable fat pad or unsightly scars, and adversely affect neurovascular structures leading to persisting pain or anesthesia of the digit.

For the incision and drainage of felons, the area of maximal fluctuance should guide where the incision is made. The two incision types recommended are either a high lateral incision to avoid the digital nerve and artery running lateral along the digit or a palmar longitudinal incision that does not cross the flexion crease, in order to avoid the underlying flexor digitorum profundus tendon attaching to the distal phalanx (see Fig. 31–3).

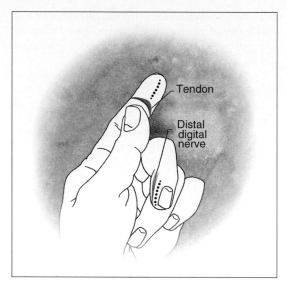

Fig. 31–3. Courtesy of Retsu Takahashi.

Lateral and AP radiographs of the involved digit should be ordered if there is suspicion for an underlying osteomyelitis or foreign body. Tetanus status should be investigated and tetanus booster given if indicated.

For the incision and drainage of a felon, a digital block should provide appropriate anesthesia as described previously. When the digit is adequately numb, a rubber drain such as a Penrose may be applied at the base of the digit to provide a relatively bloodless field if desired. An #11 scalpel blade is used at the site of maximal fluctuance to incise the abscess. Purulent fluid and/or bloody pink fluid should be expressed. Gram stain and culture are not indicated routinely unless the patient is at risk for resistant organisms (i.e., health care workers, IV drug abusers, immunocompromised patients, long-term hemodialysis, chronic antibiotic use). The tip of a curved hemostat should be used to probe the abscess cavity and break up any loculations present, being careful to avoid contact with the digital vessels. One should irrigate the cavity with sterile saline using an 18-gauge angiocath attached to a 5 or 10 mL syringe. Pack the cavity with iodoform gauze and apply a bulky dressing. The digit should be splinted and elevated above the level of the heart. Elevation can be aided with a sling. Oral antistaphylococcal antibiotics such as penicillinase-resistant penicillins (i.e., dicloxicillin) or first-generation cephalosporins (i.e., cephalexin) should be prescribed for 7–10 days. Nonsteroidal anti-inflammatories with oral opiods for breakthrough pain should be given for pain management (11–14).

Disposition

Simple felons can be discharged home. Referral for a reexamination with either a hand specialist or the emergency department should be scheduled within 24–48 h to remove the packing and inspect the finger. When the patient returns for a wound check, the packing should be replaced for another 24–48 h if there is continuous drainage. If needed, repeated irrigation of the abscess cavity with sterile saline can be done to break up loculations. Once the packing is removed, the patient can be encouraged to soak the digit for 15 minutes in warm water 3–5 times a day to speed healing (14).

There is an increasing incidence of methicillin-resistant *Staphylococcus aureus* (MRSA) so patients who return to the emergency department after felon drainage with worsening erythema or pain to the finger, increasing purulent drainage, difficulty in using the finger or who have failed to show improvement after 24–48 h should have Gram stain and cultures sent of any drainage, be admitted for IV antibiotics, consultation with a hand surgeon, and presumptively treated for MRSA with the first-line agent, vancomycin (10).

TENOSYNOVITIS

Pathophysiology/Microbiology

The double-walled flexor tendon sheaths of the hand provide an ideal environment for acute infection to set up and spread. The visceral layer adheres to the tendon and the parietal layer extends from the mid-palmar crease to just proximal to the DIP. The flexor tendon sheath of the thumb runs continuous with the radial bursa of the palm and the fifth finger's tendon sheath runs continuous with the ulnar palmar bursa. This allows for acute synovial space infections to travel from the distal digit to the ulnar and radial bursa rapidly. Usually, infections within the flexor tendon sheath result from adjacent pulp infections or local trauma to the flexor tendon sheath; however, they do less commonly occur from hematogenous spread.

The most common organism generally isolated from acute flexor tenosynovitis is *S. aureus*. However, there may be some variation in the distribution of gram-positive organisms in different populations. A study from Cook County hospital investigated patients with serious surgical issues of the hand during a 3$^1/_2$-year period. Among patients with flexor tenosynovitis, *Streptococcus* species were the most commonly isolated organisms (15).

Less common causes of bacterial tenosynovitis should be considered, including disseminated *Neisseria gonor-rhea*. One-third of patients with disseminated gonococcal infections will present with tenosynovitis alone, often in the extensor tendons of the dorsum of the hands and wrists (16). Some authors have suggested treating all high-risk patients with tenosynovitis as disseminated gonorrhea until final culture results are available (6).

Chronic flexor tenosynovitis is usually caused by mycobacterium or fungal infections and should be referred to a hand surgeon for biopsy and culture.

Clinical Presentation/ Management/Disposition

The four cardinal symptoms and signs of flexor tenosynovitis described by Dr. Kanavel are:

1. Exquisite tenderness over the course of the tendon sheath, limited to the sheath
2. Flexion of the finger at rest
3. Exquisite pain on extending the finger
4. Symmetrical swelling of the entire finger (fusiform swelling) (see Fig. 31–4) (17)

All flexor tenosynovitis cases require hospital admission and consultation with a hand surgeon due to the risk of ischemic complications. Radiographs may be helpful if a foreign body, osteomyelitis, or subcutaneous gas are suspected. Early cases (presenting within 48 h) can be managed with intravenous antibiotics, splinting, and elevation of the extremity. However, if no benefit is noted within 24 h or the patient presents after 48 h, surgery is

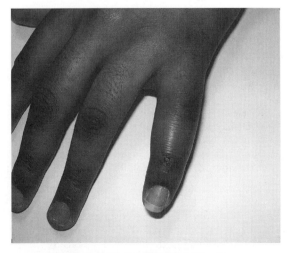

Fig. 31–4. Courtesy of Dr. Mark Silverberg.

needed to prevent complications to the tendon. Ischemic complications to the tendon can occur if pressures exceed 30 mm Hg. Any infection producing pus in the tendon sheath must be drained operatively to prevent poor outcome (18).

SPECIAL CONSIDERATIONS

All cases of paronychias, felons, and flexor tenosynovitis should consider possible unusual etiologies of the infection especially if there is any suspicion of a bite injury. Toothpick injuries have been known to cause pyogenic tenosynovitis and should be treated similarly to bite wounds (19; see Chapter 32)). If the patient was exposed to fresh water or salt water with the preceding abrasion or laceration, aeromonas species or *Vibrio vulnificus*, respectively, should be considered potential infecting bacterial pathogens. Additionally, if the patient has a history of working as a butcher, fish or clam handler, or veterinarian, *Erysipelothrix rhusiopathiae* may be the infecting organism (20).

CASE OUTCOME

The patient was diagnosed with an acute septic flexor tenosynovitis and taken to surgery. Prior to surgery, rectal, cervical, and pharyngeal culture on Thayer–Martin media were collected. The patient was treated with nafcillin and ceftriaxone. In surgery, copious cloudy fluid was obtained from the flexor tendon sheath, which grew *N. gonorrhea* as did the pharyngeal culture. The patient was discharged on a 10-day course of cefixime and doxycycline. She was also given counseling on safe sexual practices. On follow-up, she had full ROM of the digit with no complications.

REFERENCES

1. Roberge RJ, Weinstein D, Thimons MM: Perionychial infections associated with sculptured nails. *Am J Emerg Med* 17(6):581–582, 1999.
2. Brook I: Paronychia: A mixed infection. Microbiology and management. *J Hand Surg [Br]* 18(3):358–359, 1993.
3. Singer AJ, Hollander JE (eds.): *Lacerations and Acute Wounds: An Evidence-Based Guide, 1st ed.* Philadelphia, F.A. Davis Company, 2003, p 209.
4. Denkler K: A comprehensive review of epinephrine in the finger: To do or not to do. *Plast Reconstr Surg* 108(1): 114–124, 2001.
5. Wilhelmi BJ, Blackwell SJ, Miller JH, et al.: Do not use epinephrine in digital blocks: Myth or truth? *Plast Reconstr Surg* 107(2):393–397, 2001.
6. Hausman MR, Lisser SP: Hand infections. *Orthop Clin North Am* 23(1):171–185, 2001.
7. Hochman LG: Paronychia: More than just an abscess. *Int J Dermatol* 34(6):385–386, 1995.
8. Daniel CR, 3rd, Daniel MP, Daniel CM, et al.: Chronic paronychia and onycholysis: A thirteen-year experience. *Cutis* 58(6):397–401, 1996.
9. Tosti A, Piraccini BM, Ghetti E, et al.: Topical steroids versus systemic antifungals in the treatment of chronic paronychia: An open, randomized double-blind and double dummy study. *J Am Acad Dermatol* 47(1):73–76, 2002.
10. Connolly B, Johnstone F, Gerlinger T, et al.: Methicillin-resistant *Staphylococcus aureus* in a finger felon. *J Hand Surg [Am]* 25(1):173–175.
11. Canales FL, Newmeyer, WL, 3rd, Kilgore ES Jr.: The treatment of felons and paronychias. *Hand Clin* 5(4):515–523, 1989.
12. Jebson PJ: Infections of the fingertip. Paronychias and felons. *Hand Clin* 14(4):547–555, viii, 1998.
13. Kilgore ES, Jr., Brown LG, Newmeyer WL, et al.: Treatment of felons. *Am J Surg* 130(2):194–198.
14. Palivos, LR: In Reichman EF, Simon RF (ed.): *Emergency Medicine Procedures.* New York, McGraw-Hill, pp 821–828.
15. Weinzweig N, Gonzalez M: Surgical infections of the hand and upper extremity: A county hospital experience. *Ann Plast Surg* 49(6):621–627, 2002.
16. Schaefer, R.A., Enzenauer RJ, Pruitt A, et al., Acute gonococcal flexor tenosynovitis in an adolescent male with pharyngitis. A case report and literature review. *Clin Orthop* 281:212–215, 1992.
17. Kanavel AB: *Infections of the Hand, 5th ed.* Philadelphia, Lea & Febiger, 1925, p 495.
18. Canale ST (ed.): *Campbell's Operative Orthopedics, 10th ed.* St. Louis, Mosby Inc, 2003.
19. Chang MC, Huang YL, Liu Y, et al.: Infectious complications associated with toothpick injuries of the hand. *J Hand Surg [Am]* 28(2):327–331, 2003.
20. Swartz MN: Clinical practice. Cellulitis. *N Engl J Med* 350(9):904–912, 2004.

32

Animal Bites and Rabies

Robert A. Green
Wallace A. Carter

HIGH YIELD FACTS

1. Immunocompromised patients are at higher risk of developing infection after bite wounds. In addition, bites wounds to the hands are prone to infection. Both these groups of patients are candidates for prophylactic antibiotics when they present to the emergency department for care with bite wounds.

2. Commonly prescribed antibiotics for nonbite wounds such as first-generation cephalosporins (cephazolin) and antistaphylococcal penicillinase-resistant penicillins (dicloxacillin) are not the preferred choice for animal bite wounds. Combinations of beta-lactamase inhibitor and penicillin-based regimens (amoxicillin-clauvulanic acid or ampicillin-sulbactam) offer the best empiric single-agent coverage of the commonly implicated bacterial organisms in bite wounds.

3. Rabies, while a relatively rare disease, is uniformly fatal. A meticulous history along with knowledge of local epidemiology will be vital in making an accurate assessment. If an accurate assessment cannot be made it is well established that the disease has been transmitted as a result of relatively innocuous contacts and a low threshold for offering post-exposure prophylaxis is prudent.

CASE PRESENTATION

Case 1

A 56-year-old male presents to the emergency department after being bitten on his finger by his neighbor's dog. The dog wandered into his yard and when attempting to carry the dog back to his neighbors, the dog bit him on his right hand. He has two linear lacerations of his second digit of the right hand. After careful inspection there is no evidence of neurovascular injury.

He has a significant past medical history of alcohol-related cirrhosis. The neighbor stated that the dog has been healthy but never received his rabies vaccine.

Case 2

A 27-year-old female presents to the emergency department with a 2×2 cm area of induration and fluctuance of the right lateral lower extremity, 4 cm proximal to the lateral malleolus. The wound was the site of a bite wound the day earlier from her cat after accidentally stepping on its tail walking down her staircase. Twelve hours after the bite she noticed the beginning of redness, swelling, and pain. The patient is nontoxic appearing with a normal blood pressure and pulse. She has no comorbid medical conditions.

INTRODUCTION/EPIDEMIOLOGY

Animal bites account for up 0.4–1% of all emergency department (ED) visits in the United States (1, 2). In 2002, this represented one million ED visits of the 110 million estimated total visits (3). However, it is estimated that this represents only 17% of the total number of bite incidents, the majority of victims not requiring or seeking care (4).

Patients typically present to the ED for one of three main reasons. Very commonly, the patient has suffered a bite recently (<8 h) and leads to seeking care in the ED. Dog bites account for an estimated 80% of these injuries, with cat bites responsible for another 10% and then human bites following as the third most common animal bite (5). Children account for up to 42% of patient visits due to dog bite injuries (6). Dog bite wounds were found to occur frequently to the arm/hand (45.3%) but in very young children, bites to the head/neck region predominate (73%) (1).

These patients typically do not have clinically evident infections due to their bite wound. Dog bites more commonly present with lacerations and cat bites frequently present with puncture type wounds although the two are not mutually exclusive.

The second most common reason patients present to the ED are for signs and symptoms of infection, which typically occurs 1 or 2 days after a bite wound. Some infections can develop as early as 8–12 h after the bite. Wound infections can manifest as abscess, purulent wound, or cellulitis/lymphangitis.

Estimated bacterial infection rates after a dog bite range from 5.5% to up to 16% in two meta-analysis studies of dog bite wounds (7,8) Cat bites result in infection in up to 50% of cases. This is very likely due to their sharp teeth and puncture wound mechanism that deposits bacteria deep into tissue and renders irrigation procedures difficult.

Thirdly, patients come to the EDinquiring about the need for rabies vaccine or tetanus vaccine. These patients typically have less severe injuries and the focus of their concern is the long-term infectious complications. Minor-appearing bite wounds may be misleading so these patients require the same full-wound evaluation and management as the more significant injuries. Rabies infection results in a rapidly progressive and fatal viral encephalomyelitis that is transmitted in the saliva of an infected animal. Rabies progresses over 7–14 days, and the mean time between initial presentation and death is 16.2 days. Described for centuries and felt by many historical scholars to be the oldest communicable disease of humans, it remains in the 21st century a disease that results in tremendous worldwide mortality and costs for postexposure prophylaxis (PEP) and prevention strategies (9, 10).

In the 19th century rabies was a large public health problem, particularly in Europe. There were reports during this period that people either killed themselves, or were killed, if even a dog suspected of being rabid bit them. In 1885 Louis Pasteur administered the first postexposure prophylaxis to prevent rabies (11–14).

Although there is no treatment for rabies once the infection is established, effective vaccine regimens have been developed to prevent the disease. The development of human rabies vaccines and immunoglobins, combined with animal control and vaccination, has resulted in rabies becoming rare in humans in the United States. However, it remains a huge public health problem in other parts of the world. The World Health Organization (WHO) ranks death from rabies as number 10 in all infectious disease worldwide, with 50,000 to 60,000 annual deaths, and that approximately 10 million people require postexposure treatment each year (15).

Worldwide the dog remains the main culprit. In Africa, Asia, and South and Latin America 90% of cases result from canine bites. In the United States there is an average of 1–2 cases of human rabies reported per year. In the vast majority of these cases the infection was contracted while traveling outside the United States. There are over 35,000 persons in the United States who receive postexposure treatment that the Centers for Disease Control and Prevention (CDC-P) estimates may cost as much as $1 billion annually (16, 17).

PATHOPHYSIOLOGY/MICROBIOLOGY

The bacteriology of infected dog, cat, and human bite wounds have been extensively described by Talan et al.

One study confirmed the polymicrobial nature of infected mammalian bite wounds with the finding of an average of four or five organisms per infected wound. Another study demonstrated that there was little difference in the spectrum of bacterial isolates between those seen early with uninfected wounds and those presenting to the ED with established infection (18).

Pasteurella species were found in 75% of cat bite wound infections and 50% of dog bite infections. Eikenella corrodens was found in 30% of human bite wound infections. *Staphylococcus* species and *Streptococcus* species were commonly found in bites wounds from dogs, cats, and humans as were anaerobes such as *Prevotella*, *Fusobacterium*, *Bacteroides*, and *Peptosteptococcus*. In the absence of randomized clinical trials examining the best antibiotic for use in the prevention and/or treatment of bite wound infections, these studies form the basis for the rationale choice of antibiotics.

Capnocytophagia

Capnocytophagia canimorsus is a gram-negative bacillus causing a wide variety of severe infections in humans following a dog bite. First described in 1976 in a patient with septicemia and meningitis (19), this organism can cause severe sepsis, disseminated intravascular coagulation (DIC), and death (20–24). Most cases are immunocompromised patients, specifically those with alcoholism or asplenia. Sepsis occurs after 3–7 days following a dog bite with the patient presenting with fever, malaise, myalgia, vomiting, diarrhea, abdominal pain, dyspnea, confusion, headache, and skin manifestations (21). Awareness of this syndrome is important as proper treatment requires aggressive supportive therapy and intravenous antibiotics that include coverage of this organism.

Capnocytophagia canimorsus is susceptible to penicillin, amoxicillin, second- and third-generation cephalosporins, erythromycin, azithromycin, clarithromycin, fluoroquinolones, clindamycin, and doxycyline. First-generation cephalosporins, aztreonam, and the aminogylcosides are not preferred coverage for *Capnocytophagia* due to their lack of in vitro efficacy (25, 26).

Pasteurella multocida and Other Pasteurella Species

Pasteurella species are gram-negative coccobacilli and are implicated in 75% and 50% of cat and dogs wound infections respectively (27). These bacteria often cause clinical infection earlier than most bacterial organisms; signs and symptoms can appear as early as 7–24 h after the bite (27, 28). Although various localized infections have been described including bone and joint infections, meningitis, endocarditis, and intraabdominal infections, the most frequent clinical manifestation of the *Pasteurella* infection involves the skin and soft tissue (28). Initial symptoms include tenderness, induration, and inflammation. Abscesses, purulent wounds, and cellulitis occur in 19, 39, and 42%, respectively, of cases (27). Pasteurella species are susceptible to penicillin, ampicillin, amoxicillin, second- and third-generation cephalosporins, azithromycin, and the fluoroquinolones. First-generation cephalosporins, erythromycin, and dicloxacillin are not recommended.

Eikenella Corrodens

Eikenella corrodens is commonly found in human gingival plaque (29). It is uniquely prevalent in humans as opposed to other mammalian oral flora. *Eikenella corrodens* is a gram-negative rod that is a facultative anaerobe and is reported to be the infecting organism in 30% of infected human bites (30). These bacteria are susceptible to penicillin, amoxicillin, second- and third-generation cephalosporins, azithromycin, and the fluoroquinolones. First- generation cephalosporins, erythromycin, clindamycin, and dicloxacillin are not reliably effective.

Clenched Fist Injury

Patients presenting to the emergency department with small lacerations overlying the MCP joint require special attention. Inquiry into the details of the occurrence is critical as often the patient is not aware that this may represent a bite wound, or may be reluctant to disclose that the injury resulted from an altercation. These injuries are referred to as clenched fist injuries and can present with a minor appearing laceration without evidence of infection, or more commonly presents the day after injury with an established infection (Fig. 32–1). These injuries are sustained usually after a punch to another person's face, striking teeth. Fractures, joint space disruption, and foreign bodies can complicate these cases.

The innocuous lesion from a clenched fist injury often leads to delay in ED presentation and results in increased complications (31). Careful examination is essential as lacerations of the extensor tendon are often missed as the tendon moves proximally after the clenched fist is placed in neutral position during the exam in the emergency department. Viewing the tendon in the clenched fist position is essential to better evaluate these injuries. Radiographic

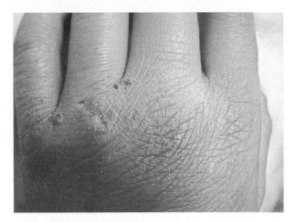

Fig. 32–1. Image reproduced with permission from EMedHome. com: www.EMedHome.com.

examination is necessary to evaluate for foreign body, fractures, or air in the joint space.

These injuries require antibiotic prophylaxis that covers the typical oral pathogens in addition to coverage of *E. corrodens*. Wound infections from human bites are typically polymicrobial with an average of four organisms per infected wound. *Staphylococcal aureus*, Streptococcal species, *E. corrodens*, Prevotella, and Fusobacterium were frequently isolated (30). Patients who present with established infection with such signs as swelling, inflammation, discharge, or fever frequently require admission to the hospital for IV antibiotics, hand elevation, surgical consultation, and possibly surgical intervention.

Animal Rabies

The rabies virus is well studied in the United States and shows distinct differences based on the geographical region in the infected animals. Six cases were identified among travelers outside the United States bitten by dogs (32). Due to vigorous animal immunization policies the incidence of rabies in domestic animals has decreased dramatically since the 1950s, while wild animals remain the primary vector. In 2001 there were 7437 case of animal rabies reported to the CDC from 49 states (Hawaii, District of Columbia, and Puerto Rico reported zero). Wild animals accounted for 93% of these cases. Raccoons were the most frequently reported species at 37%, followed by skunks at 30%, bats at 20%, and foxes at 6%. Domesticated species accounted for the remaining 7% with its presence in cats increasing but decreasing in other domesticated species. Recent reports show the incidence in dogs is decreasing by 22%. Pennsylvania and New York reported the largest number of domestic animal rabies cases (16, 33).

Bats present a particular problem since there has been a number of reports that human rabies has occurred without a "known" contact. The silver-haired bat appears to be the most frequently identified species. It has been suggested that the viral strain from this species has increased virulence, which may result in disease transmission with seemingly innocuous contact. In another analysis in 2002 by Kreb et al., it was found that since 1990, 24 of 26 human rabies cases came from genetic variants found in bats. Of these, only two have a clear history of a bite. In 2001 the 1281 cases of rabies in bats represented an increase from previous years. They were reported in 47 of the 48 contiguous states with Texas, California, and New York reporting the most cases. Puerto Rico, Hawaii, and Alaska reported no cases of rabies in bats (14, 32, 33).

While assurance of a 0% chance of acquiring rabies is never possible, it has been stated that bites from squirrels, hamsters, guinea pigs, gerbils, chipmunks, rats, mice, and domesticated rabbits have so rarely been found to be rabid that PET is not indicated except for the most unusual circumstances (16).

Human Rabies

In the United States, human deaths from rabies have declined dramatically from the early part of the 20th century. From 1980 to 1986, the CDC obtained reports on 32 cases of human rabies. Of these, one quarter reported having no definite history of animal bite. Six patients had dog bites outside the United States. Seventeen (53%) were associated with rabies virus variants found in Infectovorous bats. This high number is worrisome since previously bats were thought to account for only 20% of the wildlife species reported to be rabid (32–34).

Worldwide, rabies continues to be a significant source of illness. The WHO received reports of 33,209 cases of human rabies in 1996. Since most of the rabies cases occur in underdeveloped countries with poorly developed reporting systems, it is widely believed that the number is a gross underestimate. Some authorities believe that a more accurate number is 100,000 deaths annually (11).

Rabies infection occurs by the fusing of the rabies virus envelope to the host cell in either the nervous system or muscle. The rabies virus, part of the Rhabdovirus species, may enter the peripheral nervous system directly. This occurs by binding to a ganglioside and then to the cell adhesion molecule. The replicated virus will then migrate to the central nervous system (CNS). The rabies virus may also replicate in muscle tissue prior to CNS infection. It can remain sequestered at or near the entry site in mus-

cle tissue bound to nicotinic acetylcholine receptors. It will replicate and ascend to the CNS at a variable rate of 8–20 mm per day. This may partially explain the wide variation in incubation periods and the commonly held belief that distal inoculation may delay infection due to the greater distance that needs to be traversed to reach the CNS. Once it reaches the CNS it will spread centrifugally to other organs (35).

At post mortem exam the virus has been isolated in the skin, salivary glands, cornea, kidney, pancreas, and myocardium. However, the saliva has been found to contain the highest concentration of virions. This explains why bites and saliva contact are the main means of transmission. Systemically, one of the more notable abnormalities is the presence of myocarditis. Negri bodies have been recovered from the hearts of patients who have died from rabies. This entity resembles those myocarditides associated with hyperadrenergic physiology and may be a pathway for the terminal event in patients who are infected with the rabies virus (36).

How rabies damages the CNS is unclear. Gross examination of the brain in patients who have rabies appear grossly unremarkable. Histologically, the appearance is similar to encephalitis. There is monocellular infiltration with hemorrhage and demyelination that occurs mostly in the gray matter. Microscopy reveals the presence of Negri bodies. These are described as round eosinophilic cytoplasmic inclusions that contain viral nucleocapsids with a tendency to concentrate in hippocampal pyramidal cells. Paralytic rabies often referred to as "dumb rabies," which is the clinical presentation in approximately 20% of the patients, will affect the spinal cord. Microscopic examination will reveal severe inflammation and necrosis. These findings account for the ascending flaccid paralysis characteristic of this variant (36).

Since the early symptoms of rabies are occult it is important to understand who is at risk for acquiring the infection.

When considering who will acquire rabies there are several variables that should be considered (Table 32–1). Saliva, as previously described, is the major depot for this virus. Therefore, any wound that is exposed to a significant amount of saliva will greatly increase the likelihood of transmission. Intuitively, a bite on exposed skin or through a preexisting wound or multiple bites will increase the disease likelihood. Because of the way the virus spreads there is reason to believe that bites of the head and neck pose a greater risk than do those of distal extremities. While limited, there are data to suggest that the virus can be spread via aerosolized contact with mucous membranes of the respiratory tract. Incubation period should also be considered when performing this risk analysis.

Table 32–1. Important Historical Questions for Rabies Assessment

Biting situation
  Type and breed of animal
  Immunization status of animal
  Circumstances of bite (provoked/unprovoked)
  What type of clothing were you wearing
    (multiple layers?)
  Where did the animal come in contact with you?
  Is the animal captured so it can be observed?
Patient
  What treatment was administered before you came
    to the hospital?
  Rabies immunization status
  Allergies
  Current medications
  Currently immunocompromised by disease or therapy?

While widely variable with reports ranging from a few days to years, 75% will become ill within 90 days of exposure (35).

The symptoms in the initial phase are very nonspecific and often attributed to other syndromes (Table 32–2). In one series, physicians considered rabies in only 14% of patients during their first visit to the health care providers even with some of the patients having an exposure history. Symptoms in this phase may include headache, malaise, fever, personality changes, insomnia, and anxiety. Other symptoms such as nausea, vomiting, anorexia, and abdominal pain along with URI symptoms have been reported (37).

Neurologic symptoms are also described as subtle. Paresthesia at the wound site occurs in only half of the patients and is often interpreted as expected sequelae of a bite wound (13). Changes in sleep patterns, irritability, and depression may be present. Minor changes in cognition and personality are reported but often difficult to find in a prospective fashion especially in the emergency department setting.

The finding of myoedema on physical exam has been reported by multiple authors. This is described as mounding of the muscle that is struck with a reflex hammer, which then resolves. It may be present early in the prodromal phase and persist throughout the course of the disease (38).

Unlike the incubation phase, which may last for years, the prodrome phase is relatively short, typically lasting 4 days before more specific signs and symptoms appear (35).

Rabies in humans can take one of two forms, furious (encephalitic) or paralytic (dumb). Human cases are predominantly the furious form characterized by hydrophobia, delirium, and agitation. It is this form that the lay public associates with the clinical presentation of this disease. The paralytic form, which is marked by severe ascending flaccid paralysis, manifests minimal central nervous system involvement until the terminal phase of the illness. In both forms the prodromal stays can range from 2 to 7 days before coma. Death will occur on average in 18 days and once symptoms appear intensive support will prolong, but not alter the outcome (13, 14, 16, 37).

In furious rabies, hyperactivity is the *sine qua non.* Increasing agitation, violent thrashing, and seizures are seen commonly. Hydrophobia, which stems from a combination of an increased reflex of the respiratory tract as well as pharyngeal spasm, is a striking manifestation. Initially, this reaction is triggered by the patient attempting to drink water, but in later stages it may be triggered simply by the

Table 32–2. Stages of Rabies

Stage Type	Duration(%)	Symptoms
Incubation	≥30 days (25) 30–90 days (50) 90 days–1 year (20) >1 year (5)	None
Prodrome	2–10 days	Nonspecific viral-like symptoms Paresthesia at bite site(<50%) Subtle neurologic changes (personality/sleep)
Acute		
Furious	2–10 days	Hyperactivity agitation, hydrophobia, seizure, hydrophobia, autonomic instability
Paralytic	2–10 days	Ascending flaccid paralysis, clear sensorium
Terminal	Up to 18 days	Coma that progresses to death (irreversible)

sight of liquid. This hyperactivity may progress to a point where the pharyngeal muscle spasm is triggered by gentle streams of air that contact the patient's face and is known as aerophobia. As the central infection progresses, pituitary gland dysfunction may result in disorders of water metabolism (Diabetes Insipidus, SIADH). Eventually the respiratory center will be affected. Autonomic dysfunction may be present in the form of increasing salivation and sweating and pupillary dilation. Cardiac arrhythmia may occur due to either brainstem dysfunction or myocarditis (11, 13, 15, 39).

Paralytic or dumb rabies as the name implies in the initial phase will have none of the manifestation of hyperactivity seen in the furious form. Increasing lethargy and poor coordination may be present. A clear sensorium with meningeal signs that eventually lapses into coma has been described. The hallmark neurologic finding in this form is that of an ascending flaccid paralysis. This can further cloud diagnosis because it may be confused with other syndromes such as Guillian-Barre. This form represents a real risk to health care workers because the diagnosis of rabies may not be entertained, which may lower the threshold of some care givers to exercise extreme caution when handling salvia and respiratory secretions which as previously mentioned are a potent depot for the rabies virus.

RABIES LABORATORY/ DIAGNOSTIC TESTING

The utility of wound cultures has been unclear given the polymicrobial nature of infections. However, with the current antibiotic resistance patterns, cultures may be of some utility for wounds failing to respond to empiric treatment.

The diagnosis of rabies is made easily in patients who present with typical symptoms of hyperactivity, hydrophobia, and aerophobia following the bite of a rabid animal. Unfortunately, at this point the diagnosis becomes one of epidemiological importance because the patient's eventual outcome is almost assured.

It is important to remember that during the incubation period diagnostic studies are not helpful. Rather, it is much more important during this phase to take a detailed history and, if even a remote possibility exists that the patient may have come in contact with an infected animal, to offer immediate postexposure treatment.

Since laboratory tests are not uniformly sensitive, a battery of tests appears to be the best approach (40). Collection of tissue and fluid that are known to harbor the virus, is recommended. Serum, saliva, and cerebrospinal fluid

are easily obtained. Due to the viruses' predilection for highly innervated tissue, a skin biopsy from the nape of the neck that is above the hairline and captures numerous hair follicles may have diagnostic yield. Laboratory methods such as direct fluorescent antibody staining and reverse transcriptase polymerase chain reaction tests have been utilized (40). Some experts advocate the polymerase chain reaction test because it allows for precise identification of a particular rabies virus strain. Due to the infrequent nature of this disease it is expected that most local and hospital laboratories may not be adequately prepared to perform these tests rapidly, especially during nights, weekends, and holidays. It is recommended that if there is a clinical suspicion, the clinician should immediately notify their local public health agency and infectious disease expert to organize an effective and expeditious testing strategy.

MANAGEMENT

Wound Inspection, Radiography, Cleansing, Debridement, and Tetanus Prophylaxis

The initial evaluation of the patient after a bite wound should include a thorough history of the events of the bite. Radiographs should be obtained if there is suspicion of foreign body, fracture, or joint penetration. Wounds should be anesthetized and explored for evidence of foreign bodies such as teeth, soft tissue injuries such as laceration of tendons, or joint penetration. Positive findings may result in surgical specialty consultation for operative intervention.

After anesthesia, the wound should be irrigated with normal saline. This process facilitates clot removal as well as removal of foreign debris and contaminating bacteria. One practical option is to use a 20- or 30-cc syringe attached to an 18-gauge angiocath. With moderate pressure this stream of irrigation is strong enough to dislodge contaminated material by the resultant hydraulic force acting on particulate matter. Irrigation with several hundred cc's of saline should be sufficient for all but heavily contaminated wounds.

Some bacteria and spores flourish in the anaerobic environment of devitalized tissue. After the wound is irrigated, devitalized tissue along the wound edges and partially avulsed fat globules should be carefully excised from the wound. This will promote healing at the same time as decreasing infection (42). These wounds are all considered "tetanus prone" wounds and require appropriate tetanus prophylaxis as indicated based on the patients' history of prior immunization (see Chapter 33).

Suturing Wounds

Many providers are concerned about suturing animal bite wounds because of their concern for increased infection rate. This concern is understandable since one is introducing a foreign body material into a contaminated field in addition to impeding the egress of drainage from the wound. The literature, however, does supply some reassurance that suturing certain bite wounds does not result in increased risk of infection. Maimaris and Quinton published their results in 1988, where 169 discreet dog bite lacerations were randomized to receive either sutures or no sutures (43). None of the 96 patients received antibiotics. There was no significant difference in the overall infection rate of 7.7% between the two groups, although patients with bite wounds to their hands did better if their wounds were not sutured (16% infection rate in the sutured group versus 8% in the nonsutured group). It was evident from this study that bite wounds to hands should be left open and that perhaps certain bite wounds can be safely sutured. Chen et al. reported a 5.5% infection rate in 145 patients after primary closure of noninfected bite wounds from dogs, cats, and humans (44). This relatively low rate of infection is within the range of infection rates from nonbite wounds reported in the literature. Eighty-six percent of these patients were sent home on prophylactic antibiotics, which likely improved their clinical outcomes.

It is these authors' recommendation that sutures should not be placed in patients who have been determined to possess significant risk factors for wound infection after a bite injury (Table 32–3). These wounds should be left open and either undergo delayed primary closure or heal by secondary intent. Bite wounds to the face and those to patients without significant risk factors for wound infection can be sutured after copious irrigation and with scheduled follow-up in 2 or 3 days. These patients should be placed on appropriate prophylactic antibiotics.

Table 32–3. High Risk of Infection after Bite Wounds

All nontrivial cat bites
Human bites including clenched fist injuries
Bites to the hand—any animal
Immunosuppressed patients
    Diabetes
    Cirrhosis or chronic alcohol use
    Asplenia
    Steroid use or post chemotherapy
    Elderly
    Peripheral vascular disease

Antibiotic Prophylaxis for Animal Bites

Antimicrobial prophylaxis has been demonstrated to decrease the incidence of infection when administered prior to certain surgical procedures. Administration of antibiotics after a bite wound is often termed "prophylactic" in the sense that an established infection has not yet been identified. High-risk wounds warrant prophylactic treatment (45).

Clear evidence and recommendations regarding the use of prophylactic antibiotics after bite wounds have been lacking. Randomized studies are few, contain small numbers of patients, and utilize dissimilar antibiotics, many of which have subsequently been determined to be poor empiric choices. Meta-analysis reviews have been done but are limited by the same paucity of original research. A review by Medirios et al. looked at eight of the randomized studies and found little evidence that prophylactic antibiotics changed the outcome in wounds other than those to the hand or those resulting from human or cat bite (7). Lack of evidence of the efficacy of prophylactic antibiotics after dog bite wounds to nonhand areas found in this study was not found in an earlier meta-analysis study by Cummings. In this study, there was a statistically significant relative risk reduction of 44% in the use of antibiotics after dog bites (8).

In a recent study of the bacteriologic analysis of infected dog and cat bite wounds, *Pasturella* species was present in 50% and 75% of dog and cat wounds, respectively, confirming previous data of the importance of this pathogenic organism in wounds of this nature (27). Streptococci, staphylococci, and oral anaerobes were also found in many of these wounds. Many of the earlier studies on the efficacy of antibiotics after bite wounds used antibiotics not efficacious against the main pathogenic organism found to be present in infected wounds. Until this is fully resolved, it remains good clinical practice to empirically treat the patient's with substantial wounds for 3–5 days if they have risk factors for infection (Table 32–3). All patients with nontrivial cat bite wounds and bite wounds to the hand including the clenched fist injury should receive prophylactic antibiotics.

The antibiotic choice should be based on the available evidence of the sensitivities to various antibiotics of the pathogens commonly found in infected bite wounds (Table 32–4) (46). Coverage of *Pasturella* sp., *Staphylococcus* sp., Streptococcal sp., and oral anaerobes should ideally be included. First-generation cephalosporins, dicloxacillin, and erythromycin are not ideal choices. Amoxicillin/clauvulanic acid, combination penicillin plus dicloxacillin, fluoroquinolones such as levofloxacin,

Table 32–4. Antimicrobial Susceptibilities of Bacteria Frequently Isolated from Animal Bite Wounds*

	Percentages of Isolates Susceptible					
Agent	Staphlococcus Aureus	Eikenella Corrodens	Anaerobes	Pasteurella Multocida	Capnocytophaga Canimorsus	Staphlococcus Intermedius
Penicillin	10	99	50/95$	95	95	70
Dicloxacillin	99	5	50	30	NS	100
Amoxicillin/clavulanic acid	100	100	100	100	95	100
Cephalexin	100	20	40	30	NS	95
Cefuroxime	100	70	40	90	NS	NS
Cefoxitin	100	95	100	95	95	NS
Erythromycin	100	20	40	20	95	95
Tetracycline	95	85	60	90	95	NS
TMP-SMX	100	95	0	95	V	NS
Ciprofloxacin	100	100	40	95	100	100
Levofloxacin	100	100	60	100	100	100
Trovafloxacin	100	100	85&	100	100	100
Moxifloxacin	100	100	85&	100	100	100
Azithromycin	100	80	70&#	100	100	NS
Clarithromycin	100	60	70&#	70	100	NS
Ketolides (HMR 3647)	100	100	85&	100	NS	100
Clindamycin	95	0	100	0	95	95

Goldstein E: Bites, in G. Mandell, J. Bennett and R. Dolin, (Eds): Reprinted from Principles and Practice
of Infectious Diseases, 5th Ed. Philadelphia, 2000; p 3203 with permission from Elsevier.
*Data are compiled from various studies
$Percentage of human bite isolates/percentage of animal bite isolates.
&Many fusobacteria are resistant.
#Some peptostreptococci are resistant.
Abbreviations: NS, Not studies; TMP-SMX, trimethoprim-sulfamethoxazole; V, variable

azithromycin, or second-generation cephalosporins such as cefuroxime or cefoxitin would be appropriate (Table 32–5).

Treatment of Infected Bite Wounds

Once infected, bite wounds require meticulous attention and treatment. Standard treatment of the more serious

Table 32–5. Antibiotic Choice for Oral Prophylaxis or Oral Treatment of Bites Wounds

Oral regimens
Amoxicillin/clauvulanic acid
Cefuroxime axetil
Penicillin plus dixcloxacillin
Levofloxacin
Azithromycin

complications of wound infections should be initiated. Patients at high risk for sepsis should be identified and treated appropriately but all patients should be considered for systemic complications of the local wound. Wound abscesses require incision and drainage and may result in admission to the hospital. Intravenous antibiotics should be instituted if admission is warranted after wound cultures and, in the setting of suspicion of bacteremia, blood cultures should be obtained (Table 32–6). Particular care and

Table 32–6. Antibiotic Choice for IV Treatment of Infected Wounds

Ampicillin/sulbactam
Cefoxitin
Levofloxacin plus clindamycin
Azithromycin

attention are in order when attending to hand infections. Infection spreads quickly through the tendon sheaths and can rapidly spread proximally. Surgical treatment is mandatory for bacterial tenosynovitis or other purulent complication of hand infections. Intravenous antibiotics and elevation of the affected part is often the less invasive alternative if the infection has not progressed to the point requiring operative intervention.

Immunizations/Prevention of Rabies

Preexposure prophylaxis

This option is limited to those people who, by profession or hobby, have a high likelihood of being repetitively exposed to the rabies virus. This group would also include travelers whose itinerary will bring them to endemic areas. While an important arm of therapy it is beyond the scope of this chapter. Due to a regimen that requires a series of injections and may include determination of antibody response it is usually beyond the scope of most emergency departments. These patients should be referred to local health care practitioners or the local health department (47, 48).

Postexposure treatment

The cornerstone of this therapy is to remember that postexposure prophylaxis is a medical urgency and never a medical emergency. As such, adherence to the well-established principle of triage and the primary and secondary survey to rule out life-threatening conditions remains the emergency physician's first action. In addition to performing a risk assessment for rabies exposure, the clinician must also offer appropriate care for animal bites as described earlier in the chapter. Tetanus prophylaxis must also be considered. If the exposure includes a wound, then the well-established principle of wound preparation should be considered a vital first step in prophylaxis. Appropriate care and irrigation methods to reduce the size of the innoculum are essential (49).

Once those methods have been employed the health care provider must evaluate the need for postexposure prophylaxis. A careful analysis of the situation must be performed and should include the following elements (50).

Type of exposure. Rabies virus must be introduced by a bite wound or through disrupted skin or less commonly via mucous membranes. The patient who presents with any skin penetration by teeth or saliva contamination, especially proximate to disrupted skin, constitutes an exposure and therefore carries a risk. It must be remembered that not all bites, especially those by bats, are apparent. Patients who present with an aerosolized exposure to rabies virus should also be considered for postexposure treatment. Isolated contact with a rabid animal through petting or contacting its blood, feces, or urine does not constitute exposure. If these circumstances are not met then the need for postexposure treatment is exceedingly low and unless extenuating circumstances exist is not warranted.

Animal epidemiology. In order to evaluate this variable, knowledge of local rabies rates and involved species is needed and may be obtained from your local health department (Table 32–7). Since the patient may have traveled from their point of exposure a careful travel history is appropriate. Rabies has been found in bats in all of the 49 continental states and now represents the largest reservoir in the United States. These animals present a challenge to the clinician because they may cause relatively small and innocuous wounds. Consequently, if there is "reasonable probability" that an exposure occurred, for example, in someone who has been sleeping in a room that was occupied by a bat, then postexposure treatment might be appropriate.

- Wild carnivores. Bites by raccoons, skunks, foxes, and coyotes must be assumed to constitute an exposure and treatment should be offered.

- Rodents. Animals such as squirrels, hamsters, guinea pigs, gerbils, chipmunks, rats, mice, rabbits, and hares have not been known to transmit rabies to humans. Since there are exceptions in the rodent family, such as woodchucks, the local health department should be consulted to determine local patterns prior to offering prophylaxis.

- Dog and cats. These animals have a varying likelihood of transmitting rabies. Prevalence among dogs varies by region and should be considered when making the decision for postexposure treatment. Cats represent a greater risk with more cats infected with rabies than dogs. The roaming habits of cats along with fewer immunizations and other laws regarding this species may account for this difference. In either case if the biting animal can be captured, a 10-day period of observation by a veterinarian is indicated. If any signs suggestive of rabies develop then the animal should be immediately euthanized and its head refrigerated and shipped to a qualified laboratory. If the animal cannot be captured and observed, then postexposure treatment should be offered especially if the attack appears unprovoked (32–34, 51).

Table 32–7. Rabies Postexposure Prophylaxis Guide—United States, 1999

Animal Type	Evaluation and Disposition of Animal	Postexposure Prophylaxis Recommendations
Dogs, cats, and ferrets	Healthy and available for 10 days observation	Persons should not begin prophylaxis unless animal develops clinical signs of rabies[a]
	Rabid or suspected rabid	Immediately vaccinate
	Unknown (e.g., escaped)	Consult public officials
Skunks, raccoons, foxes and most other carnivores; bats	Regarded as rabid unless unless animal proven negative by laboratory tests[b]	Consider immediate vaccination
Livestock, small rodents, lagomorphs (rabbits and hares large rodents (wood-chucks and beavers), and other mammals	Consider individually	Consult public health officials. Bites of squirrels, hamsters, guinea pigs, gerbils chipmunks, rats, mice, other small rodents, rabbits and hares almost never require antirabies postexposure prophylaxis

[a]During the 10-day observation period, begin postexposure prophylaxis at the first sign of rabies in a dog, cat, or ferret that has bitten someone. If the animal exhibits clinical signs of rabies, it should be euthanized immediately and tested.
[b]The animal should be euthanized and tested as soon as possible. Holding for observation is not recommended. Discontinue vaccine if immunoflourescence test results of the animal are negative.
Source: Adapted from Centers for Disease Control and Prevention.

The L and M proteins that comprise the ribonucleoprotein complex will accumulate in the cytoplasm of rabies-infected neurons and compose Negri bodies, which is the pathognomonic microscope finding in rabies infection. The G proteins form the visible protrusions on the virion envelope and are the only rabies virus protein known to induce neutralizing antibodies, which can confer immunity. However, this process is unpredictable and may not be protective in humans. The nucleocapsid proteins induce antibodies that are not protective but are useful in certain diagnostic tests (11, 40).

Postexposure therapy is targeted at the virus during the period of local replication before it infects the nervous system. Once the virus enters the peripheral nervous system current treatment is ineffective in preventing further replication and spread to multiple organ systems (52).

Once the decision to treat has been made there are two types of products that are commercially available. Vaccines induce an active response that produces neutralizing antibodies and need 7–10 days to develop protective levels. Rabies Immune Globulin (RIG) provides a passive immunity that persists for approximately 21 days. The postexposure prophylaxis protocol mandates that both products be used (Table 32–8) (47).

There are four formulations of three inactive rabies vaccines. The vaccine most widely available in the United States is Human Diploid Dell Vaccine (HDCV). This vaccine, which produces active immunity, should always be administered in the deltoid to avoid infiltration into the fat, which will prevent the production of antibodies. It should never be mixed in the same syringe as the Immune Globulin. The dose is 1 mL intramuscular with the first dose being counted as day 0. This dose is repeated on days 3, 7, 14, 28. The dose is the same regardless of size or age (47).

Passive immunity is achieved by administering Human Rabies Immune Globulin (HRIG). It contains 150 IU of neutralizing antibody per milliliter and is given as a single dose of 20 IU/kg-body weight. As much of this dose, as anatomically possible, should be infiltrated into and around the wound. This includes wounds that are to be sutured. Care should be exercised when infiltrating digits to avoid elevating compartment pressure with tissue necrosis. In the event of multiple bites, especially in children, if the dose does not appear to be sufficient to infiltrate all wounds the vaccine can be diluted two- to threefold with sterile saline to assure adequate infiltration volume. If there is additional volume, it should be administered intramuscularly at a site far from where the vaccine is to be given to avoid passive immunization inactivating the vaccine (Table 32–9) (47).

Adverse reactions are generally mild and well tolerated. Between 30 and 74% of patients will have local

Table 32–8. Rabies Biologics—United States, 1999

Human Rabies Vaccine	Product Name	Manufacturer
Human diploid cell vaccine (HFCV)		Pasteur-Meriux Serum et Vaccins, Connaught Laboratories Inc. Phone: (800) 822-2463
Intramuscular	Imovax Rabies	
Intradermal	Imovax Rabies I.D.	
Rabies vaccine absorbed (RVA)	Rabies Vaccine	Bioport Corporation
Intramuscular	Absorbed (RVA)	Phone: (517) 335-8120
Purified chick embryo cell vaccine (PCEC)	RabAvert	Chiron Corporation Phone: (800) 244-7668
Intramuscular		
Rabies immune globulin (RIG)	Imogam Rabies-HT	Pasteur-Meriux Serum et Vaccins, Connaught Laboratories Inc. Phone: (800) 244-7668

Source: Adapted from Centers for Disease Control and Prevention.

Table 32–9. Rabies Postexposure Prophylaxis Schedule—United States, 1999

Vaccination Status	Treatment	Regimen[a]
Not previously vaccinated	Wound cleansing	All postexposure treatment should begin with immediate thorough cleansing of all wounds with soap and water. If available, a virucidal agent such as a povidone-iodine solution should be used to irrigate wounds
	RIG	Administer 20IU/kg body weight. If anatomically feasible, the full dose should be infiltrated around the wound(s) and any remaining volume should be administered IM at an anatomical site distant from vaccine administration. Also, RIG should not administered in the same syringe as vaccine. Because RIG might partially suppress active production of antibody, no more than the recommended dose should be given
	Vaccine	HDCV, RVA, or PCEC 1.0 mL. IM (deltoid area[b]), one each on days 0 and 3, 7, 14, 28
Previously vaccinated[c]	Wound cleansing	All postexposure treatment should begin with immediate thorough cleansing of all wounds with soap and water. If available, a virucidal agent such as a povidone-iodine solution should be used to irrigate wounds
	RIG	RIG should not be administered
	Vaccine	HDCV, RVA or PCEC 1.0 mL. IM (deltoid area[b]), one each on days 0 and 3

[a] These regimens are applicable for all age groups, including children.
[b] The deltoid area is the only acceptable site of vaccination for adults and older children. For younger children, the outer aspect of the thigh may be used. Vaccine should never be administered in the gluteal area.
[c] Any person with a history of preexposure vaccination with HDCV, RVA or PCEC; or prior postexposure prophylaxis with HDCV, RVA or PCEC; or previous vaccination with any other type of rabies vaccine and a documented history of antibody response to the prior vaccination.
HDCV = human diploid cell vaccine; PCEC = purified chick embryo cell vaccine; RIG = rabies immune globulin; RVA = rabies vaccine absorbed; IM = intramuscular.
Source: Adapted from Centers for Disease Control and Prevention.

reaction with HDCV that may include pain, erythema, and itching and swelling. Headache, nausea, abdominal pain, and dizziness have been reported at a lower rate of 5–40%. Also reported is an immune complex-like reaction; however, this occurs in approximately 6% of persons who receive booster doses and less frequently in persons receiving the primary series. Once the vaccine series has begun it should not be stopped or delayed due to mild local or systemic reactions. Antinflammatory and antipyretic agents are usually sufficient to control these symptoms. In the rare case of a patient with a known severe hypersensitivity to rabies vaccine the vaccinations should be considered lifesaving. Advice should be sought from the local state health department or CDC to assist the physician in planning a prudent course of action.

It must be stressed that the well-established recommendations by the CDC be followed without deviation in all cases of suspected rabies. This includes meticulous attention to wound care. Thoroughly washing and irrigating all bites or scratches using accepted techniques is a critical part of therapy. Wounds should be thoroughly scrubbed if possible and not simply flushed. The current CDC recommendations include the addition of a virucidal agent to the solution. There have been no treatment failures reported in the United States since HDCV became available and the protocol followed. However, there have been treatment failures internationally, all of which were associated with protocol deviation.

Special Circumstances

Immunosupression. Inability to mount an adequate immune response presents a challenge in exposures for these patients. The CDC's Advisory Committee on Immunization Practice identifies the following group as being immunocompromised: human immunodeficiency virus (HIV) infection, aplastic anemia, leukemia, and lymphoma and systemic malignancies. Patients on immunosuppressive drugs such as corticosteroids, antimalarials, and alkylating and antimetabolite agents are also considered immunosuppressed. Postexposure therapy should be offered to these patients utilizing the standard regimens. These patients should be monitored closely for antibody response. During the treatment schedule all immunosuppressive drugs should be withheld, if possible, to avoid the possibility of an incomplete immunologic response.

Previous immunization

This group comprises patients who have received a complete course of one of the preexposure or postexposure CDC recommended regimens. In immunocompetent patients an amnestic response to booster injection is expected so HRIG is not needed. These patients should receive two doses of one of the three approved vaccines.

Pregnancy

Since rabies is uniformly fatal and there is no evidence that adverse pregnancy outcomes or congenital abnormalities are associated with rabies vaccination, pregnancy is never considered a contraindication to postexposure treatment (47).

DISPOSITION

Most patients without evidence of infection can be discharged home unless the traumatic injury dictates admission. Routine 24–48-h follow-up should be instituted whether or not patients were given antibiotics or sutured. Careful attention to the early development of infection is necessary. If evidence of infection is present on follow-up evaluation, sutures should be removed to allow drainage of the wound. Antibiotics should be initiated or adjusted based on the initial decision and treatment.

Patients presenting with infection especially of the extremities or who themselves are immunocompromised should be considered for hospital admission. Wound cultures, IV antibiotics, surgical consultation, and elevation of the affected body part should be instituted. If discharged, arrangements should be made for follow-up within 24–48 h for the reevaluation of the infection and the response to antibiotics.

CASE OUTCOME

Case 1

The patient was administered a digital block and the wound was explored. No evidence of tendon injury, foreign body, or vascular injury was evident. The wound was irrigated with normal saline using a 20-cc syringe and an 18-gauge angiocath. The wound was not closed with sutures. He was given a dose of amoxicillin/clauvulanic acid 875 mg po early during the care in the ED. A prescription was given for the same 875 mg BID for 3 days. The patient was instructed to elevate the hand as much as possible. No rabies vaccine was given. The dog was observed for 10 days without any evidence of illness.

Case 2

The physician incised the small superficial abscess with a #15 blade with the expression of a small amount of grayish discharge. The patient was given one dose of IV ampicillin/sulbactam and discharged with a prescription for amoxicillin/clauvulanic acid 875 mg for 7 days. The culture returned growing *Pasteurella multocida* that was sensitive to penicillin and amoxicillin. The patient recovered uneventfully.

REFERENCES

1. Weiss H, Friedman D, Coben J: Incidence of dog bite injuries treated in emergency departments. *JAMA* 279:51–53, 1998.
2. Goldstein E: Bite wounds and infection. *Clin Infect Dis* 14:633–638, 1992.
3. McCaig LF: National Hospital Ambulatory Medical Care Survey: 2002 Emergency Department Summary. *Advance Data from Vital and Health Statistics - CDC* 340:1–36, 2004.
4. Sacks J, Kresnow M, Houston B: Dog bites: How big a problem? *Injury Prev* 2:52–54, 1996.
5. Weber D, Hansen A: Infections resulting from animal bites. *Infect Dis Clin North Am* 5:663–680, 1991.
6. Nonfatal dog bite-related injuries treated in hospital emergency departments–United States, 2001. *MMWR Morbid Mortal Wkly Rep* 52:605–610, 2003.
7. Medeiros I, Saconato H: Antibiotic prophylaxis for mammalian bites. *Cochrane Database Syst Rev* :1–19, 2001.
8. Cummings P: Antibiotics to prevent infection in patients with dog bite wounds: A meta-analysis of randomized trials. *Ann Emerg Med* 23:535–540, 1994.
9. Haupt W: Rabies—risk of exposure and current trends in prevention of human cases. *Vaccine* 17:13–14, 1999.
10. World Health Organization. *World Survey of Rabies No. 32 for the Year 1996.* Geneva, World Health Organization, 1998.
11. Black T, Rupprecht C: Rabies virus, in Mandell GL, Bennett JE, and Doling R (eds.): *Principles of Infectious Diseases, 5th ed.* Philadelphia, Churchill Livingstone.
12. Baer G: Rabies—an historical perspective. *Infect Agents Dis* 3:168–180, 1994.
13. Weiss E: Acquired zoonoses, in PS Auerbach (ed.): *Wilderness Medicine, 4th ed.* St. Louis, Mosby, 2001.
14. Weber E: Rabies, in Marx JA (ed.): *Emergency Medicine Concepts and Clinical Practices, 5th ed.* St. Louis, Mosby, 2002.
15. World Heath Organization: *Media Center Fact Sheet: Rabies.* Geneva, World Heath Organization.
16. Weber D: Rabies, in Tintinalli JE (ed.), *Emergency Medicine, A Comprehensive Study Guide, 6th ed.* New York, McGraw Hill, 2004.
17. Krebs J: *J Public Health Manag Pract* 4:56–62, 1998.
18. Goldstein E, Citron D, Finegold S: Dog bite wounds and infection: A prospective clinical study. *Ann Emerg Med* 9:508–512, 1980.
19. Bobo RA, Newton EJ: A previously undescribed gram-negative bacillus causing septicemia and meningitis. *Am J Clin Pathol* 65:564–569, 1976.
20. Krol-van Straaten MJ, Landheer JE, de Maat CE: Beware of the dog: Meningitis in a splenectomised woman. *Neth J Med* 36:301–303, 1990.
21. Pers C, Gahrn-Hansen B, Frederiksen W: Capnocytophaga canimorsus septicemia in Denmark, 1982–1995: Review of 39 cases. *Clin Infect Dis* 23:71–75, 1996.
22. Parenti DM, Snydman DR: Capnocytophaga species: Infections in nonimmunocompromised and immunocompromised hosts. *J Infect Dis* 151:140–147, 1985.
23. Hantson P, Gautier PE, Vekemans MC, et al.: Fatal capnocytophaga canimorsus septicemia in a previously healthy woman. *Ann Emerg Med* 20:93–94, 1991.
24. Saab M, Corcoran JP, Southworth SA, et al.: Fatal septicaemia in a previously healthy man following a dog bite. *Int J Clin Pract* 52:205, 1998.
25. Verghese A, Hamati F, Berk S, et al.: Susceptibility of dysgonic fermenter 2 to antimicrobial agents in vitro. *Antimicrob Agents Chemother* 32:78–80, 1988.
26. Bremmelgaard A, Pers C, Kristiansen JE, et al.: Susceptibility testing of Danish isolates of Capnocytophaga and CDC group DF-2 bacteria. *APMIS* 97:43–48, 1989.
27. Talan D, Citron D, Abrahamian F, et al. (Emergency Medicine Animal Bite Infection Study Group): Bacteriologic analysis of infected dog and cat bites. *N Engl J Med* 340:85–92, 1999.
28. Weber D, Wolfson J, Swartz M, et al.: *Pasteurella multocida* infections. Report of 34 cases and review of the literature. *Medicine* 63:133–154, 1984.
29. Goldstein EJ, Tarenzi LA, Agyare EO, et al.: Prevalence of *Eikenella corrodens* in dental plaque. *J Clin Microbiol* 17:636–639, 1983.
30. Talan DA, Abrahamian FM, Moran GJ, et al.: Clinical presentation and bacteriologic analysis of infected human bites in patients presenting to emergency departments. *Clin Infect Dis* 37:1481–1489, 2003.
31. Faciszewski T, Coleman DA: Human bite wounds. *Hand Clin* 5:561–569, 1989.
32. Noah D, Drenzek C, Smith J, et al.: Epidemiology of human rabies in the United States, 1980 to 1996. *Ann Intern Med* 128:922–930, 1998.
33. Krebs J, Noll H, Rupprecht C, et al.: Rabies surveillance in the United States during 2001. *J Am Vet Med Assoc* 221:1690–1701, 2002.
34. Krebs J, Wheeling J: Rabies surveillance in the United States during 2002. *J Am Vet Med Assoc* 223, 2003.
35. Smith J, Fishbein D, Rupprecht C, et al.: Unexplained rabies in three immigrants in the United States. A virologic investigation. *N Engl J Med* 324:205–211, 1991.
36. Esiri N, Kennedy P: Virus diseases, in Adams JH Duchen LW (eds.): *Greenfield's Neuropathology, 6th ed.* New York, Oxford University Press, 1992.
37. Anderson L, Nicholson K, Tauxe R, et al.: Human rabies in the United States, 1960 to 1979: Epidemiology, diagnosis, and prevention. *Ann Intern Med* 100:728–735, 1984.
38. Hemachudha T, Phanthumchinda K, Phanuphak P, et al.: Myoedema as a clinical sign in paralytic rabies. 1:1210, 1987.

39. Fishbein D, Bernard K: Rabies virus, in Mandell GM, Bennett JE, Dolin R (eds.): *Principles and Practices of Infectious Diseases, 5th ed.* New York, Churchill Livingstone, 1994.

40. Center for Disease Control/National Center for Infectious Diseases: Rabies.

41. Crepin P, Audry L, Rotivel Y, et al.: Intravitam diagnosis of human rabies by PCR using saliva and cerebrospinal fluid. *J Clin Microbiol* 36:1117–1121, 1998.

42. Zook E, Miller M, Van Beek A, et al.: Successful treatment protocol for canine fang injuries. *J Trauma–Injury Infect Critl Care* 20:237–243, 1980.

43. Maimaris C, Quinton D: Dog-bite lacerations: A controlled trial of primary wound closure. *Arch Emerg Med* 5:156–161, 1988.

44. Chen E, Hornig S, Shepherd S, et al.: Primary closure of mammalian bites. *Acad Emerg Med* 7:157–161, 2000.

45. Antimicrobial prophylaxis for surgery. *Med Lett* 2:27–32, 2004.

46. Goldstein E: Bites, in Mandell G , Bennett J, Dolin R (eds.): Reprinted from *Principles and Practice of Infectious Diseases, 5th ed.* Philadelphia, 2000; p 3203 with permission from Elsevier.

47. Human Rabies Prevention – United States 1999. Recommendations of the Advisory Committee on Immunization Practices (ACIP). *Morb Mortal Wkly Rep* 48, 1999.

48. Fu Z: Rabies and rabies research: Past, present and future. *Vaccine* 15:S20–S24, 1997.

49. Stone S, Carter W: Wound preparation, in Tintinalli JE (ed.): *Emergency Medicine, A Comprehensive Study Guide, 6th ed.* New York, McGraw-Hill, 2004.

50. Myers J: Bite wound infections, in Tom JS (ed.): *Expert Guide to Infectious Diseases.* Philadelphia, American College of Physicians, 2002.

51. Rupprecht C, Smith J, Fekadu M, et al.: The ascension of wildlife rabies: A cause for public health concern or intervention? *Emerg Infect Dis* 1:107–114, 1995.

52. Murphy F, Harrison AK, Winn W, et al.: Comparative pathogenesis of rabies and rabies-like viruses: Infection of the central nervous system and centrifugal spread of virus to peripheral tissues. *Lab Invest* 29:1–16, 1973.

33

Tetanus

Roma Hernandez
Sean Henderson

HIGH YIELD FACTS

1. Tetanus is a clinically based diagnosis and should be suspected in every presentation of generalized spasms.

2. *Clostridium tetani* is a ubiquitous organism that can affect a variety of injuries, ranging from superficial abrasions to corneal abrasions to burns. An injury or portal of entry is not necessary for tetanus to develop. Tetanus prophylaxis should not be based on the presence of a specific type of injury alone.

3. Prevention is key, especially in the young, immunocompromised, and the elderly. Lack of immunization remains the greatest risk factor for developing tetanus.

4. Early and aggressive management of the airway in patients infected with moderate or severe tetanus takes priority in definitive treatment.

5. Having a history of tetanus does not confer immunity to the disease. Active immunization with tetanus toxoid (Td) should be administered to patients recovering from tetanus as recurrent attacks may occur.

CASE PRESENTATION

A 25-year-old recent immigrant male from Mexico presents with superficial abrasions to the knuckles of his left hand. He has no past medical or surgical history. He is not on any medications and denies any known allergies to medications. He has never received any vaccinations or immunizations. Because of the minor nature of his wound, he did not seek medical attention at the time of injury.

Now a week out from his acute injury, the patient complains mainly of rigidity in his jaw, mild dysphagia, and back spasms. He does not remember exactly when he obtained the superficial cuts on his left hand. While waiting in the emergency department, he notices left upper extremity spasms near the abrasions, progressing to his lower extremities. These spasms are described as very painful.

The patient's physical exam is remarkable for superficial abrasions to his left hand, an inability to fully open his jaw, and hyperactive tendon reflexes. The motor exam reveals spasms in his back and lower extremities, provoked by stimulation of his muscles during the physical examination. His mental status remains essentially normal. Within a few hours, the patient deteriorates, develops labile hypertension, tachydysrhthymias, and respiratory failure. He is intubated, using vecuronium and midazolam, and is transferred to the ICU for further management.

INTRODUCTION/EPIDEMIOLOGY

Tetanus is a devastating, potentially lethal disease. It is characterized by generalized muscle spasms, rigidity, autonomic instability, and impending respiratory failure. Despite the availability of effective immunization, the disease has not been completely eradicated and mortality and morbidity remains high, even in the setting of optimal treatment. Tetanus carries a mortality rate exceeding 50% in the elderly and a global fatality rate estimated to be 30–50% (1–3). Neonatal tetanus, accounting for some 50% of worldwide cases, has a 90% fatality rate (4, 5). However, in the United States, only two cases have been reported since 1989 (6). Such a discrepancy in the frequency of tetanus subtypes epitomizes the health care disparity between industrialized and underdeveloped countries. Although the advent of immunization programs and improved wound management has decreased the incidence of tetanus dramatically in industrialized countries, it continues to be a major worldwide public health problem.

Since tetanus toxoid was introduced in the late 1940s as part of routine immunization schedules, the number of reported tetanus cases in the United States has declined steadily. In 2002, there were only 25 cases of tetanus reported to the CDC in the United States, as compared to 126 cases documented in 1997, and 500–600 cases reported during the 1940s (6–8). However, it has been suggested that the actual true number of tetanus cases is underestimated and the number of cases in the United States may actually be 2–4 times greater than reported (3).

Classically, there were several well-defined high-risk groups that included individuals older than 50 years, women, African-Americans from the South, and persons without any previous military experience (5, 9, 10). Over the past several years, those classical at-risk groups have been replaced. According to a recent CDC surveillance summary from 1998–2000, the highest average annual incidence of tetanus cases occurred in persons older than 60 years (0.35 case/million population), people of Hispanic ethnicity (0.37 case/million population), and in the elderly with diabetes (0.70 case/million population) (7). Most recently, another at-risk group has emerged, namely the immunocompromised.

Of the variables contributing to tetanus susceptibility, the lack of immunization poses the greatest risk. In a series of studies, those not immunized, partially immunized, or who completed a primary series but failed to get scheduled boosters, were among the highest percentage of patients who contracted tetanus (7, 11–14). Serologic surveys showed that only 28–50% of those between ages 65 and 70 were adequately immunized (2). It should be noted that there have been case studies documenting that fully immunized patients may still contract tetanus, despite having adequate tetanus antibody titers (1).

The percentage of reported cases among individuals younger than 40 years during 1991–1995 was 28%, a number that increased to 42% by 1996–2000 (6–8). This increase is thought to be due to a rise in the number of tetanus cases in young injection drug users, especially in California. Up to 84% of the tetanus cases found in IV drug users during 1998–2000 were from California (7).

Ethnic differences in immunity also exist. In a national population-based seroprevalence survey conducted from 1988 to 1991, only 58% of Mexican-Americans were found to have protective levels of antibody against tetanus as compared to 73% in non-Hispanic whites and 68% in non-Hispanic blacks (6, 7). In contrast to historical epidemiological reviews, a retrospective case series review documented that 91% of total tetanus cases in an inner-city health-care facility in Southern California occurred in the Hispanic population; 72% of the cases were seen in patients younger than 50 years; and only one case of tetanus occurred in a female patient (14).

Although IV drug use and acute trauma are known to facilitate an anaerobic environment prone to causing tetanus, abscesses, skin abrasions, and gangrene can also result in the development of tetanus. Wounds that are contaminated, more than 6-h old, stellate, greater than 1 cm in depth, have devitalized tissue, or those secondary to missile injury, crush injury, or burns are particularly at high risk for contracting *C. tetani* (2, 9, 15, 16). Tetanus has also been reported following otitis media, diabetic complications, foreign bodies, corneal abrasions, dental procedures, septic abortions, unhygienic childbirth, and unsanitary circumcision practices (2). Of the type of injuries associated with tetanus, puncture wounds (50%) are found to be the most common, followed by lacerations (33%) and abrasions (9%) (7). Injuries to the lower

extremities are reported to be more common portals of infection as compared to upper extremities, the trunk, or the head. More importantly, in up to 6–8% of tetanus cases, no etiology of tetanus was found (4, 24). In 30% of documented cases of tetanus, there is no apparent portal of entry (17). Therefore, the lack of a known wound, injury, or history of acute trauma should not exclude the diagnosis of tetanus.

PATHOPHYSIOLOGY/MICROBIOLOGY

Clostridium tetani is an anaerobic, gram-positive bacillus that forms spores. It is ubiquitous in nature and found in soil, dust, rust, and the feces of animals and humans. These spores are highly resilient to extremes of temperature, moisture, and chemical substances, such as ethanol, phenol, and formalin. Once exposed to anaerobic conditions, such as the environment associated with wounds, tissue necrosis, or foreign bodies, the spores can germinate. Although ubiquitous, tetanus is not contagious from person to person.

Proliferating bacteria produce exotoxins, tetanolysin, and tetanospasmin. Tetanolysin has no proven clinical significance whereas tetanospasmin causes tetanus. Tetanospasmin is a zinc metalloprotease that cleaves synaptobrevin, a protein essential for neurotransmitter release. When released it inhibits the release of gama-aminobutyuric acid (GABA) and glycine neurotransmitters, both of which are inhibitory neurotransmitters. Once internalized in presynaptic cells, the metalloprotease is transported to the central nervous system through retrograde intra-axonal transport. The incubation period for tetanus ranges from 24 h to 3 weeks, but is usually 7–14 days (1). Injury sites closer to the central nervous system correlate with shorter incubation period. Disinhibition of the motor and autonomic nervous system results in sustained excitatory discharge. The resultant muscle rigidity, uncontrolled spasms, and autonomic hyperactivity are clinical manifestations of tetanus (13).

CLINICAL PRESENTATION

Traditionally, there are four classifications of tetanus: neonatal, cephalic, local, and generalized tetanus. Although neonatal tetanus is rare in the United States secondary to tetanus prophylactic measures, worldwide, it remains the most common form (5). This stems as a consequence of improper obstetric care, unhygienic circumcision practices, or infection of umbilical stumps (4, 18).

Neonatal tetanus is found in the setting of an unimmunized mother since passive transmission of maternal antibodies usually protects the newborn. Clinical disease occurs by the second week of life and common manifestations include generalized weakness, a poor sucking reflex, or irritability. Over time, tetanic spasms develop, producing the characteristic opisthotonic posturing of tetanus (arching of the back caused by sustained contraction of back muscles). Without optimal treatment, autonomic dysregulation is the main cause of death.

Cephalic tetanus is a rare form of the disease but remains a severe variant of localized tetanus, occurring on the head or face. It commonly presents as trismus (lockjaw), peripheral facial nerve weakness, such as Bell palsy, or as dysphagia. Although a localized variant, cephalic tetanus has a higher mortality (17). It is often associated with concurrent chronic otitis media or prior head injury (19). Progression to generalized tetanus has been implicated as a poor prognostic factor.

Localized tetanus is the least severe type of the disease. The hallmark of localized tetanus is fixed muscle rigidity and pain, at, or adjacent to, the site of injury. Muscle rigidity may range from mild to intense and can persist for several months without any progression. This disorder is usually self-limiting, lasting less than 2 weeks. Prognosis is generally excellent with spontaneous resolution (3).

In the United States, generalized tetanus is most common. Clinical presentation is characterized by muscle rigidity, stiffness, spasms, and autonomic instability. Spasms can be uncontrollable, leading to respiratory arrest. Tetanic seizures can occur in the generalized subtype. In up to three-fourths of generalized tetanus cases, trismus is the initial manifestation (19). Other symptoms and signs include dysphagia, risus sardonicus (a grimace with sustained contraction of facial muscles), opisthotonos, vertebral fractures, or abdominal rigidity. Short incubation periods of *C. tetani* correlate with severe disease and poorer prognosis. In a recent retrospective study, generalized tetanus and incubation periods of less than or equal to 1 week were associated with a mortality rate of 75% (20).

LABORATORY/DIAGNOSTIC TESTING

The diagnosis of tetanus is clinical. Although tetanus may be evident by the presenting symptoms and signs of a patient, early tetanus remains a challenge to diagnose, especially in areas where the disease is uncommon.

Traditionally, labs for evaluating tetanus included a CBC, CK level, wound cultures, and serum antitoxin levels. Wound cultures yield unreliable results and are of low yield. CBC and CK levels are nonspecific. Serum antitoxin levels prove to be impractical as the results are not immediately available to the emergency medicine physician. Cerebral spinal fluid is usually normal and electroencephalograms do not show specific changes (19). Based on several literature studies, the accepted therapeutic level of tetanus antitoxin is 0.01 IU/mL (1, 2, 4, 21). Although such a level is considered to be the minimum protective value against contracting tetanus, some authors indicate that this does not guarantee immunity to the disease. Tetanus has been documented in patients with higher levels of antibody, up to 0.16 IU/mL (1).

Because there are no specific laboratory studies for detecting tetanus, the history and physical exam play important roles in making the correct diagnosis. A complete immunization history of the patient should be documented. Clues lie mainly in the clinical presentation of the patient. Trismus is usually the first symptom. Upper and lower extremity spasms follow early in the disease. Generalized spasms, if not aggressively treated, can progress to respiratory failure and the need for mechanical ventilation. Autonomic instability, resulting from a surge of catecholamines, ranges from tachycardia, cardiac ischemia, dysrhythmias, labile hypertension, hyperthermia, and diaphoresis. Such autonomic dysregulation is associated with a poor prognosis if not aggressively treated (22).

Since tetanus has nonspecific signs and symptoms, various causes of generalized spasms should be ruled out before initiating treatment for tetanus. Strychnine poisoning closely mimics the symptoms of tetanus except that trismus and abdominal rigidity are usually absent. Seizure disorder or status epilepticus may imitate tetanus; however, tetanic "seizures" are not associated with a loss of consciousness and are extremely painful. Other similar clinical presentations include alveolar abscess, drug-induced dystonia (phenothiazines and metoclopramide), encephalitis, rabies, meningitis, metabolic abnormalities, such as hypocalcemia or hypomagnesemia, and acute abdominal processes.

MANAGEMENT

Early recognition of the disease and aggressive management are essential in insuring a positive outcome. The goals of therapy are to (1) insure appropriate prophylaxis, (2) stabilize and resuscitate patient, (3) neutralize tetanus toxin, (4) eliminate the source of *C. tetani* with antibiotics and carefully debride wound, (5) treat existing muscle spasms and manage autonomic instability, and (6) control pain.

Priority in the initial treatment of severe tetanus should focus on stabilizing and resuscitating the patient *in extremis*. The most common cause of death from tetanus, particularly in underdeveloped areas, is respiratory failure. It can occur either as a complication of generalized tetanus, failure to treat spasms expeditiously, or as a side effect of medications, such as benzodiazepines.

Given the duration of intubation common with this disease, percutaneous tracheostomy is usually performed in the ICU, following intubation, or after the first generalized seizure. This type of airway prevents further stimulus for provoking reflex spasms in the patient (17).

After securing the airway, the next step in managing acute tetanus is administering the appropriate drugs according to the phase and severity of the disease. A list of updated drugs used in managing tetanus is outlined in Table 33–1.

Once the diagnosis is tetanus is suspected, HTIG should be given to neutralize the tetanospasmin toxin. HTIG works by inactivating free neurotoxin only; it does not cross the blood brain barrier, rendering it ineffective against intra-axonal neurotoxin. Doses of 500–10,000 IU have been reported in the treatment of tetanus (2–4). Since having had the disease does not guarantee immunity, active immunization with Td should be administered simultaneously to those with acute tetanus. This enhances both short-term (passive) immunity and long-term humoral and cellular (active) immunity. Differing sites and separate syringes should be used to inject Td and HTIG, if both are needed simultaneously.

Following the neutralization of tetanospasmin, antibiotics should be administered to eliminate its source. Traditionally, benzyl penicillin, 1.2 million units IV q6 h × 10 days, has been reported as the recommended antibiotic for tetanus treatment. Because penicillin also acts as a GABA antagonist, it is thought to contribute synergistic effects to tetanospasmin in producing muscle spasms (19). However, metronidazole, 500–600 mg IV every 8 h, is currently the antibiotic of choice for treating tetanus. Metronidazole is superior to penicillin in terms of shortened recovery time and lower mortality rate (2–4). In a recent randomized controlled trial, intramuscular benzathine penicillin, intravenous benzyl penicillin, and metronidazole were shown to be equally effective (23). In cases where there are contraindications to metronidazole or penicillin use, third-generation cephalosporins, macrolides, or tetracyclines have been reported to be safe alternatives (3).

Aside from antibiotic therapy, eliminating the source of the toxin necessitates effective wound debridement. In patients with deep or high risk wounds, thorough excision removes any toxin-producing organisms and creates an aerobic environment that will hinder the growth of *C. tetani* spores. Debridement should be done only after the administration of Td since tetanospasmin is released into the bloodstream with each procedure. Cultures need to be sent at the time of surgical excision and proper follow-up should be arranged for appropriate wound care.

In severe cases of tetanus, muscle spasms and rigidity predominate during the early phase of the disease. Supportive and aggressive measures should be utilized to control muscle spasms and autonomic instability. Benzodiazepenes remain the drug of choice for spasm treatment, secondary to their sedative and GABA-agonist properties. Diazepam has been traditionally used for its wide safety margin and range of intake routes. Midazolam, although a more expensive alternative, is not suspended in cardiotoxic propylene glycol, and therefore may be preferred for prolonged use (20). After resolution of symptoms, benzodiazepenes should be slowly weaned to prevent withdrawal symptoms.

When muscle spasms are refractory to benzodiazepine use, neuromuscular blocking agents are necessary to control muscle spasms. Traditionally pancuronium has been used. Pancuronium has recently fallen out of favor because it may exacerbate autonomic instability by inhibiting catecholamine uptake and inducing tachycardia and hypertension. Vecuronium has been reported to be less cardioactive and is ideal for immediate and long-term control of refractory spasms (2).

During the early phase of tetanus, succinylcholine can be used but the possibility of hyperkalemia limits its utility (2). Rocuronium remains as another alternative for its longer acting properties (17).

Other reported treatments of muscle spasms resistant to benzodiazepenes and/or neuromuscular blocking agents include intrathecal baclofen or dantrolene. Intrathecal baclofen is a specific GABA-B agonist. Side effects include respiratory depression, warranting mechanical ventilation (19). Dantrolene acts as a muscle relaxant and has been reported to be successful in controlling challenging muscle spasms. In one particular study, the patient's condition improved with dantrolene, without the use of paralysis (17).

In severe tetanus, managing autonomic instability has been problematic. A universally effective therapeutic regimen is lacking. Beta blockers have been recommended as first line therapy to control autonomic hyperactivity. However, pure beta blockers, such as propranolol, can worsen reflex tachycardia from unopposed alpha blockade. Therefore, labetalol is currently recommended as a better choice for providing hemodynamic control (4, 19). Clonidine may be used as a safe alternative and has been

Table 33–1. Drugs Used in the Management of Tetanus (2, 11)

Drug/Class	Indication	Dosage	Route
I. Benzodiazepines (BZ)	Spasm control and sedation		
1) Diazepam (BZ)		5–20 mg prn	IV
2) Midazolam (BZ)		5–15 mg/h	IV infusion
II. GABA-B agonist	Spasm control refractory to BZ		
1) Intrathecal baclofen		500–1000 ug/24 h	IV bolus
		1–2 mg/24 h	IV infusion
III. Muscle relaxant	Spasm control alternative		
1) Dantrolene		1–1.5 mg/kg	IV load dose
		0.5–1 mg/kg q4–6 h	IV infusion × <25 days
IV. Neuromuscular blocking agents	Spasm control refractory to BZ Minimize sedation		
1) Vecuronium		6–8 mg/h	IV
2) Pancuronium		0.01 mg/kg	IV
3) Succinylcholine	Used only in initial phase because of hyperkalemia	2 mg/kg	IV
V. Antibiotics	Elimination of *C. Tetani* toxin		
1) Metronidazole	First-line antibiotic	500–600 mg q8h	IV or PO × 10 days
2) Benzyl penicillin		1.2 million units q6h	IV × 10 days
3) Benzathine penicillin		1.2 million units	IM × 1
VI. Alpha and Beta blocker	Control of autonomic dysfunction		
1) Labetalol		0.25–1.0 mg/minute	IV infusion
VII. Alpha 2 agonist	Control of autonomic dysfunction		
1) Clonidine		0.2–0.4 mg/24 h	IV or PO
VIII. Other			
2) Magnesium sulfate		4 g	IV bolus
		2–3 g/h	IV infusion
IX. Opioid	Control of pain and peripheral vasodilation		
1) Morphine sulfate		2–10 mg	IV
X. Detoxified Exotoxin	Active immunization		
1) DTaP	Ages 7 years or younger	0.5 mL	IM
2) Tetanus toxoid	Ages older than 7 years	0.5 mL	IM × 1 q10 years
XI. Human immunoglobulin	Passive immunization Neutralizes free exotoxin		
1) HTIG	Treatment of tetanus	500–6000 units	IM
	Postexposure	250 units	IM

reported to lower mortality (17). High-dose magnesium sulfate has also been documented to produce stabilizing effects in severe tetanus (4, 19). Magnesium sulfate has been reported to be more effective as an adjunct in controlling autonomic instability when given with appropriate sedation than when used alone (13). High doses of

atropine, up to 100 mg/h IV, have been found to achieve muscarinic and nicotinic blockade (17).

Because muscle spasms, rigidity, and seizures associated with tetanus have been described as excruciatingly painful, analgesia is essential in effectively treating tetanus. Morphine sulfate not only provides adequate pain cessation but also aids in autonomic stabilization via peripheral vasodilation (4, 19, 24). Fentanyl may be an alternate choice for pain management.

Complications of tetanus include fractures and dislocations from severe muscle contractions, labile hypertension, and dysrhythmias resulting from autonomic dysregulation, deep-vein thrombosis or pulmonary embolus secondary to prolonged immobility, stress ulceration, contractures, and gastrointestinal bleeding. Residual neurologic sequelae are rare (13). Preventing the sequelae of long-term critical illness is necessary for insuring positive outcomes.

Most patients who survive the disease have the potential to regain full activity and mobility with aggressive physical therapy. Since having had tetanus does not confer immunity to the disease, recovering patients should be actively immunized.

DISPOSITION

After patients with tetanus have been stabilized in the emergency department, transfer to an ICU setting for further management is necessary because of potential rapid decompensation in these patients. They should be monitored in a dark, quiet area to minimize precipitation of reflex tetanic spasms. When transport to another facility for higher level of care is warranted, ACLS-trained personnel must accompany transport.

PREVENTION

Prevention of tetanus is the key to long-term management and overall elimination of the disease. Emergency medicine physicians have the opportunity to decrease incidence, morbidity, and mortality associated with tetanus by insuring that patients have updated immunization.

The Advisory Committee of Immunization Practices provides routine vaccination schedules according to age, type of wound, and either primary or booster immunizations. Recommendations for primary immunization depend on the age of the patient. Two pediatric formulations for childhood immunizations exist, namely DTaP (diphtheria and tetanus toxoids and acellular pertussis vaccine) and DTP (diphtheria and tetanus toxoids with pertussis vaccine). Either DTaP or DTP is the vaccine used for children up to 7 years old. In the United States, the schedule for the four doses is given at 2, 4, 6, and 15–18 months of age, followed by a booster shot by age 5. Thereafter,

boosters are given every 10 years, unless postexposure prophylaxis warrants administration sooner (21, 25, 26).

When patients older than 7 years present for a primary immunization series, they should receive two intramuscular doses of Td (adult formulation). These doses are given at least 4 weeks apart, followed by a third dose 6–12 months later, regardless of whether they have incomplete primary immunization. Td boosters should follow every 10 years thereafter (25, 26). Written documentation of administered immunizations facilitates appropriate wound care.

For postexposure cases, the patient's immunization status and type of wound define subsequent treatment. Patients who are older than 7 years and have completed the primary immunization series (>three doses) should receive a booster dose of Td, given the last dose was administered when the patient was older than 5 years and the wound is dirty or tetanus-prone (Table 33–2). A similar patient with a clean wound and either an incomplete primary immunization series or an unknown immunization status needs to be treated with Td. Patients with incomplete or unknown immunization series who have a dirty wound need both Td and HTIG. Td is replaced with DTaP or DT (if pertussis vaccine is contraindicated) for use in patients who are less than 7 years old (2, 25, 26).

Both Td and HTIG can be given to pregnant women and patients with AIDS. Neonatal tetanus can be entirely prevented by vaccinating unimmunized mothers. Although Td is considered safe for the fetus, immunizations should be avoided during the first trimester of pregnancy. Td is only prohibited in pregnancy if the mother has contraindications to active immunization, such as a severe allergic reaction. HIV infection associated with pregnancy and concomitant polyclonal hyperimmunoglobulinemia can limit the transfer of protective maternal antibodies to the fetus (17). In HIV patients with a CD4 lymphocyte count less that or equal to 300×10^6/L, there is a reduced antibody response to tetanus vaccination (12, 17). Liberal use of HTIG may be warranted in AIDS patients, that is, more frequent dosing, regardless of primary immunization (2).

CASE OUTCOME

Our patient subsequently developed generalized tetanus, manifesting opisthotonos and abdominal rigidity once in the ICU. Serum obtained for an antitetanus toxoid antibody titer revealed no immunity. His serum and urine samples to rule out strychnine and other illicit drug use were negative. To exclude a dystonic reaction, he was

Table 33–2. Active and Passive Tetanus Immunization in Specific Wounds

If the Wound Is:	And the Patient Has Completed Primary Immunization, then:	If the Patient Has Received Either Incomplete Primary Immunization or Has an Unknown History of Immunization, then:
Dirty	Give Td[a] unless last Td booster < 5 years	Give Td and HTIG[b]
Clean	None unless last Td booster > 10 years	Give Td
Unknown	Give Td if last Td booster > 5 years and tetanus-prone wound[c]	Give Td and HTIG if tetanus-prone wound[c]

[a]Replace Td with DTaP or DT (if pertussis is contraindicated) in patients who are less than 7 years old.
[b]Simultaneous administration of Td and HTIG must be given at different sites and separate syringes.
[c]Tetanus-prone wounds include wounds that are older than 6 h, deeper than 1 cm, contaminated with soil or feces, stellate, infected, denervated, or ischemic.

given benzotropine, which had no effect. His muscle spasms and abdominal rigidity were aggressively controlled with heavy benzodiazepene use. After a prolonged course the patient underwent an elective tracheostomy.

During the third week of his hospitalization, he developed sinus tachycardia and labile hypertension, controlled with appropriate use of labetalol. The patient recovered, was weaned off benzodiazepines. Once free of spasms, his tracheostomy was replaced with a fenestrated tube and then capped. The patient had a full recovery with aggressive physical therapy in a rehabilitation center.

Overall, tetanus is a preventable disease with significant morbidity and mortality. Appropriate attention to immunization status, especially in the course of wound management, is mandatory for emergency physicians. Because tetanus is diagnosed based on clinical evidence, therapy should be initiated promptly to prevent unexpected complications, morbidity, and mortality.

REFERENCES

1. Gareau AB, Eby RJ, McLellan BA, Williams DR: Tetanus immunization status and immunologic response to a booster in an emergency department geriatric population. *Ann Emerg Med* 19(12):1377–1322, 1990.
2. Hsu SS, Groleau G: Tetanus in the emergency department: A current review. *J Emerg Med* 20(4):357–365, 2001.
3. Richardson JP, Knight AL: The management and prevention of tetanus. *J Emerg Med* 11:737–742, 1993.
4. Bleck TP: Tetanus: Pathophysiology, management, and prophylaxis, in *Disease-a-Month*. Littleton MA, Mosby, Inc., 1991; vol. 37, pp 547–602.
5. Galazka A, Gasse F: The present status of tetanus and tetanus vaccination. *Curr Top Microbiol Immunol* 195:31–53, 1995.
6. Centers for Disease Control: Tetanus surveillance—United States, 1995–1997. *Morb Mortal Wkly Rep* 39:37–41, 1990.
7. Centers for Disease Control: Tetanus surveillance—United States, 1998–2000. *Morb Mortal Wkly Rep* 52:1–12, 2003.
8. Centers for Disease Control: Summary of notifiable diseases—United States, 2000. *Morb Mortal Wkly Rep* 49(53):1–102, 2002.
9. Gergen PJ, McQuillen GM, Kiely M, Ezzati-Rice TM, Sutter RW, Virella G: A population-based survey of immunity to tetanus in the United States. *N Engl J Med* 332:419–423, 1995.
10. Henderson SO, Wakim N: Tetanus, in Rakel RE, Bope ET (eds.): *Conn's Current Therapy*. Philadelphia, PA, W.B. Saunders, 2002; vol. 69, pp 292–301.
11. Furste, W: Tetanus prophylaxis in the United States, 1992. *Bull Am Coll Surg* 77(8):22–26, 1992.
12. Furste W: Four keys to 100 per cent success in tetanus prophylaxis. *Am J Surg* 128:616–623, 1974.
13. Groleau G: Tetanus. *Emerg Med Clin N Am* 10(2):351–360, 1992.
14. Henderson SO, Mody T, Groth D, Moore JJ, Newton E: The presentation of tetanus in an emergency department. *J Emerg Med* 16(5):705–708, 1998.
15. Edlich RF, Wilder BJ, Silloway KA, Nichter LS, Bryant CA: Quality assessment of tetanus prophylaxis in the wounded patient. *Am Surg* 52:544–547, 1986.
16. Giangrasso J, Smith KR: Misuse of tetanus immunoprophylaxis in wound care. *Ann Emerg Med* 14(6):574–579, 1985.

17. Farrar JJ, Yen LM, Cook T, et al.: Tetanus. *J Neurol Neurosurg Psychiatry* 69:292–301, 2000.

18. Davies-Adetugbo AA, Torimoro SEA, Ako-Nai KA. Prognostic factors in neonatal tetanus. *TM&IH* 1998;3: 9–13.

19. Ernst ME, Klepser ME, Fouts M, Marangos M: Tetanus: Pathophysiology and management. *Ann Pharmacother* 31:1507–1513, 1997.

20. Saltoglu N, Tasova Y, Midikli D, Burgut R, Dundar IH: Prognostic factors affecting deaths from adult tetanus. *Clin Microbiol Infect* 10(3):229–233, 2004.

21. Robles NL, Walske BR: Current concepts of tetanus prophylaxis. *Am J Surg* 118:835–838, 1969.

22. Bassin SL: Tetanus. *Curr Treat Options Neurol* 6(1):25–34, 2004.

23. Ganesh KAV, Kothari VM, Krishnan A, Karnad DR: Benzathine penicillin, metronidazole and benzyl penicillin in the treatment of tetanus: A randomized, controlled trial. *Ann Trop Med Parasitol* 98(1):59–63, 2004.

24. Abrahamian FM: Management of tetanus: A review. *Curr Treat Opt Infect Dis* 2:209–216, 2001.

25. American College of Emergency Physicians: Policy statement: Tetanus immunization for adults and children in the emergency department. Information paper revised by the Public Health Committee, March 2000.

26. Centers for Disease Control: Diphtheria, tetanus, and pertussis: Recommendations for vaccine use and other preventive measures: Recommendations of the Advisory Committee on Immunization Practices. *Morb Mortal Wkly Rep* 40:1–28, 1991.

34

Bioterrorism: Anthrax, Smallpox, Plague, and Tularemia

Kerry King

INTRODUCTION

The threat of modern day biological terrorism within our communities became a reality in America in October 2001 when deliberately contaminated mail resulted in 22 cases of clinical anthrax (1). Although the "attack" was unsophisticated and the number of documented cases was small, emergency departments throughout the country were inundated with requests for information and with patients concerned for possible exposure with substantial psychological and economic impact on our society and health care system (2, 3). These incidents occurring in the wake of the September 11 attacks have resulted in heightened awareness of our vulnerability to future biological terror events with the very real potential for large numbers of victims. Likewise, there has been much focus and effort on improving our ability to prevent, detect and respond to a future biological incident. Paramount to this effort has been the education and training of medical and emergency response personnel with regard to biological agents and the respective clinical disease processes that most have never encountered. The Centers for Disease Control and Prevention (CDC) along with the United States Department of Defense, Department of Homeland Security, national and regional medical and public safety organizations have developed an extensive resource of educational materials and guidelines directed at medical preparedness and response to a biological terror event (4). As in all disaster medicine, emergency medicine has and will be at the forefront of this effort.

In 1999 the CDC directed a working group which identified agents of concern that could be used in a biological terror event. A subgroup of these agents was designated Category "A." These are the agents of highest potential threat based on characteristics such as mortality, ease of dissemination, person to person transmission, and ability to incite panic and social disruption (5). Four of the agents at the top of the Category "A" list are Bacillus anthracis, Yersinia pestis, Francisella tularensis, and Variola major.

ANTHRAX

History and Background

Anthrax has been recognized for centuries as a disease with potential for significant morbidity and mortality. What is believed to be the earliest known recorded description is found in the Book of Genesis which refers to the fifth plague killing Egyptian cattle in 1491 BC. Much later in the 17th century an epidemic of the "black bane" swept through Europe killing both people and livestock (6). The causative agent, *Bacillus anthracis*, played a leading role in the development of modern day clinical microbiology and immunology. It was the first disease for which a definitive microbial origin was established by Robert Koch in 1876 and the first disease for which an effective live bacterial vaccine was developed by Luis Pasteur in 1881 (6, 7). The inhalation form of anthrax was first described in England in the late 19th century among mill workers handling raw wool, hence the common name of "Wool sorters' Disease (8)." The potential to induce a rapidly progressive and fatal disease by exposure to highly stable aerosolized spores has motivated more than 80 years of research and development on anthrax as a biological weapon by at least five countries including Japan, the United States, and the United Kingdom (1, 6, 9–11). More recently the former Soviet Union is known to have had a major anthrax weapons program including the development of antibiotic resistant strains. In 1995, it was confirmed that Iraq also had produced and weaponized *B. anthracis* (1, 12, 13). The anthrax attacks in the United States in 2001 demonstrate the significant public health and economic impact that can be produced with a relatively limited and unsophisticated event (14). Estimates of the impact of a large scale release over a metropolitan area suggest the number of deaths to be from 100,000 to 3,000,000 with an equally catastrophic economic impact (14–16). The potential availability, ease of dissemination, high morbidity, mortality and recent history of use as a domestic bioterror agent identify *Bacillus anthracis* as one of the primary agents of concern.

Epidemiology

Anthrax is a zoonosis which occurs in mammals, most commonly grazing herbivores such as goats, sheep, cattle, horses, and swine. It is prevalent throughout the world and has been linked with human cases from Africa, Asia, Europe, and the Americas (1, 6) The incidence of naturally occurring disease world wide is about 2000 cases per year. In the United States the reported incidence is

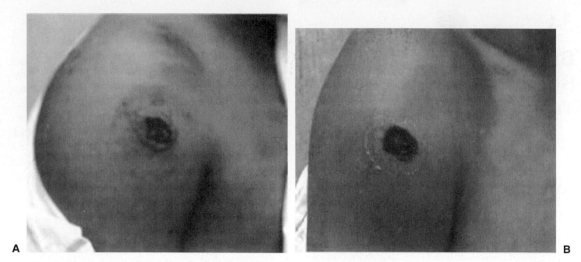

Fig. 34–1. (A) Ulcer and vesicle ring and (B) black eschar. *Source:* Courtesy of the Centers for Disease Control (Public Domain).

approximately one case per year and there has not been a naturally occurring case of inhalation anthrax reported since 1976 (14).

In 2001, 22 cases of anthrax were identified in the United States (11 inhalation and 11 cutaneous) as a result of the intentional distribution of *B. anthracis* spores sent in at least five letters through the U.S. Postal Service. The spores in the letters were identified as coming from the same strain (Ames); however, the specific source of the culture(s) used to create the spore-containing powder remains unknown (14). In the setting of this intentional release, epidemiologic data indicate that infection may occur from secondary aerosolization of spores carried away from the site of the initial release on cross contaminated material such as envelopes. Similarly, in 1979, an accidental release of spores from a biologic weapons facility in the city of Sverdlovsk in the then Soviet Union resulted in cases of inhalation anthrax up to 4 km down wind from the point of release and fatalities in animals more than 50 km away (12).

The disease is initiated by contact with infectious spores which are extremely hardy and can remain viable in soil for decades. Naturally occurring infection in humans usually results from contact with contaminated animals or animal products such as hides, hair, or poorly cooked meat. Although spores are highly infective, the vegetative bacillus is not and there are no known cases of human-to-human transmission (1, 8). Infection typically occurs through one of three routes, inhalation, cutaneous, or gastrointestinal. Naturally occurring inhalation and gastrointestinal anthrax are rare and 95% or more of

cases are cutaneous (1, 6, 8). Following an intentional release, inhalation anthrax is expected to account for the most significant morbidity and mortality. However, data from the 2001 events suggest that up to 50% of patients may present with cutaneous disease (14). As a result of these recent events and the rarity of naturally occurring disease, the identification of a single patient presenting with clinical signs and symptoms suspicious for any form of anthrax would require immediate notification of public health authorities.

Microbiology and Pathophysiology

B. anthracis is an aerobic, gram-positive, nonmotile spore forming bacillus. It is readily cultured on standard laboratory media such as sheep blood agar with colony morphology and microscopic characteristics that are similar to other nonvirulent bacillus species such as *B. cereus* which is commonly encountered as a contaminant in clinical cultures. Spores will germinate into the rapidly multiplying vegetative bacillus when exposed to a nutrient-rich environment such as blood or animal tissue. Conversely, the vegetative bacillus will form spores if nutrients are exhausted or if exposed to ambient environmental conditions (1, 6, 7, 9). Viable spores have been documented to persist for decades in contaminated soil (17).

Anthrax infections are initiated by endospores which enter the body through a break in the skin or mucosa and via inhalation. With skin or mucosal entry spores will germinate into the vegetative bacillus and begin multiplying at the entry site resulting in local tissue edema and

Table 34–1. CDC Category a Agents

Agent	Clinical Disease
Variola major	Smallpox
B. anthracis	Anthrax
Y. pestis	Plague
F. tularensis	Tularemia
Clostridium botulinum toxin	Botulism
Filoviruses (Ebola, Marburg)	Hemorrhagic fever
Arenaviruses (Lassa, Junin)	Hemorrhagic fever

Source: Adapted from *Morb Mortal Wkly Rep* 49(RR-4):1–14, 2000.

necrosis. Inhaled spores and occasionally those that enter through skin or mucosa will be ingested by macrophages where they then germinate, begin to multiply, and are carried to regional lymph nodes. Vegetative bacilli are then released from the macrophages, continue to multiply in the lymphatic system and eventually enter the bloodstream resulting in as many as 10^7–10^8 organisms per milliliter of blood (1, 9). A number of factors contribute to the virulence of *B. anthracis*. Foremost among these is the production of three factors which combine to form two exotoxins, edema toxin, and lethal toxin and the production of a capsule that inhibits phagocytosis of the vegetative forms (1, 6, 7, 9, 18–20). The protective factor enables the toxins to bind to the host cell surface and enter the cytoplasm. The edema toxin is a calmodulin-dependent adenylate cyclase that is believed to increase cellular levels of cyclic AMP and disrupt water homeostasis resulting in cellular edema. It is also known to impair neutrophil function (1, 6, 9). The lethal toxin is a zinc metalloprotease that inhibits immune cell and cytokine response early in infection and stimulates the release of tumor necrosis factor and interleukin-1β from macrophages which is believed to be responsible for the overwhelming toxicity and sudden death associated with anthrax (1, 9, 18–20). In inhalation anthrax, spores are deposited in the alveolar spaces, ingested by macrophages and carried to mediastinal lymph nodes where they germinate, multiply and begin toxin production (1, 6, 9). Once vegetative bacilli begin replicating and releasing toxins there is rapid development of hemorrhagic lymphadenitis, hemorrhagic mediastinitis, systemic toxicity, shock and death (1, 6, 9, 12). Autopsies of 42 victims of inhalation anthrax from the Sverdlovsk incident identified hemorrhagic mediastinitis and pleural effusions in all cases. None had evidence of an infiltrative pneumonic process though 11 of the 42 did have focal necrotizing pneumonic lesions (21).

Clinical Presentation

Historically the incubation period from exposure to symptom onset for cutaneous anthrax has been quoted as 3–5 days (1, 6). Data available for the cases of cutaneous anthrax diagnosed in 2001 indicate a median incubation time of 5 days with a range of 1–10 days (14, 22). Following exposure through the skin, bacterial proliferation and toxin release produce local tissue edema and necrosis. The lesion begins as a pruritic macule or papule which resembles an insect bite (1, 6, 7) Over 1–2 days it develops into one or more 2–3 cm vesicles which may be hemorrhagic and then rupture leaving a round necrotic ulcer which is usually painless. This is followed by development of a depressed black eschar which may be associated with significant local edema. The eschar dries and sloughs off after 1–2 weeks.

Systemic symptoms of fever and malaise may be present. Lymphangitis with painful lymphadenopathy and systemic toxicity occur in a minority of patients. Antibiotics do not hasten resolution of the local lesion and eschar but they do prevent systemic spread and toxicity. Untreated, the mortality of cutaneous anthrax is as high as 20%; however, with appropriate antibiotics administration death is a rare occurrence (1, 6, 7). The differential diagnosis of cutaneous anthrax includes brown recluse spider bite, ulceroglandular tularemia, scrub typhus, rat bite fever, ecthyma gangrenosum, accidental vaccinia, and necrotic herpes simplex (1, 22). Gastrointestinal anthrax is a rare form of anthrax seen primarily in underdeveloped areas following ingestion of contaminated poorly cooked meat (6, 9). It can involve any segment of the GI tract but is typically described as having two distinct clinical presentations, abdominal and oropharyngeal. The abdominal form presents with nonspecific symptoms of nausea, vomiting, anorexia, fever and abdominal pain. With progression, hematemesis and bloody diarrhea develop followed by systemic toxicity, shock and death (1, 6, 9). Although autopsy reports show evidence of gastrointestinal involvement in patients dying from inhalation anthrax it has never been documented as an isolated presentation in the United States nor were there cases of isolated gastrointestinal anthrax diagnosed in the 2001 incident or in the Sverdlovsk incident of 1979 (12, 14, 21, 23). In the oropharyngeal form, edema and lymphadenopathy occur in the cervical area. An inflammatory lesion similar to that described for cutaneous anthrax is seen with pseudomembranous ulcerations usually involving the posterior pharyngeal wall, the hard palate, or the tonsils. The main clinical features are sore throat, dysphagia, fever, lymphadenopathy, and toxemia. Most affected patients die of toxemia and sepsis

Table 34–2. Symptoms and Signs of Inhalational Anthrax, Laboratory-Confirmed Influenza, and Influenza-Like Illness (ILI) from Other Causes

Symptom/Sign	Inhalational Anthrax (n = 11)	Laboratory-Confirmed Influenza	ILI from Other Causes
Elevated temperature	70%	68–77%	40–73%
Fever or chills	100%	83–90%	75–89%
Fatigue/malaise	100%	75–94%	62–94%
Cough (minimal or nonproductive)	90%	84–93%	72–80%
Shortness of breath	80%	6%	6%
Chest discomfort or pleuritic chest pain	60%	35%	23%
Headache	50%	84–91%	74–89%
Myalgias	50%	67–94%	73–94%
Sore throat	20%	64–84%	64–84%
Rhinorrhea	10%	79%	68%
Nausea or vomiting	80%	12%	12%
Abdominal pain	30%	22%	22%

Courtesy: Centers for Disease Control (Public Domain)
Source: Adapted from *MMWR Morb Mortal Wkly Rep* 50(44):984–986, 2001.

though less severe cases with full recovery have been reported in pediatric patients (6, 9).

With inhalation anthrax onset of symptoms is as rapid as 2–3 days following exposure although clinical data from the Sverdlovsk incident suggest that spores may remain dormant for a variable period of time with symptom onset delayed up to 43 days (6, 7, 9, 12). In experimental inhalation infection in monkeys fatal disease occurred up to 58 days after exposure (23). Historically presentation has been described as initial nonspecific symptoms of fever, chills, malaise, and fatigue usually associated with a nonproductive cough. This is then followed in hours to days by the development of dyspnea, respiratory failure and shock with mortality rates approaching 90% (6, 7, 9, 24). Data from the 11 cases of inhalation anthrax identified in the 2001 incident document a similar presentation (1, 14, 22, 25). Average incubation from known exposure to symptoms was 4 days (range 4–6 days). Fever, chills, malaise, drenching sweats, and profound fatigue were encountered in all patients (22). Minimal or nonproductive cough, nausea, vomiting, and chest discomfort were symptoms reported by most patients (22, 25). Rhinorrhea and productive cough were uncommon. Six of 11 patients (55%) survived with aggressive supportive care and multidrug antibiotic regimens including a fluoroquinolone. All four patients presenting with fulminant symptoms died. There are insufficient data available to identify factors associated with improved prog-

nosis; however, early identification and initiation of antibiotics is suggested (25). Unless there is a preexisting suspicion of anthrax exposure, patients presenting with early symptoms of inhalation illness are likely to be misdiagnosed as an influenza-like illness (ILI) or community acquired pneumonia (CAP). Guidelines provided by the CDC to assist in clinically distinguishing ILI from inhalation anthrax demonstrate a significant overlap in symptoms; however, the presence of rhinorrhea, nasal congestion, and sore throat favor ILI (26). Conversely the presence of shortness of breath, pleuritic chest pain, nausea, and vomiting would suggest consideration for a more significant diagnosis such as CAP, atypical pneumonia, or anthrax. Table 34–2 compares some common clinical features of inhalation anthrax versus ILI (26).

Diagnosis

As previously discussed the diagnosis on the basis of clinical grounds may be difficult with significant overlap of presenting symptoms with more commonly encountered disease processes. Additionally, definitive laboratory testing is not readily available in most centers and must be obtained through the CDC or at certain laboratories in the Laboratory Response Network (LRN) in coordination with public health officials (27, 28). Although it is possible that chest x-ray may be normal with early presentation, all 11 patients with inhalation anthrax from 2001 had abnormalities evident to include mediastinal widening (7), infiltrates (7) and pleural effusions (1, 9, 29). Pleural effusions were an eventual complication in all 11 patients (22). Other more subtle findings were the presence of paratracheal fullness or hilar fullness. All eight patients who underwent evaluation with chest CT had abnormal results with pleural effusions (8), mediastinal widening (7) and infiltrates (6, 25). The presence of mediastinal widening with pleural effusions and hyper-dense lymphadenopathy on CT in an acutely ill patient is highly suggestive of inhalation anthrax. However, these findings are not specific for anthrax as a number of pulmonary processes may present with similar imaging to include histoplasmosis, tuberculosis, lymphoma, sarcoid, autoimmune, and metastatic disease (22, 30). As such, definitive diagnostic testing will still be required.

Routine laboratory data which although nonspecific may provide suggestive evidence include presence of hyponatremia, hypoalbuminemia, elevated bilirubin or transaminase levels and hemoconcentration with increased hematocrit (25, 31). In acutely toxic appearing patients with anthrax infection bacilli may be visible on Gram stain of peripheral blood. The standard blood culture appears to be the most useful and readily available means of definitive diagnosis. Growth is usually evident within 24 h and all eight patients from 2001 who had blood cultures obtained prior to initiation of antibiotics had positive blood cultures at 24 h (25). Blood appears to be sterilized after even one or two doses of antibiotics, underscoring the importance of obtaining cultures prior to initiation of antibiotic therapy (1). Laboratory personnel must be notified of the suspicion for anthrax both for appropriate handling and processing of specimens and because *B. anthracis* may be incorrectly identified as the isolation of Bacillus species in routine cultures most often represents growth of the common contaminant *Bacillus cereus* (32). Sputum Gram stain and culture are unlikely to be helpful due to the fact that although *B. anthracis* infection may cause necrotic, hemorrhagic infiltrates, it is not typically a pneumonic process and in 2001 only one patient had a positive sputum Gram stain (25). Nasal swab is not recommended as a clinical screening test as the predictability remains unknown (33). Gram stain and culture from vesicular fluid of skin lesions may be helpful if obtained prior to antibiotics. If the Gram stain is negative or the patient is taking antibiotics already, punch biopsy should be performed, and specimens sent to a laboratory with the ability to perform immunohistochemical staining or polymerase chain reaction assays (1, 34).

Patients presenting with altered mental status or signs of meningeal irritation should have CSF obtained for Gram stain and culture as historical data suggest as many as 50% of patients with inhalation anthrax will develop meningitis (6, 7). All patients with a suspected or presumptive diagnosis should have specimens submitted to the CDC or LRN for confirmation. Public health officials will provide guidance on appropriate collection, handling, and submission of specimens. Confirmatory tests include enzyme-linked immunosorbent assay (ELISA) for detection of antibodies against protective antigen and anticapsular antibodies, *B. anthracis*-specific polymerase chain reaction (PCR), and direct fluorescent immunohistochemical staining for *B. anthracis* cell wall and capsular antigens (22, 28, 30, 33). A number of rapid PCR tests have recently been developed and are currently under investigation for use in clinical screening and to detect *B. anthracis* in environmental samples (35–37).

Treatment

The first clinical or laboratory suspicion of an anthrax illness must lead to early initiation of antibiotic treatment pending confirmed diagnosis along with immediate notification of the local and state public health officials (1, 25, 38). Although the CDC has published recommendations for antibiotics for the treatment of anthrax, there is limited human data available and recommendations are based primarily on animal studies and in vitro sensitivity testing (39). Studies investigating in vitro susceptibilities of 50 historical isolates, 119 endemic isolates from Europe and Africa and all 15 isolates of *B. anthracis* from the 2001 incident have revealed good sensitivity to the fluoroquinolones, tetracycline, doxycycline, vancomycin, rifampin, imipenem, meropenem, chloramphenicol, clindamycin, and clarithromycin. There was intermediate susceptibility to erythromycin, azithromycin, and ceftriaxone with significant resistance noted to cefepime and trimethoprim-sulfamethoxazole (39–44). Although all 15 isolates from 2001 were sensitive to penicillin, both beta-lactamase positive and beta-lactamase negative penicillin resistance has been identified as well as cephalosporinase producing strains (39, 40, 42). For inhalation anthrax in adults, current recommendations are for initial treatment with IV ciprofloxacin (400 mg Q12) or doxycycline (100 mg Q12). Although there are no controlled studies supporting a multidrug regimen, it is recommended that at least one other agent with good in vitro sensitivity be given (25, 39). Combinations of ciprofloxacin, rifampin, and vancomycin; and ciprofloxacin, rifampin, and clindamycin were used successfully in 2001. Available in vitro data suggest that other fluoroquinolones (gatifloxacin, ofloxacin, and levofloxacin) should be effective also (44). Penicillins and cephalosporins are not recommended for initial treatment due to evidence of resistance and isolates with beta lactamase and cephalosporinase activity (39, 40, 42). If meningitis is suspected, ciprofloxacin is recommended over doxycycline due to better CSF levels plus augmentation with chloramphenicol, rifampin, or penicillin (25, 39). Fluoroquinolones are associated with arthropathy in children and adolescents and tetracyclines have resulted in retarded skeletal growth and discoloration of teeth in children under 9 years of age (45). Despite these concerns, pregnancy or breastfeeding is not considered a contraindication to the use of ciprofloxacin or doxycycline for inhalation anthrax due to the significant morbidity and mortality associated with the infection (1, 25, 33, 39, 46, 47). Ciprofloxacin is recommended as first line therapy with doxycycline as an alternative (25, 39). This is also the recommendation for infants and children as expert consensus opinion is that the benefit outweighs the theoretical risk. In children the recommended dose of ciprofloxacin is 10 mg/kg/dose every 12 h intravenously (maximum 400 mg/dose) or 15 mg/kg/dose every 12 h orally (maximum 500 mg/dose). The recommended dose of doxycycline is 2.2 mg/kg/dose every 12 h intravenously or orally (maximum 100 mg/dose) (1, 25, 33, 39, 46). Patients may be switched to oral agents following clinical improvement and treatment should be continued for at least 60 days (1, 25, 39). There are no data identifying an optimal oral regimen. Ciprofloxacin and rifampin were used successfully during the 2001 events. In a mass casualty scenario, first line treatment with oral ciprofloxacin, 500 mg Q12 as a single agent is recommended with doxycycline, 100 mg Q12 or ampicillin 500 mg Q8 as alternatives, preferably guided by sensitivity testing. The treatment of gastrointestinal anthrax is the same as that for inhalation disease (25, 39).

For cutaneous anthrax, ciprofloxacin or doxycycline is first-line therapy in adults (1, 25, 39). Intravenous therapy with a multidrug regimen as for inhalation disease is recommended for signs of systemic involvement, extensive edema, or lesions on the head and neck. Single drug oral therapy at standard doses is acceptable for isolated cutaneous lesions. Ciprofloxacin or doxycycline is also recommended as the initial treatment of localized cutaneous anthrax in infants, children, pregnancy, and breast feeding mothers (39, 46). Ciprofloxacin is the preferred first line agent with doxycycline as an alternative. Amoxicillin has been recommended as a suitable alternative in pregnancy, breast feeding, age younger than 18 years, or antibiotic intolerance (25). Intravenous therapy with multiple antimicrobial agents as for inhalation disease is recommended for systemic involvement, extensive edema, or lesions on the head or neck (25, 39, 46). Uncomplicated cutaneous anthrax is typically treated for 7–10 days; however, in the setting of a suspected aerosolized exposure or bioterrorist

attack, antimicrobial therapy should be continued for 60 days (25, 39). Amoxicillin is recommended to complete treatment of cutaneous disease in children, pregnancy, and breast feeding once susceptibility to penicillin is documented. The dose of amoxicillin is 80 mg/kg/day orally divided every 8 h (maximum 500 mg/dose) (25, 39, 46, 47). Some authorities have also recommended the use of corticosteroids as adjunct therapy for patients with inhalation disease, meningitis, or cutaneous disease associated with significant edema (1, 39).

Infection Control and Decontamination

As noted previously, laboratory personnel should be notified for appropriate specimen handling and precautions. Standard hospital disinfection solutions such as hypochlorite are adequate for cleaning surfaces contaminated by blood or body fluids (1, 7, 9). The extent to which environmental decontamination following a B. anthracis release is necessary remains unclear. In the Sverdlovsk incident no new cases were identified beyond 43 days despite limited decontamination efforts (12). Exposure to aerosolized spores immediately following initial release is believed to pose the greatest threat; however, multiple factors can impact the duration that spores remain airborne to include environmental conditions as well as characteristics of the spore source preparation (1, 7). Epidemiologic data and environmental studies following the 2001 attacks do suggest concern for secondary or "re-aerosolization" of spores from contaminated surfaces (1, 14). In a large airborne release, the cost of environmental cleanup may be prohibitive. Chlorine dioxide was used to decontaminate buildings in the Washington DC area following the 2001 events at a cost of 27 million dollars (2). The total cost of decontamination from this relatively small event is estimated in excess of 100 million dollars (3). Individuals who have potentially been exposed to B. anthracis spores should wash thoroughly with soap and water (1, 9). There are no definitive recommendations for readily available sporicidal decontamination agents for general use on clothes, floors, etc.; however, a 5% solution of sodium hypochlorite (bleach) is suggested and in one study under specific conditions demonstrated 99.9% sporicidal effect (48, 49).

Prevention and Prophylaxis

The efficacy of antibiotic prophylaxis with ciprofloxacin, doxycycline or penicillin following exposure to aerosolized B. anthracis has been demonstrated in primates and these agents have been approved by the FDA for prophylaxis following B. anthracis exposure (23, 50). Oral ciprofloxacin is the agent of choice following known

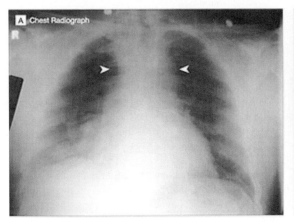

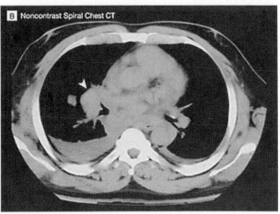

Fig. 34–2. (A) Portable chest radiograph of 56-year-old man with inhalational anthrax depicts a widened mediastinum (white arrowheads), bilateral hilar fullness, a right pleural effusion, and bilateral perihilar air-space disease. (B) Noncontrast spiral CT scan depicts an enlarged and hyperdense right hilar lymph node (white arrowhead), bilateral pleural effusions (black arrowheads), and edema of the mediastinal fat (Mayer TA, Bersoff-Matcha S, Murphy C, et al. Clinical presentation of inhalational anthrax following bioterrorism exposure. *JAMA* 286:2549–2553, 2001).

or suspected exposure to aerosolized *B. anthracis* in all patient populations (25, 39, 46, 47, 51). Doxycycline is an acceptable alternative in adults if ciprofloxacin is not available or is contraindicated. Amoxicillin is the preferred alternative for children and pregnant women when *B. anthracis* is known to be susceptible to penicillin. Prophylaxis should be continued for 60 days. *B. anthracis* infection is not known to spread from person to person and standard barrier precautions for blood and body fluids are sufficient (1, 6, 7, 9). Prophylaxis is not indicated for individuals in whom the only exposure is to an infected patient (1). Anthrax vaccine adsorbed (AVA), also known as BioThrax, is the only FDA-approved vaccine currently available in the United States. It was developed in the early 1950s and initially licensed by the FDA in 1970 primarily for protection against cutaneous anthrax in veterinarians, lab personnel, and individuals handling animal hides or hair (1, 25, 52–54). Although it has been used by the U.S. military since 1991, it was not FDA approved for prevention of inhalation anthrax until December of 2003 (55). AVA is a killed, cell free, supernatant of a toxigenic, noncapsulated strain of *B. anthracis* (52). Human and animal data have demonstrated that preexposure prophylaxis with AVA induces production of antibodies to protective antigen (PA) and animal data indicate that anti-PA antibody confers protection from cutaneous and inhalation anthrax infection (7, 53, 54, 56). Anti-PA antibodies are believed to block the effects of edema toxin and lethal toxin, thereby not only preventing tissue destruction but also preventing these factors from inhibiting the immune response to both spores and the vegetative bacillus (52, 57). The current FDA-approved immunization series requires six injections given at 0, 2, and 4 weeks and then at 6, 12, and 18 months followed by an annual booster. Although there has been much controversy surrounding the use of AVA by the U.S. military, recent reviews by the FDA, the Institute of Medicine, and the CDC have determined that the vaccine provides effective preexposure prophylaxis for *B. anthracis* exposure by any route and appears to be safe with a side effect profile similar to other commonly used vaccines (53, 55, 58). Currently the CDC is recommending preexposure prophylaxis only for specific personnel employed in Bioterrorism Level B laboratories or above, or workers who will be making repeated entries into known *B. anthracis*-spore contaminated areas after a terrorist attack (59). There is evidence from primate studies supporting postexposure prophylaxis in combination with antibiotic treatment (23). An expert consensus panel has recommended the use of AVA for postexposure prophylaxis and an Investigational New Drug (IND) protocol is available through the CDC for the use of an abbreviated three injection series in conjunction with antibiotic therapy (1, 59). A recombinant protective antigen vaccine (rPA) has been developed and the Department of Health and Human Services announced plans in March 2004 to obtain an initial 75 million doses for use in the event of a bioterror attack (60). Research is also being conducted with the use of human monoclonal anti-PA antibodies for postexposure prophylaxis (Abthrax™, Human Genome Sciences and MDX-1303, Medarex Inc.) with favorable results in animal studies (61, 62).

SMALLPOX

History and Background

Prior to its eradication as a naturally occurring disease, smallpox had been a major cause of morbidity and mortality throughout recorded medical history. Hippocrates described fevers that were "pustular" and dreadful to behold around 400 BC and it is believed that epidemics of smallpox occurred in China around 1122 BC (63). Epidemics were severe in western Europe during the 17th and 18th centuries, killing 20–40% of the population. In the 20th century alone it is estimated that this disease was responsible for more than 300 million fatalities. The introduction of smallpox into a nonimmune population is predicted to have devastating effects and historically has resulted in the death of more than 80% of vulnerable populations. The last recorded case of naturally occurring smallpox was in Somalia in 1977 (63–65). Routine vaccination for smallpox was discontinued in the United States in 1972 and all civilian immunization programs were stopped in the early 1980s when endemic smallpox was declared eradicated by the World Health Organization (WHO) in 1980 (64–66). Today the diagnosis of a single case of smallpox would be considered a public health emergency. There have been reports from individuals who participated in the biological weapons program of the former Soviet Union that massive amounts of smallpox have been produced since 1980 as part of an ongoing biological weapons development. There are also reports of attempts at genetic engineering to enhance the weapons potential of the organism and that other countries may now have stockpiles of the virus (13, 64). Although there has not been a single case of variola infection identified for more than 25 years, there are two known sources of the virus still in existence. One is at the Centers for Disease Control in Atlanta and the second at the Russian State Research Center of Virology and Biotechnology in Koltsovo, Russian Federation (64, 65). Concern for clandestine availability, person to person transmissibility, high morbidity and mortality, and potential for catastrophic economic and social disruption make the possibility of the use of variola major as a biological terror agent a priority concern.

Epidemiology

Humans are the only known host for the variola virus, the causative agent of smallpox and there is no known animal reservoir (64–66). The most common means of transmission is person to person via the respiratory route following close face to face contact (less than 2 m). The virus can also be spread through infectious fomites on clothing or linens (64–67). Infected individuals are considered contagious from onset of rash until resolution of all lesions. Mortality estimates for variola major in unvaccinated individuals vary widely but is generally in the range of 20–40%. Mortality rate in vaccinated individuals is 1–3% (64–66).

Microbiology and Pathophysiology

Variola, the causative agent of smallpox, is a DNA virus belonging to the orthopox virus genus. It occurs in at least two strains, variola major and variola minor which causes a milder form of the disease with much less associated morbidity and mortality. Other members of this family include cowpox and monkeypox as well as vaccinia, the agent that is used in the smallpox vaccination. Both are highly transmissible from person to person via respiratory droplets. Although smallpox may be spread by contact with contaminated clothing or bedding, it is predominantly passed by close (less than 2 m) face to face contact (64–66). After exposure the virus replicates in the epithelium of the upper respiratory tract and then migrates to regional lymph nodes. This is followed in 3–4 days by an initial viremia that often is asymptomatic. Symptoms that do occur at this time suggest a nonspecific viral illness. Another cycle of viral replication then takes place in lymph nodes, spleen, and bone marrow followed by a second viremia at 7–17 days postexposure. This is accompanied by the usual signs and symptoms of toxemia followed by the development of the characteristic rash within 48 h. Death usually occurs in 1–2 weeks following the onset of clinical illness and is believed due to the overwhelming viremia, associated toxemia, and secondary bacterial sepsis (64–68).

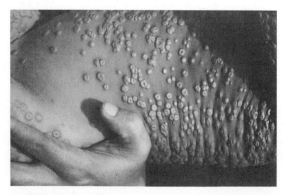

Fig. 34–3. Small pox lesions on skin of trunk. *Source:* Courtesy of Centers for Disease Control and Prevention (Public Domain).

Clinical Presentation

Early symptoms are nonspecific and if patients present prior to the development of rash, the initial case(s) are very likely to be misdiagnosed. As noted, patients will present with symptoms 7–17 days after exposure and are considered infectious with onset of rash (6, 65, 67). Classic presentation is abrupt onset of a fever of 101°F (38°C) or higher which is followed in 1–2 days by rash. Other symptoms include headache, backache, rigors, vomiting, pharyngitis, delirium, and seizures (64–68). Rash is usually noted first on the oral mucosa and pharynx followed in succession by the head, face, proximal extremities, distal extremities, and trunk. The palms and soles are usually involved. (Note the contradistinction with the rash of varicella which begins on the trunk then spreads to the face and extremities and rarely involves palms or soles.) Initially, lesions are maculopapular and may be morbilliform in appearance. Within 1–2 days they develop into vesicles, which after an additional 1–2 days become umbilicated pustules. Two days later pustules begin to scab over and then slough after 8–17 days leaving deep hypopigmented scars.

Lesions on one area of the body will all be in the same stage of development, unlike varicella which may have papules, vesicles, pustules, and dried lesions all in the same area (64–68). Eschar from scabs contains active viral particles and patients are considered infective until all lesions have healed (65–66). There can be significant variability in the severity of symptoms and rash ranging from fever only with mild symptoms and no skin lesions (Variola sine eruptione) to diffuse confluent lesions covering the entire body. Mortality increases along with severity of symptoms and rash (65,68). Previously immunized individuals may have an atypical presentation with less sever symptoms, nonvesicular rash, fewer lesions, and more rapid resolution. Rare variants include a hemorrhagic form which can be seen in any age or sex but is more common in pregnant women and has a very high fatality of 95%. Another highly virulent form is known as malignant or "flat" type because of the diffuse velvety eruption that covers the entire skin and also involves mucosal surfaces. It is complicated by diffuse sloughing of skin and mucosa much like a Stevens-Johnson syndrome and likewise has a very high mortality (68).

Diagnosis

Initial diagnosis will be clinical as there are no readily available laboratory tests for confirmation. The presence of orthopox virus can be identified by electron microscopy of vesicle fluid. Aggregates of viral particles called Guarenieri bodies can also be seen by light microscopy (64, 65, 67). Neither method can discriminate variola from other orthopox agents however. Definitive diagnosis will require culture and/or PCR which can be obtained in 8–24 h and is only available from CDC and Laboratory Response Network (LRN) reference laboratories in coordination with local public health authorities. Clearly, it will be imperative to differentiate smallpox from other disease entities which may present with fever and vesicular exanthems such as varicella, syphilis, erythema multiforme, and cutaneouos drug reactions. The CDC has established major and minor criteria for the clinical diagnosis of smallpox and applied these to the development of a clinical algorithm for the evaluation and management of suspected cases (69).

High-risk cases requiring immediate public health involvement are defined as patients presenting with classic lesions which are in the same stage of development in any given area of the body and which were preceded by a febrile prodrome for 1–4 days.

A suspected high-risk case of smallpox is a public health emergency. Smallpox surveillance in the United States includes detecting a suspected case or cases, making a definitive diagnosis with rapid laboratory confirmation at CDC, and preventing further transmission. A high-risk suspected case should be reported immediately by telephone to state and local public health officials and advice should be obtained regarding isolation and laboratory specimen collection. State or local health officials should notify the CDC immediately if a high-risk suspected case of smallpox is reported (65–69).

Treatment

Once the diagnosis is suspected or made, treatment will be primarily supportive. There are no antiviral agents that have been proven effective or are FDA approved for the treatment of smallpox (64, 65, 67). Cidofivir has been shown to be effective in vitro against variola major and a number of other orthopox agents (65). An IND protocol has been established for its use in the event of a smallpox outbreak (68, 70). With an isolated outbreak and a small number of cases, hospitalized patients should be placed in negative pressure isolation rooms and tended only by health care personnel who have been vaccinated with in the last 3 years. Because of the problem of health-care-associated smallpox transmission, if the patient's condition allows, medical and public health authorities should consider isolation and observation outside a hospital setting to prevent health-care-associated smallpox transmission and overtaxing of medical resources (64, 65, 68).

Health care workers must strictly adhere to standard precautions of gowns, masks, and gloves, as well as airborne and contact precautions. With a large number of cases, patients may need to be quarantined in designated "smallpox" facilities. Quarantine policy guidelines have been developed by the CDC to be used by state and local public health and safety officials in developing quarantine policy and procedures (71). Severe cases to include hemorrhagic and flat type will need hospitalization in an intensive care setting for burn-level care and probable associated sepsis (68).

Infection Control and Decontamination

In a biological terror incident employing the intentional release of variola, the first cases of smallpox are not likely to be identified for 7 days or more due to the incubation period. By the time the first case is identified, it will not be necessary to employ decontamination procedures as the agent in the initial release is unlikely to be active. Based on studies with vaccinia, it is anticipated that the virus would be inactive after 24–48 h of environmental exposure although it may persist longer in conditions of low humidity (<20%) and low ambient temperature (<10°C). Vaccinia, which was released at ambient temperatures of greater than 31°C and humidity of 80% was completely destroyed in 6 h. Although virus has been recovered in the lab from scab eschar for months and in one report from a specimen held for 13 years, based on epidemiological data, the risk of transmission from these sources is considered to be very low (65). It has been documented that transmission can occur by handling contaminated clothes and linen and it is believed that the virus maintains infectivity for a much longer period in this environment (64, 65, 67, 68). All such material should be handled as biohazardous waste and either autoclaved or washed in hot water and bleach. Standard hospital disinfectants such as hypochlorite or quaternary ammonia are effective for cleaning contaminated surfaces (65, 67). Once a case is identified, much of the management will focus on prevention of spread to contacts and care givers. It is estimated that each patient with active disease will expose 10–20 additional individuals (65). All contacts and care givers who have not been vaccinated within the last 3 years should receive the vaccinia vaccine as this has been shown to both prevent disease and lessen the severity of symptoms if given up to 4 days after exposure (64, 67, 68). If possible all household contacts and anyone with face to face contact of 2 m or less should be isolated for 17 days and at a minimum they should be closely monitored for this same time period and immediately isolated if they develop a fever or other symptoms (65, 70).

Vaccine

The exact duration of protection from smallpox following vaccinia vaccination has not yet been determined. Neutralizing antibodies and evidence of cell mediated immunity may persist for up to 30 years but it is not known how this would correlate with protection against clinical disease (66, 72). Epidemiological data indicate some level of protection is still present after more than 20 years (66). Currently best estimates are that a high level of protection persists for at least 3 years, with a substantial but decreasing level of immunity for 10 years or more (66, 73). With household contact or close face to face exposure (less than 2 m) to a documented case or in the event of a large scale outbreak, it is recommended that vaccination be provided to all exposed or at risk individuals not immunized with in the last 3 years (64–66, 68, 73).

There is currently sufficient supply of smallpox vaccine in the National Pharmaceutical Stockpile (NSP) to immunize the entire population of the United States (73). This includes 14.8 million doses of the original FDA-approved vaccine, DryVax (Wyeth) along with 85 million doses of a vaccine produced by Aventis that could be used under an IND protocol. Recent evidence indicates that these vaccines may be diluted 1:5 with no significant decrease in efficacy (73–75). Additionally there are more than 200 million doses of two new vaccines produced by Accambis-Baxter which are currently undergoing clinical trials and appear to be at least as effective as DryVax (73). Each of these vaccines utilizes the New York City Board of Health (NYCBH) vaccinia strain that is used in the DryVax product. There are two other potential vaccines utilizing highly attenuated strains of vaccinia (Modified Vaccinia Ankara and Lister) that are currently under development and which are likely to have a much lower adverse side effect profile (73).

Strict adherence to CDC guidelines for vaccinia use is required with specific attention to handling, preparation, indications, and contraindications (66, 73, 76). Historically, the incidence of serious adverse reactions to vaccinia vaccine is low but not insignificant with approximately one serious non-life-threatening reaction such as inadvertent inoculation or erythema multiforme per 1000 vaccinees. Life-threatening adverse reactions such as postvaccinia encephalitis or progressive vaccinia occurred in approximately 5 per100,000 vaccinees with death occurring in approximately 1 per 1,000,000 (66, 76).

As preexposure prophylaxis, vaccinia vaccine would be contraindicated in anyone who either has or lives with someone who has immune suppression for any reason (HIV, chemotherapy, steroid use or immune suppressant drugs, leukemia), history of eczema or atopic dermatitis, active exfoliative skin disorder, or pregnancy (66, 73, 76). Contraindications for the vaccinee only but not close contacts include vaccine-component allergies, women who are breastfeeding, those taking topical ocular steroid medications, those with moderate-to-severe intercurrent illness, and persons under age 18 years. The incidence of adverse events is significantly lower in repeat versus first-time vaccines (73). In the event of a known exposure to smallpox there are no absolute contraindications to the use of vaccinia vaccine as those at increased risk for vaccine complications are also at increased risk for life-threatening complications of smallpox (66, 73, 76). Careful consideration must be given to the risk of vaccination versus the risk of the disease. A limited supply of vaccinia immune globulin (VIG) is available from the CDC for the treatment of life-threatening adverse reactions (76).

PLAGUE

History and Background

Yersinia Pestis, the etiologic agent of plague, was first identified by Alexandre Yersin in Hong Kong in 1894 (77). It is believed to have been responsible for three devastating pandemics in recorded history with combined death toll estimates exceeding 100 million (78–80). The first pandemic began in Egypt in AD 541 eventually spreading throughout all of the known world with population losses of between 50% and 60% (81). The second pandemic originated in Europe in 1346 and lasted more than 130 years. The third pandemic began in China in 1855 and although in sharp decline it continues today with small outbreaks occurring throughout the world and endemic disease on every continent except Australia (81, 82).

What is believed to be the first attempted use of *Y. pestis* as a biological weapon occurred in the Crimean War during the siege of the port city of Caffa in 1346 (78). The besieging Tartar army was suffering an epidemic of plague and catapulted the corpses of victims into the city. Although plague did subsequently spread through the city, it was most likely due to the local rat and flea population rather than as a result of these grisly projectiles. During World War II, Unit 731, one of the Japanese army's biological warfare research units, conducted dozens of experiments on the use of plague as a biological weapon (83). Although the bacteria proved to lack the hardy

survivability necessary to maintain infectivity following an airborne release, they were successful at initiating epidemics in many Chinese cities and villages by aerial release of infected fleas which spread the disease to the local rat population. The United States conducted research on the use of plague as a biological weapon in the 1950s and 1960s but they were unsuccessful at developing a suitably stable form of *Y. pestis* prior to the termination of their offensive weapons program in 1970 (78, 80). In 1992 it was reported that the former Soviet Union was successful in developing and producing large quantities of a genetically engineered highly stable strain of *Y. pestis* that could be effectively delivered through aerial munitions (13, 84). The World Health Organization has estimated that in a worse-case scenario, the release of 50 kg of such an agent over a metropolitan area with a population of 5 million could result in 150,000 cases of pneumonic plague with a fatality rate in excess of 20% (85). Given the availability of naturally occurring *Y. pestis* around the world, capacity for its mass production and aerosol dissemination, difficulty in preventing such activities, high fatality rate of pneumonic plague, and potential for secondary spread of cases during an epidemic, the possible use of *Y. pestis* as a biological weapon is of great concern (80).

Epidemiology

Plague, also known as the "Black Death" is a naturally occurring zoonotic infection with some epidemiological and clinical similarities to tularemia. As was previously noted, it is present throughout the majority of the world with an average of 1700 cases reported annually over the last 50 years (81). Rats, prairie dogs, chipmunks, marmots, and ground squirrels along with more than 200 other species of animals are responsible for maintaining endemic areas of *Y. pestis* and more than 80 species of fleas are involved in transmission between animal hosts (78–81). In naturally occurring disease humans are an incidental host with the usual mode of transmission being from the bite of an infected flea. Less common means of transmission include exposure to or ingestion of infected animal tissues and body fluids. Pneumonic plague can be spread directly from some animals such as cats as well as person to person via respiratory droplets (78, 79, 86, 87). Although most authorities agree that *Y. pestis* does not persist in the environment outside of the animal or insect host, there is some evidence indicating that it may remain viable for a week or more under moist cool conditions (88). Plague was first documented in the United States in 1900 (89). Today the disease is endemic to 17 western states with a total of 112 cases reported from 11 states during 1988–2002 with the vast majority (87%) of cases from New Mexico, Arizona, Colorado, and California (90). The major risk for a bioterror event is believed to be an intentional aerosol release. A sudden clustered presentation of pneumonic and/or septicemic forms of plague would suggest a bioterror event and concern for *Y. pestis* (80, 91). In a series of 390 cases reported from 1947 to 1966 the overall mortality rate was 15%. Of the three principle forms of the disease, bubonic plague accounted for 84% of cases with a 14% mortality, primary septicemic plague for 13% of cases with a 22% mortality and primary pneumonic plague for 2% of cases with a 57% mortality (92). In the preantibiotic era of the early 1900s, the overall mortality rate for plague in the United States was 66% (89). More recent data suggest a similar mortality for untreated bubonic plague of 60% and 100% for the pneumonic and septicemic forms (93).

Microbiology and Pathophysiology

Y. pestis is a gram-negative, nonmotile, nonsporulating, bacillus, or coccobacillus that shows characteristic bipolar ("safety pin") staining with Wright, Giemsa, or Wayson stain. It is a member of the Enterobacteriaceae family which includes *Y. enterocolitica* (78, 79). The virulence of *Y. pestis* requires a number of plasmid-encoded protein factors. These include the fraction 1 (F1) antigen that forms a protein capsule and inhibits phagocytosis, the V and W antigens that also have antiphagocytic function as well as promoting other virulence factors and a plasminogen activator protease which is necessary for systemic spread of infection (78, 80, 88).

Bacteria proliferate in the flea gut following a blood meal from an infected animal and then typically are inoculated into the subcutaneous tissue of a human or other host when they are regurgitated during a subsequent blood meal (78–81). Only after they are introduced to the animal host environment do they begin producing the virulent factors necessary to initiate and sustain infection (78, 80, 88). From the inoculation site they are carried to the regional lymph nodes where they proliferate and produce a severe lymphadenitis forming the classic "bubo." If untreated, infection will spread systemically resulting in secondary septicemia with involvement of almost every organ system, shock, and death. Tissues most commonly involved include the spleen, liver, lungs, kidney, skin, and mucous membranes. Cardiac involvement with interstitial myocarditis and CNS infection with meningitis may also occur (78–81, 94, 95). Systemic spread to the lungs results in secondary pneumonic plague which may be seen in up to 12% of naturally occurring cases (81). *Y. pestis* endotoxin and coagulase activity are believed to contribute to

the development of shock and DIC with acral cyanosis and ischemic tissue death (78–80).

About 13% of naturally occurring cases will present with systemic infection without the development of localized adenopathy. This is referred to as primary septicemic plague which has a mortality nearly twice that of patients presenting with bubonic plague (92). Primary pneumonic plague is initiated by the inhalation of infectious aerosol and is the most rapidly fatal form of the disease (78, 80). Naturally occurring cases usually arise from exposure to patients with bubonic, septicemic, or pneumonic plague who are expelling respiratory droplets containing the fully virulent organism (78–80, 93). Primary pneumonic infection also occurs following exposure to infected domestic animals such as cats (86, 87). Patients and animals do not have to have pulmonary symptoms to be infectious as asymptomatic pharyngeal carriage has been reported with bubonic plague (93, 96). Inhalation of these fully virulent organisms produces a much more rapidly progressive infection than secondary pneumonic plague from systemic spread (78). Primary pneumonic plague is the predominant form that would be expected following an intentional release of a bioterror agent (78, 80, 91). In both primary and secondary plague pneumonia, the usual pathologic findings are diffuse pulmonary congestion, edema, hemorrhagic necrosis, and scant neutrophilic infiltration (79).

Clinical Presentation

If aerosolized *Y. pestis* were used as a biological warfare agent, the expected clinical manifestations would be a rapidly progressive pneumonia and/or septicemia. If infected fleas were disseminated, bubonic and to a lesser extent septicemic plague would be the most likely presentation (78, 80, 89, 92).

Bubonic plague typically presents after a 1–8 day incubation period following inoculation from an infected flea. Initial symptoms are nonspecific and include fever, chills, malaise, headache, myalgias, arthralgias, nausea, vomiting, and lethargy. This is followed within hours by the development of painful adenopathy in the inguinal, axillary or cervical lymph nodes depending on the area of inoculation. Buboes become visible within 24 h of symptom onset and are intensely painful, tender, and firm to palpation with surrounding edema, erythema, and warmth (77–81, 88). Skin lesions in the area of the buboes are typically absent although one series from Vietnam noted the presence of a pustule, vesicle, or eschar in up to 25% of patients (93). Rarely buboes will become fluctuant with suppuration and spontaneous drainage. Differential diagnosis will include tularemia, cat scratch disease,

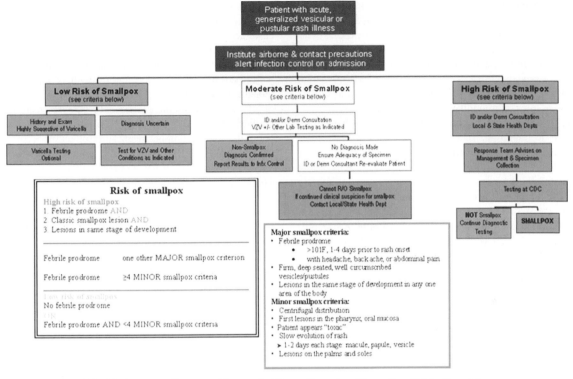

Fig. 34–4. *Source:* Courtesy of Centers for Disease Control and Prevention (Public Domain).

chancroid, lymphogranuloma venereum, staphylococcal, or streptococcal adenitis, tuberculosis, scrub typhus, acute filarial lymphadenitis, and strangulated inguinal hernia. The bubo of plague can be differentiated from most other causes of regional adenitis by the rapid onset, associated exquisite pain and tenderness in the presence of toxemia and with a notable absence of lymphangitis (79). If untreated, the majority of patients will develop septicemia typically within 2–6 days (78).

In naturally occurring disease septicemic plague may present primarily without the presence of buboes in approximately 13% of patients (92). Mortality data from the preantibiotic era of the early 1900s indicate that two-thirds or more of all patients will develop septicemia if untreated (89). Along with the typical constitutional symptoms of bubonic plague patients will present with or soon develop signs of gram-negative sepsis with a rapidly progressive endotoxemia including hypotension, tachycardia, confusion, and oliguria (77–81, 88, 92, 94, 95). Abdominal pain is more common in septicemic patients (40% vs. 10% in bubonic) and is likely due to the presence of splenomegaly (95). A common complication is the onset of disseminated intravascular coagulation (DIC) producing diffuse purpura with acral ischemia and gan-

grene, hence the name "Black Death (77–80, 88)." Early differential diagnosis should include sepsis from a variety of bacterial sources, tularemia, toxic shock, typhoid fever, brucellosis, malaria, and rickettsiosis.

Pneumonic plague occurs secondarily from hematogenous dissemination in bubonic or septicemic plague or primarily following inhalation of infectious aerosols (77–81, 88). It is the most rapidly progressive and lethal form of plague and is invariably fatal when antibiotic therapy is delayed more than 1 day after the onset of illness. It is also the predominant form expected following airborne release in a bioterror incident (77–80, 91, 92). Primary pneumonic plague accounts for less than 2% of cases of naturally occurring disease (92). It is estimated that 5–15% of bubonic cases may develop secondary plague pneumonia (79, 81). For primary pneumonia, the time from aerosol exposure to onset of symptoms is 1–6 days (80, 96, 97). Patients typically have rapid onset of fever, dyspnea, and cough productive of watery or mucoid sputum that is often bloody. In contrast, patients with secondary pneumonic plague typically present with a pulmonary picture similar to adult respiratory distress syndrome (ARDS) with scant or no sputum production (79). Both forms are associated with signs of toxemia and constitutional symptoms previously described for bubonic and septicemic plague (77–81, 88, 91). Regardless of the source it is a very aggressive process with progressive dyspnea, tachypnea, and rapid development of respiratory failure. In the absence of buboes, early differential diagnosis is broad and will include tularemia, anthrax, ARDS, SARS, and hantavirus as well as typical and atypical community acquired pneumonias.

Other less common presentations of *Y. pestis* infection include meningitis and pharyngitis. In a series of 390 patients from the United States there were 12 cases of meningitis (3%) all of which occurred in patients being treated for bubonic plague (92). There are no defining characteristics that distinguish *Y. pestis* meningitis from that caused by more common bacterial agents. Likewise isolated plague pharyngitis is believed to be a rare presentation which would be difficult to distinguish from more common etiologies of exudative pharyngitis with cervical lymphadenopathy (92, 98). Asymptomatic pharyngeal carriage of *Y. pestis* has been documented during outbreaks of plague and would suggest the possibility of occult respiratory transmission (99).

Diagnosis

Since plague is an infrequently encountered disease in most parts of the world, it is not likely to be considered in the differential diagnosis by physicians encountering sporadic naturally occurring cases or in the initial cases seen following an intentional release. In the latter event, the first suspicion is likely to follow the recognition of a sudden cluster of cases of a rapidly progressive painful adenitis or severe pneumonia with sepsis in previously healthy patients (78, 80, 91, 92). In one series of 27 cases of endemic plague only 10(37%) received the correct initial clinical diagnosis with the remainder being diagnosed as upper respiratory infection 5(19%), nonspecific febrile illness 5(19%), gastrointestinal or urinary tract infection 4(15%), and meningitis 3(10%) (94). The first suspicion of plague regardless of presumed etiology should prompt immediate consultation with infectious disease and epidemiology consultants along with notification of public health officials (80, 91). Laboratory personnel should be notified before submitting any specimens or as soon as plague is suspected to ensure appropriate handling for staining and culture and for coordination with local state and CDC reference laboratories for definitive testing (78, 80, 91, 92). Additionally there are reported cases of *Y. pestis* infection acquired through handling of laboratory specimens (100). Only labs equipped for biosafety level 2 should be utilized (80, 91). The CDC has published clinical and laboratory guidelines to aid in the identification of potential plague cases (101, 102).

Suspected plague should be considered if the following conditions are met:

1. Clinical symptoms that are compatible with plague, that is, fever and lymphadenopathy in a person who resides in or recently traveled to a plague-endemic area.

2. If small gram-negative and/or bipolar-staining coccobacilli are seen on a smear taken from affected tissues, e.g.:
   - Bubo (bubonic plague)
   - Blood (septicemic plague)
   - Tracheal/lung aspirate (pneumonic plague)

Presumptive plague should be considered when one or both of the following conditions are met:

1. If immunofluorescence stain of smear or material is positive for the presence of Yersinia pestis F1 antigen.

2. If only a single serum specimen is tested and the anti-F1 antigen titer by agglutination is >1:10.[a]

Confirmed plague is diagnosed if one of the following conditions is met:

1. If a culture isolate is lysed by specific bacteriophage

2. If two serum specimens demonstrate a fourfold anti-F1 antigen titer difference by agglutination testing[a]

3. If a single serum specimen tested by agglutination has a titer of >1:128 and the patient has no known previous plague exposure or vaccination history[a]

---

[a]Agglutination testing must be shown to be specific to *Y. pestis* F1 antigen by hemagglutination inhibition
Source: Courtesy of Centers for Disease Control and Prevention (Public Domain).

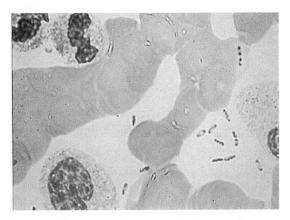

Fig. 34–5. Wayson stain of *Yersinia pestis*. Note the characteristic "safety pin" appearance of the bacteria. *Source:* Courtesy of Centers for Disease Control and Prevention (Public Domain).

Gram stain and culture of buboes, blood, sputum, CSF, pharynx and skin lesions should be obtained as appropriate (78–81, 91, 92). In suspected cases of plague, several samples of blood should be collected for culture during a 45-minute period before initiation of antibiotic treatment, unless such a delay is contraindicated by the patient's condition (92). In the setting of fulminant pneumonia, the presence of Gram negative bacilli or coccobacilli in blood or sputum of previously healthy patients would be suggestive of *Y. pestis* (79, 803). If buboes are present an aspirate should be obtained using a 20-gauge needle and 1–2 cc of sterile saline. If suspicious organisms are seen on Gram stain of any specimens, repeat stains with Wright, Giemsa, or Wayson stain may show characteristic bipolar or "safety pin" staining pattern (77–81, 88, 101). Of note is that this staining pattern is not specific to *Y. pestis*

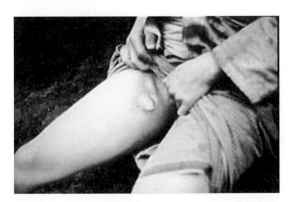

Fig. 34–6. Inguinal buboes in patient with bubonic plague. *Source:* Courtesy of Centers for Disease Control and Prevention (Public Domain).

and may be seen in other species such as pasturella, *E. coli,* and klebsiella (79, 102). In one series of 27 cases of endemic plague, blood cultures and cultures of bubo aspirate were positive in 96 and 77% of patients, respectively (94). Cultures should be grown on standard media at both 27°C and 37°C for optimal identification and are usually positive by 24–48 h (79, 80, 102). In the United States, in coordination with public health officials, specimens should also be sent to local state or CDC reference laboratories for *Y. pestis* identification utilizing direct fluorescent antibody (DFA) staining, passive hemagglutination or ELISA for F1 capsular antigen identification along with acute phase serum sample for F1 antibody titers (77–80, 91, 92, 101). A number of new rapid assays are currently under investigation but are not yet widely available. These include a PCR directed at the plasminogen activator gene and a rapid ELISA capable of detecting as little as 4 ng/mL of F1 antigen (103–105). Another promising technology is the use of a monoclonal antibody to the F1 antigen in a rapid dip stick test which can detect as little as 0.5 ng/mL of F1 antigen and appears to be both highly sensitive and specific in preliminary investigations (106). With regard to routine laboratory studies, white blood cell count is usually elevated with a predominance of immature and mature neutrophils. Particularly in children there may be an acute luekemoid reaction with counts as high as 50,000–100,000 per microliter. Hemoglobin and platelets will usually be normal unless DIC is present. With systemic disease transaminase levels and bilirubin are often increased due to liver involvement (77–81). Chest radiographic findings in pneumonic plague are variable and include isolated hilar adenopathy, segmental infiltrate, bilateral interstitial and alveolar infiltrates, and localized or diffuse bronchopneumonia (78–80, 87, 91, 102, 107). Diffuse bilateral alveolar infiltration similar to ARDS is the most consistent finding in secondary pneumonic plague where as primary pneumonic plague more typically presents with rapidly progressive segmental infiltrate(s) or bronchopneumonia (79, 87, 102).

Treatment

Currently the only FDA-approved agents for the treatment of plague are streptomycin, tetracycline and doxycycline (78–80, 91, 92). Historically, the agent of choice has been streptomycin. Although not FDA approved for use in plague, gentamicin is more readily available and appears to be equally efficacious based on animal models, in vitro data and anecdotal clinical evidence. There are no controlled clinical studies comparing the efficacy of tetracycline and doxycycline to streptomycin or gentamicin;

however, anecdotal clinical data, animal data, and in vitro studies support their use with doxycycline demonstrating slightly better activity than tetracycline (91, 92, 94, 108–110). There are no clinical data on the use of fluoroquinalones in humans; however, animal and in vitro data suggest that ciprofloxacin, levofloxacin, and ofloxacin would be as efficacious as streptomycin or gentamicin with some data suggesting better activity than the tetracyclines (108–110, 111–113). Although in vitro data have demonstrated good activity with penicillin derivatives and third-generation cephalosporins, (108, 109) data from a murine model of primary pneumonic plague suggest that all of the beta lactam antibiotics tested (cefazolin, cefotetan, ceftriaxone, ceftazidime, aztreonam, and ampicillin) are significantly inferior to streptomycin (113). Chloramphenicol has been used successfully in the treatment of plague and has been recommended in the setting of meningitis due to its ability to cross the blood brain barrier (78–80, 114). Based on the recommendations of The Working Group on Civilian Biodefense, the CDC has established recommendations for the treatment of plague (80). These recommendations are based on consensus expert opinion and do not imply FDA approval. Recommendations apply to all forms of plague and the minimum recommended duration for all agents is 10 days. The preferred agents for adults are streptomycin 1 g IM twice daily or gentamicin 5 mg/kg IM or IV daily or 2 mg/kg loading dose followed by 1.7 mg/kg three times daily. Alternatives are doxycycline 100 mg IV twice daily or 200 mg IV once daily, ciprofloxacin 400 mg IV twice daily or chloramphenicol 25 mg/kg IV four times daily. The agent of choice during pregnancy and breastfeeding is gentamicin with doxycycline or ciprofloxacin as alternatives. In children the preferred agents are streptomycin 15 mg/kg IM twice daily or gentamicin 2.5 mg/kg IM or IV three times a day. Alternatives are doxycycline 2.2 mg/kg IV twice daily, ciprofloxacin 15 mg/kg IV twice daily, or chloramphenicol 25 mg/kg IV four times a day. The maximum dose of each of these agents in children should never exceed the recommended adult dose. In the event that parenteral treatment is not possible or practical such as in a mass casualty situation, oral treatment is an alternative. Preferred agents in adults, including during pregnancy and breast feeding are doxycycline 100 mg twice daily or ciprofloxacin 500 mg twice daily with chloramphenicol 25 mg/kg four times a day as an alternative. In children the oral agents of choice are doxycycline 2.2 mg/kg twice daily or ciprofloxacin 20 mg/kg twice daily. Alternative for children aged 2 years or older is chloramphenicol 25 mg/kg four times a day. The maximum dose of each of these agents in children should never exceed the recommended adult dose.

Infection Control and Decontamination

Special environmental decontamination procedures are usually not indicated. In the setting of a clandestine release of plague bacilli, the aerosol would have dissipated long before the first case of pneumonic plague occurred. *Y. pestis* is very sensitive to the action of sunlight and heating and does not survive long outside the host (80, 115). A recent study did show that under controlled conditions some organisms can maintain viability on environmental surfaces for up to 5 days; however, there is no evidence to suggest that residual plague bacilli pose an environmental threat following the dissolution of the primary aerosol (116). Routine hospital infection control measures utilizing standard procedures and cleaning agents for equipment, linen, and surface decontamination are sufficient (115). All patients suspected of having pneumonic plague should be maintained under respiratory droplet precautions for 48 h after antibiotic treatment begins. Persons who have confirmed cases of pneumonic plague should be kept under droplet precautions until sputum cultures are negative. Special care must be taken in handling all secretions, blood, and bubo discharge. If pneumonic plague is present, then strict, rigidly enforced respiratory isolation procedures must be followed, including the use of gowns, gloves, and eye protection (80, 115).

Prevention and Prophylaxis

Once it was known or strongly suspected that pneumonic plague cases were occurring, anyone with fever or cough in the presumed area of exposure should be isolated and immediately treated with antimicrobials for presumptive pneumonic plague. Delaying therapy until confirmatory testing is performed would greatly decrease survival (80). Hospital, household or other close contacts (less than 2 m) of persons with untreated or suspected pneumonic plague should receive postexposure antibiotic prophylaxis for 7 days (80, 115). The agents recommended for prophylaxis are the same as those recommended for oral therapy in the setting of a mass casualty. Prophylaxis following exposure to bubonic plague patients usually is not indicated unless the exposed individuals live in the same household with a possibility of vector contact, i.e., fleas (79). With regard to preexposure prophylaxis, there is currently no proven efficacious vaccine available. A formaldehyde-killed whole cell vaccine which was used predominantly by the United States military has not been manufactured since 1999 and is no longer available. Although this vaccine may have been beneficial against bubonic plague, it is not protective against primary pneumonic disease (115, 117). A number of potential vaccine candidates are currently under investigation with very promising results in animal studies using F1 and V antigen subunit vaccines and a vaccine using plasmid DNA which codes for the F1 subunit (117–120).

TULAREMIA

History and Background

Francisella tularensis, the causative agent of tularemia is an aerobic gram negative coccobacillus that was first identified in Tulare County in the state of California in 1911. In 1921 Dr. Edward Francis was the first to describe transmission of disease via a deer fly and to use the term tularemia to describe the clinical disease (121). It has been recognized as a potential biological weapon for more than 60 years beginning with Unit 731, a Japanese biological warfare unit during World War II, which conducted experiments on prisoners and Chinese civilians with tularemia as well as plague and anthrax (10, 11). The United States offensive biological weapons program is believed to be the first to actually develop weaponized *F. tularensis* in the 1950s and 1960s (11). The former Soviet Union began experimenting with *F. tularensis* as a biological weapon at about the same time and is believed to have continued weapons production into the 1990s to include the development of antibiotic resistant strains (13). In 1969, the WHO estimated that 50 kg of *F tularensis* released over a city of 5 million would result in 250,000 victims with incapacitating illness and more than 19,000 deaths. A recent estimation by the CDC is that such an intentional release would cost more than 5 billion dollars for every 100,000 exposures (122, 123). *F. tularensis* is considered to be a dangerous potential biological weapon because of its extreme infectivity, ease of dissemination, and substantial capacity to cause illness and death.

Epidemiology

Tularemia, also known as "rabbit fever" and "deer fly fever" is a naturally occurring zoonotic infection resembling plague and brucellosis. *F. tularensis* can be found throughout most of the world and in the United States it has been identified in all 50 states except Hawaii (122, 123). Sporadic outbreaks still occur in the United States with an average of less than 200 cases reported per year (123, 124). Humans are incidentally infected via varied environmental exposures most commonly by skin or mucous membrane contact with tissues or body fluids of infected animals, bites of infected ticks, deer flies, or mosquitoes. Less commonly transmission occurs via inhalation of contaminated dusts or ingestion of contaminated foods or water. It is not transmitted person to person (121, 123). *F. tularensis* can remain viable for weeks in water, soil, dead animals, hides and for years in frozen meat. Voles, mice, rats, rabbits, and squirrels are common natural reservoirs. The major risk for a bioterror event in the United States is believed to be aerosol release. A sudden clustered presentation of the pneumonic and/or typhoidal forms of tularemia would suggest a bioterror event and concern for *F. tularensis* (123). Case fatality rate for natural disease in the United States is 1.4%; however, the fatality rate for untreated inhalation induced infection is expected to be as high as 30–60% (121).

Bacteriology and Pathophysiology

F. tularensis is a gram-negative, non-spore forming coccobacillus and facultative intracellular aerobe which occurs in two strains or subspecies. Type A (biovar tularensis) is the predominant strain found in North America and is highly virulent. Type B (biovar palaearctica) is found predominantly in Asia and Europe and is a much less virulent organism. As few as 10 organisms of type A can cause infection via the inhalation route (121, 125). After introduction through skin, mucous membrane, gastrointestinal tract, or lungs, the bacteria are taken up by macrophages where they begin dividing intracellularly. The initial tissue reaction, regardless of portal of entry, is localized suppurative necrosis which produces edematous, inflamed ulcers in skin and mucosa and if untreated will eventually lead to granuloma formation (121, 123). Inhalation exposure in humans has been shown by bronchoscopy to produce ulcers, inflammation, and hemorrhagic edema similar to that seen in skin and exposed mucous membranes (126).

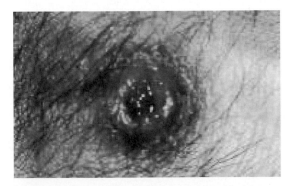

Fig. 34–7. Cutaneous ulcer of tularemia. *Source:* Courtesy of William Beisel, M.D., Colonel, Medical Corps, U.S. Army (Ret).

Untreated it will spread to local lymph nodes, multiply, and disseminate throughout the body.

Clinical Presentation

Six distinct clinical presentations of tularemia have been described which may be seen singly or in combination. These are ulceroglandular, glandular, oculoglandular, oropharyngeal, pneumonic, and typhoidal (123–125). A more practical and clinically relevant scheme has been suggested based on pathogenesis, clinical management, and prognosis with only two categories, ulceroglandular (includes glandular, oculoglandular, and pharyngeal), and typhoidal (includes pneumonic and systemic) (121). The overall severity of presentation will depend on a number of factors including virulence of the organism, route of exposure, and size of inoculum as well as host factors such as immune suppression or concomitant illness. Onset of illness is usually abrupt following a 3–6 day incubation period. Incubation may be as brief as 1 day and as long as 21 days (121, 123). Constitutional symptoms include fever, myalgias, back pain, fatigue, headache and rigors. Nonproductive cough and chest pain suggest bronchial or pulmonary involvement. Sore throat, nausea, vomiting, and diarrhea may also be present. Pulse-temperature dissociation with relative bradycardia has been sited as suggestive of tularemia but is present in less than half of the patients (125). Without treatment symptoms may persist for months and any of the localized forms of the disease may spread systemically via hematogenous dissemination with resultant sepsis, shock and involvement of any organ system. Untreated mortality for naturally occurring disease is as high as 15% versus a mortality of 1.4% with treatment (123).

Ulceroglandular tularemia is the most common form and is seen in 75% of cases of naturally occurring disease. It is initiated by inoculation of skin or mucous membranes with infected blood or body fluids or from the bite of an infected insect. It begins as a tender papule which progresses over 2–3 days to a painful indolent ulcer with regional lymphadenopathy and is usually accompanied by typical abrupt onset of constitutional symptoms (121, 123, 125, 127). Differential diagnosis will include pyogenic infections, cat scratch disease, syphilis, bubonic plague, and chancroid. Up to two-thirds of patients may have additional dermatologic findings such as urticaria, erythema multeforme, or erythema nodosum (128).

Glandular tularemia presents with the same signs and symptoms except for the absence of an ulcerated skin or mucous membrane lesion.

The oculoglandular form involves inoculation via the conjunctiva and is characterized by a purulent unilateral conjunctivitis with significant chemosis, periorbital edema, preauricular and/or cervical adenopathy. Small ulcers are frequently present on the palpebral conjunctiva.

The oropharyngeal form is caused by inoculation of the pharynx by ingestion or inhalation. It presents as ulcerative, exudative, and/or membranous pharyngitis with painful cervical adenopathy.

Pneumonic and typhoidal tularemia may occur by hematogenous dissemination of localized ulceroglandular involvement or as an isolated entity (121, 123, 125). This would be the predominant presentation expected following an aerosol-inhalation exposure though ulceroglandular presentations may still be seen.

Pneumonic tularemia typically presents with the abrupt onset of fever, rigors, dyspnea, nonproductive cough, and chest pain. Pulmonary findings are variable and are not specific to tularemia (121, 123). Clinically it is indistinguishable from other typical and atypical pneumonias. Sites of extrapulmonary manifestations may be present and suggest the diagnosis. Isolated pneumonia caused by an inhalation exposure would not be expected to present with peripheral adenopathy. Although up to 80% of typhoidal tularemia develop pneumonia, 50–75% of inhalation exposures may initially present with rapid onset of systemic signs but no pulmonary symptoms (123). Untreated mortality is 30–60% and this is significantly reduced to 1–3% with appropriate antibiotic treatment (121). In addition to community acquired pneumonia, differential diagnosis for a sudden cluster of cases would include the possibility of anthrax and plague. In general, the progression of disease would be much less rapid than that expected with either of these entities. Anthrax is a more fulminating illness with rapid development of respiratory insufficiency and shock. Primary plague pneumonia likewise would be expected to have a rapid onset of severe pneumonia with purulent or bloody sputum with rapid development of respiratory insufficiency and shock (1).

Typhoidal tularemia is the presence of systemic signs with toxicity and no evidence of cutaneous or mucosal involvement. It accounts for 5–15% of naturally occurring disease and occurs mainly after inhalation of contaminated dust or infectious aerosol; however, systemic involvement can also occur from hematogenous spread of localized infection. As previously noted, the majority of inhalation exposures may initially present with a typhoidal picture and up to 80% will eventually develop evidence of pneumonia (121, 123, 125). Differential diagnosis includes typhoid fever, typhus, brucellosis, malaria, rickettsiosis, toxic shock, and sepsis.

Diagnosis

Since tularemia is an infrequently seen disease, it is not likely to be considered in the initial differential diagnosis by most clinicians and rapid diagnostic testing is not yet widely available. Initial recognition following an intentional release is likely to be made by public health officials due to an unusual clustering of pneumonic or typhoidal cases (121, 123, 129). Differential diagnosis will include other typhoidal syndromes (salmonella, rickettsia, malaria) and both typical and atypical pneumonia (*S., mycoplasma*, plague, legionella). Initial chest x-ray will be abnormal in up to 50% of patients presenting with typhoidal or pneumonic symptoms but findings are variable, nonspecific, and may show bronchopneumonia, lobar pneumonia, interstitial disease, effusions, granuloma, and hilar adenopathy. Other routine laboratory tests are usually not helpful in the acute setting and presumptive diagnosis is established based on the clinical grounds with subsequent confirmation by serology at 2–4 weeks in sporadically occurring cases (121, 123, 124). The presence of leukocytosis is a variable finding with WBC in the range of 5–22,000. A predominant lymphocytosis may be seen as the disease progresses. Platletts and hematocrit are normal unless the situation is complicated by sepsis and/or DIC. Mild elevations in LDH and transaminases are often seen with typhoidal symptoms. Occasionally rhabdomyolysis may complicate the course with typical findings of urinary myoglobin and elevated CPK (121, 123, 125). Gram stain is of limited value due to the poor staining qualities of the organism; however, thorough evaluation of stains of sputum or necrotic material frequently demonstrates poorly staining gram-negative coccobacilli (123, 129). Growth of *F. tularensis* in culture is the definitive means of confirming the diagnosis. It is only occasionally isolated from the blood but tissue biopsy or scraping is the best source for both Gram stain and culture (123). Organisms can also be grown from pharyngeal washings, sputum specimens, and fasting gastric aspirates in a high proportion of patients with inhalation tularemia. *F. tularensis* is a virulent laboratory hazard which has historically caused disease in lab personnel and should only be handled in laboratories equipped for biosafety level 2 (BSL-2) (129, 130). Laboratory personnel need to be alerted to the possibility of tularemia and public health officials must be notified for suspicion of inhalation disease (129). Although *F. tularensis* will grow in routine culture media, standard blood culture broth or agar enhanced with cystiene will provide optimal growth and recovery. Direct fluorescent antibody staining and enzyme linked immunoassay identification is available through LRN reference laboratories and results can be obtained within a few hours of specimen receipt with proper notification and involvement of public health authorities (123). Recent studies have shown excellent results with rapid identification utilizing PCR and this technique is becoming more widely available (131, 132).

Treatment

Streptomycin and gentamicin are the preferred agents for treatment in all age groups and in pregnancy (123). Historically streptomycin has been the first line agent recommended for tularemia in doses of 10–15 mg/kg up to a maximum of 1 g given IM every 12 h (121, 123, 127). Gentamicin in doses 5 mg/kg/day is also effective and given the development of streptomycin-resistant strains is now recommended in place of streptomycin. Fluoroquinolones, in particular ciprofloxacin, has shown good activity against *F tularensis* and is considered an alternative first line therapy in doses of 15 mg/kg up to a maximum of 400 mg given IV twice daily. Doxycycline in doses of 2.2 mg/kg to a maximum of 100 mg IV twice a day and chloramphenical 15 mg/kg IV four times a day are also acceptable alternatives but may be associated with a slightly higher incidence of treatment failure and relapse (123, 127). Fluoroquinolones, doxycycline, and chloramphenicol are acceptable alternatives in all age groups. Chloramphenicol is not recommended in pregnancy. Regardless of the agent, treatment should be continued for a minimum of 10–14 days. Patients can be converted from parenteral treatment to oral with ciprofloxacin or doxycycline in standard doses once systemic symptoms have resolved (121, 123).

Infection Control and Decontamination

There is no definitive information on the duration of viability of *F. tularensis* following aerosol release. The organism can survive for long periods in cool moist conditions but it is expected that there would be a much more rapid loss of viability due to dessication, solar radiation, oxidation, and other environmental factors with limited risk from secondary exposure or dispersal (123). Standard levels of chlorine in municipal water should protect against waterborne infection and make wide-spread disease from contamination of municipal water supplies an unlikely event (121, 123). For suspected acute exposures, external decontamination with soap and water is sufficient. Contaminated surfaces may be cleaned with household bleach solution diluted 10:1 with water. *F. tularensis* is not transmitted person to person and standard hospital infection control practices are sufficient. Isolation of patients is not required (121, 123).

Prevention and Prophylaxis

There is currently no readily available vaccine for tularemia. An attenuated vaccine has been used in the former Soviet Union since 1930 in areas where tularemia is endemic (121, 123). Live attenuated vaccine is associated with a significant decrease in incidence of inhalation tularemia in laboratory workers (133). In volunteer studies the vaccine did not protect all participants from aerosol challenges (134). An attenuated vaccine is currently under review by the FDA and available via an IND protocol for laboratory workers (135). There is currently ongoing private and federally funded research to develop a safe effective tularemia vaccine (136, 137). Vaccine would not be indicated for postexposure prophylaxis as immunity takes 2 weeks or more to develop and it would not be expected to prevent disease. Prophylaxis with antibiotics would only be indicated in the unlikely event of a recognized acute aerosol exposure. Oral ciprofloxacin or doxycycline as a 2-week course is the recommended agents for prophylaxis. Prophylaxis is not recommended after symptomatic clustered cases are recognized or for possible natural exposure (123).

REFERENCES

1. Inglesby TV, Toole T, et al.: Anthrax as a biological weapon, 2002 updated recommendations for management. *JAMA* 287:2236–2252, 2002.
2. Abrams J: *Anthrax Cleanup Cost $27 Million*. Associated Press, 2003.
3. Shane S: *Cleanup of Anthrax Will Cost Hundreds Of Millions Of Dollars*. Baltimore Sun.
4. Centers for Disease Control and Prevention: Agents, diseases and other threats. Available at http://www.bt.cdc.gov
5. Centers for Disease Control and Prevention: Biological and chemical terrorism: Strategic plan for preparedness and response. *Morb Mortal Wkly Rep* 49(RR-4):1–14, 2000.
6. Lew DP: Bacillus anthracis (anthrax), in *Mandell: Principles and Practice of Infectious Diseases, 5th ed.* New York, Churchill Livingston, Inc, 2000, pp. 2215–2220.
7. Friedlander AM: Anthrax, in: Sidell FR, Takafuji ET, Franz DR (eds.): *Medical Aspects of Chemical and Bilogical Warfare.* Washington DC, TMM Publications, 1997, pp. 467–478.
8. LaForce FM: Woolsorters' disease in England. *Bull NY Acad Med* 54:956–963, 1978.
9. Dixon TC, Meselson M, et al.: Anthrax. *N Engl J Med* 341(11):815–826, 1999.
10. Nicolas DK: *Unlocking A Deadly Secret, New York Times,* 1995.
11. Christopher GW, Cieslak TJ, Pavlin JA, Eitzen EM Jr.: Biological warfare. A historical perspective. *JAMA* 278(5): 412–417, 1997.
12. Meselson M, Guillemin J, Hugh-Jones M, et al.: The Sverdlovsk anthrax outbreak of 1979. *Science* 266:1202–1208, 1994.
13. Alibek K: *Biohazard.* New York, Random House Inc, 1999.
14. Jernigan DB, Raghunathan PL, Bell BP, et al.: Investigation of bioterrorism-related anthrax, United States, 2001: Epidemiologic findings. *Emerg Infect Dis* 8(10):1019–1028, 2002.
15. Wein LM, Craft DL, Kaplan EH: Emergency response to an anthrax attack. *Proc Natl Acad Sci USA* 100(7) 4346–4351, 2003.
16. Kaufmann AF, Meltzer MI, Schmid GP: The economic impact of a bioterrorist attack: Are prevention and postattack intervention programs justifiable? *Emerg Infect Dis* 3(2):83–94, 1997.
17. Manchee RJ, Broster MG, Stagg AJ, Hibbs SE: Formaldehyde solution effectively inactivates spores of *Bacillus anthracis* on the Scottish island of Gruinard. *Appl Environ Microbiol* 60:4167–4171, 1994.
18. Hanna P: Anthrax pathogenesis and host response. *Curr Top Microbiol Immunol* 225:13–35, 1998.
19. Moaveri M, Leppla SH: The roles of anthrax toxin in pathogenesis. *Curr Opin Microbiol* 7(1):19–24, 2004.
20. Little SF, Ivins BE: Molecular pathogenesis of Bacillus anthracis infection. *Microbes Infect* 1(2):131–139, 1999.
21. Abramova FA, Grinberg LM, Yamploskaya O, et al.: Pathology of inhalation anthrax in 42 cases from the Sverdlovsk outbreak. *Proc Natl Acad Sci USA* 90:2291–2294, 1993.
22. Bell DM, Kozarsky PE, Stephens DS: Clinical issues in the prophylaxis, diagnosis, and treatment of anthrax. *Emerg Infect Dis* 8(2):222–225, 2002.
23. Friedlander AM, Welkos SL, Pitt ML, et al.: Postexposure prophylaxis against experimental inhalation anthrax. *J Infect Dis* 167(5):1239–1242, 1993.
24. Brachman P, Friedlander A: Inhalation anthrax. *Ann NY Acad Sci* 353:83–93, 1980.
25. Jernigan JA, Stephens DS, Ashford DA, et al.: Bioterrorism-related inhalational anthrax: The first 10 cases reported in the United States. *Emerg Infect Dis* 7(6): 933–944, 2001.
26. Centers for Disease Control and Prevention: Notice to readers: Considerations for distinguishing influenza-like illness from inhalational anthrax. *MMWR Morb Mortal Wkly Rep* 50(44):984–986, 2001.
27. Centers for Disease Control and Prevention: Anthrax: Diagnosis/Evaluation (Signs and Symptoms). Available at http://www.bt.cdc.gov/agent/anthrax/diagnosis/index.asp. Accessed 11 Mar 2004.
28. Centers for Disease Control and Prevention: Laboratory Information. Available at http://www.bt.cdc.gov/ LabIssues/index.asp. Accessed 11 Mar 2004.
29. Barakat LA, Quentzel HL, Jernigan JA , et al. Fatal inhalational anthrax in a 94-year-old Connecticut woman. *JAMA* 287(7):863–868, 2002.
30. Hansell D, Padley S: Imaging, in *Albert: Comprehensive Respiratory Medicine.* St Louis, Mosby, Inc., 1999.

31. Kuehnert MJ, Doyle TJ, Hill HA et al.: Clinical features that discriminate inhalational anthrax from other acute respiratory illnesses. *Clin Infect Dis* 36(3):328–333, 2003.

32. Penn C, Klotz S: Anthrax, in Gorbach S, Bartlett J, Blacklow N (eds.): *Infectious Diseases.* Philadelphia, PA, WB Saunders Co, 1998; pp 1575–1578.

33. Swartz, MN: Recognition and management of anthrax—an update. *N Engl J Med* 345(22):1621–1626, 2001.

34. Centers for Disease Control and Prevention: Investigation of bioterrorism-related anthrax and interim guidelines for clinical evaluation of persons with possible anthrax. *MMWR Morb Mortal Wkly Rep* 50(43):941–948, 2001.

35. Williams DD, Benedek O, Turnbough CL: *Appl Environ Microbiol.* 69(10):6288–6293, 2003.

36. Kwan SK, Jong-Man K, Jong-Wan K, et al.: Identification of *Bacillus anthracis* by rpoB Sequence analysis and multiplex PCR. *J Clin Microbiol* 41(7):2908–2914, 2003.

37. Hurtle H, Bode E, Kulesh DA, et al.: Detection of the *Bacillus anthracis* gyrA gene by using a minor groove binder probe. *J Clin Microbiol* 42(1):179–185, 2004.

38. Fine AM, Wong JB, Fraser HS, et al.: Is it influenza or anthrax? A decision analytic approach to the treatment of patients with influenza-like illnesses. *Ann Emerg Med* 43(3):318–328, 2004.

39. Centers for Disease Control and Prevention: Update: Investigation of bioterrorism-related anthrax and interim guidelines for exposure management and antimicrobial therapy, October 2001. *MMWR Morb Mortal Wkly Rep* 50(42):909–19, 2001.

40. Mohammed MJ, Marston CK, Popovic T, et al.: Antimicrobial susceptibility testing of Bacillus anthracis: Comparison of results obtained by using the National Committee for Clinical Laboratory Standards broth microdilution reference and Etest agar gradient diffusion methods. *J Clin Microbiol* 40(6):1902–1907.

41. Frean J, Klugman KP, Arntzen L, Bukofzer S: Susceptibility of *Bacillus anthracis* to eleven antimicrobial agents including novel fluoroquinolones and a ketolide. *J Antimicrob Chemother* 52(2):297–299, 2003.

42. Coker PR, Smith KL, Hugh-Jones ME: Antimicrobial susceptibilities of diverse *Bacillus anthracis* isolates. *Antimicrob Agents Chemother* 46(12):3843–3845, 2002.

43. Bakici MZ, Elaldi N, Bakir M, et al.: Antimicrobial susceptibility of *Bacillus anthracis* in an endemic area. *Scand J Infect Dis* 34(8):564–566, 2002.

44. Esel D, Doganay M, Sumerkan B: Antimicrobial susceptibilities of 40 isolates of *Bacillus anthracis* isolated in Turkey. *Int J Antimicrob Agents* 22(1):70–72, 2003.

45. Physicians Desk Reference: *Thompson PDR*, 58th *ed*. 2004.

46. American Academy of Pediatrics Committee on Drugs: The transfer of drugs and other chemicals into human milk. *Pediatrics* 108:776–789, 2001.

47. Centers for Disease Control and Prevention. Notice to readers: Update: Interim recommendations for antimicrobial prophylaxis for children and breastfeeding mothers and treatment of children with anthrax. *MMWR Morb Mortal Wkly Rep* 50(45)1014–1016, 2001.

48. Sagripanti JL, Bonifacino A: Comparative sporicidal effects of liquid chemical agents. *Appl Environ Microbiol* 62(2):545–551, 1996.

49. Whitney EA, Beatty ME, Taylor TH, et al.: Inactivation of *Bacillus anthracis* spores. *Emerg Infect Dis* 9(6), 2003.

50. Food and Drug Administration: Prescription drug products; doxycycline and penicillin G procaine administration for inhalational anthrax (postexposure). *Fed Reg* 66(55)679–682, 2001.

51. Centers for Disease Control and Prevention: Notice to readers: Updated recommendations for antimicrobial prophylaxis among asymptomatic pregnant women after exposure to *Bacillus anthracis*. *MMWR Morb Mortal Wkly Rep* 50(43):960, 2001.

52. Welkos S, Little S, Friedlander A, et al.: The role of antibodies to *Bacillus anthracis* and anthrax toxin components in inhibiting the early stages of infection by anthrax spores. *Microbiology* 147(6):1677–1685, 2001.

53. Joellenbeck LM, Zwanziger LL, Durch JS, Strom BL (eds.): *The Anthrax Vaccine: Is It Safe? Does It Work?* Washinngton, DC, National Academy Press, 2003.

54. Friedlander AM, Pittman PR, Parker GW: Anthrax vaccine: Evidence for safety and efficacy against inhalational anthrax. *JAMA* 282:2104–2106, 1999.

55. FDA Statement: FDA Issues Final Rule and Final Order Regarding Safety and Efficacy of Certain Licensed Biological Products Including Anthrax Vaccine. Available at http://www.fda.gov/bbs/topics/NEWS/2003/NEW01001.html

56. Pitt M, Little S, Ivins B, et al.: In vitro correlate of immunity in a rabbit model of inhalational anthrax. *Vaccine* 19(32):4768–4773, 2001.

57. Leppla SH, Robbins JB, Schneerson R, Shiloach J: Development of an improved vaccine for anthrax. *J Clin Invest* 110(2):141–144, 2002.

58. Centers for Disease Control and Prevention: Surveillance for adverse events associated with anthrax vaccination—U.S. Department of Defense, 1998–2000. *MMWR Morb Mortal Wkly Rep* 49(16):341–345, 2000.

59. Centers for Disease Control and Prevention: Notice to readers: Use of anthrax vaccine in response to terrorism: Supplemental recommendations of the Advisory Committee on Immunization Practices. 51(45):1024–1026, 2002.

60. Center for Infectious Disease Research and Policy: HHS to buy up to 75 million doses of new anthrax vaccine. Mar 2004. Available at http://www.cidrap.umn.edu/cidrap/content/bt/anthrax/news/mar1204anthrax.html.

61. Center for Infectious Disease Research and Policy: FDA grants fast-track status for anthrax drug. Available at http://www.cidrap.umn.edu/cidrap/content/bt/anthrax/news/aug2703abthrax.html.

62. Center for Infectious Disease Research and Policy: Antibody may prove to be anthrax prophylactic and therapeutic agent. Available at http://www.cidrap.umn.edu/cidrap/content/bt/bioprep/btwatch/btwatch-oct-2003.html.

63. Cunha BA. Smallpox and measles: Historical aspects and clinical differentiation. *Infect Dis Clin N Am* 18(1), 2004.

64. McClain DJ: Smallpox, in Sidell FR, Takafuji ET, Franz DR (eds.): *Medical Management of Biological Casualties*. Washington, DC, TMM Publications, 1998; pp 539–559.

65. Henderson DA, Inglesby TV, Bartlett JG, et al.: Smallpox as a biological weapon: Medical and public health management. Working Group on Civilian Biodefense. *JAMA* 281(22):2127–2137, 1999.

66. Centers for Disease Control and Prevention: Vaccinia (smallpox) vaccine: Recommendations of the Advisory Committee on Immunization Practices (ACIP). *MMWR Morb Mortal Wkly Rep* 50(RR10):1–25, 2001.

67. Breman JG, Henderson DA: Diagnosis and management of smallpox. *N Engl J Med* 346:1300–1308, 2002.

68. Centers for Disease Control and Prevention. Smallpox: Disease, Prevention, and Intervention: Available at http://www.bt.cdc.gov/agent/smallpox/training/overview/index.asp.

69. Centers for Disease Control and Prevention: Acute, generalized vesicular or pustular rash illness testing protocol in the United States. Available at http://www.bt.cdc.gov/agent/smallpox/diagnosis/rashtestingprotocol.asp.

70. Darling RG, Catlett CL, Huebner KD, Jarrett DG: Threats in bioterrorism. I: CDC category A agents. *Emerg Med Clin North Am* 20(2):273–309, 2002.

71. Centers for Disease Control and Prevention: Isolation and quarantine guidelines "Guide C" in the smallpox response plan and guidelines. Available at http:// www.bt.cdc.gov/agent/smallpox/healthofficials.asp#infectioncontrol.

72. El-Ad R, Roth Y, Winder A: The persistence of neutralizing antibodies after revaccination against smallpox. *J Infect Dis* 161:446–448, 1990.

73. Bartlett J, Borio L, Radonovich L, et al.: Smallpox vaccination in 2003: Key information for clinicians. *Clin Infect Dis* 36(7):883–902, 2003.

74. Frey SE, Newman FK, Cruz J, et al.: Dose-related effects of smallpox vaccine. *N Engl J Med.* 346(17):1275–1280, 2002.

75. Frey SE, Couch RB, Tacket CO, et al. for National Institute of Allergy and Infectious Diseases Smallpox Vaccine Study Group: Clinical responses to undiluted and diluted smallpox vaccine. *N Engl J Med* 346(17):1265–1274, 2002.

76. Centers for Disease Control and Prevention: Smallpox vaccination and adverse reactions guidance for clinicians. *Morb Mortal Wkly Rep* 52(RR4):1–28, 2001.

77. Butler T. *Yersinia* species (including plague), in Mandell GL, Bennett JE, Dolin R (eds.): *Principles and Practice of Infectious Diseases*. New York, NY, Churchill Livingstone; 2000, pp 2406–2414.

78. McGovern TW, Friedlander AM: Plague, in Sidell FR, Takafuji ET, Franz DR (eds.): *Medical Aspects of Chemical and Biological Warfare*. Washington DC, TMM Publications; 1997. pp 479–502.

79. Dennnis DT, Gage KL. Plague, in Cohen J, Powderly WG (eds.) *Infectious Diseases, 2nd ed.* Amsterdam, Elsevier, 2004; pp 1641–1648.

80. Inglesby TV, Dennis DT, Henderson DA, et al.: Plague as a biological weapon. Medical and public health management. *JAMA* 283(17):2281–2290, 2000.

81. Perry RD, Fetherston JD: *Yersinia pestis*—etiologic agent of plague. *Clin Microbiol Rev* 10(1):35–66, 1997.

82. Ampel NM: Plagues—what's past is present: Thoughts on the origin and history of new infectious diseases. *Rev Infect Dis* 13(4):658–665, 1991.

83. Williams P, Wallace D: *Unit 731: Japan's Secret Biological Warfare in World War II*. New York, The Free Press, 1989.

84. Barry J: Planning a plague. *Newsweek*. Feb 1:40–41, 1993.

85. WHO: Aspects of *Chemical and Biological Weapons* Geneva, World Health Organization, 1970, pp 98–109.

86. Werner SB, Weidmer CE, Nelson BC, et al.: Primary plague pneumonia contracted from a domestic cat in South Lake Tahoe, California. *JAMA* 251:929–931, 1984.

87. Gage KL, Dennis DT, Orloski KA, et al.: Cases of cat-associated human plague in the Western US, 1977–98. *Clin Infect Dis* 30:893–900, 2000.

88. Cobbs CG, Chansolme DH: Plague. *Dermatol Clin* 22(3): 303–312, 2004.

89. Caten JL, Kartman L: Human plague in the United States: 1900–1966. *JAMA* 205(6):81–84, 1968.

90. Centers for Disease Control and Prevention: Imported plague—New York City, 2002. *MMWR Morb Mortal Wkly Rep* 52(31):725–728, 2003.

91. Centers for Disease Control and Prevention: Recognition of illness associated with the intentional release of a biologic agent. *MMWR Morb Mortal Wkly Rep* 50(41);893–897, 2001.

92. Centers for Disease Control and Prevention: Fatal human plague—Arizona and Colorado, 1996. *MMWR Morb Mortal Wkly Rep* 46(27):617–620, 1997.

93. Legters LJ, Cottingham AJ Jr., Hunter DH: Clinical and epidemiologic notes on a defined outbreak of plague in Vietnam. *Am J Trop Med Hyg* 19(4):639–652, 1970.

94. Crook LD, Tempest B: Plague—a clinical review of 27 cases. *Arch Intern Med* 152:1253–1256, 1992.

95. Hull HF, Montes JM, Mann JM: Septicemic plague in New Mexico. *J Infect Dis* 155:113–118, 1987.

96. Speck RS, Wolochow H. Studies on the experimental epidemiology of respiratory infections: VIII. Experimental pneumonic plague in *Macaccus rhesus*. *J Infect Dis* 100(1):58–69, 1957.

97. Finegold MJ, Petery JJ, Berendt RF, Adams HR: Studies on the pathogenesis of plague. *J Infect Dis* 53:99–114, 1968.

98. Conrad FG, LeCocq FR, Krain R: A recent epidemic of plague in Vietnam. *Arch Intern Med* 122(3):193–198, 1968.

99. Marshall JD, Quy DV, Gibson FL: Asymptomatic pharyngeal plague infection in Vietnam. *Am J Trop Med Hyg* 16(2):175–177, 1967.

100. Burmeister RW, Tigertt WD, Overholt EL: Laboratory-acquired pneumonic plague. *Ann Intern Med* 56:789–800, 1962.

101. Centers for Disease Control and Prevention: Laboratory test criteria for diagnosis of plague. Available at

http://www.cdc.gov/ncidod/dvbid/plague/lab-test-criteria .htm, accessed 21 Aug 2004.

102. Alsofrom DJ, Mettler FA Jr., Mann JM: Radiographic manifestations of plaque in New Mexico, 1975–1980. A review of 42 proved cases. *Radiology.* 139(3):561–565, 1981.

103. Hinnebusch J, Schwan TG: New method for plague surveillance using polymerase chain reaction to detect *Yersinia pestis* in fleas. *J Clin Microbiol* 31(6):1511–1514, 1993.

104. Splettstoesser WD, Rahalison L, Grunow R, et al.: Evaluation of a standardized F1 capsular antigen capture ELISA test kit for the rapid diagnosis of plague. *FEMS Immunol Med Microbiol* 41(2):149–155, 2004.

105. Loïez C: Detection of *Yersinia pestis* in sputum by real-time PCR. *J Clin Microbiol* 41(10):4873–4875, 2004.

106. Chanteau S, Rahalison L, Ralafiarisoa L, et al.: Development and testing of a rapid diagnostic test for bubonic and pneumonic plague. *Lancet* 361(9353):211–216, 2003.

107. Sites VR, Poland JD: Mediastinal lymphadenopathy in bubonic plague. *Am J Roentgenol Radium Ther Nucl Med* 116(3):567–570, 1972.

108. Smith MD, Vinh DX, Nguyen TT, et al.: In vitro antimicrobial susceptibilities of strains of *Yersinia pestis*. *Antimicrob Agents Chemother* 39(9):2153–2154, 1995.

109. Bonacorsi SP, Scavizzi MR, Guiyoule A, et al.: Assessment of a fluoroquinolone, three beta-lactams, two aminoglycosides, and a cycline in treatment of murine *Yersinia pestis* infection. *Antimicrob Agents Chemother* 38(3): 481–486, 1994.

110. Hernandez E, Girardet M, Ramisse F, et al.: Antibiotic susceptibilities of 94 isolates of *Yersinia pestis* to 24 antimicrobial agents. *J Antimicrob Chemother* 52:1029–1031, 2003.

111. Frean J, Klugman KP, Arntzen L, Bukofzer S: Susceptibility of *Yersinia pestis* to novel and conventional antimicrobial agents. *J Antimicrob Chemother* 52(2):294–296.

112. Russell P, Eley SM, Fulop MJ, et al.: The efficacy of ciprofloxacin and doxycycline against experimental tularaemia. *J Antimicrob Chemother* 41(4):461–465, 1998.

113. Byrne WR, Welkos SL, Pitt ML, et al.: Antibiotic treatment of experimental pneumonic plague in mice. *Antimicrob Agents Chemother* 42(3):675–681, 1998.

114. World Health Organization: Plague manual: Epidemiology, distribution, surveillance, and control. Available at http://www.who.int/emc-documents/plague/whocdscsredc992c. htm.

115. Centers for Disease Control and Prevention: Prevention of plague. Recommendations of the Advisory Committee on Immunization Practices (ACIP). *MMWR Morb Mortal Wkly Rep* 45(RR-14):1–15, 1996.

116. Rose LJ, Donlan R, Banerjee SN, Arduino MJ: Survival of *Yersinia pestis* on environmental surfaces. *Appl Environ Microbiol* 69(4):2166–2167, 216.

117. Williamson ED, Eley SM, Stagg AJ, et al.: A single dose sub-unit vaccine protects against pneumonic plague. *Vaccine* 19(4-5):566–571, 2000.

118. Jarrett CO, Sebbane F, Adamovicz JJ, et al.: Flea-borne transmission model to evaluate vaccine efficacy against naturally acquired bubonic plague. *Infect Immun* 72(4):2052–2056, 2004.

119. Titball RW, Williamson ED: Vaccination against bubonic and pneumonic plague. *Vaccine* 19(30):4175–4184, 2001.

120. Grosfeld H, Cohen S, Bino T, et al.: Effective protective immunity to *Yersinia pestis* infection conferred by DNA vaccine coding for derivatives of the F1 capsular antigen. *Infect Immun* 71(1):374–383, 2003.

121. Evans ME, Friedlander AM: Tularemia, in: Sidell FR, Takafuji ET, Franz DR (eds.): *Medical Aspects of Chemical and Biological Warfare.* Washington DC, TMM Publications, 1997; pp. 503–512.

122. Kaufmann AF, Meltzer MI, Schmid GP: The economic impact of a bioterrorist attack: Are prevention and postattack intervention programs justifiable? *Emerg Infect Dis* 3(2):83–94, 1997.

123. Dennis DT, Inglesby TV, Henderson DA, et al. for Working Group on Civilian Biodefense: Tularemia as a biological weapon: medical and public health management. *JAMA* 285(21):2763–2773, 2001.

124. Feldman KA, Enscore RE, Lathrop SL, et al.: An outbreak of primary pneumonic tularemia on Martha's Vineyard. *N Engl J Med* 345(22):1601–1606, 2001.

125. Evans ME, Gregory DW, Schaffner W, McGee ZA: Tularemia: A 30-year experience with 88 cases. *Medicine (Baltimore)* 64:251–269, 1985.

126. Syrjala H, Sutinen S, Jokinen K, et al.: Bronchial changes in airborne tularemia. *J Laryngol Otol* 100(10):1169–1176, 1986.

127. Cross JT, Penn RL: *Francisella tularensis* (tularemia), in: Mandell GL, et al. (eds.): *Principles and Practice of Infectious Diseases.* Philadelphia, PA, Churchill Livingstone, 2000; pp 2393–2402.

128. McGovern TW, Christopher GW, Eitzen EM: Cutaneous manifestations of biological warfare and related threat agents. *Arch Dermatol* 135(3):311–322, 1999.

129. Centers for Disease Control and Prevention: Level A laboratory procedures for the identification of Francisella tularensis. Available at http://www.bt.cdc.gov/Agent/Tularemia/ftu_la_cp_121301.pdf.

130. Overholt EL, Tigertt WD, Kadull PJ, et al.: An analysis of forty-two cases of laboratory-acquired tularemia. *Am J Med* 30:785–806, 1961.

131. Emanuel PA, Bell R, Dang JL, et al.: Detection of *Francisella tularensis* within infected mouse tissues by using a hand-held PCR thermocycler. *J Clin Microbiol* 41(2):689–693, 2003.

132. Versage JL, Severin DD, Chu MC, Petersen JM: Development of a multitarget real-time TaqMan PCR assay for enhanced detection of *Francisella tularensis* in complex specimens. *J Clin Microbiol* 41(12):5492–5499, 2003.

133. Burke DS: Immunization against tularemia: Analysis of the effectiveness of live *Francisella tularensis* vaccine in prevention of laboratory-acquired tularemia. *J Infect Dis* 135(1):55–60, 1977.

134. Saslaw S, Eigelsbach HT, Prior JA, et al.: Tularemia vaccine study: II. Respiratory challenge. *Arch Intern Med* 107:702–714, 1961.

135. Center for Infectious Disease Research and Policy: Tularemia vaccine. Available at http://www.cidrap.umn.edu/ cidrap/content/bt/tularemia/biofacts/tularemiafactsheet. html#_Tularemia_Vaccine.

136. Center for Infectious Disease Research and Policy: NIAID funds tularemia research at New York school. CIDRAP News, Dec 9, 2003. Available at http://www.cidrap.umn.edu/ cidrap/content/bt/tularemia/news/dec0903tularemia.html.

137. Press release: Dynport wins 750,000 award to develop tularemia vaccine candidate. Available at http://www. dynport.com/press.htm.

35

Occupational Exposure in Health Care Personnel

Joanne T. Maffei

HIGH YIELD FACTS

1. Management of occupational exposure to blood, and other potentially infectious bodily fluids, requires local wound care to the injury, reporting of the incident, obtaining baseline studies of the source patient and the health care personnel (HCP), assessing the need for postexposure prophylaxis (PEP) by evaluating the exposure and the source patient for risk of transmission of human immunodeficiency virus (HIV), hepatitis B virus or hepatitis C virus, prescribing PEP medications if needed, and follow-up of the HCP.

2. Occupational postexposure prophylaxis (PEP), including HIV PEP, should be considered an urgent medical concern and initiated as soon as possible. The Emergency Department should have procedures in place, and medications for PEP readily available for use. HIV PEP should be administered, ideally within 2 h, and continued for 4 weeks when prescribed.

3. Expert consultation is advised for HIV PEP for delayed exposure report, unknown source, pregnancy (known or suspected) in the exposed person, resistance of the source virus to antiretrovirals, and toxicity of the PEP regimen. Consult local experts and/or the National Clinicians' PEP Hotline 1-(888)-HIV-4911 or 1-(888)-448-4911 in these situations.

4. Nevirapine is generally not recommended for occupational HIV PEP, due to reports of serious adverse events, including two cases of life-threatening hepatotoxicity.

5. For health care personnel (HCP) who are pregnant, avoid efavirenz, indinivir shortly before delivery, didanosine [ddI] and stavudine [d4T], liquid amprenavir, atazanavir, and delaverdine in HIV PEP regimens. Expert consultation is advised.

6. Human bites must be evaluated to include the possibility that both the person bitten and the person who inflicted the bite were exposed to bloodborne pathogens.

7. Extended follow-up HIV testing for 12 months is recommended for HCP who become infected with HCV following exposure to a source coinfected with HIV and HCV.

CASE PRESENTATION

A 24-year-old female respiratory therapist presents to the emergency department after a needle-stick while drawing an arterial blood gas. The exposure occurred when the source patient moved while the needle was in his arm. The syringe had blood in it and blood was on the needle. The source patient is a 27-year-old male who is being evaluated for atypical pneumonia with hypoxia. He describes cough, fever, and weight loss and physical examination reveals clear lungs, oral thrush, and generalized lymphadenopathy. His HIV status is unknown. Baseline laboratory studies were drawn on both the source patient and the health care personnel for hepatitis B virus (HBV), hepatitis C virus (HCV), and human immunodeficiency virus (HIV). The respiratory therapist is frantic. This is her first needle-stick exposure.

INTRODUCTION/EPIDEMIOLOGY

Introduction

Prevention of occupational exposures to bloodborne pathogens by using standard precautions, proper sharps (needles and other sharp devices) disposal, safety devices, needleless systems, and promoting education and safe work practices for handling sharps is the best way to protect health care personnel (HCP) from bloodborne infections. Despite these measures, each year in the United States, it is estimated that 600,000–800,000 needle-stick and percutaneous exposures occur, and about half of them go unreported (1).

The major pathogens transmitted by blood and body fluid exposures are HBV, HCV, and HIV. The latest guidelines for managing occupational exposures to these pathogens were published in June 2001 in the Morbidity and Mortality Weekly Report (2). Since occupational exposures are considered urgent medical concerns, most emergency physicians will see these cases in their practice. Complete and timely evaluation of the exposure, source patient, and the HCP is required in order to make a determination on the need for postexposure prophylaxis (PEP) and appropriate follow-up.

Epidemiology

Occupational transmission risk and seroconversion

Hepatitis B—Risk Assessment for Hepatitis B Transmission

The risk of seroconversion from a percutaneous exposure for the unvaccinated HCP if a source patient is hepatitis B surface antigen-positive and hepatitis Be antigen-negative is 23–37%. If the source is hepatitis B surface antigen-positive and hepatitis Be antigen-positive the risk is almost double at 37–62% (2).

Occupationally Acquired Hepatitis B

Occupationally acquired HBV has declined in recent years due to the immunization of HCP against HBV, and to the use of Standard (Universal) Precautions and other measures to prevent exposures to blood and body fluids as required in the Occupational Safety and Health Administration (OSHA) bloodborne pathogens standard. In 1983, an estimated 17,000 new HBV infections occurred in HCP. In 1995 that estimate decreased by 95% to 800 new HCP HBV infections (1).

Hepatitis C—Risk Assessment for Hepatitis C Transmission

The average risk for seroconversion in a percutaneous exposure to a source patient with HCV is 1.9% (range 0–22.2%) (3). This is between the risk for seroconversion from an exposure to an HBV positive source (23–63%) and an HIV positive source (0.3%).

Occupationally Acquired Hepatitis C

The number of HCP who have acquired HCV occupationally is unknown. However, it is estimated that 2–4% of the acute HCV conversions per year (ranging from 100,000 in 1991 to 36,000 in 1996) occur in HCP after blood exposure in the workplace (1). Parenteral exposures account for the majority of occupational HCV conversions; however, there are anecdotal reports of HCV seroconversion following mucosal exposures (3–6).

Human Immunodeficiency Virus—Risk Assessment for HIV Transmission

In prospective studies of HCP seroconversion, the average risk for transmission of HIV in a percutaneous exposure

to a source patient with HIV is 0.3% (95% confidence interval (CI) = 0.2–0.5%) (7). The risk for transmission of HIV following a mucous membrane exposure is 0.09% (95% CI = 0.006–0.5%) (8). HIV transmission after non-intact skin exposure has been documented (9), but the average risk is estimated to be less than that for mucous membrane exposures (10). The risk for transmission of HIV by exposure to fluids or tissues other than blood is unknown, but is likely considerably lower than for blood exposures (11).

Several factors may influence the risk of transmission of HIV after an occupational exposure. A retrospective case-controlled study of percutaneous exposures of HCP to HIV-infected source patients found that significant risk factors for seroconversion were as follows: (1) deep injury, (2) injury with a device that was visibly contaminated with blood, (3) a procedure that involved a needle placed in the source patient's artery or vein, and (4) an exposure to a source patient who died of AIDS within 2 months after the exposure (12). It is thought that these risk factors may be a surrogate for high viral inoculum (large amount of blood and high viral titer), but this has not been proven. There may be other factors influencing the risk of transmission of HIV in an occupational exposure including the strain of the HIV virus of the source patient and the host immune response to the exposure (2).

The utility of the source patient's HIV viral load measurement in assessing risk for HIV transmission in an exposure has not been established. A lower viral load (e.g., <1500 RNA copies/mL), or one that is below the limits of detection, does not rule out the possibility of transmission of HIV in an exposure. There may be latently infected cells that can transmit HIV in the absence of viremia (2). Occupational transmission of HIV has been documented in a source patient with an undetectable viral load (13).

Occupationally Acquired HIV

As of December 2001, there were a total of 57 HCP with documented occupationally acquired HIV infections and 138 possible occupationally acquired HIV infections in the United States. The HCP with possible occupationally acquired HIV infections had a history of occupational exposure to blood, body fluids, or laboratory specimens containing HIV, without other risk factors for HIV infection, but HIV seroconversion in temporal association with a specific occupational exposure was not documented (14).

Of the 57 documented occupationally acquired HIV infections, 49 (86%) of the HCP were exposed to blood, 3 were exposed to concentrated HIV in a laboratory, 1 was exposed to exudates from a visibly bloody skin lesion, and 4 were exposed to body fluids that were not specified. The major route of exposure was percutaneous. Forty-eight (84%) of the HCP sustained 49 percutaneous injuries (one HCP sustained two percutaneous injuries within 10 days). Other routes of exposure included two concurrent percutaneous and mucocutaneous exposures, six mucocutaneous exposures, and one unknown route of exposure in a laboratory worker. The sharp objects involved in 51 percutaneous injuries (including one health care worker that sustained two percutaneous injuries and two health care workers who sustained both a percutaneous and mucocutaneous injury) include 45 (88%) hollow-bore needles, two broken pieces of glass from blood-collection tubes, two scalpels, and two unknown sharp devices/objects. Of the 55 known source patients, 38 (69%) had AIDS, 2 (4%) were symptomatic for HIV, and 6 (11%) were asymptomatic. The clinical status of nine (16%) source patients is unknown (14).

Data regarding the timing of seroconversion and clinical characteristics in HCP are limited. Health care personnel with occupationally acquired HIV infection, for which data are available, presented with a syndrome consistent with primary HIV infection in 81% of cases with a median of 35 days after exposure (15). In 51 HCP, the estimated median time interval from exposure to seroconversion was 46 days (mean of 65 days). An estimated 95% of HCP seroconverted within 6 months. There were two delayed HIV seroconversions occurring between 6 months and 1 year after the exposure. In one unusual case, the HCP was exposed to an HIV/HCV coinfected source patient, developed both HIV and HCV from this exposure, and had a rapidly fatal HCV disease course (16, 17).

PATHOPHYSIOLOGY/MICROBIOLOGY

Hepatitis B Postexposure Prophylaxis—Efficacy

Newborns given hepatitis B immune globulin (HBIG) and hepatitis B vaccine at birth for perinatal exposure to a hepatitis B surface antigen-positive/hepatitis Be antigen-positive mother is 85–95% effective in preventing HBV infection in the neonate. Multiple doses of HBIG given to HCP within 1 week following percutaneous exposure to hepatitis B surface antigen-positive blood are estimated to provide 75% protection from HBV infection. Although not studied in occupational exposures, the combination of HBIG and hepatitis B vaccine should have an increased efficacy over HBIG alone, as in the perinatal setting. The hepatitis B vaccine series should be started on any unvac-

cinated HCP presenting with an occupational exposure, since they are at continued risk for HBV exposure (2).

Hepatitis B Postexposure Prophylaxis—Safety

Hepatitis B vaccines have been administered to 100 million persons in the United States as of the year 2000. The most common side effects of the hepatitis B vaccine are fever and pain at the injection site. These side effects were no more frequently observed in vaccine recipients than in placebo recipients. The estimated incidence of anaphylaxis is 1 in 600,000 hepatitis B vaccine recipients (2).

Hepatitis B immune globulin is prepared from plasma containing a high titer of antibody to hepatitis B surface antigen (anti-HBs), and precautions are taken to eliminate HBV, HCV, and HIV from the final product. Rare serious adverse events from HBIG such as angioedema, urticaria, and anaphylaxis have occurred. Local pain and tenderness at the HBIG injection site have also occurred. Neither hepatitis B vaccine nor HBIG is contraindicated in pregnancy or lactation (2).

Hepatitis C Postexposure Management

Hepatitis C postexposure prophylaxis with either immune globulin, or antiviral agents (such as interferon with or without ribavirin) is not recommended for several reasons: (a) hepatitis C infection does not produce a protective antibody response, (b) animal studies with immunoglobulin containing hepatitis C antibodies failed to prevent transmission of HCV after exposure, (c) current immunoglobulin products no longer contain antibodies to HCV because plasma donors are eliminated from the donor pool if they are HCV positive, (d) no clinical trials have been conducted to assess the efficacy of using antiviral agents (such as interferon with, or without, ribavirin) for HCV PEP, and (e) interferon may not be an effective treatment for HCV unless the infection is already established (2, 3).

Rather than PEP for HCV exposures, early identification and referral for possible treatment of a seroconversion is the goal. There are still unresolved issues regarding treatment of HCV seroconversions. The therapy for HCV (interferon with, or without, ribavirin) is long (6–12 months) and is associated with significant toxicities. Since 15–25% of patients with acute HCV infection spontaneously resolve their infection, early treatment may be unnecessary for some exposed HCP. There is no information on treating acute HCV infection without evidence of disease. Early treatment of chronic disease might be as effective as treatment of acute infection. The appropriate regimen for treatment of acute HCV is unknown (2).

HIV Postexposure Prophylaxis

Rationale for HIV postexposure prophylaxis

Animal models of primary HIV infection and PEP, along with human data in the prevention of maternal-fetal transmission of HIV, and occupational PEP form the rationale for HIV PEP.

Pathogenesis of primary HIV infection

A primate model of mucosal exposure to simian immunodeficiency virus (SIV) demonstrated that SIV is picked up by dendritic-like cells at the inoculation site within the first 24 h, and then migrates to the regional lymph nodes within 24–48 h. Within 5 days the virus is detectable in blood (18). This model suggests that there may be a window of opportunity between exposure and systemic infection to abort or prevent the infection with antiretrovirals.

Animal models of HIV postexposure prophylaxis

Several animal models suggest that antiretrovirals have efficacy when used as PEP. They also suggest that there is decreased efficacy of PEP when there is a larger viral innocula, delayed initiation of PEP, shortened duration of PEP, or decreased dose of PEP (individual drugs or combinations) (2).

Data in HIV postexposure prophylaxis in humans

Prevention of Maternal-fetal Transmission of HIV

The Pediatric AIDS Clinical Trials Group conducted a landmark trial (Protocol 076) to assess the safety and efficacy of zidovudine (AZT) treatment to reduce mother-to-infant transmission of HIV. This study was a randomized, double blind, placebo controlled, and prospective trial of zidovudine given to the mother during pregnancy, labor, and delivery, and to the infant for 6 weeks after birth. The zidovudine treatment group had a 67% relative reduction in the risk of HIV transmission as compared to the placebo group (19). Only a small part of the protective efficacy of zidovudine treatment could be explained by the reduction in viral load in the maternal blood, suggesting that there may be another mechanism of protective efficacy of zidovudine (20). Maternal-fetal transmission of HIV is different from occupational transmission in many ways, so the extent to which this information is applicable to the prevention of occupational transmission of HIV is uncertain.

Data in occupational HIV postexposure prophylaxis

There are no data from prospective, randomized, and controlled trials of antiretrovirals in PEP of occupational exposures to HIV. Since seroconversion is infrequent, a prospective trial would require enrolling thousands of HCP to achieve statistical power to demonstrate efficacy. The CDC's retrospective case-control study of HIV seroconversion in HCP following percutaneous exposure to HIV-infected blood demonstrated that zidovudine is protective. Zidovudine is associated with 81% reduction (95% CI = 43–94%) in the risk of occupational HIV infection (12).

Failure of HIV postexposure prophylaxis

There have been 21 instances of failure of HIV PEP reported in the United States and abroad. In 16 cases zidovudine was used alone, in two cases zidovudine and didanosine (ddI) were used in combination, and three cases had a combination of three or more drugs used for PEP. The source patients were antiretroviral experienced in 13 cases. Seven cases had antiviral resistance testing of the source patient's HIV strain performed, and in four of those cases, there was reduced susceptibility to zidovudine and/or other antiretrovirals used for PEP. In addition to possible exposure of the HCP to a resistant HIV strain, other contributing factors to failure of PEP may have included a high titer and/or large inoculum of HIV in the exposure, delayed initiation, and/or shortened duration of PEP. Possible host factors such as poor cellular immunity, and source patient's virus factors may have also contributed to the failure of PEP (2).

HIV postexposure prophylaxis toxicity in health care personnel

Antiretrovirals used in occupational PEP include the nucleoside reverse transcriptase inhibitors (NRTIs), nonnucleoside reverse transcriptase inhibitors (NNRTIs), and protease inhibitors (PIs). All of these medications have side effects and toxicities, and several have significant drug interactions. Data from the National Surveillance System for Health Care Workers (NaSH) and the HIV Postexposure Prophylaxis Registry indicate that nearly half of HCP experience adverse symptoms while taking PEP, and approximately 33% stop the medications due to adverse signs or symptoms. Commonly reported symptoms included nausea, fatigue, malaise, headache, vomiting, diarrhea, myalgias, and arthralgias. Some data indicate that three-drug combination PEP has more side effects and discontinuations than two-drug combination PEP regimens (2, 21).

Serious Adverse Events Associated with Occupational Postexposure Prophylaxis

Serious adverse events, although rare, have been reported in HCP taking antiretrovirals for occupational PEP. Serious adverse events include "almost intractable vomiting," nausea, involuntary eye movements, nephrolithiasis, high fever, rash, hepatitis, pancytopenia, and hyperglycemia (2, 21, 22). One case report from France described sudden bilateral hearing loss associated with dizziness and tinnitus less than 2 weeks after the completion of stavudine, lamivudine, and nevirapine for PEP (23).

Serious Adverse Events Associated with Nevirapine Use in Postexposure Prophylaxis

There were 22 serious adverse events associated with nevirapine when used as HIV PEP reported to the Food and Drug Agency (FDA) between March 1997 and September 2000. Twelve cases of hepatotoxicity were reported, two of which were life threatening, and one of those required a liver transplant. There were 14 skin reactions which included one documented and two possible cases of Stevens-Johnson syndrome. One case of rhabdomyolysis was reported. There were four cases of both hepatotoxicity and skin reaction, and one case of both rhabdomyolysis and skin reaction (24). In light of these reports, nevirapine is generally not recommended for use in occupational PEP (2).

CLINICAL PRESENTATION

In most health care institutions the emergency department plays a major role in providing occupational PEP on a 24-h basis. Health care personnel will usually present shortly after the exposure. An evaluation of the circumstances surrounding the exposure, the source of the exposure, and the HCP's medical condition needs to be performed in order to make decisions about PEP. In many instances they will follow up with their primary provider, or occupational health consultant, after the initial emergency department visit.

Exposure Evaluation

Percutaneous injury is defined as an exposure that may place a HCP at risk for HBV, HCV, or HIV (e.g., a needlestick or cut with a sharp object), or contact of mucous membrane or nonintact skin (e.g., exposed skin that is chapped, abraded, or afflicted with dermatitis) with blood, tissue, or other body fluids that are potentially infectious. Potentially infectious fluid or tissue includes blood and body fluids containing visible blood, semen and vaginal secretions, cerebrospinal fluid, synovial fluid, pleural fluid, peritoneal fluid, pericardial fluid, amniotic fluid, and concentrated virus in a research laboratory or production facility. Of note, feces, nasal secretions, saliva, sputum, sweat, tears, urine, and vomitus are not considered potentially infectious unless they contain blood (2).

Human bites must be evaluated to include the possibility that both the person bitten and the person who inflicted the bite were exposed to bloodborne pathogens (2).

For each type of exposure, an estimate of the severity of the exposure needs to be obtained. For mucous membrane or nonintact skin exposures, an example of a small-volume exposure would be a few drops, and an example of a large-volume exposure would be a major blood splash. An example of a less severe percutaneous injury would be a superficial injury caused by a solid needle. A more severe percutaneous injury is one that involves a large-bore hollow needle, deep puncture wound, visible blood on the device, or a needle that was used in a patient's artery or vein (2).

Source Patient Evaluation

The person whose blood or body fluid is the source of the exposure needs to be evaluated for HBV, HCV, and HIV. This information may be obtained from the medical record, or from the source patient himself. The source should be informed of the exposure and tested for serologic evidence of bloodborne pathogens. Follow local and state laws regarding procedures (including informed consent) for testing source patients and maintain confidentiality of the source patient at all times. Any source patient who is found to be positive for HBV, HCV, or HIV should be referred for appropriate counseling and treatment (2).

In many instances the HBV, HCV, and HIV status of the source is unknown. The source patient's past medical history, including blood transfusion history, current medical condition, and social history including injecting-drug use history, and sexual history should be obtained if possible. Recent sexual contact, or the sharing of needles during illicit drug use, of the source patient with a known

HBV, HCV, or HIV positive person should be noted if possible (2).

Evaluate the source patient for the possibility of primary HIV infection where the HIV testing may be falsely negative. There is a "window period" from the time of infection until the HIV antibody is detectable by enzyme immunoassay (EIA) or Western blot. Presenting signs and symptoms of primary HIV infection include fever, fatigue, rash (usually maculapapular/morbilliform), headache, lymphadenopathy, pharyngitis, myalgias, arthralgias, nausea, vomiting, diarrhea, night sweats, aseptic meningitis, oral ulcers, genital ulcers, thrombocytopenia, leucopenia, and elevated liver enzymes. The acute illness may start days to weeks after exposure to HIV, and usually lasts for less than 14 days. Patients with primary HIV have high plasma viral RNA levels (25).

For a source patient who is known to be HIV positive, obtain available information about the source patient's stage of infection (symptomatic, asymptomatic, or acquired immunodeficiency syndrome (AIDS)), the most recent CD4+ T-cell count and viral load result, the antiretroviral history, and current antiretroviral use. HIV-positive class 1 patients are asymptomatic or have a known low viral load (< 1500 RNA copies/mL). HIV-positive class 2 patients are symptomatic for HIV, have AIDS, acute seroconversion (primary HIV), or known high viral load. Any information on phenotypic or genotypic viral resistance testing should be obtained if available. There may be a need to alter PEP if there is known or suspected antiretroviral resistance in the source patient. If this information on antiretroviral resistance is not readily available, do not delay the initiation of PEP, if indicated. The PEP regimen can be changed later, if needed (2).

If the source of the exposure is unknown, such as a needle in a sharps container, evaluate the circumstance around the exposure, the setting of the exposure, and the prevalence of bloodborne pathogens in the population where the exposure occurred. It is not recommended to test needles or sharps for the presence of HBV, HCV, or HIV. The reliability of the test results in this instance is unknown, and it is hazardous for personnel to handle the sharp instrument (2).

Health Care Personnel Evaluation

Assess the HCP's past medical history and current medical condition, including a complete list of medications. Pay particular attention to the presence of renal insufficiency, liver disease, pregnancy, or breastfeeding in the HCP. These conditions may alter the choice of PEP for the HCP. The hepatitis B vaccination status of the HCP and response to the vaccine if known should be assessed (2).

LABORATORY/DIAGNOSTIC TESTING

Source Patient

Test the source patient for hepatitis B surface antigen (HBsAg), hepatitis C antibody (anti-HCV), and antibody to HIV by enzyme immunoassay (EIA) as soon as possible. Repeatedly reactive results by EIA for anti-HCV should be confirmed by another test such as recombinant immunoblot assay (RIBA) or HCV polymerase chain reaction (PCR). Consider using a rapid HIV-antibody test kit for occupational exposures. A positive EIA or rapid HIV test will need to be confirmed with a Western blot or immunofluorescent antibody before informing the source patient of the result. If the source patient is negative for HIV by EIA or a rapid HIV test and has no clinical evidence of HIV or AIDS, no further testing is indicated. It is unlikely that the source patient will be in the "window period" without symptoms of primary HIV. Direct virus assays for HIV and HCV (HIV p24 antigen EIA, HIV RNA, HCV RNA) for routine screening of the source patient are not recommended. Do not test needles or sharps for the presence of bloodborne pathogens (2).

Health Care Personnel

Perform baseline testing of the HCP for anti-HBs, anti-HCV, alanine amino transferase (ALT), and HIV-antibody. Offer pregnancy testing to women of childbearing potential. For those HCP who will be started on PEP, perform baseline complete blood count, renal and hepatic function tests, glucose, and urinalysis (2).

MANAGEMENT

Exposure management involves local wound care to the injury, reporting of the incident, obtaining baseline studies of the source patient and the HCP, assessing the need for PEP by evaluating the exposure and the source patient for risk of transmission of HIV, HBV, or HCV, prescribing PEP medications if needed, and follow-up of the HCP.

Local Wound Care

Immediate first aid to the HCP's wound should be administered. Wash the HCP's wounds and skin that have been in contact with blood or body fluids with soap and water.

There is no evidence that the use of antiseptics or squeezing the wound to express fluid from the site reduces the risk of transmission of bloodborne infections. Antiseptic use is not contraindicated, however. The use of caustic agents such as bleach, or the injection of antiseptics or disinfectants into the wound is not recommended (2). Mucous membranes (nose and mouth) should be vigorously flushed with water. Eyes should be irrigated with clean water, saline, or sterile eye irrigants. Routine wound decontamination and repair should be implemented as usual. Human bite wounds may require antibiotic prophylaxis, depending on the site and severity. Tetanus prophylaxis may be indicated (26).

Report the Incident

Report the incident according to institutional, federal (including the Occupational Safety and Health Administration (OSHA)), and state regulations. The exposure report should contain the date and time of the exposure, and details of where and how the exposure occurred. If a sharp device is involved in an exposure, report the type and brand of the device, and when in the course of using the device the exposure occurred. Details of the exposure including the type of exposure (percutaneous or mucocutaneous), severity of the exposure, and available information on the source of the exposure should also be included in the report (2).

Hepatitis B Virus Postexposure Prophylaxis

Any health care personnel who may be exposed to blood, body fluids, or contaminated sharp objects should be vaccinated against hepatitis B, ideally prior to any exposure. The hepatitis B vaccine series is a three-dose series, and HCP should be tested for anti-HBs 1–2 months after completion of the series. A nonresponder is a HCP with an inadequate response to vaccination (i.e., anti-HBs <10 mIU/mL). Persons who do not respond to the primary vaccine series should complete a second three-dose series, since they have a 30–50% chance of responding to the second series. Nonresponders should also be tested to see if they are hepatitis B surface antigen-positive. Any HCP requiring a second series should be tested for anti-HBs after completion of the second series (2).

The hepatitis B vaccine series should be started for any blood or body fluid exposure in an unvaccinated HCP. Hepatitis B virus PEP depends on the vaccination status and vaccine-response status of the exposed HCP, and the hepatitis B surface antigen status of the source patient. When HBIG and/or hepatitis B vaccine is indicated, they should be given as soon as possible (preferably within 24 h) after the exposure. Hepatitis B vaccine should always be administered in the deltoid muscle. When HBIG and hepatitis B vaccine are to be given at the same time, always give them in separate sites (see Table 35–1 for management recommendations (2)).

Hepatitis C Virus Postexposure Management

No PEP with immunoglobulin, interferon, or ribavirin is recommended at the present time for HCV exposures. After baseline testing of the source patient and HCP is performed, arrange for follow-up of the HCP. There are no definitive recommendations on management of HCV-exposed HCP. Several strategies are outlined below. Each institution needs to formulate a plan so that HCP exposed to HCV who seroconvert are referred to local experts experienced in HCV therapy for evaluation and treatment if appropriate. Further study is needed in order for definitive recommendations on management of HCP HCV exposures.

Strategy 1—Conventional Approach

Perform follow-up testing at 4–6 months for anti-HCV and ALT. If earlier diagnosis of HCV infection is desired, test for HCV RNA at 4–6 weeks following the exposure. All anti-HCV (EIA) results should be confirmed by a supplemental anti-HCV test such as a recombinant immunoblot assay (RIBA). Refer HCP to an expert in HCV management if seroconversion occurs (2).

Strategy 2—Preemptive Therapy of Early HCV Infection

Monitor HCP exposed to HCV at 2-week intervals after exposure by using PCR for HCV RNA. If the HCP has a documented seroconversion, by having a repeatedly positive HCV RNA PCR assays, start interferon therapy at that time (3).

Strategy 3—Watchful Waiting

Monitor HCP exposed to HCV at 2-week intervals after exposure by using PCR for HCV RNA, and perform anti-HCV antibody tests at 3-month intervals after exposure, or when HCV RNA is detected by PCR. If seroconversion is detected by PCR, follow the HCP by checking ALT and HCV RNA by PCR over time. Treat individuals who remain positive for HCV RNA by PCR and have elevated ALT two to four months after diagnosis of seroconversion.

Table 35–1. Hepatitis B Postexposure Prophylaxis

Vaccination and Antibody Response Status of Exposed Workers[a]	Treatment Recommendations		
	Source Hepatitis B Surface Antigen (HBsAg) Positive	**Source Hepatitis B Surface Antigen (HBsAg) Negative**	**Source Unknown or Not Available for Testing**
Unvaccinated	Hepatitis B immune globulin (HBIG) X 1 and initiate the hepatitis B vaccine series	Initiate hepatitis B vaccine series	Initiate hepatitis B vaccine series
Previously vaccinated Known responder who has adequate levels of serum antibody to HbsAg (i.e., serum anti-HBs ≥ 10 mIU/mL)	No treatment	No treatment	No treatment
Previously vaccinated Known nonresponder who has inadequate response to vaccination (i.e., serum anti-HBs < 10 mIU/mL)	HBIG X 1 and initiate revaccination for nonresponders who have not completed the second three-dose vaccine series OR HBIG X 2 for those that did not respond to the second vaccine series. The first dose of HBIG should be given as soon as possible following the exposure. The second dose of HBIG should be given one month later.	No treatment	If known high risk source, treat as if source were HBsAg positive
Previously vaccinated Antibody response unknown	Test exposed person for antibody to hepatitis B (anti-HBs) 1. If adequate antibody response (anti-HBs ≥ 10 mIU/mL), no treatment is needed 2. If inadequate antibody response (anti-HBs < 10 mIU/mL) give HBIG X 1 and hepatitis B vaccine booster	No treatment	Test exposed person for antibody to hepatitis B (anti-HBs) 1. If adequate antibody response (anti-HBs ≥ 10 mIU/mL), no treatment is needed 2. If inadequate antibody response (anti-HBs < 10 mIU/mL) give hepatitis B vaccine booster and recheck titer in 1–2 months

[a](Persons who have previously been infected with HBV are immune to reinfection and do not require postexposure prophylaxis).
HBIG dose is 0.06 mL/kg intramuscularly

Source: Adapted from Updated U. S. Public Health Service guidelines published in 2001 (reference 2).

This strategy is designed to avoid treating HCP who spontaneously resolve their infection. The optimal treatment regimen is not specified (3).

HIV Postexposure Prophylaxis

After assessment of the risk of HIV transmission for a particular exposure, discuss with the HCP the risks and benefits of PEP. (Note: The antiretrovirals have been FDA-approved for treatment of HIV infection, but have not been FDA-approved for PEP.) The PEP "basic" regimen consists of two nucleoside reverse transcriptase inhibitors (NRTIs) zidovudine (ZDV, or AZT) and lamivudine (3TC), or lamivudine and stavudine (d4T), or didanosine (ddI) and stavudine. Most HIV exposures will warrant the two-drug regimen. A third drug is added to the regimen to form an "expanded" regimen when there is an exposure with an increased risk for transmission of HIV, or the source patient's virus is known or suspected to be resistant to one or more drugs in the PEP regimen. Antiretrovirals for PEP should be chosen based on the likelihood that the source patient's virus should be susceptible to the regimen. Expert consultation is advised in the selection of antiretrovirals for PEP for source patients with antiviral resistance issues. However, prompt initiation of PEP should not be delayed if expert consultation and antiviral resistance information about the source patient's virus are not readily available. There is a 24-h, seven-days-a-week National Clinician's Post-Exposure Prophylaxis Hotline (PEPline) at (888) 448-4911 that provides consultation for questions related to occupational exposures to bloodborne pathogens. The PEP regimen can be altered if needed after it has been started. The PEP "expanded" regimen consists of the "basic regimen" plus one of the following: indinavir (IDV), nelfinavir (NFV), efavirenz (EFV), or abacavir (ABC). Abacavir has been associated with a severe hypersensitivity reaction that can be fatal, so this author recommends abacavir use in PEP only with expert consultation. Other antiretrovirals that should be used only with expert consultation include ritonavir (RTV), saquinivir soft-gel formulation (SQV), amprenavir (AMP), delaverdine (DLV), and lopinavir/ritonavir. Nevirapine (NVP) is generally not recommended for use in PEP due to the adverse events reported previously (2).

The HIV Postexposure Prophylaxis table (Table 35–2) outlines the recommendations for PEP use based on the infection status of the source and the exposure type and severity. The term "consider PEP" means that PEP is optional and the decision should be made between the treating clinician and the exposed HCP based on the circumstances surrounding the exposure. For exposures due to an unknown source or a source of unknown HIV status, consider basic two-drug PEP if the source has risk factors for HIV, or if the setting where the exposure occurred suggests a risk for HIV. No PEP is warranted for exposures to an HIV-negative source. If PEP is started, and the source patient is later found to be HIV negative, discontinue PEP. Consider basic two-drug PEP for small-volume mucous membrane exposure to an HIV-positive class 1 source. Basic two-drug PEP is recommended for less severe percutaneous injuries from HIV-positive class 1 source patients, large-volume mucous membrane exposures to an HIV-positive class 1 source, and small-volume mucous membrane exposures to an HIV-positive class 2 source.

Three-drug expanded regimen is recommended for more severe percutaneous exposures to an HIV-positive class 1 source, any percutaneous exposure to an HIV-positive class 2 source, or large-volume mucous membrane exposures to an HIV-positive class 2 source (2). See HIV postexposure prophylaxis table (Table 35–2) and antiretrovirals used for HIV postexposure prophylaxis table (Table 35–3). An outstanding resource is the Guidelines for the Use of Antiretroviral Agents in HIV-Infected Adults and Adolescents which may be found on the AIDSinfo website http://aidsinfo.nih.gov/ (27). Other resources for clinicians managing occupational exposures are listed in Table 35–4.

HIV PEP should be considered an urgent medical concern and initiated as soon as possible. The emergency department should have medications for PEP readily available for use. PEP should be administered for 4 weeks when prescribed (2).

SPECIAL CIRCUMSTANCES

Expert consultation is advised for HIV PEP for delayed exposure report, anunknown source, pregnancy (known or suspected) in the exposed person, resistance of the source virus to antiretrovirals, and toxicity of the PEP regimen. Consult local experts and/or the National Clinicians' PEP Hotline (888) 448-4911 in these situations (2). Nonoccupational HIV postexposure prophylaxis is briefly discussed in this section.

Delayed Exposure Report

In animal studies, PEP is much less effective when started later than 24–36 h after the exposure. In humans, there are no data on the time interval after an exposure after which PEP is ineffective. If an exposure occurs over 36 h prior to the HCP's presentation to the ED, and the exposure warrants PEP, PEP should be prescribed. The interval after which PEP has no benefit is undefined (2).

Table 35–2. HIV Postexposure Prophylaxis

Infection Status of Source	Mucous membrane and nonintact skin (evidence of compromised skin integrity (e.g., dermatitis, abrasion, or open wound)) Small volume exposure (i.e., a few drops)	Mucous membrane and nonintact skin (evidence of compromised skin integrity (e.g., dermatitis, abrasion, or open wound)) Large volume exposure (i.e., major blood splash)	Percutaneous Less severe exposure (i.e., solid needle and superficial injury)	Percutaneous More severe exposure (e.g., large-bore hollow needle, deep puncture, visible blood on device, or needle used in a patient's artery or vein)
HIV-positive class 1 Asymptomatic HIV infection, or known low viral load (e.g., < 1500 RNA copies/mL).[a]	Consider basic two-drug PEP[b]	Recommend basic two-drug PEP	Recommend basic two-drug PEP	Recommend expanded three-drug PEP
HIV-positive class 2 Symptomatic HIV infection, AIDS, acute seroconversion, or known high viral load.[a]	Recommend basic two-drug PEP	Recommend expanded three-drug PEP	Recommend expanded three-drug PEP	Recommend expanded three-drug PEP
Unknown source or source of unknown HIV status	Generally, no PEP warranted; however, consider basic two-drug PEP[b] for source with HIV risk factors[c], or in settings where exposure to HIV-infected persons is likely	Generally, no PEP warranted; however, consider basic two-drug PEP[b] for source with HIV risk factors[c], or in settings where exposure to HIV-infected persons is likely	Generally, no PEP warranted; however, consider basic two-drug PEP[b] for source with HIV risk factors[c], or in settings where exposure to HIV-infected persons is likely	Generally, no PEP warranted; however, consider basic two-drug PEP[b] for source with HIV risk factors[c], or in settings where exposure to HIV-infected persons is likely
HIV Negative	No PEP warranted	No PEP warranted	No PEP warranted	No PEP warranted

[a]If drug resistance is a concern, obtain expert consultation. Initiation of postexposure prophylaxis (PEP) should not be delayed pending expert consultation.

[b]The designation "consider PEP" indicates that PEP is optional and should be based on an individual decision between the exposed person and the treating clinician.

[c]If PEP is offered and taken and the source is later determined to be HIV negative, PEP should be discontinued.

Source: Adapted from Updated U. S. Public Health Service guidelines published in 2001 (reference 2).

Table 35–3. Antiretrovirals Used for HIV Postexposure Prophylaxis

Antiretroviral	Dose	Side Effects	Drug Interactions	Comments
		Basic Regimen		
Zidovudine (RETROVIR™; ZDV; AZT)	300 mg twice daily	Macrocytic anemia, neutropenia, GI intolerance, headache, insomnia, asthenia, lactic acidosis with hepatic steatosis (rare but potentially life-threatening toxicity associated with the use of NRTIs)		Can be given as a single tablet (COMBIVIR™) twice daily
Plus				
Lamivudine (EPIVIR™. 3TC)	150 mg twice daily			Take with or without food Dosage adjustment in renal insufficiency
Lamivudine (3TC)	150 mg twice daily	Lactic acidosis with hepatic steatosis (higher incidence with d4T than other NRTIs), peripheral neuropathy, lipodystrophy, pancreatitis, hyperlipidemia		Take with or without food Dosage adjustment in renal insufficiency
Plus				
Stavudine (ZERIT™; d4T)	40 mg twice daily Note: if body weight is <60 kg, 30 mg twice daily			
Didanosine (VIDEX™EC, delayed-release capsule; ddI)	400 mg once daily Note: if body weight is <60 kg mg once daily	Serious toxicity (e.g., neuropathy, pancreatitis, or hepatitis) can occur. Fatal and nonfatal pancreatitis has occurred in HIV-positive, treatment-naive patients. Patients taking ddI and d4T should be carefully assessed and closely monitored for pancreatitis, lactic acidosis, and hepatitis. Nausea, diarrhea		Take didanosine 1 h before or 2 h after a meal Dosage adjustment in renal insufficiency.
Plus				
Stavudine (ZERIT™; d4T)	40 mg twice daily Note: if body weight is <60 kg, 30 mg twice daily			

(continued)

Table 35–3. Antiretrovirals Used for HIV Postexposure Prophylaxis (*Continued*)

Antiretroviral	Dose	Side Effects	Drug Interactions	Comments
		Expanded Regimen—Basic regimen plus one of the following:		
Indinavir (CRIXIVAN™, IDV)	800 mg every 8 h	Serious toxicity (e.g., nephrolithiasis) can occur; GI intolerance, nausea, indirect hyperbilirubinemia, headache, asthenia, rash, hyperglycemia, fat maldistribution, hyperlipidemia	Concomitant use of astemizole, terfenadine, dihydroergotamine, ergotamine, ergonovine, methylergonovine, rifampin, cisapride, St. John's Wort, lovastatin, simvastatin, pimozide, midazolam, or triazolam is not recommended.	Take 1 h before or 2 h after a meal. May take with skim milk or low fat meal. Must drink eight glasses of fluid per day to prevent nephrolithiasis. Dosage adjustment in hepatic insufficiency. Hyperbilirubinemia common; must avoid this drug during late pregnancy
Nelfinavir (VIRACEPT™, NFV)	750 mg (5–250 mg tablets) three times daily, with meals or snack, or 1250 mg (2–625 mg tablets) twice daily	Diarrhea, hyperlipidemia, hyperglycemia, fat maldistribution, serum transaminase elevation	Concomitant use of astemizole, terfenadine, dihydroergotamine, ergotamine, ergonovine, methylergonovine, rifampin, cisapride, St. John's Wort, lovastatin, simvastatin, pimozide, midazolam, or triazolam is not recommended. Might accelerate the clearance of certain drugs, including oral contraceptives (requiring alternative or additional contraceptive measures for women taking these drugs).	Take with a meal or snack

Drug	Dose	Adverse Effects	Drug Interactions	Comments
Efavirenz (SUSTIVA™; EFV)	600 mg daily, at bedtime	Drug is associated with rash (early onset) that can be severe and might rarely progress to Stevens–Johnson syndrome. Nervous system side effects (e.g., dizziness, somnolence, insomnia, and/or abnormal dreaming) are common. Severe psychiatric symptoms are possible (dosing before bedtime might minimize these side effects). Increased transaminase levels	Concomitant use of astemizole, cisapride, midazolam, triazolam, ergot derivatives, or St. John's Wort is not recommended because inhibition of the metabolism of these drugs could create the potential for serious and/or life-threatening adverse events (e.g., cardiac arrhythmias, prolonged sedation, or respiratory depression)	Should not be used during pregnancy because of concerns about teratogenicity
Abacavir (ZIAGEN™; ABC)	300 mg twice a day	Severe hypersensitivity reactions can occur, usually within the first 6 weeks of treatment. They can be fatal. Symptoms may include fever, rash, nausea, vomiting, malaise or fatigue, loss of appetite, respiratory symptoms such as sore throat, cough, shortness of breath		available as TRIZIVIR™ (a combination of ZDV, 3TC, and ABC) one tablet twice a day. Take with or without food Expert Consultation advised due to the possibility of severe hypersensitivity reaction

NRTIs—Nucleoside Reverse Transcriptase Inhibitors

Source: Adapted from (2) (MMWR 2001), and (27) Guidelines for the Use of Antiretroviral Agents in HIV-Infected Adults and Adolescents. MMWR 2002;51 (No.RR-7) Updated as a Living Document on October 29, 2004 [tables 10-12 page 58-62]. Located on the AIDSinfo website http://aidsinfo.nih.gov/.

Table 35–4. Occupational Exposure Resources for Clinicians

- CDC. Updated U.S. Public Health Service guidelines for the management of occupational exposures to HBV, HCV, and HIV and recommendations for postexposure prophylaxis. MMWR 2001;50(No. RR-11):1-52. http://www.cdc.gov/mmwr/preview/mmwrhtml/rr5011a1.ht
- National Clinicin's Post-Exposure Prophylaxis Hotline (PEPline) 24 hours a day/7 days a week
  - (888)-HIV-4911 or (888)-448-4911
- Needlestick! an interactive website for exposure case management located at www.needlestick.mednet.ucla.edu
- Any serious adverse events with antiretrovirals used in HIV PEP should be reported to the FDA's MedWath Program at
  - (800) FDA-1088 or (800) 332-1088 or www.fda.gov/medwatch
- Guidelines for the Use of Antiretroviral Agents in HIV-Infected Adults and Adolescents. MMWR 2002;51 (No.RR-7) Updated as a Living.

An Unknown Source

"Needle found down" is a common scenario. The decision to use PEP should be made on a case-by-case basis based on the circumstances of the exposure. It is not recommended to test needles or other sharps involved in exposures because the reliability of the test is unknown, and the person handling the sharps may be at risk for injury (2).

Known or Suspected Pregnancy in Health Care Personnel

Hepatitis B virus postexposure prophylaxis

Neither hepatitis B vaccine or HBIG are contraindicated in pregnancy or lactation (2).

Hepatitis C virus postexposure management

Although there is no recommendation for postexposure prophylaxis for exposures to HCV, the treatment of HCV infection is problematic in pregnant patients and anyone with reproductive potential. Ribavirin is teratogenic and must not be used for treatment of hepatitis C if there is a possibility of pregnancy in the HCP or the sexual partner of the HCP. Pregnancy must be avoided in the HCP or the sexual partner of the HCP during therapy with ribavirin and for 6 months after completion of treatment.

HIV postexposure prophylaxis

Evaluate the exposure, risk of transmission of HIV, and need for PEP as with any other HCP. The risks and benefits to both the HCP and the fetus should be discussed with the HCP and her health care providers. Efavirenz (Sustiva) should be avoided in pregnancy. It has been shown to be teratogenic in primates. There are recent reports of fatal and nonfatal lactic acidosis in HIV-infected pregnant women on didanosine (ddI) and stavudine (d4T), therefore this combination should be avoided, and prescribed only when the potential benefits outweigh the risk. Indinavir should not be given to pregnant women shortly before delivery, because of the hyperbilirubinemia risk in the neonate. In France, there were two cases of progressive neurologic disease and death due to mitochondrial dysfunction in infants exposed to zidovudine (AZT) and lamivudine (3TC). There have been no reports of deaths in the United States perinatal HIV cohorts due to mitochondrial dysfunction from zidovudine (AZT) and lamivudine (3TC) (2, 28).

Other antiretrovirals not recommended in pregnancy include the following: zalcitabine (ddC), which is potentially teratogenic in animal models; delaverdine, which is potentially teratogenic and carcinogenic; amprenavir oral solution which contains high levels of propylene glycol that may not be metabolized adequately in pregnancy; and a newer agent, atazanavir, which has a potential for hyperbilirubinemia in the neonate. The AIDSinfo website http://aidsinfo.nih.gov/ contains information on antiretroviral use in pregnancy in the Guidelines for the Use of Antiretroviral Agents in HIV-Infected Adults and Adolescents (29).

Antiretroviral Resistance in the Source Patient's Virus

Antiretroviral resistance (known or suspected) in the source patient's virus is a concern for those who prescribe

PEP. Surveys have shown that source patient's virus isolates have had resistance to antiretrovirals, and that occupational transmission of resistant virus has occurred (2).

The source patient's antiretroviral history and resistance testing results may not be available for review at the time the HCP presents to the emergency department for PEP evaluation. The clinician should suspect antiretroviral resistance in the source patient if he is having clinical progression of disease, increasing viral load, and/or decreasing CD4 T-cell count while on therapy. Antiretroviral resistance testing of the source patient at the time of the exposure will not help with the choice of empiric PEP medications, because most resistance testing turnaround time is 2 weeks or more. Expert consultation with local experts, and/or the National Clinicians' PEP Hotline (888) 448-4911 is warranted in this situation to select the drugs to which the source patient's virus is unlikely to be resistant. However, do not delay PEP initiation while awaiting expert consultation. The expanded regimen (three-drug PEP) is generally used in cases of suspected antiretroviral resistance. The PEP regimen can be altered after initiation, if more information is obtained about the source patient's virus at a later date (2).

Toxicity of the Postexposure Prophylaxis Regimen

Health care personnel who are prescribed PEP should be closely followed for signs of toxicity. Gastrointestinal side effects of nausea, vomiting, and diarrhea can usually be managed symptomatically without changing the PEP regimen. More severe side effects such as hyperglycemia, nephrolithiasis, pancreatitis, rash, and liver abnormalities may warrant modification of the antiretroviral regimen. Any serious adverse events should be reported to the FDA's MedWatch Program at (800) FDA-1088 or (800) 332-1088 or www.fda.gov/medwatch.

Nonoccupational HIV Postexposure Prophylaxis

Patients present to the emergency department after nonoccupational exposure to blood or body fluids following sexual assault, unsafe sexual practices, injection drug use, or percutaneous injuries with needles found outside of a hospital setting. There is no national consensus on management of nonoccupational HIV exposures. The 1998 Public Health Service Statement on management of nonoccupational exposures gave no recommendation for or against nonoccupational HIV PEP, but outlined the major issues to consider if this treatment is undertaken. Recommendation was made that if nonoccupational HIV PEP is going

to be given, that it should not be used for low risk exposures, or if the patient presents later than 72 h after the exposure. The patient should be counseled on the risk and benefit of HIV PEP, and informed consent should be obtained because nonoccupational HIV PEP is of unproven efficacy. Nonoccupational HIV PEP should not be used as a "morning-after pill" for primary HIV prevention. If nonoccupational HIV PEP is prescribed, it should be continued for 4 weeks, and the patient should be counseled on the importance of taking the entire regimen. Careful follow-up and monitoring of the patient for drug toxicities and for HIV seroconversion should take place, analogous to occupational HIV PEP follow-up (30).

According to the 2002 CDC Sexually Transmitted Diseases (STD) Treatment Guidelines—Sexual Assault and STDs, nonoccupational HIV PEP should be considered in cases in which the risk for HIV during the assault is likely high. Factors determining an increased risk of HIV transmission when an assailant's HIV status is unknown include the following: (1) whether oral, vaginal, or anal penetration occurred, (2) whether ejaculation occurred on mucous membranes, (3) whether multiple assailants were involved, (4) whether mucosal lesions are present in the assailant or survivor, and (5) other characteristics of the assault, survivor, or assailant (31).

The HIV transmission risk per encounter in a nonoccupational setting is not well established. The risk for HIV transmission from needle sharing in injection drug use is estimated to be 0.6–3% per encounter, and the risk for HIV transmission per episode of receptive penile-anal sexual exposure is 0.1–3% (32). The risk for HIV transmission per episode of receptive vaginal exposure is estimated at 0.1–0.2% (33). The risk for HIV transmission per episode of insertive anal exposure is 0.03–0.06% (32, 34). The risk for HIV transmission for insertive vaginal exposure is 0.03–0.09% (32). The risk for HIV transmission for receptive oral intercourse with ejaculation with an HIV-positive partner or a partner with unknown HIV status is 0.04% (34). The risk for HIV seroconversion per encounter in insertive oral exposure, and in female-to-female sex is unknown but is not zero.

DISPOSITION

Most emergency departments provide immediate evaluation for an exposure to bloodborne pathogens, but do not provide the follow-up care. It is essential that a HCP who needs HIV PEP get the first dose of medications as quickly as possible, has a way to get the subsequent doses without interruption, and has a medical provider who will follow him closely. This provider is usually located in an Occupational Health or Employee Health Department. Systems should be in place to handle this need for the HCP. Consult the administration in your institution if this need is not met. At the end of the emergency department visit, the HCP should be told where and when to report for follow-up, and have ready access to PEP medications.

HCP Counseling and Education

For HCP exposed to hepatitis B or hepatitis C infected blood or body fluids, there is no need to take any special precautions to prevent secondary transmission during the follow-up period. There is no need to modify sexual practices, avoid becoming pregnant, or discontinue breastfeeding. However, they should not donate blood, plasma, organs, tissue, or semen. HCP exposed to HIV-infected blood or body fluids should use the following measures to prevent secondary transmission during the follow-up period: exercise sexual abstinence or use condoms to prevent sexual transmission and avoid pregnancy; refrain from donating blood, plasma, organs, tissue, or semen; and discontinue breastfeeding since HIV can be transmitted through breast milk, and some antiretrovirals may pass into breast milk (2).

There is no need to modify the patient care responsibilities of HCP exposed to HBV-, HCV-, or HIV-infected blood or body fluids to prevent transmission to patients during the follow-up period (2). There is no need to admit the HCP following an exposure.

The emotional impact is substantial for HCP exposures, especially for exposures to HIV-infected blood or body fluids. The HCP seems to get conflicting information because he is told that the risk of seroconverting to HIV is low from the exposure, but he needs to take precautions to prevent secondary transmission of HIV just in case he seroconverts. It is important that exposed HCPs are counseled thoroughly about the risks and benefits of postexposure prophylaxis, and secondary prevention measures, and have an opportunity to have their questions answered (2).

HIV Postexposure Prophylaxis Medication Counseling

The importance of taking the entire 4-week regimen should be stressed. The HCP should be informed that knowledge about the efficacy of PEP is limited, and combination regimens are recommended because of the possibility of drug-resistant virus. The HCP should also be told that information on toxicity of antiretrovirals in pregnant persons and people who are not HIV infected is limited. Although side effects from antiretrovirals are usually minor, there have been serious adverse events in HCP taking PEP, so the HCP should be told to report any side effects of the medications right away. The HCP may decline PEP or stop PEP medications, and this should be documented in the exposure record. For those HCP exposures where PEP is not recommended, the HCP should be informed that the risk of the PEP medications outweighs the negligible risk of transmission of HIV from the exposure (2).

The HCP needs to have instruction on the significant drug–drug interactions and side effects of antiretrovirals. The HCP needs follow-up for monitoring drug toxicities of antiretrovirals. The AIDSinfo website has drug information handouts in technical and nontechnical formats and can be accessed at http://aidsinfo.nih.gov/.

The HCP should be instructed to seek medical attention for any acute illness that occurs during the follow-up period. Fever, rash, myalgias, fatigue, malaise, or lymphadenopathy may indicate HIV seroconversion, or may be symptoms of a drug reaction, or other illness (2).

Laboratory Monitoring During the Follow-up Period

Exposures to hepatitis B virus infected source

HCP who receive the hepatitis B vaccine as part of PEP, or as a routine vaccination series should be tested 1–2 months after completing the vaccine series for antibody to hepatitis B (anti-HBs). HCP who are nonresponders after a second three-dose vaccine series need to be counseled on preventative measures to avoid blood and body fluid exposures and the need for two doses of HBIG 1 month apart for any exposures to HBsAg-positive source (2).

Exposures to hepatitis C virus infected source

Baseline Testing of the Exposed HCP for Anti-HCV and ALT

Perform follow-up testing at 4–6 months for anti-HCV and ALT. If earlier diagnosis of HCV infection is desired, test for HCV RNA at 4–6 weeks following the exposure. All anti-HCV (EIA) results should be confirmed by a supplemental anti-HCV test such as a recombinant immunoblot assay (RIBA). See the HCV Postexposure Management for alternative testing schedules (2).

Exposures to HIV-infected source

Perform the following on baseline testing and again at 2 weeks after starting PEP: complete blood count, chemistries to include renal and liver function tests, glucose, and urinalysis in order to monitor for side effects of PEP. Other testing may be indicated depending on the PEP regimen and the HCP's medical condition (2).

Follow-up HIV Testing Perform

EIA at 6 weeks, 12 weeks, and 6 months after the exposure, regardless of whether the HCP received PEP medications. Extended follow-up HIV testing for 12 months is recommended for a HCP who becomes infected with HCV following exposure to a source coinfected with HIV and HCV. HIV testing (EIA) should be performed on any HCP who has an illness compatible with acute retroviral syndrome (primary HIV infection), regardless of the interval since exposure (2).

CASE OUTCOME

The source patient's presenting illness is suggestive of an undiagnosed HIV positive patient presenting with *Pneumocystis jiroveci* pneumonia (formerly known as *Pneumocystis carinii* pneumonia or PCP). Further questioning of the patient revealed that he has risk factors for HIV (multiple sexual partners, and sex with men). A rapid HIV test was done and was positive for HIV. If the rapid test for HIV was not available, HIV PEP should not have been delayed in this case, since the clinical picture was consistent with an HIV-positive source patient presenting with an opportunistic infection. Before informing the source patient of his HIV status, the patient's primary care physician obtained confirmation with an ELISA, and Western blot, which took several days. The source patient was negative for serologic evidence of HBV and HCV infections.

The exposure was a more severe exposure because the needle was hollow bore, in an artery, and there was blood on the needle. The source patient was HIV positive, class 2 because he was an HIV-positive patient presenting with an opportunistic infection, and had a low CD4 count and very high viral load at the time of the exposure. Since the source patient was unaware of his HIV diagnosis, he had not been on antiretrovirals, which makes it likely that he had the "wild-type" virus without antiretroviral resistance.

Before prescribing HIV PEP, the respiratory therapist was assessed for the possibility of pregnancy. She had regular periods, denied sexual encounters within the last 3 months, and had a negative pregnancy test. The therapist had no underlying medical conditions and was on no medications.

The respiratory therapist was prescribed the expanded regimen of zidovudine (AZT), lamuvidine (3TC), and indinavir (IDV) for 4 weeks. She took the first dose in the emergency department within 2 h of the exposure. She was counseled on the side effects of the medications, drug interactions, and instructed to keep hydrated to prevent kidney stones while on indinavir. She was followed-up by the Employee Health Department of her hospital. She tolerated the PEP medications and had no side effects. She was HIV negative at her final 6-month follow-up visit.

REFERENCES

1. NIOSH alert: *Preventing Needlestick Injuries in Health-care Settings.* Cincinnati, National Institute for Occupational Safety and Health, 1999 (DHHS publication (NIOSH) 2000-108).
2. CDC: Updated U.S. Public Health Service guidelines for the management of occupational exposures to HBV, HCV, and HIV and recommendations for postexposure prophylaxis. *Morb Mortal Wkly Rep* 50(RR-11):1–52, 2001 (http://www.cdc.gov/mmwr/preview/mmwrhtml/rr5011a1.htm)
3. Henderson DK: Managing occupational risks for hepatitis C transmission in the health care setting. *Clin Microbiol Rev* 16(3):546–568, 2003.
4. Rosen, HR: Acquisition of hepatitis C by a conjunctival splash. *Am J Infect Control* 25:242–247, 1997.
5. Sartori, M, La Terra G, Aglietta M, Manzin A, Navino C, Verzetti G: Transmission of hepatitis C via blood splash into conjunctiva. *Scand J Infect Dis* 25:270–271, 1993.
6. Ippolito G, V. Puro, N. Petrosillo, et al.: Simultaneous infection with HIV and hepatitis C virus following occupational conjunctival blood exposure (Letter). *JAMA* 280:28, 1998.
7. Bell DM: Occupational risk of human immunodeficiency virus infection in healthcare workers: An overview. *Am J Med* 102(Suppl. 5B):9–15, 1997.
8. Ippolito G, Puro V, De Carli G, and the Italian Study Group on Occupational Risk of HIV Infection: The risk of occupational human immunodeficiency virus infection in health care workers: Italian Multicenter Study. *Arch Intern Med* 153: 1451–1458, 1993.
9. CDC: Update: human immunodeficiency virus infections in health-care workers exposed to blood of infected patients. *Morb Mortal Wkly Rep* 36:285–289, 1987.
10. Fahey BJ, Koziol DE, Banks SM, Henderson DK: Frequency of nonparenteral occupational exposures to blood and body fluids before and after universal precautions training. *Am J Med* 90:145–153, 1991.
11. Henderson DK, Fahey BJ, Willy M, et al.: Risk for occupational transmission of human immunodeficiency virus type 1 (HIV-1) associated with clinical exposures: A prospective evaluation. *Ann Intern Med* 113:740–746, 1990.

12. Cardo DM, Culver DH, Ciesielski CA, et al.: A case-control study of HIV seroconversion in health care workers after percutaneous exposure. *N Engl J Med* 337:1485–1490, 1997.

13. Chiarello LA, Gerberding JL: Human immunodeficiency virus in health care settings, in Mandell GL, Bennett JE, Dolin R (eds.): *Principles and Practice of Infectious Diseases, 5th ed.* Philadelphia, Churchill Livingstone, 2000; pp 3052–3054.

14. Do AN, Ciesielski CA, Metler RP, et al.: Occupationally acquired human immunodeficiency virus (HIV) infection: National Case Surveillance Data During 20 Years of the HIV Epidemic in the United States. *Infect Control Hosp Epidemiol* 24:86–96, 2003.

15. Beltrami EM: The risk and prevention of occupational human immunodeficiency virus infection. *Semin Infect Control* 1(1):2–18, 2001.

16. Busch MP, Satten GA: Time course of viremia and antibody seroconversion following human immunodeficiency virus exposure. *Am J Med* 102(5B):117–124, 1997.

17. Ridzon R, Gallagher K, Ciesielski C, et al.: Simultaneous transmission of human immunodeficiency virus and hepatitis C virus from a needle-stick injury. *N Engl J Med* 336:919–922, 1997.

18. Spira AI, Marx PA, Patterson BK, et al.: Cellular targets of infection and route of viral dissemination after an intravaginal inoculation of simian immunodeficiency virus into rhesus macaques. *J Exp Med* 183:215–225, 1996.

19. Connor EM, Sperling RS, Gelber R, et al.: Reduction of maternal-infant transmission of human immunodeficiency virus type 1 with zidovudine treatment. *N Engl J Med* 331:1173–1180, 1994.

20. Sperling RS, Shapiro DE, Coombs RW, et al.: Maternal viral load, zidovudine treatment, and the risk of transmission of human immunodeficiency virus type 1 from mother to infant. *N Engl J Med* 335:1621–1629, 1996.

21. Wang SA, Panlilio AL, Doi PA. et al.: Experience of healthcare workers taking postexposure prophylaxis after occupational HIV exposures: Findings of the HIV postexposure prophylaxis registry. *Infect Control Hosp Epidemiol* 21:780–785, 2000.

22. Gerberding JL: Occupational exposure to HIV in health care settings. *N Engl J Med* 348:826–833, 2003.

23. Rey D, L'Heritier A, Lang JM. Severe ototoxicity in a health care worker who received postexposure prophylaxis with stavudine, lamivudine, and nevirapine after occupational exposure to HIV. *Clin Infect Dis* 34:418–419, 2002.

24. CDC: Serious adverse events attributed to nevirapine regimens for postexposure prophylaxis after HIV exposures—Worldwide, 1997–2000. *Morb Mortal Wkly Rep* 49(51 & 52): 1153–1156, 2001.

25. Kahn JO, Walker BD: Acute human immunodeficiency virus type 1 infection. *N Engl J Med* 339(1):33–39, 1998.

26. Gerberding JL, Henderson DK: Management of occupational exposures to bloodborne pathogens: Hepatitis B virus, hepatitis C virus, and human immunodeficiency virus. *Clin Infect Dis* 14:1179–1185, 1992.

27. Guidelines for the Use of Antiretroviral Agents in HIV-Infected Adults and Adolescents. *Morb Mortal Wkly Rep* 51(RR-7), 2002. Updated as a Living Document on October 29, 2004 [tables 10–12, pp 58–62]. Located on the AIDSinfo website http://aidsinfo.nih.gov/

28. Blanche S, Tardieu M, Rustin P, et al.: Persistent mitochondrial dysfunction and perinatal exposure to antiretroviral nucleoside analogues. *Lancet* 354:1084–1089, 1999.

29. Guidelines for the Use of Antiretroviral Agents in HIV-Infected Adults and Adolescents. *Morb Mortal Wkly Rep* 51(RR-7), 2002. Updated as a Living Document on October 29, 2004 [table 29 pp 93–95]. Located on the AIDSinfo website http://aidsinfo.nih.gov/

30. CDC: Management of possible sexual, injecting-drug-use, or other nonoccupational exposure to HIV, including considerations related to antiretroviral therapy: Public Health Service Statement. *Morb Mortal Wkly Rep* 47(RR-17):1–14, 1998.

31. CDC: Sexually transmitted disease treatment guidelines, 2002. *Morb Mortal Wkly Rep* 51(RR-6):69–71, 2002.

32. Hirschhorn L, Kunches L, Mayer K: Nonoccupational postexposure prophylaxis: Evolving clinical practice. *AIDS Clin Care* 12(1):6–12, 2000.

33. Mastro TD, de Vicenti I: Probabilities of sexual HIV-1 transmission. *AIDS* 10(Suppl. A):S75–S82, 1996.

34. Vittinghoff E, Douglas J, Judson F, et al.: Per-contact risk of human immunodeficiency virus transmission between male sexual partners. *Am J Epidemiol* 150:306–311, 1999.

36

Sexually Transmitted Diseases

Stephanie N. Taylor
David H. Martin

HIGH YIELD FACTS

1. Sexually transmitted diseases (STDs) and subsequent complications are commonly encountered by emergency department physicians.

2. Prompt and effective treatment of sexually transmitted diseases results in prevention of complications and reduction in transmission of STDs and HIV.

3. Syndromic management of genital ulcer disease, urethral discharge, vaginal discharge, and lower abdominal pain is a useful approach in the emergency room setting.

4. The Centers for Disease Control (CDC) STD Guidelines should be available in the emergency department for the most recent STD management and treatment recommendations.

CASE PRESENTATION

A 22-year-old man presents to the emergency department with urethral discharge, scrotal pain, and subjective fever without chills. The patient reports that the discharge began 1 week prior to presentation and he had taken a few penicillin tablets provided by a friend. His past history was significant for two previous episodes of gonorrhea and he had no drug allergies.

On physical examination, the patient is in mild distress secondary to scrotal pain. His blood pressure is 122/80, his pulse is 90, and his temperature is 100.4°F. Genital exam reveals a cloudy urethral discharge and an erythematous and swollen scrotum with a painful right testicle. There are no genital lesions or skin rashes.

INTRODUCTION/EPIDEMIOLOGY

Sexually transmitted diseases will occur in an estimated 15 million Americans annually or one in four Americans in a lifetime (1). STDs are caused by a variety of organisms that have been associated with enhanced transmission of HIV, pelvic inflammatory disease (PID), cervical cancer, and other complications (2, 3). Historically, a significant number of these infections, especially in adolescents, have been treated in emergency room settings. Results from the 1992–1998 National Hospital Ambulatory Medical Care survey revealed that 1.2 million adolescent emergency room visits had a discharge diagnosis of a sexually transmitted infection (4). In the 1992–1994 survey, PID was the most common gynecologic disorder seen in emergency departments (342,000 visits per year), and lower genital infection in women was the second most common gynecologic disorder seen (5). Despite many programs and attempts to deter the use of emergency rooms as primary care facilities, many people, especially inner-city populations with high STD rates, still use emergency rooms for this purpose (6). It is therefore very important that emergency room physicians be aware of the various STD clinical presentations and know the Center for Diseases Control (CDC) STD treatment recommendations (7). Having copies of the most recently published CDC STD Treatment Guidelines in the emergency department is necessary for reference purposes. In addition, emergency room physicians should have a high index of suspicion and low threshold for empiric therapy in patients who present with STD-related complaints (8).

The economic cost of STDs and subsequent complications is very high, with direct and indirect health care costs estimated at $10 billion a year (9). The Institute of Medicine report, *The Hidden Epidemic: Confronting Sexually Transmitted Diseases*, points out how the control of STDs has been neglected in the United States, leaving us with the highest prevalence of STDs in the developed world (9). STD surveillance reports for the year 2002 for the United States and selected U.S. cities are presented in Table 36–1 (10, 11). The actual number of cases in the U.S. population is actually greater than those presented in the surveillance reports due to incomplete diagnosis and reporting. In fact, it is estimated that more than 4 million chlamydia infections occur annually, but only 834,555 cases are reported to the CDC. In addition, though genital herpes and human papilloma virus (HPV) infections are not reportable, the number of initial office visits annually is estimated to be 200,000 and 300,000, respectively (10). In *The Hidden Epidemic* report, it is estimated that 45 million Americans are infected with herpes simplex type 2 virus and 20 million with HPV (9). It is also estimated that 5 million cases of trichomonas vaginitis occur each year (9).

Table 36–1. STD Cases and Rates per 100,000 Patients—United States and Selected U.S. Cities in 2002

	Syphilis All Stages Cases* Rate**	Syphilis (1 and 2)	Chlamydia	Gonorrhea
United States	32,871*	6,862	834,555	351,852
	11.7**	2.4	296.5	125.0
Philadelphia, PA	556	67	14,458	7,006
	37.3	4.4	952.7	461.7
Baltimore, MD	398	121	6,267	4,873
	61.1	18.6	962.0	748.4
New Orleans, LA	101	9	4,340	2,685
	20.8	1.9	895.0	554.0
Atlanta, GA	827	257	5,560	3,810
	101.3	31.5	681.4	446.9
Richmond, VA	25	3	2,108	1,507
	12.6	1.5	1,065.8	761.9
Detroit, MI	878	384	11,374	6,845
	92.3	40.4	1,195.7	719.0
San Francisco, CA	604	315	3,345	2,136
	77.8	40.6	430.6	275.0

Source: From CDC STD Surveillance 2002.

PATHOPHYSIOLOGY/MICROBIOLOGY

Syphilis is caused by the spirochete, *Treponema pallidum.* The organism is a spiral shaped, obligate human bacteria with no environmental or animal reservoirs. It is too small to be visualized with light microscopy but is visible by dark-field or phase-contrast microscopy. In addition, this organism is one of the few pathogens that has not been cultivated in vitro successfully and must be propagated in rabbit testicles in order to perform experimental studies (12).

T. pallidum is acquired by sexual contact and perinatal transmission (congenital syphilis). Accidental direct inoculation of medical personnel and transfusion-associated syphilis have been virtually eliminated due to universal precautions, serologic screening of donated blood, and use of blood components that have been stored at 4°C (*T. pallidum* is killed at this temperature).

It is estimated that the rate of acquisition of syphilis following a single sexual exposure to a patient with primary disease is 30% (13). The organism enters the body through direct inoculation of abraded skin or mucous membranes. Once inside the tissues, local replication occurs along with simultaneous escape of the organism from the local site and dissemination to the lymphatics and the bloodstream.

This sets the stage for the secondary and tertiary stages of syphilis.

The only known hosts for the DNA viruses *herpes simplex virus types 1 and 2 (HSV-1 and HSV-2)* are humans. HSV-2 is classically the etiologic agent of sexually transmitted genital herpes and HSV-1 is responsible for oral herpes infections, but both types can cause infection at either location. Contact with contaminated genital secretions is responsible for the acquisition of genital herpes. The virus is inoculated into abraded skin or susceptible mucous membranes and viral replication occurs in cells of the dermis and epidermis. During the initial infection, HSV ascends peripheral sensory nerves and enters the sensory or autonomic nerve root ganglia where latent HSV infection is established. Herpes infections are characterized by periods of latency and reactivation of clinical HSV outbreaks. Despite host immunity, these recurrences occur spontaneously or in response to stimuli such as trauma, fever, menstruation, and emotional stress. Immune mechanisms will usually rapidly limit viral replication and spread so that recurrent episodes are generally less severe than the primary infections (14).

Chancroid is a genital ulcer disease caused by *Haemophilus ducreyi,* a small, fastidious, gram-negative rod. The organism is very difficult to grow on artificial media requiring special media and conditions, and has not been isolated from nonhuman sources. *H. ducreyi* is spread from person to person by sexual contact and there is no role for fomites. This organism also requires a break in the epithelial barrier to initiate disease. Although the organism causes significant inguinal adenopathy, it remains confined to the genital area and there have been no cases of systemic disease reported, even in patients with AIDS (15).

Gonorrhea is caused by *Neisseria gonorrhoeae* and humans are the only known reservoir. Mucous membranes lined with columnar, cuboidal, or noncornified genitourinary tract epithelial cells such as those found in the urethra, cervical canal, epididymis, fallopian tubes, and the Bartholin glands are most often infected with this organism. Other mucosal sites such as the pharynx, rectum, and conjunctiva may also be infected and hematogenous dissemination to nonmucosal sites occurs. The initial phase of gonococcal infection includes adherence of the organism to cells, which is mediated by pili and other surface proteins (16). Ciliary motion is also inhibited by gonococcal endotoxin and contributes to the destruction of the surrounding cells. In addition, *N. gonorrhoeae* occasionally may evade the immune system and cause disseminated disease.

Chlamydia trachomatis is a sexually transmitted, obligate intracellular organism that is the most common reportable bacterial disease in the United States. The biology of *C. trachomatis* is unique among sexually transmitted organisms due to the two-part life cycle that includes elementary and reticulate body stages. The elementary body is metabolically inactive with a protective cell wall that allows it to survive extracellularly. The reticulate body is metabolically active and is found only within cells. Infection is initiated when an elementary body binds to a cell surface and enters the cytoplasm by endocytosis. In this location the organism is able to evade the host's cellular defense system and begins to replicate as reticulate bodies. As the inclusion grows, the reticulate bodies undergo transformation back to elementary bodies; 100–1000 infectious elementary bodies are released via cell rupture 48–72 h after initial infection (17).

Vaginitis is defined as inflammation or infection of the vagina leading to vaginal irritation and discharge. The most common causes of vaginitis are vulvovaginal candidiasis, bacterial vaginosis, and trichomonas. *Candida albicans* is responsible for 85–90% of yeast strains isolated from women (18). Although other strains such as *Candida glabrata* or *C. tropicalis* can cause vaginitis,

C. albicans is capable of adhering to vaginal epithelial cells in significantly higher numbers (19). The organism gains access to the vagina from the adjacent perianal area and germination of the organism enhances colonization and facilitates tissue invasion (20–22). The exact mechanism of the inflammatory reaction to this organism has not been completely delineated, but it appears that cell damage is caused by direct epithelial invasion by the organism; proteases and other hydrolytic enzymes may play a role (18, 23).

Trichomonas vaginalis is a flagellated protozoan that is the etiologic agent of trichomonas vaginitis. In addition to vaginitis, this organism also causes nongonococcal urethritis in men. The pathogenesis of *T. vaginalis* human infection has not been completely elucidated. There is an element of cellular destruction that occurs via direct cell contact and cytotoxicity (23). In addition, at least four specific binding adhesins and a cytotoxin that causes detachment and clumping of cultured cells have been identified (24).

Bacterial vaginosis (BV) is the most common cause of vaginal symptoms and discharge in women of childbearing age. Vaginal inflammation and true infection of tissues are not characteristic of this disorder and is the reason the term vaginosis is preferred instead of vaginitis. BV is caused by the overgrowth and replacement of normal vaginal flora (*Lactobacillus*) with mixed flora such as *Gardnerella vaginalis, Mycoplamsa hominis, Mobiluncus* sp., and anaerobes. The reason for the overgrowth of these organisms is the subject of ongoing investigation. The presence of *Lactobacillus* appears to inhibit the overgrowth of these organisms and this process may be mediated by the production of H_2O_2. To date, no host factors that predispose to the development of bacterial vaginosis have been identified. The role of sexual transmission remains controversial and currently BV is not considered a sexually transmitted disorder.

Other viral STDs include human papilloma virus (HPV) and molluscum contagiosum. HPV is a DNA virus that causes sexually transmitted genital warts or condyloma acuminata. There are over 100 types of HPV and at least 35 of them primarily infect genital epithelial cells. HPV types 6 and 11 are most commonly associated with genital warts, while types 16 and 18 are commonly associated with the development of cervical cancer. In order to cause infection, HPV must gain entry to the basal layer of the epithelium through small or microscopic abrasions. This leads to transformation of one or more basal cells and the expression of viral DNA in the basal layer, which is thought to be responsible for the proliferation of blood vessels and keratinocytes that result in the formation of a wart.

Molluscum contagiosum is caused by the molluscum contagiosum virus (MCV), which is a member of the poxvirus family. Both sexual and nonsexual transmission of this virus occurs. In children, the nonsexual form includes lesions of the face, trunk, and upper extremities and appears to be spread by direct contact of infected individuals or fomites (25). MCV infection only occurs in the epidermis and dissemination has not been demonstrated, even in profoundly immunocompromised patients. Transmission results from inoculation of the virus through microscopic abrasions. A host-derived growth factor may be involved as well and it is thought that lack of this factor is responsible for the limited ability to culture the virus in vitro. Focal areas of epidermal hyperplasia surrounding cyst-shaped lobules with debris and molluscum bodies are seen on biopsy of the lesions.

Ectoparasites are also sexually transmitted but not all cases are acquired in this manner. *Sarcoptes scabiei*, the human itch mite, is the ectoparasite that causes scabies. The female mite uses her head as a tool to burrow into the skin where eggs are laid. Saliva, other body secretions, and feces diffuse into the dermis and initiate an inflammatory immune response. The mite induces IgE antibodies and also causes an immediate hypersensitivity reaction. A cellular infiltrate of T cells, macrophages, and B cells can be found in the dermis and demonstrate the important role that cellular immune response plays in the pathogenesis of scabies infestation.

Phthirus pubis, the pubic louse, is the etiologic agent of pediculosis pubis. They are transmitted by intimate contact and survive by sucking blood from human hosts through bites. In addition, the claws of pubic lice match the diameter of pubic and axillary hairs, and therefore the organisms may be found in the axilla, on beards, eyelashes, or eyebrows. Individuals vary in their sensitivity and response to louse bites from very mild itching or stinging to severe itching and skin irritation and excoriation.

CLINICAL PRESENTATION

Syphilis is known as the "Great Imitator" due to its variety of clinical presentations, and it is said that "He who knows syphilis, knows medicine." Syphilis is characterized by different stages of disease and patients are most infectious in the early stages. Table 36–2 presents the clinical manifestations of the various stages of syphilis. Classically, primary syphilis is characterized by a single, painless, indurated, and clean-based ulcer with well-defined borders at the site of the initial infection (Fig. 36–1). The chancre begins as a papule 14–21 days after inoculation that rapidly ulcerates. It is usually associated with nontender regional adenopathy and the differential diagnosis includes herpes, chancroid, trauma, fixed drug eruption, or staphylococcal or streptococcal infection. In the absence of treatment, this lesion will resolve spontaneously in 3–6 weeks. Clinicians should know that the classical clinical presentation of primary syphilis is only seen in about two-thirds of cases (26).

Secondary syphilis results from hematogenous dissemination of the organism and occurs 4–10 weeks after an untreated primary syphilis chancre resolves, though primary

Table 36–2. Clinical Manifestations of Genital Ulcer Diseases

Syphilis	
Primary	Painless, clean-based, indurated ulcer or chancre on penis, labia, vagina, anus, cervix, lips, mouth, etc.
Secondary	Generalized maculopapular rash including palms and soles, adenopathy, fever, patchy alopecia, condyloma lata, mucous membrane patches, neurologic (headache, meningismus, meningitis, etc.)
Latent	No physical manifestations or evidence of infection but patients have reactive serologic tests for syphilis
Tertiary	Aortitis, aortic aneurysm, neurosyphilis (tabes dorsalis, paresis, psychosis, dementia, meningitis, CVA), gummas (skin bones, subcutaneous tissue, etc.)
Herpes	Crops of small vesicles on an erythematous base that rapidly evolve into tiny, shallow ulcers that may coalesce to form larger ulcers. Other findings may include fever in primary cases, dysuria, urethritis and rarely urinary retention
Chancroid	Painful ulcer with irregular borders and purulent, exudative base. Associated with tender, suppurative lymphadenopathy in 50% of patients

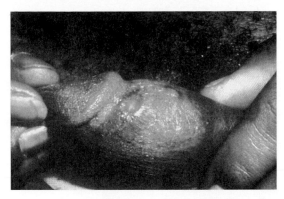

Fig. 36–1. Primary syphilis chancre or ulcer (from Martin DH, Mroczkowski TF: Dermatologic manifestations of STDs other than HIV. *Infect Dis Clin North Am* 8:535, 1994, permission pending).

lesions occasionally persist into the secondary stage. Figs. 36–2 to 36–4 demonstrate the classic maculopapular rash of the trunk and extremities that involves the palms and soles. Patients often complain of "flu-like illness" with low-grade fever, malaise, arthralgias, and myalgia. Other

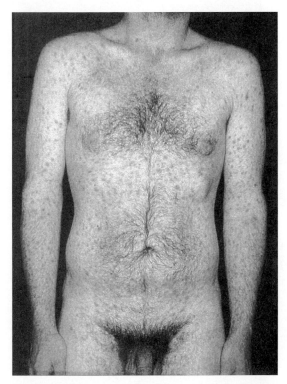

Fig. 36–2. Maculopapular rash of secondary syphilis (CDC STD slide file).

clinical findings of secondary syphilis include condyloma lata (Fig. 36–5), patchy alopecia, generalized lymphadenopathy, and mucous patches. The differential diagnosis includes pityriasis rosea, tinea versicolor, drug eruptions, viral exanthems, lichen planus, erythema multiforme, seborrheic dermatitis, psoriasis, and scabies. Given this broad differential diagnosis, it is recommended that serological tests for syphilis be included in the evaluation of all sexually active individuals with generalized skin rashes.

Untreated secondary syphilis also will resolve spontaneously in 3–12 weeks. This is followed by latent syphilis, which is characterized by reactive serologic tests for syphilis and no clinical manifestations of infection. It is arbitrarily divided into early (<1 year duration) and late latent syphilis. The latent phase may persist for the patient's lifetime, but after 5–30 years, as many as one-third may go on to develop findings of tertiary syphilis with destructive lesions of the aorta, central nervous system, and skin or bone as outlined in Table 36–2.

Herpes lesions occur after 7–10 days incubation in a primary case and appear as a cluster of painful vesicles on an erythematous base that rapidly erode to form tiny, shallow ulcers that may coalesce into larger ulcers (Table 36–2; Figs. 36–6 and 36–7). The primary or initial episode is usually more severe than recurrent episodes and may be associated with systemic symptoms such as fever, headache, malaise, or myalgias. Primary HSV may also be associated with urethral discharge and/or dysuria in a substantial number of men. Both internal and external dysuria (from urine touching HSV lesions) occur frequently in women. Following the initial outbreak, the virus remains latent in the regional dorsal root ganglia. Reactivation or recurrent outbreaks occur secondary to numerous factors including local trauma, fever, emotional stress, or menstruation. These outbreaks are usually less severe and of shorter duration than primary episodes. It is also important to note that asymptomatic shedding of HSV occurs in the absence of lesions and can result in transmission of herpes during times of apparent disease inactivity.

Chancroid has an incubation period of approximately 7 days and it classically presents as one or more, nonindurated, painful ulcers with a purulent base and ragged, undermined borders (Table 36–2). There is no prodromal phase associated with chancroid and the lesion begins as a painful papule that becomes pustular and then erodes to become an ulcer. Unilateral tender inguinal lymphadenopathy is also characteristic in 50–60% of patients (Fig. 36–8). This process may progress into the development of buboes (fluctuant node masses) that may rupture

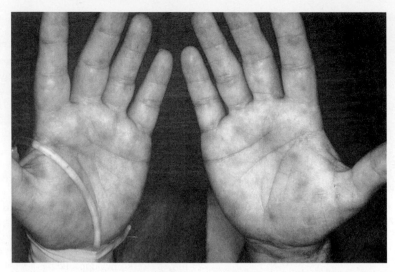

Fig. 36–3. Secondary syphilis—rash of the palms (from Martin DH, Mroczkowski TF: Dermatologic manifestations of STDs other than HIV. *Infect Dis Clin North Am* 8:538, 1994, permission pending).

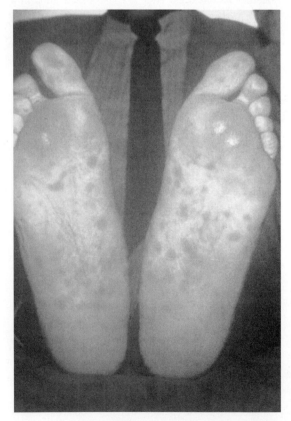

Fig. 36–4. Secondary syphilis—rash of soles (CDC STD slide file).

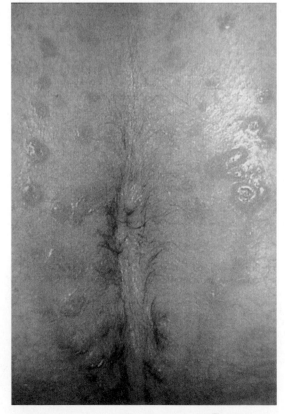

Fig. 36–5. Secondary syphilis—condyloma LATA (CDC STD slide file).

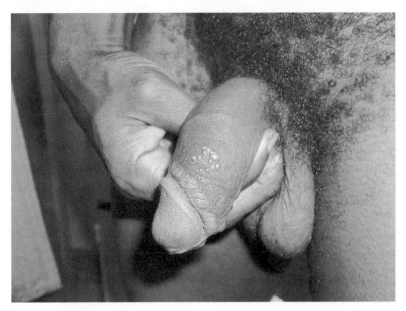

Fig. 36–6. Genital herpes (provided courtesy of Stephanie N. Taylor, MD).

spontaneously or require drainage. Despite many distinguishing features, there is considerable overlap between the clinical appearance of chancroid, syphilis, and herpes simplex virus (HSV) (26). In addition, it is estimated that 10% of patients with chancroid may also be co-infected with either HSV or *T. pallidum* or both (15).

The clinical manifestations and complications of gonorrhea and chlamydia are presented in Tables 36–3 and 36–4, respectively. The clinical manifestations of these infections are very similar except that chlamydial infections tend to be characterized by milder symptoms and less abrupt onset. A high percentage of patients infected with these organisms are asymptomatic. This is especially true of *C. trachomatis.* Both organisms prefer infecting columnar or transitional epithelial cells of the cervix and urethra with extension to the endometrium, fallopian tubes,

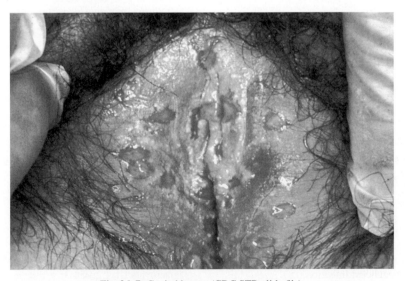

Fig. 36–7. Genital herpes (CDC STD slide file).

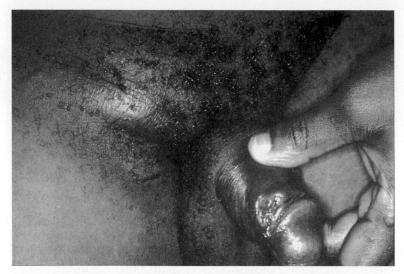

Fig. 36–8. Chancroid—ulcer with right inguinal buboe (from Martin DH, Mroczkowski TF: Dermatologic manifestations of STDs other than HIV. *Infect Dis Clin North Am* 8: 550, 1994, permission pending).

epididymis, peritoneum, and rectum (27). Both organisms also cause conjunctivitis and rarely, systemic manifestations such as perihepatitis and reactive arthritis. The most common clinical manifestations, however, are mucopurulent cervicitis and urethritis. The gonococcal discharge is usually more copious and purulent (Fig. 36–9) when compared with the modest, clear, or gray discharge of chlamydia or nongonococcal urethritis (Fig. 36–10). It is important to note, however, that these cannot always be distinguished based upon clinical presentation alone. Finally,

Table 36–3. Clinical Manifestations of *Neisseria gonorrhoeae*

Men
    Urethritis
    Epididymitis
    Proctitis
    Conjunctivitis
    Periurethral abscess
    Penile lymphangitis
    Disseminated gonococcal infection (DGI)
Women
    Cervicitis
    Bartholin glands abscess
    Perihepatitis (Fitz-Hugh-Curtis syndrome)
    Pelvic inflammatory disease (PID)
    Infertility
    Conjunctivitis
    Endometritis
    Tubo-ovarian abscess
    Ectopic pregnancy
    Ophthalmia neonatorum
    Disseminated gonococcal infection (DGI)

Table 36–4. Clinical Manifestations of *Chlamydia trachomatis*

Men
    Urethritis [nongonococcal urethritis (NGU)]
    Epididymitis
    Conjunctivitis
    Proctitis
    Reiter syndrome (urethritis, conjunctivitis, arthritis, characteristic skin lesions)
    Lymphogranuloma venereum (lymphotrophic serovars L1, L2, & L3)
Women
    Cervicitis
    Pelvic inflammatory disease (salpingitis, endometritis)
    Acute urethral syndrome (urethritis)
    Conjunctivitis
    Bartholinitis
    Perihepatitis
    Reiter syndrome
    Lymphogranuloma venereum (lymphotrophic serovars L1, L2, & L3)

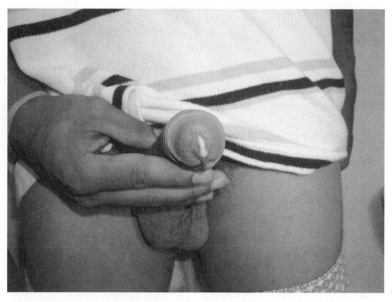

Fig. 36–9. Gonococcal urethritis (provided courtesy of Stephanie N. Taylor, MD).

gonorrhea can also present as disseminated disease. Disseminated gonococcal infection (DGI) results from gonococcal bacteremia and is characterized by acute arthritis, tenosynovitis, migratory arthralgias, and necrotic pustules on an erythematous base (Fig. 36–11). There are usually less than 30 pustules located primarily on the extremities.

Ascension of infection into the upper genital tract occurs in a significant number of women infected with the gonococcus and chlamydia and may cause pelvic inflammatory disease (PID). Extensive tubal inflammation and scarring has also been demonstrated in the absence of symptoms. PID is therefore often "silent" and occurs three

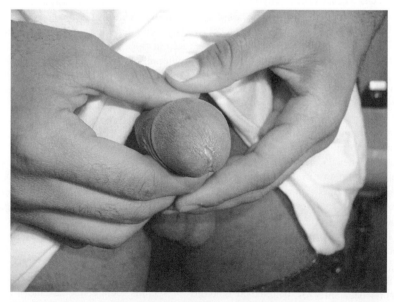

Fig. 36–10. Nongonoccocal urethritis (provided courtesy of Stephanie N. Taylor, MD).

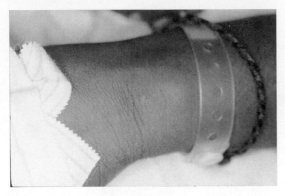

Fig. 36–11. Disseminated gonococcal infection (provided courtesy of Stephanie N. Taylor, MD).

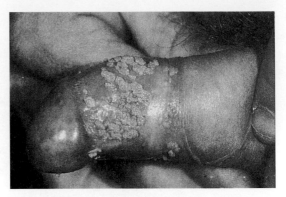

Fig. 36–12. Genital warts (CDC STD slide file).

times as often as symptomatic PID. Unfortunately, the complications of silent PID, ectopic pregnancy and infertility, remain the same as its symptomatic counterpart and are the reason for screening and treatment of asymptomatic chlamydial infection. Criteria for the diagnosis of PID include lower abdominal pain, cervical motion tenderness, bilateral or unilateral adnexal tenderness, combined with temperature ≥38°C, white blood cell count (WBC) ≥10,500, purulent endocervical discharge, erythrocyte sedimentation rate >15 mm/h, and the presence of *N. gonorrhoeae or C. trachomatis* in the endocervix (28). Fever and elevated white blood cell counts often are missing, especially in cases caused by chlamydia.

Another infection caused by both chlamydia and gonorrhea is epididymitis in men. A few men with chlamydial or gonococcal infections develop this upper genital tract infection that is considered the female equivalent of PID. Epididymitis presents most commonly with unilateral scrotal pain, swelling, and fever in a young man with associated urethritis.

Vaginitis is one of the most common reasons why women seek medical attention. Symptoms of vaginitis include vaginal discharge, pruritus, and complaints caused by inflammation such as soreness, irritation, dysuria, and dyspareunia. It is also important to remember that both cervicitis and vaginitis can cause vaginal discharge and the distinction can be difficult. Therefore it is essential that the cervix be evaluated in women with the complaint of vaginal discharge. Table 36–5 outlines the classic clinical manifestations of the most common causes of vaginitis.

Genital warts appear as verrucous, cauliflower-like lesions or fleshy outgrowths on the skin or mucous membranes of the genital area (Fig. 36–12). Though there is no reason to initiate therapy for these in the emergency room

setting, it is important that the emergency room physician be able to recognize these lesions and arrange referral for treatment and follow-up of these patients. In men genital warts commonly appear on the penis, scrotum, perianal area and urethral meatus. In women they are commonly seen on the introitus, vulva, perineum, and perianal area.

Molluscum contagiosum presents as smooth, dome-shaped, flesh-colored or pearly lesions (Fig. 36–13). They are 3–5 mm in size and have a characteristic umbilicated center from which caseous material can be expressed. Occasionally "giant molluscum" lesions 10–15 mm in size are seen. Ten to twenty lesions are present in normal hosts, but hundreds of lesions can be seen in immunocompromised hosts.

Scabies presents as excoriated papular, pruritic lesions typically found in the finger web spaces, periumbilical area, genitalia, nipples, or axilla. Burrows may also be seen in these areas or on the wrists and elbows. Patients with pubic lice also present with intense pruritis in the genital area. Patients have often noticed the organism or the eggs on hair shafts. Though difficult to see upon examination, pubic lice form characteristic "blue spots" in the skin at the site of louse bites.

LABORATORY/DIAGNOSTIC TESTING

Syphilis diagnosis depends upon the combination of physical findings, history, serologic testing, and darkfield microscopy of primary or secondary lesions. Though not available in most emergency room settings, darkfield microscopy can make a rapid and accurate diagnosis of primary syphilis at a time when serologic studies may be falsely negative. There are two types of serologic tests for syphilis, nontreponemal and treponemal. Serologic tests such as the RPR (rapid plasma reagin) and VDRL

Table 36–5. Findings in Women with Vaginitis Compared to Normal Women

Etiologic Agent	Common Symptoms	Discharge Characteristics	Microscopy	pH	Amine or Fishy Odor with KOH
Normal	None	Scant; clear or white	Normal epithelial cells and lactobacilli	≤4.5	None
Candida vaginitis	*Candida albicans* and other *Candida* sp.	Vulvar itching, burning, or irritation	White, clumped and adherent; vulvar and vaginal erythema	WBCs, epithelial cells, yeast, and pseudohyphae	≤4.5	None
Bacterial vaginosis	*G.vaginalis, Mycoplasma* sp. and anaerobes	Malodorous discharge	White or gray, homogeneous	Clue cells, coccobacillary flora, absence of WBCs and lactobacilli	>4.5	Present
Trichomonas vaginitis	*Trichomonas vaginalis*	Malodorous discharge with pruritus	Profuse and yellow; vaginal erythema with "strawberry cervix"	Motile Trichomonads, many WBCs	often >5	May be present

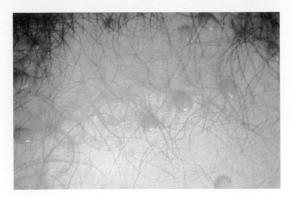

Fig. 36–13. Molluscum contagiosum (CDC STD slide file).

(Venereal Disease Research Laboratory) are nontreponemal tests and detect the presence of nonspecific antibodies to cardiolipin that are formed during infection with syphilis and some other medical conditions. RPR or VDRL serologic studies are reported as an antibody titer. In most cases of early syphilis, titers decline following successful treatment and therefore are useful in following patients over time. Titers should become negative in most individuals adequately treated for early syphilis but low-titer positive tests will persist in some. These patients are referred to as being "serofast."

Treponemal serologic tests such as the FTA-ABS (fluorescent treponemal absorbed), MHA-TP (microhemagglutination antibody to *T. pallidum*), or IgG/IgM syphilis ELISA assays detect specific treponemal antibody and are more sensitive and specific than nontreponemal studies. Because of their increased specificity and sensitivity they are used to confirm positive nontreponemal tests that can occur in a variety of medical conditions. These include lupus, pregnancy, intravenous drug use, chronic liver disease, and viral hepatitis among others. Treponemal tests are not reported as titers and remain positive for the lifetime of most patients. For this reason, these tests cannot be used to follow disease activity or to monitor response to treatment.

In the emergency room setting, the results of these tests will usually not be readily available though the RPR card test can be done on a "stat" basis. Because ER patients are easily lost to follow-up, patients with findings suspicious for early syphilis, such as ulcers or rashes, should have serologic studies submitted and should also be treated empirically while serologic results and follow-up are pending.

The diagnosis of herpes in the emergency medicine setting is primarily based upon the clinical presentation of characteristic lesions. Viral cultures remain the gold standard for diagnosis and isolation rates are 90% when blister fluid is cultured compared to 30% for crusted lesions. Though serologic tests are widely available, none have reliably differentiated HSV-1 from HSV-2 until recently. These tests are available only through reference laboratories and are of no practical use in emergency departments.

Laboratory diagnosis of chancroid is not widely available because the organism is difficult to isolate and requires special growth conditions and culture media. DNA amplification tests are available for use in research settings only. A clinical diagnosis of chancroid should be suspected if a patient has one or more painful, purulent ulcers with undermined borders. The probability of chancroid is increased for any genital ulcer by a negative darkfield examination or serologic test for syphilis, and a negative test for HSV. However, rarely are these tests of exclusion available in the emergency department. Therefore it is recommended that empiric treatment for both syphilis and chancroid be administered to patients with genital ulcers in communities where *H. ducreyi* is present (15). Emergency department physicians should contact their local health department if they feel they have seen a case of chancroid to determine if other cases of the disease are being seen locally and if not, to alert them to the possibility of the first case.

Gonorrhea and chlamydia cultures are still considered the gold standard for laboratory diagnosis of these infections, but they are of limited utility due to cumbersome, time-consuming, and labor-intensive laboratory methods, specimen handling challenges, expense, and limited availability. Urethral smear Gram stain is still valuable for rapid diagnosis and is 95–98% sensitive for gonorrhea in symptomatic men. Other stains such as methylene blue alone or combined with gentian violet, safranin, or acridine orange have been used with equivalent sensitivity, but have not been as extensively studied. Automated methods for the detection and/or amplification of gonococcal and chlamydial DNA or RNA represent exciting developments in the arena of diagnostic testing for these organisms. These methods can be used on cervical, urethral, and urine specimens from both men and women. Although the organisms can be detected by other nonculture means such as enzyme-linked immunoassay and direct immunofluorescence, amplification methods have surpassed them all as the screening tests of choice because of increased sensitivity and excellent specificity. In addition, amplification tests have revolutionized the approach to gonococcal and chlamydial screening and prevention of high-risk asymptomatic individuals by allowing the use of nonconventional specimens such as patient-collected vaginal swabs and urine.

Patients suspected of having disseminated gonococcal infection should have standard GC cultures taken from the cervix/urethra, pharynx, and rectum because blood cultures are only positive 20–30% of the time and joint fluid cultures are rarely positive. Documented infection at a mucosal site is extremely helpful in confirming the diagnosis. However, Gram stain and cultures of unroofed pustules and joint fluid are still important as conditions such as endocarditis and septic arthritis may mimic the presentation of DGI and these tests may help with the correct diagnosis of these cases.

The mainstay of laboratory diagnosis of vaginitis is microscopic evaluation of a saline wet prep and a KOH prep of vaginal discharge. Table 36–5 outlines the microscopic findings used in the diagnosis of candida vaginitis, bacterial vaginosis, and trichomonas vaginitis. In addition, for a more reliable clinical diagnosis of bacterial vaginosis, at least three of the following four signs should be present: (1) homogeneous, white, and adherent discharge; (2) vaginal fluid pH greater than 4.5; (3) positive amine test with release of fishy odor upon addition of 10% KOH; and (4) at least 20% vaginal squamous cells manifested as clue cells by light microscopy.

The diagnosis of genital warts, molluscum contagiosum, and ectoparasites relies upon clinical presentation. Rarely are laboratory studies or histopathology of biopsy specimens used to confirm the diagnosis. Occasionally, the diagnosis of scabies or pubic lice can be confirmed with microscopic examination of skin scrapings for evidence of scabies, and examination of hair samples for eggs/nits or the organism for pubic lice but this requires expertise acquired through practice.

MANAGEMENT

Early and effective diagnosis and treatment of sexually transmitted diseases prevent serious complications and reduce the transmission of STDs and HIV. The most recent Centers for Disease Control STD treatment guidelines and recommendations are presented in Tables 36–6 through 36–16. Clinical management of patients with STD complaints in the emergency department, however, is often met with the challenge of not having results of STD laboratory studies readily available and poor patient follow-up. In addition, in busy emergency departments, microscopy may not be available, and if it is, lack of time and microscope experience present serious challenges and difficulties to emergency room physicians. For these rea-

Table 36–6. Treatment Regimens for Syphilis

Primary, secondary, and early latent
    Benzathine penicillin 2.4 MU IM
    PCN allergic–doxycycline 100 mg p.o. BID for
      14 days
Late latent
    Benzathine penicillin 2.4 MU IM q wk. × 3 injections
      (total 7.2 MU IM)
    PCN allergic—doxycycline 100 mg p.o.
      BID × 4 weeks
Neurosyphilis
    Aqueous crystalline PCN 3-4 MU IV q 4 h
      10–14 days—PCN allergic patients need to be
      desensitized and treated with PCN
Special circumstances
    Pregnant and PCN allergic—desensitize and treat
      with PCN
    HIV—same treatment for stage of syphilis in
      non-HIV patients

Source: Adapted from the *2002 CDC Sexually Transmitted Diseases Treatment Guidelines*

sons, a low threshold for syndromic treatment is recommended.

Syndromic management means basing the treatment regimen on the patient's presenting syndrome, or combination of signs and symptoms that are indicative of certain

Table 36–7. Treatment Regimens for Herpes

Initial outbreak—duration of therapy 7–10 days
    Acyclovir 400 mg p.o. TID
             or
    Famciclovir 250 mg p.o. TID
             or
    Valacyclovir 1000 mg p.o. BID

Recurrent episodes—duration of therapy 3–5 days
    Acyclovir 400 mg p.o. three times daily × 5 days
             or
    Acyclovir 800 mg p.o. twice daily × 5 days
             or
    Famciclovir 125 mg p.o. twice daily × 5 days
             or
    Valacyclovir 500 mg p.o. twice daily × 3–5 days
             or
    Valacyclovir 1 g p.o. daily × 5 days

Source: Adapted from the *2002 CDC Sexually Transmitted Diseases Treatment Guidelines.*

Table 36–8. Treatment Regimens for Chancroid

Azithromycin 1 g orally
or
Ceftriaxone 250 mg IM in a single dose
or
Ciprofloxacin 500 mg p.o. twice daily × 3 days
or
Erythromycin base 500 mg p.o. TID × 7 days

Source: Adapted from the *2002 CDC Sexually Transmitted Diseases Treatment Guidelines.*

sexually transmitted diseases. This approach can be used for genital ulcers, urethral discharge in men, vaginal discharge, and lower abdominal pain in women. Treatment is provided to cover the major organisms causing these syndromes. For example, a young sexually active man presenting with urethral discharge and/or epididymal tenderness would be treated for both gonorrhea and chlamydia. Women with vaginal discharge would be treated for yeast, trichomonas, and bacterial vaginosis if the speculum exam revealed a normal cervix. If cervical discharge or a friable cervix is seen on speculum exam, the patient would also be treated for gonorrhea and chlamydia.

Table 36–9. Treatment Regimens for Gonococcal Infections

Gonococcal urethritis/cervicitis (MPC)
  Cefixime 400 mg p.o. single dose
  Ceftriaxone 125 mg IM single dose
  Ciprofloxacin 500 mg, ofloxacin 400 mg, or
    levofloxacin 250 mg p.o. single dose (except in CA, Hawaii, patients from Asia or the Pacific, and men who have sex with men (MSM) in the United States. Due to increased quinolone resistance in these patients, ceftriaxone 125 mg IM, cefixime 400 mg, or sectinomycin 2 g IM is currently recommended)
  Add azithromycin 1 g or Doxy 100 mg BID × 7 days for concomitant *Chlamydia trachomatis* infection
Alternatives
  Spectinomycin 2 g IM single dose
  Cefoxitin 2 g IM plus probenecid 1 g p.o.
Disseminated gonococcal infections (DGI)
  Ceftriaxone 1 g IM or IV qd (plus chlamydia therapy) until clinical improvement—finish 7-day course with cefixime or ciprofloxacin, ofloxacin, or levofloxacin

Source: Adapted from the *2002 CDC Sexually Transmitted Diseases Treatment Guidelines.*

Table 36–10. Treatment Regimens for Uncomplicated Chlamydial Infections or nongonococcal urethritis in men

Urethritis or cervicitis
Recommended regimens:
  Azithromycin 1 g orally in a single dose or doxycycline 100 mg orally BID for 7 days
Alternative regimens:
  Erythromycin base 500 mg orally QID for 7 days
  or
  Erythromycin ethylsuccinate 800 mg orally QID for 7 days
  or
  Ofloxacin 300 mg BID for 7 days or levofloxacin 500 mg p.o. qd for 7 days
Chlamydial infections in pregnancy
Recommended:
  Erythromycin base 500 mg orally QID for 7 days
  or
  Amoxicillin 500 mg orally TID for 7 days
Alternate regimens:
  Erythromycin base 250 mg orally QID for 14 days
  or
  Erythromycin ethlysuccinate 800 mg orally QID for 7 days or 400 mg QID for 14 days
  or
  Azithromycin 1 g orally, single dose

Source: Adapted from the *2002 CDC Sexually Transmitted Diseases Treatment Guidelines.*

Table 36–11. Treatment Regimens for Pelvic Inflammatory Disease

Criteria for hospitalization
  Cannot rule out surgical emergency
  Pregnancy
  Clinical failure of oral antimicrobials
  Inability to follow or tolerate oral regimen
  Severe illness, nausea/vomiting, high fever
  Tubo-ovarian abscess
Inpatient regimen
  Cefotetan 2 g IV q 12 h or cefoxitin 2 g IV q 6 h plus doxycycline 100 mg IV q 12 h
  Discontinue 24 h after clinical improvement then complete 14-day course with doxycycline
Outpatient regimen
  Ceftriaxone 250 mg IM single dose or cefoxitin 2 g IM and probenecid 1 g p.o. plus doxycycline × 14 days

Source: Adapted from the *2002 CDC Sexually Transmitted Diseases Treatment Guidelines.*

Table 36–12. Treatment Regimen for Epididymitis

Infection likely due to gonorrhea or chlamydia
    Ceftriaxone 250 mg IM in a single dose
                PLUS
    Doxycycline 100 mg p.o. twice daily for 10 days
Infection likely due to enteric organisms or age >35 years
    Ofloxacin 300 mg p.o. twice daily for 10 days
                or
    Levofloxacin 500 mg p.o. once daily for 10 days

Source: Adapted from the *2002 CDC Sexually Transmitted Diseases Treatment Guidelines.*

In addition, women with lower abdominal pain, without the criteria for hospitalization noted in Table 36–11, would be treated with an outpatient regimen for PID. Patients with genital ulcers would be empirically treated for both syphilis and chancroid (if the latter is being seen in the local community), unless the lesions are characteristic of classic herpes.

Table 36–13. Treatment Regimens for Vaginitis

Candida vulvovaginitis
    Intravaginal regimens
        Butoconazole, clotrimazole, miconazole, nystatin, tioconazole, terconazole
    Oral regimen
        Fluconazole 150 mg in a single dose
Trichomonas vaginitis
    Metronidazole 2 g orally in a single dose
Alternative regimen
    Metronidazole 500 mg p.o. twice a day for 7 days
Pregnancy
    Metronidazole 2 g orally in a single dose
Bacterial vaginosis
    Metronidazole 500 mg p.o. twice daily for 7 days
                or
    Metronidazole gel 0.75%, 5 g intravaginally once daily for 5 days
                or
    Clindamycin cream 5%, 5 g intravaginally qh for 7 days
Alternative regimens
    Metronidazole 2 g p.o. in a single dose
                or
    Clindamycin 300 mg p.o. twice daily for 7 days
                or
    Clindamycin ovules 100 g intravaginally qh for 3 days

Source: Adapted from the *2002 CDC Sexually Transmitted Diseases Treatment Guidelines.*

Table 36–14. Treatment Regimens for HPV

Patient applied
    Podofilox 0.5% solution or gel
                or
    Imiquimod 5% cream
Provider administered
    Cryotherapy
                or
    Podophyllin resin 10–25%
                or
    Trichloroacetic or bichloroacetic acid 80–90%
                or
    Surgical removal

Source: Adapted from the *2002 CDC Sexually Transmitted Diseases Treatment Guidelines.*

Table 36–15. Treatment Regimens for Pediculosis Pubis (Pubic Lice)

Decontaminate bedding and clothing
Recommended regimens
    Permethrin 1%
    Lindane 1% shampoo
    Pyrethrins with piperonyl butoxide
Retreatment may be necessary if symptoms persist
Treatment of sex partners within the last month

Source: Adapted from the *2002 CDC Sexually Transmitted Diseases Treatment Guidelines.*

Table 36–16. Treatment Regimens for Scabies

Recommended regimen
    Permethrin cream 5%
Alternative regimen
    Lindane 1%
                or
    Invermectin 200 μg/kg, repeat in 2 weeks
Sex partners and household contacts within the preceding month should be treated

Source: Adapted from the *2002 CDC Sexually Transmitted Diseases Treatment Guidelines.*

The advantages of syndromic management include immediate treatment, decreased numbers of untreated patients lost to follow-up, decreased transmission of STDs secondary to early treatment of infected individuals, and patient satisfaction. For these reasons syndromic management is a valuable approach to STD treatment in emergency departments and has proven to be both effective and cost-effective in resource-poor areas throughout the world (29).

DISPOSITION

Emergency medicine physicians play a critical role in public health initiatives to control STDs due to the numbers of patients using emergency rooms for primary medical care. Patients with STDs often will present initially to the emergency room where adequate treatment may help interrupt STD transmission in the community and prevent expensive complications of STDs. Emergency department physicians are encouraged to have a high index of suspicion regarding STDs and maintain a low threshold for empiric syndromic treatment of STDs. In addition, emergency room physicians should provide patients with STD risk reduction information, refer partners for therapy, and assist with STD control initiatives by reporting selected STDs to their local public health departments.

CASE OUTCOME

The patient provided a urine sample for gonorrhea and chlamydia testing by a nucleic acid amplification assay and was treated for urethritis and epididymitis with ceftriaxone 250 mg IM and doxycycline 100 mg orally bid for 14 days. Syphilis serology was also obtained. The patient was seen for follow-up at the STD clinic 1 week later and had complete resolution of the discharge and scrotal pain. Results of urine studies from the emergency room were positive for gonorrhea and chlamydia. The patient's VDRL returned positive at 1:64 with positive confirmatory syphilis serology. A negative VDRL was documented in the clinic medical record 6 months prior. The patient was treated with benzathine penicillin 2.4 million units IM for early latent syphilis and referred to public health officials to obtain information necessary to insure that all recent sexual contacts would be treated.

REFERENCES

1. Cates W: Estimates of the incidence and prevalence of sexually transmitted diseases in the United States. *Sex Transm Dis* 26(Suppl.):S2–S7, 1999.

2. Quinn T: Association of sexually transmitted diseases and infection with the human immunodeficiency virus: Biological cofactor and markers of behavioral interventions. *Int J STD AIDS* 7:17–24, 1996.

3. Grosskurth H, Mosha F, Todd J, et al.: Impact of improved treatment of sexually transmitted diseases on HIV infection in rural Tanzania: Randomized controlled trial. *Lancet* 436:530–536, 1995.

4. Beckmann KR, Melzer-Lange MD, Gorelick MH: Emergency department management of sexually transmitted infections in US adolescents: Results from the National Hospital Ambulatory Medical Care Survey. *Ann Emer Med* 43:333–338, 2004.

5. Curtis KM, Hillis SD, Kieke NA, et al.: Visits to emergency departments for gynecologic disorders in the United States, 1992–1994. *Obstet Gynecol* 91:1007–1012, 1998.

6. Mehta SD, Shahan J, Zenilman JM: Ambulatory STD management in an inner-city emergency department: Descriptive epidemiology, care utilization patterns, and patient perceptions of local public STD clinics. *Sex Transm Dis* 47:154–157, 2000.

7. Centers for Disease Control and Prevention: 2002 Sexually transmitted diseases treatment guidelines. *Morb Mortal Wkly Rep* 51(RR-6):1–80, 2002.

8. McKinzie J: Sexually transmitted diseases. *Emerg Med Clin North Am* 19:723–743, 2001.

9. Institute of Medicine: *The Hidden Epidemic: Confronting Sexually Transmitted Diseases.* Washington, DC, National Academy Press, 1997.

10. Centers for Disease Control and Prevention: *Sexually Transmitted Disease Surveillance 2002.* Atlanta, GA, U.S. Department of Health and Human Services, Centers for Disease Control and Prevention, September 2003.

11. CDC: Primary and Secondary Syphilis – United States 2002. *Morb Mortal Wkly Rep* 52:1117–1120, 2003.

12. Stamm LV: Biology of *Treponema pallidum*, in Holmes KK, Sparling PF, Mardh P-A, et al. (eds.) *Sexually Transmitted Diseases.* New York, McGraw-Hill; 1999, pp 467–472, 639.

13. Schroeter AL, Turner RH, Lucas JB, et al.: Therapy for incubating syphilis: Effectiveness of gonorrhea treatment. *JAMA* 218:711–713, 1971.

14. Corey L, Wald A: Genital herpes, in Holmes KK, Sparling PF, Mardh P-A, et al. (eds.): *Sexually Transmitted Diseases.* New York, McGraw-Hill, 1999; pp 285–312.

15. Taylor SN: Chancroid, in Rakel RE, Bope ET (eds.): *Conn's Current Therapy 2001.* Philadelphia, Mosby, 2001; pp 764–765.

16. Buchanan TM: Attachment role of gonococcal pili: Optimum conditions and quantitation of adherence of isolated to human cells in vitro. *J Clin Invest* 61:931–943, 1978.

17. Schachter J: Biology of *Chlamydia trachomatis*, in Holmes KK, Sparling PF, Mardh P-A, et al. (eds.): *Sexually Transmitted Diseases.* New York, McGraw-Hill, 1999; pp 391–405.

18. Sobel JD: Vulvovaginal candidiasis, in Holmes KK, Sparling PF, Mardh P-A, et al, (eds.): *Sexually Transmitted Diseases.* New York, McGraw-Hill, 1999; pp 629–639.

19. King RD, Lee JC, Morris AL: Adherence of *Candida albicans* and other *Candida* species to mucosal epithelial cells. *Infect Immun* 27:667–674, 1980.

20. Sobel JD, Myer P, Levison ME, et al.: *Candida albicans* adherence to vaginal epithelial cells. *J Infect Dis* 143:76–82, 1981.

21. Bertholf ME, Stafford MJ: Colonization of *Candida albicans* in vagina, rectum, and mouth. *J Family Pract* 16:919–924, 1983.

22. O'Conner MI, Sobel, JD: Epidemiology of recurrent vulvovaginal candidiasis: Identification and strain differentiation of *Candida albicans. J Infect Dis* 154:358–363, 1986.

23. Sobel JD: Vaginal infections in women. *Med Clin North Am* 74:1573–1602, 1990.

24. Krieger JN, Alderete JF: *Trichomonas vaginalis* and trichomoniasis, in Holmes KK, Sparling PF, Mardh P-A, et al. (eds.): *Sexually Transmitted Diseases*. New York, McGraw-Hill, 1999; pp 587–604.

25. Douglas JD: Molluscum contagiosum. *Trichomonas vaginalis* and trichomoniasis, in Holmes KK, Sparling PF, Mardh P-A, et al. (eds.): *Sexually Transmitted Diseases*. New York, McGraw-Hill, 1999; pp 385–389.

26. DiCarlo RP, Martin DH: The clinical diagnosis of genital ulcer disease in men. *Clin Infect Dis* 25:292–298, 1997.

27. Taylor SN: *Chlamydia trachomatis* infection, in Rakel RE, Bope ET (eds.): *Conn's Current Therapy 2004*. Philadelphia, Mosby, 2004; pp 1120–1122.

28. Sweet RL: Pelvic inflammatory disease and infertility in women. *Infect Dis Clin North Am* 1:199–215, 1987.

29. Taylor SN: Syndromic treatment of sexually transmitted diseases. *Rev Med Microbiol* 11:233–245, 2000.

37

Emerging Infections

Stephen J. Playe
Pieter V. Esterhay

OVERVIEW

Definition

Emerging infectious diseases fall into one of three categories. The first category includes diseases that have not previously occurred in humans. This is difficult to establish, and probably rare; however, SARS may be a truly new human disease. The second category involves diseases that have occurred previously but affected only small numbers of persons in isolated locations. Examples of this are AIDS and Ebola hemorrhagic fever. The third category includes diseases that have occurred throughout history, but have only recently been recognized as distinct diseases caused by an infectious agent. Lyme disease and gastric ulcers are examples of this.

Principles of Emergence

Changing human behavior that results in new or increased contact with either a reservoir or vector of pathological microbes most often causes an infectious disease to emerge. Techniques of mass food production, for example, are responsible for the large outbreaks of hemolytic uremic syndrome secondary to *Escherichia coli* O 157: H7. Air conditioning systems led to the emergence of Legionnaire disease. Building homes increasingly near woods played a role in the emergence of Lyme disease. Closer contact with rodents exposed humans to the Hantavirus. Evolving sexual practices played a role in the AIDS epidemic. Rapid international travel as well as international food distribution has been responsible for the spread of infectious diseases into previously unaffected regions.

In the minority of cases, microbial changes are responsible. Examples include the evolution of a new strain of cholera (*Vibrio cholerae* O 139), which combined increased virulence with long-term survival in the environment. The recent avian influenza (H5N1) outbreak resulted from an antigenic shift causing a virulent disease in humans. Theoretically, a coinfection with human and avian influenza could result in genetic reassortment to generate a strain which is both virulent and highly contagious among humans. This could lead to a devastating pandemic.

Role of the Emergency Physician

Much of emergency medicine is pattern recognition. In the case of an emerging infection, it is important that emergency medical providers recognize a new or unusual pattern of disease. This could be a unique individual patient presentation or unexpected clusters of similar diseases. Recent travel history can be a very important clue.

To identify and contain emerging diseases, as well as identify possible bioterrorism activities, emergency personnel must promptly notify local or state health departments whenever suspicions arise. An important recent development is the creation of EMERGEncy IDnet, an interdisciplinary, multicenter, ED-based network for identification of emerging infectious diseases (1). Information is electronically stored, transferred, and analyzed at a central receiving site that has been established in cooperation with the Centers for Disease Control and Prevention (CDC) and 11 university-affiliated, urban hospital emergency departments (1). This can help identify new patterns of disease that would not be recognized by individual practices.

Exposure Prevention

Standard precautions should be observed with all patients. When confronted with an unknown, potentially contagious disease, it is prudent to additionally observe contact precautions (preventing indirect contact via contaminated intermediate objects in the patient's environment), droplet precautions (including goggles or face shield when within 3 feet of the patient), and aerosol precautions (surgical mask on the patient, patient in a negative pressure ventilation room, and caretakers wearing individually fitted N-95 filter masks).

Diagnosis and Treatment

Diagnosis depends upon the recognition of the clinical pattern, knowledge of potential exposure, and awareness of current medical events in the region, the country, and the world.

Recently emerging diseases, including their treatment, will be described in detail in the following sections.

SEVERE ACUTE RESPIRATORY SYNDROME

Introduction

Severe acute respiratory syndrome (SARS) is a recently discovered viral illness resulting in severe febrile lower respiratory tract infection that often leads to respiratory failure. The causative virus is a coronavirus, apparently new in humans, which has been named the SARS-associated coronavirus (SARS-CoV). The Coronaviridae family is the second most common cause of common cold. SARS is the first emerging infection of the 21st century to gain a worldwide distribution. Between November 2002 and July 2003, 8437 new cases resulted in 812 deaths. Cases were primarily confirmed in China and neighboring Asian countries, although cases did occur in Canada and the United States. It is unclear at this time if the disease will reappear, but health care workers must be educated and vigilant in observing for signs and symptoms to initiate prompt public health measures to contain an outbreak (2).

As yet unconfirmed research indicates that SARS-CoV originated in livestock or small mammals, most likely in rural, southern China where humans and animals live in close proximity. Zoonotic transmission appears likely as corona viruses are known to infect pigs and birds and the three other known corona viruses include mammalian and avian viruses. Further, human coronavirus 229E and OC43 are both known to cause upper and lower respiratory tract illness. Some research indicates the animal origin of SARS-CoV may be the civet cat, a small relative of the mongoose, native to China, sold as a delicacy in markets (2).

Once SARS-CoV gained access to human hosts, it spread rapidly throughout mainland China. Initially information from that country was internally suppressed due to political and public safety concerns. It now appears at least 5327 cases were confirmed throughout the country with an additional 1755 cases in Hong Kong. Neighboring Taiwan also confirmed 671 cases. High travel corridors led to a significant outbreak in Toronto, Canada. By June 2003, 250 cases had been confirmed in that city. The United States had 29 probable cases. To date, the WHO has identified 8384 probable SARS cases with 774 deaths (a case fatality rate of 9.6%) among 29 countries (2, 6).

SARS-CoV is thought to be transmitted by close person-to-person contact. The exact mode of transmission has not been confirmed; however, the disease has been contracted from skin, and respiratory or mucous membrane contact with aerosolized droplets from infected individuals. Less evidence exists for oral–fecal transmis-

sion although SARS-CoV has been demonstrated to survive for several days in feces raising the possibility of fomite transmission (2, 3).

History

SARS is transmitted by respiratory droplets created during a cough or sneeze by an infected individual. These droplets travel several feet through the air and can be deposited on another person's mucous membranes or skin. Therefore, paramount for risk of SARS contraction is close contact to known or suspected SARS patients within 10 days of symptom onset. Contact includes any direct physical contact between bodies, exposure to secretions of the patient, or any close conversation. Lacking direct person-to-person contacted with an infected individual, SARS should only be considered if, within 10 days of onset of symptoms, the patient traveled to, or had contact with a sick individual who has traveled to, China, Hong Kong, or Taiwan; or, if the patient has a high-risk occupational exposure including health care workers caring for SARS infected individuals or laboratory personnel working with live SARS-CoV; or if the patient is part of a cluster of atypical pneumonias without an alternative diagnosis (3).

SARS follows a very nonspecific flu-like disease course. After SARS-CoV exposure, there is a 2–7-day asymptomatic incubation period. Patients then experience a 3–7-day period of fever, malaise, myalgia, headache, anorexia, and, less commonly, diarrhea. This period is very similar to influenza. Their condition deteriorates as lower respiratory effects are felt. Dry cough, wheezing, dyspnea, and/or progressive hypoxemia may lead to respiratory failure (2, 3).

The clinical course of SARS explains why international travel played such a big role and why hospital health care providers were disproportionately infected. Infected patients were able to travel during the asymptomatic incubation period as well as the early mild illness. Since SARS patients, unlike those with other viral illnesses, are most viremic and contagious *late* in the course, when they have become clinically ill and are often hospitalized, health care workers were frequently infected.

Physical Examination

The physical examination is suggestive of influenza or a respiratory tract infection. Fever and any finding of respiratory illness (i.e., cough, wheezing, dyspnea) are considered *moderate* illness. If additionally there is evidence of pneumonia or ARDS, it is considered *severe* illness.

Less common findings include chills, rigors, pharyngitis, rhinorrhea, nausea, vomiting, and diarrhea.

Laboratory/Diagnostic Testing

In general, CDC recommendations for testing for SARS depend on whether there is known outbreak in the world population. Diagnostic algorithms for both outbreak and nonoutbreak situations have been created (3).

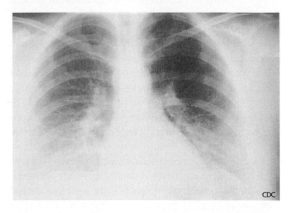

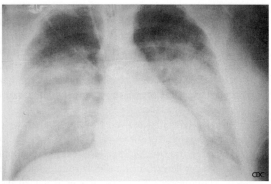

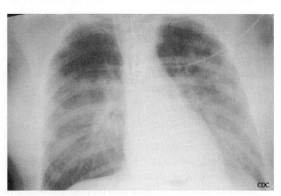

Fig. 37–1. Evolution of HPS (courtesy D. Loren Ketai).

Although not diagnostic, laboratory confirmed cases of SARS have demonstrated lymphopenia with low or normal total white blood cell counts, elevated hepatic transaminases, elevated creatine kinase, elevated C-reactive protein, prolonged activated partial thromboplastin time, or elevated lactate dehydrogenase (4).

Chest radiography is initially abnormal in only 60% of patients. However, serial radiographs became abnormal in almost all patients by 2 weeks after symptom onset. Initially, interstitial infiltrates can be observed ranging from peripheral, pleural-based ground glass to frank consolidation. During disease progression, lower lung fields tend to be affected first with widespread opacification. SARS does not appear to lead to effusion, cavitation, or lymphadenopathy (2, 3). High resolution computed tomography may prove to be a more sensitive and helpful imaging modality, especially early in the course of the disease.

Because of the need to rule out other more common causes of pneumonia, all patients with infiltrates on radiographs should have blood cultures, RSV, and influenza viral testing and urinary testing for legionella and pneumococcal antigens (3).

Specific diagnostic testing is being aggressively pursued, but no test is yet able to identify the pathogen early enough in the disease course to effect management decisions. Indirect immunofluorescence assays for SARS-CoV antibodies and polymerase chain reaction (PCR) testing of nasal swabs, sputum, serum, and stool specimens have been developed but adequate diagnostic sensitivity has not been achieved. This is especially true in the early phase of illness as, unlike many similar viral illnesses, SARS viral shedding appears to be low until 10 days following symptom onset. Serologic response does not appear until day 5 or 6 of symptomatic illness. The CDC is currently classifying a case of non-SARS only after negative serology is achieved 21 days after symptom onset. Although complicating diagnostic testing, SARS' propensity for significant viral shedding only during symptomatic phase may actually be helping to limit the outbreak since spread from asymptomatic or incubating individuals has not been reported (3, 5).

In the context of the above sensitivity limitations, CDC laboratory confirmation of SARS can only be achieved in three ways: serum antibody detection by ELISA any time from acute illness to more than 21 days postonset; PCR confirmation from one specimen on two occasions, two specimens from different sources, or two specimens from the same sources on two different days; or isolation of SARS-CoV in cell culture confirmed by PCR.

Clinician Protection

Strict droplet and contact precautions should be followed when dealing with suspected SARS patients because of the risk for droplet and fomite transmission (3).

Treatment

Treatment of SARS is supportive and includes nutrition, fluid, and, in advanced cases, mechanical ventilation. No definitive medication treatment has proven effective despite aggressive research. Many antiviral agents have been used, most commonly ribavirin. While it does not have proven anti-SARS activity there are anecdotal reports of efficacy when used in combination with steroids. Currently, screening is being pursued among thousands of existing antiviral medications to identify efficacy against SARS viral proteases. Interferon has also shown preliminary promise. Subsequent to SARS genomic sequencing, specific SARS-CoV medications and vaccine are in early development but wide availability is thought to be several years away (2).

Given its nonspecific symptoms and possible similarity to bacterial respiratory illnesses, coverage with antibiotics early in the course, prior to SARS confirmatory testing, is prudent. Antibiotics provide, however, no protection from SARS itself. Due to the contagiousness and potential for rapid deterioration, all suspected cases should be considered for hospital admission.

Differential Diagnosis

Given the nonspecific early manifestations of SARS, the differential for SARS is extensive. Any upper respiratory infection or pneumonia of any etiology including bacterial, viral, or fungal must be considered. Likewise, prior to respiratory phase onset, all causes of fever must be considered including nonrespiratory sources such as meningitis and sepsis. The key distinguishing factor for SARS is the exposure risk.

Medicolegal Implications

Any suspected SARS case must be placed on strict droplet precautions. Isolation would be prudent as well to limit contacts; likely patients will need both mechanical ventilation and ICU care. Local, state, and federal health agencies must be notified. Subsequently, attempts to identify all contacts within 2 weeks prior to symptom onset must be made. As of April 4, 2003, SARS joined cholera, diphtheria, tuberculosis, plague, smallpox, yellow fever, and viral hemorrhagic fevers on the U.S. list of quarantinable communicable diseases (2). However, even in outbreak situations, failure to consider and rule out other treatable causes of febrile and respiratory tract illness would be a mistake.

WEST NILE VIRUS

Introduction

West Nile virus (WNV) is an arthropodborne virus transmitted to humans via mosquito bites. Capable of crossing the blood-brain barrier, the virus can lead to encephalitis and/or meningitis. Infected birds, which may be asymptomatic, are the viral reservoir and they may contain high hematologic viral titers for 1–2 weeks. The virus has been identified in 111 different bird species. *Culex, Aedes,* and *Anopheles* mosquito species transmit WNV to humans after biting infected birds. A dozen other animals, including horses and dogs, may also harbor the virus but are not viremic at levels necessary for transmission (7–9).

First discovered in Uganda's West Nile district in 1937, interest in the virus renewed with the first outbreak in the United States in New York in August 1999 among birds, horses, and humans. In the subsequent 5 years, the virus has been demonstrated in human, bird, veterinary, or mosquito populations in all states with the exception of Hawaii, Alaska, and Oregon. In 2003, a total of 9862 cases were reported in the United States of which 2866 patients developed meningitis or encephalitis. There were 264 fatalities (7).

It is unclear at this time if WNV will become a significant long-term health concern in the United States. In Egypt, seropositivity in children is 50% and WNV is the most common cause of viral meningitis and encephalitis. In Asia and Africa, the illness runs a benign course in children with only rare fatalities. The North American strain is considerably more virulent. In the United States, the elderly population has been most affected and has a particularly high fatality rate. Even in outbreak areas, the likelihood of developing clinical disease after infection is less than 1% (7–9).

Although the vast majority of cases are mosquito-borne, during the 2002 epidemic 23 individuals contracted West Nile after receiving blood products from 16 separate viremic donors. Subsequently, blood collection agencies have implemented nucleic acid amplification tests. The testing provides security against transfusion infection and provides surveillance data for possible West Nile outbreak in the general population (10). WNV can also be transmitted through breast milk, pregnancy, and organ transplantation.

History

The incubation period is thought to range from 3 to 14 days. Approximately three-quarters of infections are asymptomatic. *West Nile fever (WNF)* develops in approximately 20% of infected persons. It is characterized by a febrile illness of sudden onset, often accompanied by malaise, anorexia, nausea, vomiting, eye pain, headaches, myalgia, rash, or lymphadenopathy which lasts 3–6 days. Recovery is generally complete.

Severe disease develops in approximately one person per 150 infections. While Old World outbreaks have included myocarditis, pancreatitis, and fulminant hepatitis, severe disease in the United States has been manifested by the following three types of neurological abnormalities.

West Nile meningitis (WNM) presents with meningeal inflammation, which may produce nuchal rigidity, Kernig or Brudzinski sign, photophobia, or phonophobia. Patients generally have fever (greater than 38°C) or hypothermia (less than 35°C); CSF pleocytosis with elevated protein; peripheral WBC greater than 10,000 mm^3; and magnetic residence imaging consistent with acute meningeal inflammation.

West Nile encephalitis (WNE) can be seen alone or in combination with meningeal inflammation. Encephalitis is characterized by alterations of consciousness ranging from mild lethargy to confusion, stupor, or coma. Seizures, personality changes, weakness, tremor, myoclonus, and Parkinsonism have been reported. Clinical evidence includes all of those described for WNM (above) as well as electroencephalography, which may show findings consistent with encephalitis.

West Nile Acute Flaccid Paralysis (WNAFP) presents with the acute onset of limb weakness that is rapidly progressive over 48 h. This condition includes at least two of the following features: asymmetric weakness; decreased or no reflexes of the affected limb(s); absence of pain, paresthesia, or numbness in the effected limb(s); CSF pleocytosis and elevated protein; electrodiagnostic studies consistent with an anterior horn cell process; spinal cord MRI demonstrating an abnormally increased signal in the anterior gray matter.

WNV illness typically begins with the rapid onset of fever. Headache, weakness, myalgia, rash, arthralgias, and photophobia occur variably in less than half of patients. Headache, when present, is often retro orbital and associated with photophobia (8).

Physical

Central nervous system involvement determines the extent of physical findings. Most patients demonstrate fever. In more severe cases, neurological findings include confusion, disorientation, depressed mental status, coma, or meningismus. Hepatosplenomegaly is found in 10–20% of patients. Nonexudative pharyngitis has also been observed. Internationally, truncal maculopapular rash has been seen in nearly 50% of patients, but this has not been seen with the same frequency in the United States (8, 9). Likewise, generalized or submental lymphadenopathy, and extremity weakness and paralysis have been seen. Many patients have focal neurological signs including cranial nerve deficits, ataxia, myelitis, or flaccid paralysis of an extremity. These deficits frequently result in permanent disability.

Laboratory/Diagnostic Testing

CSF analysis is the best indicator of active infection. WNV-specific IgM antibody detected by antibody-capture enzyme-immunoassay (EIA) is the most sensitive and best means of diagnosing the illness. Polymerase chain reaction methods are positive only in up to 60% of cases.

Serum tests are useful if paired acute phase (collected 0–8 days after onset of illness) and convalescent phase (collected 14–21 days after the acute specimen) demonstrate seroconversion. Antibody synthesis in immunocompromised patients may be delayed or absent.

Clinician Protection

Due to low levels of viremia, there is no risk of person-to-person transmission of WNV in the clinical setting.

Treatment

Treatment of WNV infection is supportive. High dose ribavirin and interferon alpha-2b have shown in vitro activity but no controlled studies of either or any other medication including steroids, antiepileptics, or osmotic agents have been completed (11). Hospitalization is recommended in severe cases for respiratory or symptomatic support.

Differential Diagnosis

The differential diagnosis includes all causes of encephalitis and meningitis. Enteroviral aseptic meningitis secondary to coxsackievirus is the most common cause of aseptic meningitis in the summer months, often associated with nonexudative pharyngitis, maculopapular rash, and diarrhea. The most common cause of nonseasonal aseptic meningitis in the United States is herpes simplex virus type I. Drug-induced meningitis, most commonly due to NSAIDs, should be considered (8, 9).

Other arthropodborne viral encephalitides such as Eastern Equine, Japanese, and St. Louis encephalitis should be considered in presentations with rapid onset of fever and severe headache. Finally, all systemic illnesses with potential for CNS manifestations must be considered including systemic lupus erythematosis, sepsis, mononucleosis, Rocky Mountain spotted fever, Legionnaire disease, and subacute bacterial endocarditis (8, 9).

Medicolegal Implications

Failure to consider the diagnosis in encephalitic or meningitic patients who present in summer or early fall, especially in areas with WNV activity, or to inquire about recent travel to a WNV active area could be problematic and lead to misdiagnosis (11, 12). Despite these historical clues, it is important to remember that any unexplained encephalitis or meningitis could be due to WNV infection because in some warmer areas year-round transmission is possible. Failure to consider alternative treatable diseases, such as bacterial meningitis, could be a serious mistake.

LEPTOSPIROSIS

Introduction

Leptospirosis, also known as mud fever, and swineherd's disease, is a bacterial infection caused by the spirochete *leptospiraceae*, and is the most common zoonosis worldwide. The largest primary reservoir is wild mammals with recurring transmission to domesticated animal populations. Rats and other rodents make up the core of the reservoir with dogs, cats, and livestock of importance in the United States.

Spirochete shedding occurs in a host's urine. Urinary shedding into soil, mud, or water leads to contaminated sources where the spirochetes can survive for months as long as temperatures remain greater than 71°F. These flagellated aerobes invade the host through broken skin or mucous membranes. Thus, individuals such as veterinarians, farmworkers, and outdoor enthusiasts are at higher risk (13, 15). Leptospirosis occurs worldwide but due to temperature requirements, the highest prevalence is in the tropics. In the United States, Hawaii has the highest in-

cidence with 128 cases per 100,000 individuals in 1992 (13).

Following infection, the spirochetes multiply in the lymphatics and cause vasculitis in the kidneys and liver. Interstitial nephritis and tubular necrosis may eventually result in renal failure. Hepatic effects include centrilobular necrosis with resulting jaundice. When skeletal muscle is invaded, the spirochetes may cause edema and focal necrosis. Severe disease presents as a disseminated vasculitic syndrome from diffuse capillary endothelial damage (13, 15).

The incubation period ranges from 24 h to 4 weeks although most commonly it is 5–14 days. A significant minority of patients exposed never develop disease despite seroconversion. Only 1 in 10 will develop jaundice indicative of Weil disease, the severe, icteric form of leptospirosis (13, 15).

Leptospirosis is a two-stage disease with a wide range of signs and symptoms which can progress to multiorgan failure and death. The severity depends upon the site of inoculation, the virulence of the strain, and the condition of the host. The first stage is considered the leptospiremic, or septic, stage because during its 3–8 day length, the spirochete can be cultured from blood and cerebrospinal fluid. Fever, chills, malaise, and myalgias characterize this nonspecific flu-like illness. Other symptoms may include rash, sore throat, chest pain, cough, and headache (13, 14).

Patients demonstrate improvement after the first stage with a several afebrile days before entering the second, leptospiruric or immune, stage associated with circulating antibodies. This stage lasts from days to more than a month. During this stage, the spirochetes may be recovered from the urine. Organ-specific manifestations occur including rash, uveitis, and aseptic meningitis. Approximately half of patients develop renal complications (including azotemia, hematuria, or proteinuria), pulmonary complications (such as cough), or meningeal symptoms. Encephalitis and focal nerve palsies are reported less frequently. This form is self-limited and usually nonfatal (13–15).

Weil disease, or "icteric leptospirosis," is a severe form of leptospirosis with a 5–10% mortality rate which climbs up to 35% when there is hepatorenal involvement. In these individuals, fever persists during the leptospiruric stage. Subsequent profound jaundice defines the syndrome which occurs approximately 1 week after onset of the first stage. The jaundice commonly heralds hepatic necrosis from centrilobular necrosis, renal failure from acute tubular necrosis, respiratory failure, and hemorrhagic diathesis. Less often rhabdomyolysis, myocarditis, pericarditis, or congestive heart failure develops (13–15).

History

A history of known exposure is the best key to diagnosis. Contact with either infected animal body fluid or organs, or contaminated soil or water is necessary for infection. Another clue to diagnosis is the time of presentation. Leptospirosis is often considered a disease of the summer, as the spirochetes can survive longer outside the host in warmer environments. Also, given the need for exposure to environmental sources, leptospirosis is largely an occupational disease; however, recreational exposure may occur as well. In the late 1990s, both white-water rafters in Costa Rica and triathletes in Springfield, IL contracted the disease after exposure to contaminated waters (13, 15).

Physical Examination

The physical exam may be normal in mild cases. In the leptospiremic stage, abrupt remittent fever, conjunctival suffusion without purulent discharge, lymphadenopathy, pharyngitis, hepatosplenomegaly, and, rarely, pretibial maculopapular rash can be seen. Conjunctival suffusion and muscle tenderness, especially in the calf and lumbar area, are characteristic of the disease but are seen only in a minority of cases (15).

In the leptospiruric stage, signs present in the acute, leptospiremic phase persist and are accompanied by symptoms related to specific organ involvement. Pulmonary involvement will cause crackles, hemoptysis, dyspnea, and possible respiratory failure. Cardiac involvement leads to signs of congestive heart failure or pericarditis. Hematologic involvement leads to easy bleeding, ecchymosis, petechiae, purpura, and abdominal tenderness. Neurologic involvement causes meningismus and, less often, cranial nerve palsies, encephalitis, and mental status changes. Ocular disease can present as subconjunctival hemorrhage and uveitis. In Weil disease, jaundice, hepatomegaly, abdominal tenderness, and coagulopathies can be found. Severe cases may present with shock.

Laboratory/Diagnostic Testing

Recovering the organism from cultures of blood, cerebrospinal fluid, or urine, depending on the stage of illness, is definitive evidence of infection. By definition, blood cultures will be positive in the first stage of illness, but not until approximately 4 days following the onset of symptoms. In the second stage of illness, blood cultures will often become negative. Cerebrospinal fluid cultures may be positive within the first 10 days. Urine cultures will begin growing organisms several days after initial infec-

tion and persist for up to 2 months; however, growth may take several weeks. Despite slow growth, urine is the most reliable source for culture. Polymerase chain reaction assays have been developed and could offer the advantage of confirming diagnosis during the acute, leptospiremic phase (19).

Most cases are diagnosed by serology. The microscopic agglutination test (MAT) may also be performed. A titer $\geq$1:100 is considered positive, as is a four-fold increase in titers. MAT will usually not become positive until 2 weeks following the onset of symptoms. Antibiotic treatment will decrease the sensitivity of the test. The CDC performs this test. Macroscopic slide agglutination can allow presumptive diagnosis when performed in conjunction with a high pretest probability based on symptoms; however, the test is not specific. Recent development of ELISA testing for IgM directed toward the leptospires allows diagnosis of new infections between 3 and 5 days. Dark-field examination of urine to visualize the spirochetes may be done but due to low sensitivity this test is no longer recommended (13–15,19).

General laboratory testing suggestive of leptospirosis includes increased white blood cell counts with left shift along with an elevated erythrocyte sedimentation rate. Mildly elevated liver function tests (AST and ALT approximately 200 U/L), total bilirubin, and alkaline phosphatase are possible. Urinalysis may demonstrate white and red blood cells, proteinuria, and variable casts. Cerebrospinal fluid may demonstrate increased neutrophils or monocytes with normal glucose and normal to elevated protein.

In Weil disease, serum testing consistent with renal failure and azotemia predominate. Thrombocytopenia occurs often as does elevated bilirubin without proportionately increased transaminases. Creatine phosphokinase (CPK) will be elevated often as well and higher levels are associated with greater levels of jaundice. In rare cases, chest x-ray demonstrates patchy infiltrates secondary to alveolar hemorrhage.

Clinician Protection

Person-to-person spread of the leptospirosis is extremely uncommon. The transient leptospiruria should not lead to transmission if basic body fluid precautions are observed.

Treatment

Despite severe complications, specifically renal and hepatic failure, leptospirosis is most often a nonfatal, self-limited disease. However, systemic immune response may lead to secondary end-organ damage and treatment should always be initiated when the diagnosis is made (13).

Mild disease can be treated with doxycycline (100 mg po bid × 7 days); alternatives include ampicillin or amoxicillin. Severe disease should be treated with intravenous penicillin G with alternatives of ampicillin or amoxicillin. Severe disease in penicillin allergic patients may be treated with erythromycin. Antibiotics are given for 7 days (13). Secondary complications of disease may require support, such as hemodialysis for renal failure and platelet transfusion for thrombocytopenia (14, 15).

The CDC recommends chemoprophylaxis with doxycycline at 200 mg once a week starting 1 day after initial exposure and continuing through the end of exposure (13).

Differential Diagnosis

The differential diagnosis is extensive including any influenza-like illness with headache and severe myalgia. More common causes of fever with abdominal pain, such as appendicitis, should be considered. Diseases with generalized lymphadenopathy (including mononucleosis), as well as conditions that cause hepatomegaly or hepatitis must be considered.

Likewise, less common diseases including hantavirus, dengue, and rickettsial diseases should be kept in mind (13–15).

Medicolegal Implications

Failure to consider leptospirosis especially in the face of at-risk populations such as veterinarians, farmworkers, inner-city dwellers with exposure to rodents, or outdoor enthusiasts is one pitfall. Prophylaxis for other individuals exposed to contaminated source should also be considered. Missing other life-threatening illness with entirely different specific therapy (such as bacterial meningitis, cholangitis, or hepatitis) can also be disastrous.

HANTAVIRUS PULMONARY SYNDROME

Introduction

An outbreak of a novel febrile disease leading to respiratory failure occurred in the United States in the early 1990s. It was then known as "four corners disease" because of its deadly outbreak in the area where Colorado, Utah, Arizona, and New Mexico meet. It was characterized by an influenza-like prodrome followed by respiratory failure and death in young, otherwise healthy patients.

Preferential viral effects in the lungs led to interstitial pneumonitis and alveolar fibrosis secondary to concentrated pleural and alveolar edema which eventually led to circulatory collapse. This disease was subsequently discovered to be secondary to the Sin Nombre virus (SNV) and was named hantavirus pulmonary syndrome (HPS).

Hantaviruses are a subset of the Bunyavirus family which is grouped with three other families under the term viral hemmorhagic fevers (VHF) which include Ebola, Marburg, dengue, and yellow fevers. In the United States, the primary hantaviral disease, hantavirus pulmonary syndrome (HPS), differs from other VHF in that it does not cause hemorrhage and is not transmitted by mosquitoes (16–18).

The Sin Nombre hantavirus is a zoonoses with a rodent vector. Infection occurs by inhalation of aerosolized urine or feces from host animals. This often occurs when chronically infected deer mice seek shelter in human dwellings. Although human-to-human transmission has not been documented in the United States, in South America there have been case reports suggesting this possibility (17).

On a global level, Seoul Hantavirus, Hantaan virus, and Puumala viruses are Hantaviruses which affect the retroperitoneum leading to local capillary permeability and hemorrhagic fever with renal failure. Hemmorhagic fever with renal failure syndrome (HFRS) occurs almost exclusively in the Eastern Hemisphere while HPS is almost exclusively a Western Hemisphere disease (17). Although closely related to HPS, HFRS is outside the scope of what will be discussed below.

Since its identification in 1993, most of the 366 confirmed HPS cases in the United States have been caused by the Sin Nombre virus. Thirty-one states have reported cases while half of all cases are from the original Four Corners area (16, 17). In the western United States, the deer mouse is the reservoir for the Sin Nombre virus. In the northeastern United States, the white-footed mouse harbors both the Sin Nombre and New York viruses. The virus is not pathologic to their rodent host. Disease presentation occurs year round but has spring-summer peaks in incidence.

Among cases for which history is available, 70% of infected individuals had a recent exposure to peridomestic activities, such as cleaning, in buildings with evidence of rodent infestation (18). Travel to areas where Hantavirus infection has been reported is not considered a risk factor for infection with HPS (18). The possibility of exposure to Hantavirus for campers, hikers, and tourists is very small and is reduced further if steps are taken to avoid rodent contact. The potential for occupationally acquired

SNV infections has been recognized but is historically infrequent. In addition, a recent HPS antibody seroprevalence study among farmworkers, plumbers, contractors, and park service workers found no evidence of Sin Nombre viral infection (16, 17).

History

A 3–5 day febrile prodrome develops after a 1–4-week incubation period. Nonspecific symptoms predominate early on with myalgias, fever, headache, chills, lightheadedness, dry cough, nausea, and vomiting. Some patients report malaise and diarrhea. Abdominal pain, back pain, or arthralgias are less frequent. Diagnosis in this early stage is unlikely due to nonspecific symptoms and lack of pulmonary involvement (16–18).

Dyspnea, tachypnea, and cough generally do not develop until day 5–7, marking the beginning of the cardiopulmonary phase. This phase lasts 24–48 h and is significant for rapid decline in respiratory function and possible circulatory collapse. Seventy-five percent of the patients demonstrating pulmonary edema have required mechanical ventilation (16).

Resolution of the cardiopulmonary stage is marked by significant diuresis. Convalescence is often as rapid with resolution in 1–2 days. There are minimal lasting effects including fatigue and exercise intolerance among survivors.

Physical Examination

The examination is normal during the prodrome. Pulmonary capillary leak leads to noncardiogenic pulmonary edema. Intravascular depletion and myocardial depression may lead to prerenal azotemia and finally shock.

Thus, in a vast majority of patients, fever, tachypnea, tachycardia, and crackles are found, and the physical examination is otherwise essentially normal. Hypotension is rare on initial presentation (16, 17).

Findings of petechiae, rash, conjunctival hemorrhage, conjunctivitis, sinusitis, pharyngitis, and peripheral or periorbital edema strongly suggest an alternate diagnosis.

Laboratory/Diagnostic Testing

The CDC considers a clinical scenario compatible with HPS in conjunction with serological testing, evidence of viral antigen in tissue by immunohistochemistry, or the presence of amplifiable viral RNA sequences in blood or tissue, diagnostic for HPS. Specific diagnosis of HPS is most often made by ELISA targeted to Hantavirus IgM and IgG. At the time of presentation, two-thirds of patients will have an elevated titer of one or both antibodies. The remaining third develop an increase of IgG titers during convalescence. The ELISA test is available at the CDC and many state laboratories (18).

Nonspecific laboratory testing suggestive of HPS includes an elevated hematocrit secondary to hemoconcentration, thrombocytopenia, mildly elevated transaminases, and increased lactate dehydrogenase. A platelet level below 150,000 occurred in 80% of cases. Acidosis may result in low serum bicarbonate. Unfortunately, these and other nonspecific tests often do not become abnormal until the cardiopulmonary phase has begun (18).

Neutrophilia with left shift and presence of atypical lymphocytes (myelocytes) on peripheral smear is very suggestive of HPS infection. Severe hypoalbuminemia coupled with acute respiratory deterioration is also highly suggestive of HPS. The combination of respiratory insufficiency with a plasma lactate greater than 4.0 mmol/L predicts poor outcome (18). Arterial blood gas will demonstrate hypoxemia with concurrent hypocapnia since gas exchange, not ventilation, is impaired (17).

Chest radiography typically shows noncardiogenic pulmonary edema. Kerley B lines and peribronchial cuffing will be present in the absence of cardiomegaly. Perihilar haziness is 1characteristic. Interstitial processes evolve to bilateral alveolar involvement. Pleural effusions are common. Although there is an overlap between radiographic appearance of acute respiratory distress syndrome (ARDS) and HPS, the presence of pleural effusions, interstitial edema prominence, and lack of initial peripheral distribution of airway disease is more suggestive of HPS. Figure 37–1 illustrates the radiological progression of the disease.

Clinician Protection

Since there are no confirmed cases of person-to-person transmission, protection beyond universal precautions is not necessary. Given the prolonged incubation time for HPS, it is unlikely that a patient would present wearing clothing contaminated with infected rodent urine or feces. Virions on dry surfaces have been shown to remain viable for as long as 2 days; however, they are susceptible to simple decontamination with household bleach (18).

Treatment

Treatment is supportive. Patients with severe respiratory compromise may require intensive care unit admission. Intubation, mechanical ventilation, and vasopressor

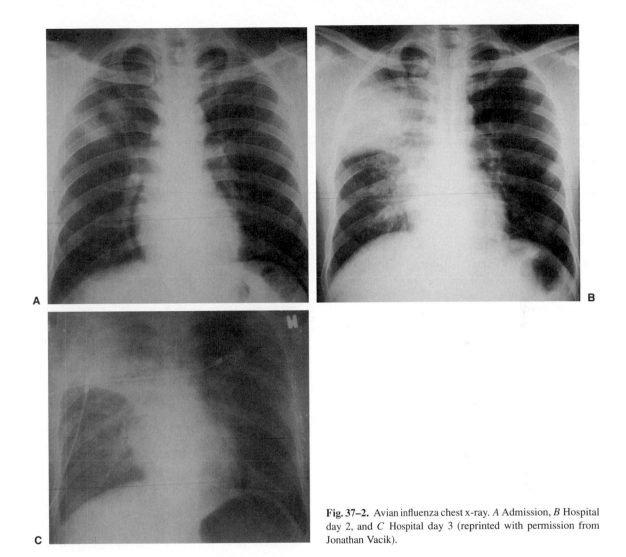

Fig. 37–2. Avian influenza chest x-ray. *A* Admission, *B* Hospital day 2, and *C* Hospital day 3 (reprinted with permission from Jonathan Vacik).

support should be initiated as needed. Despite suspicion of HPS, broad spectrum antibiotics targeting pathogens of severe community acquired pneumonia (see Chapter 10) should be considered until HPS is confirmed. Fluid volume, perfusion, electrolyte, and acid-base status must be carefully monitored (16–18).

While ribavirin antiviral therapy is indicated for the closely related HFRS, placebo-controlled trials have not been completed for HPS and it is not currently recommended (18).

Within 24 h of the onset of the cardiopulmonary phase, almost all patients develop some degree of hypotension.

Myocardial depression may also occur with resultant bradycardia or ventricular fibrillation. All patients should be admitted to the intensive care unit. Despite intensive care treatment, the case fatality is 38% (18).

Differential Diagnosis

Both cardiogenic and noncardiogenic causes of pulmonary edema must be considered. An echocardiogram could be considered to evaluate cardiac function and help differentiate ARDS as cardiac function is more significantly depressed with HPS. Drug-induced pulmonary edema, Goodpasture syndrome, and infections including influenza, Q fever, severe community-acquired pneumonia, pneumonic plague, leptospirosis, tularemia, coccidiomycosis and histoplasmosis must be considered (16, 18).

Medicolegal Implications

Pitfalls include failure to elicit a history of exposure to rodent infested areas. Hypoxia from noncardiogenic pulmonary edema in the setting of potential exposure especially with fever and myalgias but without other common viral symptoms must prompt hantaviral serologic testing (16, 18).

AVIAN INFLUENZA

Introduction

Epidemic human influenza can be caused by either of the two types: influenza A and B. Influenza A virus can be divided into subtypes on the basis of two surface antigens: hemagglutinin (H) and neuraminidase (N). Infected individuals develop immunity to the subtype of influenza that infected them. Influenza disease essentially "reemerges" every year due to antigenic "drift" which is the development of antigenic variants caused by point mutations that occurred during viral replication. Antigenic "shift" is an abrupt major change in the influenza A virus resulting in a new hemagglutinin or neuraminidase protein that has not been seen in humans for many years. If the resultant new influenza subtype is introduced into the human population, lack of immunity can lead to widespread disease and a pandemic can occur.

Wild birds are the natural hosts for influenza type A virus, harboring the infection without becoming ill. Many animals, including poultry, humans, and pigs, can be infected and become ill. In January 2003, outbreaks of highly pathogenic influenza A (H5N1) were reported in Asian poultry. By early 2004, more than 1 million domestic birds either died from the disease or were culled (killed) in an effort to contain the outbreak. The outbreaks, however, are ongoing among bird populations in a number of Asian countries and have caused, at the time of this writing, 15 human deaths in Vietnam and 8 deaths in Thailand. This "avian flu" is highly virulent but apparently not contagious among humans. The great fear is that a human could become simultaneously infected by the highly virulent avian strain and a highly contagious human strain. Genetic realignment within the patient could lead to a strain that demonstrates the dreaded combination

of being highly virulent, highly contagious, and genetically "new" to the human population. This could result in a worldwide, devastating pandemic the likes of which are seen only several times each century.

In addition to the tragedy of the human deaths, the economic implication of the loss of poultry has been devastating in Southeast Asia. In 2003 and 2004, there have been several outbreaks of avian influenza in poultry in Canada and the United States.

Much of the material in this section is based on the Centers for Disease Control and Prevention Website dealing with avian influenza. This website is frequently updated and should be referred to by emergency clinicians (www.cdc.gov).

History

Symptoms range from typical influenza-like symptoms (the abrupt onset of fever, chills, cough, sore throat, and muscle aches) to conjunctivitis, pneumonia, and acute respiratory distress. Avian influenza must be considered in any patient who has a history of travel to a country with documented avian influenza in the poultry and/or human population within 10 days of symptom onset.

Physical Examination

Patients can be toxic appearing with fever, prostration, conjunctivitis, and/or adventitial pulmonary sounds suggestive of pneumonia.

Laboratory/Diagnostic Testing

Chest radiographs can reveal single or multiple infiltrates that may progress rapidly over several days as demonstrated in Figure 2. It is recommended that testing for avian influenza A (H5N1) should be considered on a case-by-case basis in consultation with state and local heath departments for patients with a history of contact with poultry or a known or suspected human case of avian influenza A (H5N1) in a H5N1-affected country within 10 days of symptom onset and documented temperature greater than 38°C and one or more of the following: cough, sore throat, or shortness of breath.

The respiratory sample (nasopharyngeal swab or aspirate) should be tested by RT-PCR for influenza A, and if possible for H1 and H3. If such capacity is not available in the state, or if the result of local testing is positive, then CDC should be contacted and the specimen should be sent to CDC for testing. Virus isolation should not be attempted unless a biosafety level 3+ facility is available to receive and culture specimens. Optimally, an acute-(within 1 week of illness onset) and convalescent-phase (after 3 weeks of illness onset) serum sample should be collected and stored locally in case testing for antibody to the avian influenza virus should be needed. Requests for testing should come through the state and local health departments, which should contact the CDC Director's Emergency Operations Center at 770-488-7100 before sending specimens for testing.

Clinical Protection

Human influenza is transmitted primarily via large respiratory droplets and standard precautions plus droplet precautions are recommended for the care of patients potentially infected. Due to uncertainty about the exact mode by which avian influenza may be transmitted, the high risk of serious disease and mortality, and the possible emergence of a pandemic strain, the CDC recommends enhanced precautions. In addition to standard and droplet precautions, contact precautions, eye protection, and airborne precautions are advised. In addition to the respiratory hygiene and cough etiquette suggested for any patient presenting with an acute cough illness, patients suspected of avian influenza infection should be provided with a surgical mask and separated from other persons. They should be expeditiously placed in a private room with negative pressure ventilation. All caregivers should wear fit-tested N-95 filter masks when in the patient's room.

Treatment

In addition to supportive treatment, anti-influenza drugs should be given. Some of the H5N1 viruses isolated from poultry and humans in Asia have demonstrated resistance to the antiviral M2 inhibitors, amantadine, and rimantadine. Oseltamivir, a neuraminidase inhibitor, has been clinically successful and no resistance has yet been reported (75 mg po bid for 5 days in adults; 2 mg/kg up to 75 mg po bid for children aged 1–12.)

Differential Diagnosis

Human influenza A or B, more usual viral or bacterial causes of pneumonia, as well as other travel-related illnesses (including SARS) must be considered.

Medicolegal Implications

The prudent emergency physician will obtain a thorough travel history, provide appropriate transmission protection

to the ED staff and visitors, and will report suspected cases to local and state public health agencies. Suspected cases should be admitted to the hospital in strict isolation until the public health department confirms that it is safe to do otherwise.

CONCLUSION

Emergency physicians play an important role in the recognition and control of emerging infectious diseases. As in other aspects of the practice, pattern recognition is the cornerstone of diagnosis. Emergency physicians must be familiar with the clinical presentation of currently emerging infectious diseases in their region as well as nationally and internationally. To be able to promptly activate the public health system one must recognize new, different, and unusual patterns of disease presentation in the emergency department. Key components of the history that must be obtained include travel and potential occupational, dietary, or recreational exposures. The emergency physician must direct appropriate patient isolation and precautions to protect oneself, the staff, and all other persons in the treatment area.

Emerging infections are, by definition, rapidly changing. The usual sources of medical information, peer-reviewed articles and medical textbooks, generally will not provide adequate information. The practicing emergency physician must be aware of local and national news and can frequently obtain up-to-date information through the Web site of the Centers for Disease Control and Prevention (www.cdc.gov) which includes the excellent online, peer-reviewed periodical *Emerging Infectious Diseases* and the *Morbidity and Mortality Weekly Report*.

REFERENCES

1. Talan DA, Moran GJ, Mower WR, et al.:*EMERGEncy ID NET: An emergency department –based emerging infections sentinel network. *Ann Emerg Med* 32(6):703–711, 1998.
2. Oehler RL, Lorenzo N, Jani A, Cunha BA (2003, July 30): Severe acute respiratory syndrome *E-Medicine – Infectious Disease.* Retrieved on March 20, 2004 from http://www.emedicine.com/med/topic3662.htm
3. Clinical Guidance on the Identification and Evaluation of Possible SARS-CoV Disease among Persons Presenting with Community-Acquired Illness, Version 2. (2004, January 8). Retrieved on March 20, 2004 from CDC website at http://www.cdc.gov/ncidod/sars/clinicalguidance.htm
4. Wang J-T, Sheng W-H, Fang C-T, et al.: Clinical manifestations, laboratory findings, and treatment outcomes

of SARS patients *Emerg Infect Dis* [serial online] 10(5), 2004 May [date cited]. Available from: http://www.cdc.gov/ncidod/EIDvol10no5/ 03-0640.htm

5. Kemper CA: Diagnostic testing for SARS *Infect Dis Alert* 22(20):157–168, 2003.

6. Revised U.S. surveillance case definition for severe acute respiratory syndrome and update on SARS Cases—United States and Worldwide. *Morb Mortal Wkly Rep* 52:1202–1206, 2003.

7. West Nile Virus Background: Virus History and Distribution (2004, April 6). Retrieved on May 30, 2004 from CDC website at http://www.cdc.gov/ncidod/ dvbid/westnile/background.htm

8. Burke CA (2002, October 3): West Nile encephalitis. *E-Medicine – Infectious Disease*. Retrieved on March 20, 2004 from http://www.emedicine.com/med/topic3160.htm

9. Donson DA, Lai MK, Silber SH (2002, September 3): West Nile virus. *E-Medicine – Infectious Disease*. Retrieved on March 20, 2004 from http://www.emedicine.com/med/topic542.htm

10. Update: Detection of West Nile virus in blood donations—United States, 2003. *Morb Mortal Wkly Rep* 52:916, 2003.

11. West Nile Virus: Information for the Clinician (2003, September 24). Retrieved on May 30, 2004 from CDC website at http://www.cdc.gov/ncidod/dvbid/westnile/resources/fact_sheet_clinician.htm

12. Petersen LR, Marfin AA: West Nile virus: A primer for the clinician. *Ann Intern Med* 137(13):173–179, 2002.

13. Ashford D (2003): Leptospirosis. *The Yellow Book: Health Information for International Traveler 2003-2004*. Retrieved on August 29, 2004, from http://www.cdc.gov/travel/diseases/lepto.htm

14. Jezior M, Peterson CK, Morris JT (2001, Oct 14): Leptospirosis. *E-Medicine – Infectious Disease*. Retrieved on March 20, 2004, from http://www.emedicine.com/med/topic1283.htm

15. Green-McKenzie J (2001, Aug 14): Leptospirosis. *E-Medicine – Infectious Disease*. Retrieved on March 20, 2004, from http://www.emedicine.com/emerg/topic856.htm

16. Cunha B (2002, October 9): Hantavirus pulmonary syndrome. *E-Medicine – Infectious Disease*. Retrieved on March 20, 2004, from http://www.emedicine.com/med/topic3402.htm

17. Schmaljohn C, Hjelle B: Hantaviruses: A global disease problem. *Emerg Infect Dis* 3(2):95–104, 1997, Apr–Jun.

18. Hantavirus Pulmonary Syndrome Technical Information for Healthcare Providers. (n.d.). Retrieved on August 30, 2004, from the Centers for Disease Control and Prevention website: http://www.cdc.gov/ncidod/diseases/hanta/hps/noframes/phys/technicalinfoindex.htm

19. Levett PN: Leptospirosis. *Mandell, Douglas, and Bennett's Principles and Practice of Infectious Diseases*, 6th ed. Philadelphia, Elsevier Inc., 2005.

38

Tick-Borne Diseases

Julio E. Figueroa

HIGH YIELD FACTS

1. Think tick-borne diseases in any patient with influenza-like illness presenting during the warm months.

2. Presumptive therapy for the most common tick-borne infections is imperative in suspected cases.

3. Think about infection with multiple agents if one tick-borne infection is suspected.

CASE PRESENTATION

A 42-year-old man presents with fever, chills, headache, and severe muscle aches. He states that he started feeling ill three days prior to his presentation. He was seen by his primary care physician and diagnosed with a severe viral syndrome. He progressively became worse. He was evaluated in the emergency department.

The patient was previously well without major medical problems. He works for a mortgage company. He enjoys bird watching and had recently made a birding trip in Minnesota the week prior. He denied vomiting, diarrhea, urinary symptoms, rash, or sick contacts.

On examination in the emergency department, he had a temperature of 37.7°C, a pulse of 60, respiratory rate of 16, and a blood pressure of 110/60. He looked extremely ill with cool extremities. He had no meningismus, no adenopathy, clear breath sounds, no murmurs, normal abdominal examination, and normal neurological examination.

Routine laboratory tests revealed a white blood cell count of 1400 cells per mcL composed of 30% polymorphonuclear cells and 63% lymphocytes, a hemoglobin of 16 g/dL, aspartate aminotransferase (AST) of 235 U/L (normal <45), lactate dehydrogenase of 1176 U/L (normal <220), alkaline phosphatase of 136 U/L (normal <120), and a total bilirubin of 0.6 mg/dL (normal <1.3).

INTRODUCTION/EPIDEMIOLOGY

Animal- and vector-borne infectious diseases present special challenges for the emergency department physician. Recognition of these diseases frequently requires obtain-ing an extensive history from the patient for possible exposures as well as a careful examination for the presence of the insect vectors on the patient. The situation is further complicated by the protean manifestations that many of these diseases have at initial presentation to the clinic or hospital. Routine microbiologic studies frequently fail to give the appropriate diagnosis. Finally, in the case of some of these pathogens, appropriate antimicrobial therapy can reduce morbidity and mortality. Therefore, one must have a high index of suspicion and commonly must treat the patient expectantly before the final diagnosis is known. In a busy emergency department, however, the physician may find it helpful to target certain patients for extra investigation.

This chapter will review the important epidemiologic and clinical clues for a diagnosis of tick-borne diseases. In addition, it will describe the major disease entities found in North America.

Epidemiology

Patients with tick-borne diseases may present with a myriad of symptoms and signs. Most commonly, individuals will present with fever and an influenza-like syndrome. The probable etiologies of such a syndrome can be stratified initially on the basis of the following epidemiologic factors:

- Arthropod exposure
- Geographic location
- Time of year
- Occupations, hobbies, and habits

Arthropod exposure

The initial clue to the diagnosis is the potential exposure to ticks. Unfortunately, even in experienced individuals, it is difficult at times to assess whether the individual in question has had tick exposure because most tick bites go unrecognized. Therefore, one must use surrogate markers for actual tick exposure. For example, individuals may not recall or recognize exposures to ticks but may relate a history of other arthropods (e.g., mosquitoes) that may indicate risk of tick exposure. In addition, they may relate a history of ticks on household pets that spent some time outdoors. This observation may be important for two reasons. First, this fact demonstrates that ticks are in the patient's environment. Second, household pets may carry infected ticks indoors so that even individuals who have no

Table 38–1. Pathogens Carried by Specific Tick Species

Tick Genus	Pathogens
Ixodes spp.	*Borrelia burgdorferi*
	Babesia microti and *Babesia divergens*
	Anaplasma phagocytophilum
	Francisella tularensis
	Tick-borne encephalitis viruses
	Powassan encephalitis virus
	Bartonella henselae
	Tick paralysis
Amblyomma spp.	*Ehrlichia chaffeensis*
	Ehrlichia ewingii
	Borrelia lonestari
	Rickettsia parkeri
	Fransciella tularensis
	Tick paralysis
Dermacentor spp.	*Rickettsia rickettsii*
	Fransciella tularensis
	Colorado tick fever virus
	Powassan encephalitis virus
	Tick paralysis
Ornithodoros spp.	*Borrelia* spp. (*B. hermsii* in US)
	West Nile Virus?

history of outdoor activities may be at risk for tick-borne diseases.

On the other hand, the presence of tick exposure does not, in itself, predict the presence of a tick-related illness in areas where ticks are highly endemic. Belongia et al. reported in their survey of 62 patients with nonspecific febrile illness in Wisconsin that the positive predictive value of a recognized tick bite for tick-borne infections was 34% (1). The negative predictive value was 79%.

Description of the tick could potentially be useful as well. At the minimum, the distinction between soft- and hard-body ticks can be rather useful. As shown in Table 38–1, *Ornithodorus* spp. (soft-body ticks) are the major vector of tick-borne relapsing fever *Borrelia* spp. Hard-body ticks are the major vectors for most other tick-borne diseases. Although experienced individuals may be able to distinguish among the various hard ticks, it is doubtful that this would be helpful in most cases.

Geography

The major genera of ticks that are responsible for human disease have known geographic distributions (Fig. 38–1).

Moreover, certain ticks have been associated with the transmission of certain microbes (Table 38–1). Therefore, the geographic location of the potential tick exposure provides a quick differential diagnosis for the emergency department physician. In this respect, therefore, an accurate travel history is critical.

Time of year

Ticks, as other arthropods, are more active in warm weather. Moreover, mild weathers will increase tick populations during warmer months. Although there are ticks that are active during cold winter months (e.g. Winter Tick or *Dermacentor albipictus*), these ticks have never been associated with human disease. Therefore, the majority of important tick exposures will occur during the warmer (mostly summer) months. One should, however, keep in mind that the peaks of tick activity are variable depending on the tick and the geographic location.

Occupations, hobbies, and habits

The clinician can easily detect those individuals who clearly have a wilderness experience. The more challenging situations involve patients with more subtle exposures. Perhaps the most amusing association with tick-borne diseases was published by Standaert et al. (2). In a case-control study of an Ehrlichia outbreak in a Tennessee golfing community, the investigators demonstrated that case patients were more likely to play golf (relative risk = 1.9), have golf scores >100 (RR = 2.4), and to retrieve lost golf balls (RR = 3.7) than controls. Ticks surveyed from the roughs of the golf course in question were noted to be infected with *Ehrlichia chaffeensis*.

Clinical Manifestations of Tick-Borne Diseases

Several tick-borne diseases have similar initial clinical manifestations. Therefore, it is useful to categorize clinical presentations by syndromes (Table 38–2). Moreover, clinical presentations may be more severe in several sub-populations as indicated in the table. Each organism has its unique pathophysiology that usually involves dissemination and/or vascular inflammation. Recent reviews for each organism are cited in the text.

Influenza-like illness

Many of tick-borne pathogens can present with severe influenza-like syndromes. Frequently, patients present

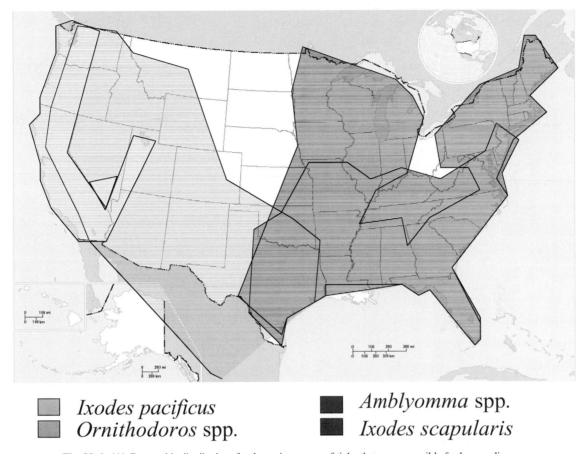

Ixodes pacificus
Ornithodoros spp.

Amblyomma spp.
Ixodes scapularis

Fig. 38–1. **(A)** Geographic distributions for the major genera of ticks that are responsible for human disease.

with fever, headaches, myalgias, and a variety of gastrointestinal symptoms. The differential diagnosis is large, including viral infections and routine bacterial infections. The distinguishing characteristics, such as skin rash, can be absent or present only after the initial illness. Therefore, one must have a high index of suspicion in any febrile illness with a generalized symptom complex. However, these organisms do have some characteristics that can help to distinguish among the possible etiologies.

Rickettsia rickettsii (Rocky Mountain spotted fever; RMSF)

Perhaps the quintessential tick-related infection, *R. rickettsia* is transmitted by the Dermacentor and Amblyomma ticks (for review, see (3–5)). The incubation period from the time of tick exposure to clinical illness is between 5–10 days. Classically, individuals with *R. rickettsia* in-

fection present with fever, headache, and a centripetal petechial rash. However, the typical petechial rash occurs usually after 6 days after the onset of illness and only in 35–60% of patients. The initial rash may actually be macular in character appearing 2–5 days after the onset of fever. These macules commonly occur on wrist, forearms, and ankles. Eventually these may become palpable petechiae. Fifty to 80% of patients have the characteristic distribution on the palms and soles. As many as 10–15% of infected individuals never develop a rash. Necrotic lesions (eschars) are very uncommon (1%).

Uncommon clinical manifestations (seen in <20%) include myocarditis, arrhythmia, pneumonitis, seizures, meningitis, encephalitis, decreased hearing, stupor, gangrene, and septic shock.

Individuals at risk for more severe disease include the elderly, African-Americans, alcoholics, and glucose-6-phosphate dehydrogenase (G6PD) deficient individuals.

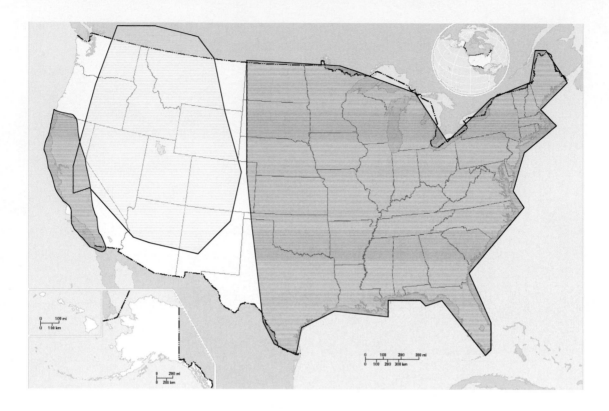

 Dermacentor andersoni   ▓ *Dermacentor variabilis*

Fig. 38–1. (B) (*Continued*)

Seen mainly in men of African or Mediterranean origin, G6PD deficiency is associated with a rapid and severe clinical syndrome. Approximately 10–14% of the black men are G6PD deficient (6).

Commonly seen laboratory abnormalities can include thrombocytopenia, elevated aspartate aminotransferase, and hyponatremia. Uncommonly, patients will have anemia, azotemia, and CSF pleocytosis.

R. parkeri

Recently described causing infection in the United States, *R. parkeri* causes an RMSF-like syndrome (7). The major distinguishing feature is the appearance of an eschar at the site of the tick bite (tache noire) or multiple eschars in addition to the macular or petechial rash. The incidence and the clinical manifestation of this bacterial infection in the United States remain to be fully elucidated.

E. chaffeensis (Human monocytic ehrlichiosis) and *Anaplasma phagocytophilum* (human granulocytic ehrlichiosis) and *Ehrlichia ewingii*

Clinical manifestations of human ehrlichiosis are similar to RMSF except for the rash (8–10). In *E. chaffeensis* infection, a maculopapular rash is seen in 1/3 of patients but can be as high as 60% in children. Petechial rash is rare. Rash is less common with other agents that cause ehrlichiosis. Severe disease is seen in immunocompromised patients especially those with corticosteroid use, cancer chemotherapy, HIV infection, and asplenia.

Common laboratory abnormalities include those seen in RMSF. In addition, patients with ehrlichiosis also frequently have leukopenia and hemoconcentration.

Borrelia burgdorferi (Lyme borreliosis)

Individuals with documented Lyme borreliosis can have a variety of clinical presentations (see (11–14) for recent

Table 38–2. Summary of Clinical Syndromes, Etiologies, and Epidemiology of Tick-Borne Diseases in the United States

Syndrome Type	Clinical Features	Etiologies in US	Unique Features	Individuals at Risk
Influenza-like illness	Fever Headache Myalgias Arthalgias Nausea	R. rickettsii	Centripedal petechial rash (80%)	Elderly Alcoholics G6PD deficiency
	Vomiting Abdominal Pain Diarrhea	R. parkeri	Eschar and macular rash	Unknown
		E. chaffeensis	Rash less common (20%)	HIV
		E. ewingii	Rash less common	HIV
		A. phagocytophilum	Rash less Common	Corticosteroid HIV asplenia
		B. burgdorferi	Erythema migrans Bell's palsy Fewer GI symptoms	
		B. lonestari	Erythema migrans	Pregnancy
		Borrelia species	Endemic relapsing fever Hemolysis	Immunocomp romised
		Babesia microti		Asplenia
		Babesia divergens		Elderly
		Francisella tularensis	Skin ulcer Adenopathy Pulse-temperature disassociation	
		Colorado tick fever virus	Biphasic "saddleback" fever hyperesthetic skin	
		B. henselae(?)		HIV
		R. rickettsii		
Acute Abdomen	Fever Severe abdominal pain with localizing signs Occasionally bloody stool or vomitus	A. phagocytophilum		
Encephalitis	Fever Headache Altered mental status	Tick-borne encephalitis viruses	Travel to Eurasia Biphasic disease	
		Powassen encephalitis virus	Paralysis	
		See etiologies causing influenza-like disease		
Paralysis		Tick paralysis (toxin-mediated seen with several tick species)	Symmetrical Normal mental status	
		Encephalitis viruses	Asymmetric Altered mental status	
		B. burgdorferi	Facial palsy	
		B. henselae	Facial Palsy	

reviews). However, the most common one in early infection is that of an influenza-like syndrome with a predominance of headache and arthralgias (usually oligoarticular or migratory). Gastrointestinal and pulmonary symptoms are not commonly seen. Occasionally, they will describe facial paresthesias or present with facial nerve palsy.

The characteristic erythema migrans rash generally appears at the site of a tick bite within 7–10 days after the exposure and is noted in up to 85% of patients. It is frequently located around the knees, axilla, and in the groins. Secondary rashes have also been noted. The presence of erythema migrans rash is helpful but not always present even in documented cases. In series of patients with a summertime influenza-like syndrome performed in endemic areas, 7–20% of patients with this syndrome had laboratory evidence of recent Borrelia infection in the absence of the rash. Steere and colleagues recently suggested that at least some of those individuals are infected with other tick-borne agents and have false positive borrelia serologies. Therefore, the clinician needs to consider this diagnosis in individuals with summertime influenza-like illnesses and do a thorough skin examination for the erythema migrans lesion. This is especially true if the major symptoms include headache and arthralgias. The lack of the rash makes it less likely but does not rule it out completely.

Patients with Lyme borreliosis can uncommonly also present with heart block, carditis, aseptic meningitis, encephalitis, neuritis, and borrelial lymphocytoma (a solitary bluish-red lesion of up to a few centimeters in and under the skin).

Coinfection with other tick-borne diseases (such as *Babesia* species) is present in 10% of patients in some series (15).

Borrelia lonestari (Southern tick-associated rash illness; STARI)

B. lonestari carried by Amblyomma ticks is the probable cause of a febrile illness associated with an erythema migrans-like rash resembling Lyme borreliosis. These patients have been described in the Southern United States (16, 17). The presenting characteristics and natural history of this syndrome is currently under investigation by the Centers for Disease Control and Prevention (see www.cdc.gov/ncidod/dvbid/stari/).

Borrelia Species Associated with Relapsing Fever

A number of *Borrelia* species (in the United States primarily *B. hermsii*) can be transmitted through tick expo-

sure and result in influenza-like illnesses that recur with some periodicity (18, 19). The initial episode usually occurs within 7 days of tick bite from the Ornithodoros (soft tick) and lasts for 1–4 days. In a recent series, the symptoms and signs frequently included headache (>90%), myalgia (>90%), chills (88%), arthralgia (>70%), nausea (>70%), vomiting (>70%), abdominal pain (>40%), confusion (38%), photophobia (25%), dizziness (25%), neck pain (24%), dry cough (27%), diarrhea (25%), and rash (18%). The rash may be petechial, macular, or papular. Patients may also have dysuria, jaundice, hepatomegaly, splenomegaly, conjunctival injection, eschar, meningitis, nerve palsies, seizures, bleeding. The febrile episode may terminate with a crisis characterized by hypotension and shock. Pregnancy seems to be a risk factor for more severe disease.

The hallmark clinical feature is the recurrence of a milder syndrome with an average interval of 7–9 days. Patients may experience malaise in between febrile episodes. The average number of relapses is 3 (ranging from 0–13).

Babesia microti and *Babesia divergens* (babesiosis)

After an incubation period of 1–4 weeks, clinically evident babesiosis presents with influenza-like illness with fever, chills, sweating, myalgias, and fatigue (see (20, 21) for review). Distinguishing characteristics include the presence of hepatosplenomegaly and hemolytic anemia.

Most infections appear to be unrecognized. More severe disease is seen in immunosuppressed, asplenic, and/or elderly individuals. In addition, infection with *B. divergens* appears to be more aggressive than those caused by *B. microti*. Coinfection with other tick-borne diseases (especially *B. burgdorferi*) should be considered. Transfusion-associated transmission has been described.

Francisella tularensis (tularemia)

Tularemia has a variety of different clinical presentations depending on the mode of infection and the host response (22–24). These include ulceroglandular, glandular, oculoglandular, pharyngeal, typhoidal, and pneumonic. The incubation period ranges between 1 and 21 days.

Most individuals experience the sudden onset of fever, chills, headache, malaise, anorexia, and fatigue. Other prominent symptoms may include cough, myalgias, chest pain, vomiting, sore throat, abdominal pain, and diarrhea. Gastrointestinal symptoms are more commonly seen in the typhoidal form. Bloody diarrhea is rarely reported.

In some individuals, a skin ulcer will be present with the regional or generalized tender adenopathy. In tick-borne disease, the ulcer can be found at the site of the bite usually on the lower extremities, perineum, or trunk. A pulse-temperature deficit has been noted in a significant minority (up to 42%) of identified patients. Without treatment, fever may last for days along with weight loss, chronic malaise, and adenopathy. Some individuals will have a milder, selflimited course due to the acquisition of a less virulent strain.

Laboratory abnormalities include elevated liver enzymes (in 75% of cases) with occasional hyperbilirubinemia and cholestasis (in more severe cases).

One should consider the possibility of a bioterrorism event if this diagnosis is made although natural localized outbreaks (most recently in Martha's Vineyard) have been described (24–26).

Colorado tick fever

Caused by a coltivirus and spread by *Dermacentor andersoni* (wood tick), Colorado tick fever typically causes an influenza-like syndrome that usually is selflimiting (27). The incubation period is approximately 3–4 days. The onset is usually abrupt with a predominance of myalgias, headaches, and hyperesthesia. Gastrointestinal and respiratory symptoms are not common. Encephalitis and aseptic meningitis can be seen in 5–10% of children. A rash reminiscent of RMSF can be seen in 10–15% of individuals. Some individuals will have a relapsing fever pattern with recurrent fever 2–3 days later. Fatigue and lassitude may persist for weeks afterwards.

The virus infects hematopoeitic cells; therefore, transfusion-related transmission has been described.

Laboratory abnormalities include neutropenia and thrombocytopenia. Liver enzyme abnormalities are uncommon.

Bartonella henselae (bartonellosis)

Recently discovered in Ixodes ticks, *B. henselae*, the agent of cat-scratch disease, should be in the differential diagnosis of anyone with a febrile illness after tick exposure (28). As of this writing, there have been no proven cases of bartonellosis transmitted through this route. Therefore, it is difficult to discuss how the presentation would differ between cat- and tick-associated transmission. In general, bartonellosis can have a variety of presentations including isolated fever, papular or pustular skin lesion with regional adenopathy, hepatitis, hepatic peliosis, encephalitis, bacil-

lary angiomatosis, isolated bacteremia, and endocarditis (29, 30).

Acute abdomen

Many of these infections will present with a wide variety of gastrointestinal symptoms (31). Occasionally, patients with either RMSF or granulocytic ehrlichiosis will present with fever and severe abdominal pain that localizes (31). In particular, patients have had exploratory laporatomy for suspected acute cholecystitis or appendicitis. Occasionally, they will present with bloody stools or vomitus indicating organism-mediated vasculitis. Bowel infarction has been reported in severe cases (31).

Encephalitis

Although many of the above entities can present with aseptic meningitis or encephalitis as part of a systemic febrile illness, these viruses present primarily as a febrile illness with altered mental status.

Tick-borne encephalitis virus and Russian spring-summer encephalitis virus

These viruses are primarily seen in Eurasia and transmitted by Ixodes ticks (32). The incubation period is usually between 7 and 14 days. Several related viruses cause a biphasic febrile illness with the influenza-like, viremic phase lasting 2–4 days. This is followed in about 1–20 days by meningitis and/or encephalitis in 20–30% of individuals. Residual neurologic sequelae are seen in 30–60% of individuals with encephalitis.

During the viremic phase, leukopenia and thrombocytopenia are common. Liver enzymes may also be mildly elevated. With the onset of neurologic disease, pleocytosis in the cerebral spinal fluid is common.

Powassan encephalitis virus

A rare cause of encephalitis, this arbovirus is the only encephalitis virus transmitted by ticks in America. Cases are primarily reported from Canada and the Northeastern United States (33). Most infections do not result in disease. However, those with clinical symptoms will have fever, headache, altered mental status, and focal neurologic signs. Frequently these individuals present similarly to those with herpes simplex encephalitis. Mortality in patients with encephalitis is high (up to 15%), and neurologic sequelae are common in survivors.

Paralysis

Tick Paralysis

Tick paralysis is a well-recognized toxinogenic disease, associated with Dermacentor, Amblyomma, and Ixodes tick feeding (34). The neurotoxin is present in the saliva of these ticks and can cause symptoms if the female tick remains feeding for 2 to 7 days. The muscle weakness progresses to ascending flaccid paralysis over a period of hours to days. Sensory function usually remains intact as does mental status. If left untreated, the paralysis can lead to respiratory failure and death (about 10%). Another presentation is acute ataxia without muscle weakness. After tick removal, recovery can be expected in hours to days. Routine laboratory studies including cerebrospinal fluid are normal.

Encephalitis Viruses

Both tick-borne encephalitis viruses and Powassan encephalitis virus can present with flaccid paralysis that can be asymmetric. Mental status is usually affected in these situations because of the encephalitic process that is involved in paralysis.

B. burgdorferi and *B. henselae*

Both of these organisms can cause syndromes of peripheral nerve palsies (predominantly facial nerve) with or without encephalitis.

DIAGNOSTIC TESTING

The diagnostic modalities that can be used in each specific tick-borne disease are noted in Table 38–3. In the vast majority of situations, diagnostic testing is most important for epidemiologic surveillance and *not* for initial treatment decisions. Most of the testing requires either acute and convalescent serology or reference laboratory methodologies that will not be available for several days in most cases. Therefore, one needs to have a high index of suspicion and treat presumptively while obtaining the tests that will confirm the diagnosis.

In addition, since one tick can transmit several infectious agents, one should also consider testing for multiple agents at one time in the appropriate clinical scenario.

MANAGEMENT OF TICK-BORNE DISEASES

The initial management of tick-borne diseases depends on the presentation involved in each case. Careful examina-

tion of the skin for ticks with careful removal is important. Furthermore, in patients with symptoms consistent with tick-borne infections, empiric antibiotic therapy should be started. Finally, a few individuals with Ixodes tick bites but no obvious signs or symptoms of infection of may benefit from a single dose of an antibiotic.

Removal of Ticks

Proper removal of ticks is important to prevent further disease transmission. Because ticks have barbed mouthparts that are buried into the dermis, extraction of these ectoparasites requires care and some expertise. Several commercial tick removal devices are available for less experienced individuals. The general principles and common misconceptions for successful removal are listed in Table 38–4 (see (34) and http://www.cdc.gov/ncidod/dvrd/rmsf/Prevention.htm). In addition, patients should be advised on methods to reduce tick exposure and prevent tick bites.

Directed treatment for individuals with syndromes consistent with tick-borne infections

Table 38–3 lists the recommended treatment strategy for each particular organism. These recommendations come from clinical experience rather than randomized controlled trials (35). Fortunately, many of the important entities respond to doxycycline. Therefore, it can be considered as a good choice for empiric therapy in individuals who have a consistent syndrome and who tolerate tetracyclines. Alternatives are mentioned as outlined. In some diseases, most notably tularemia, doxycycline is associated with a greater number of relapses, and therefore should be switched once the diagnosis of tularemia is made. Moreover, care should be taken to consider babesiosis as this infection requires completely different therapy.

An infectious disease consultation is in order in many cases. Moreover, the latest treatment guidelines are maintained at the CDC web site in several locations (http://www.bt.cdc.gov/agent/agentlist.asp, http://www.cdc.gov/ncidod/dvbid/, http://www.cdc.gov/ncidod/dvrd/branch/vrzb.htm, and http://www.dpd.cdc.gov/dpdx/HTML/Babesiosis.htm).

Empiric treatment for individuals with tick bites but without symptoms

The CDC recommendations do not include routine antibiotics for those with tick bites. Preemptive antibiotics are not cost-effective in most situations depending on the probability of infection after a tick bite. Nadelman

Table 38–3. Diagnostic and Therapeutic Options for Tick-Borne Diseases

Organism or Condition	Ticks	Diagnosis	Treatment
Anaplasma phagocytophilum	*Ixodes* spp.	Serology	Doxycycline
Babesia microti Babesia divergens	*Ixodes* spp.	Blood smear Serology	Quinine + Clindamycin OR Atovaquone + Azithromycin Exchange transfusion in severe cases
Bartonella henselae	*Ixodes* spp.	Serology PCR	Supportive care Doxycycline OR Erythromycin OR Azithromycin OR Quinolone Rifampin (in combination with another)
Borrelia burgdorferi	*Ixodes* spp.	Serology PCR	Doxycycline OR Amoxicillin OR Ceftriaxone for certain cases
Borrelia lonestari	*Amblyomma* spp.	Call the Centers for Disease Control and Prevention (CDC)	Doxycycline
Borrelia spp. (relapsing fever)	*Ornithodoros* spp.	Blood (thick and thin) smear during fever	Doxycycline Erythromycin Chloramphenicol
Colorado tick fever virus	*Dermacentor* spp.	Serology	Supportive care
Ehrlichia chaffeensis	*Amblyomma* spp.	Serology PCR Immunohistochemistry	Doxycycline
Ehrlichia ewingii	*Amblyomma* spp.	Serology PCR Immunohistochemistry	Doxycycline
Francisella tularensis	*Ixodes* spp., *Amblyoma* spp., *Dermacentor* spp.	Serology Fluorescent antibody testing Cultures (hold for longer period)	Streptomycin OR Doxycycline (higher relapse) OR Ciprofloxacin OR Chloramphenicol
Powassan encephalitis virus	*Ixodes* spp.	Serum or CSF serology	Supportive care
Rickettsia parkeri	*Amblyomma* spp.	Serology PCR Call CDC	Doxycycline
Rickettsia rickettsii	*Amblyomma* spp. *Dermacentor* spp.	Serology PCR Immunohistochemistry	Doxycycline Chloramphenicol
Tick paralysis	*Ixodes* spp., *Amblyoma* spp., *Dermacentor* spp.	None needed	Tick removal
Tick-borne encephalitis viruses	*Ixodes* spp.	Serum or CSF serology	Supportive care
West Nile virus	*Ornithodoros* spp.	Serum and CSF Serology	Supportive care

Table 38–4. Proper Approach to Tick Removal

Wear gloves to handle ticks; never use bare hands

Use blunt forceps, tweezers, or commercial removal devices; avoid sharp forceps

Grasp the tick as close to its mouth as possible

Pull tick off with a slow and steady motion

    Do not use a twisting or jerking motion to remove the tick

    Do not crush, puncture, or squeeze the tick's body

After removal, disinfect the bite area

Do not apply substances such as:

    petroleum jelly

    gasoline

    lidocaine (Xylocaine), etc., to the tick

    heat with a match or hot nail

Advise on methods to reduce tick exposure (http://www.cdc.gov/ncidod/dvrd/rmsf/Prevention.htm)

et al. studied the use of one 200-mg dose of doxycycline after tick bite in an area highly endemic for Lyme disease (36). In that cohort, 3.2% of those receiving placebo developed Lyme disease as compared with 0.4% of those who received doxycycline. The effect was particularly prominent in those with nymphal ticks that were at least partially engorged with blood (9.9% for placebo and 0% for treatment). Treatment was associated with 30.1% adverse reactions (primarily gastrointestinal in nature) while placebo-treated individuals had 11.1% adverse effects. Therefore, it may be reasonable although not mandatory to treat individuals with recent tick bites in areas of high Lyme disease endemicity with a single dose of doxycycline. No information is known for other tick-borne pathogens.

All patients with tick exposures should be warned of the potential symptoms and signs of tick-borne infections and told to return for evaluation and presumptive treatment if consistent symptoms and signs develop.

CASE OUTCOME

Because of the recent tick exposure, the patient was started on doxycycline (100 mg twice daily for 10 days. The patient's symptoms resolved within 72 h. Serologic studies confirmed an acute infection with *A. phagocytophilum*. Serologies for other tick-borne infections were negative. The patient was advised on measures to reduce tick exposure in the future.

REFERENCES

1. Belongia EA, Reed KD, Mitchell PD, et al.: Tickborne infections as a cause of nonspecific febrile illness in Wisconsin. *Clin Infect Dis* 32:1434–1439, 2001
2. Standaert SM, Dawson JE, Schaffner W, et al.: Ehrlichiosis in a golf-oriented retirement community. *N Engl J Med* 333:420–425, 1995
3. Raoult D, Roux V: Rickettsioses as paradigms of new or emerging infectious diseases. *Clin Microbiol Rev* 10:694–719, 1997
4. LaScola B, Raoult D: Laboratory diagnosis of rickettsioses: Current approaches to diagnosis of old and new rickettsial diseases. *J Clin Microbiol* 35:2715–2727, 1997
5. Sexton DJ, Kaye KS: Rocky mountain spotted fever. *Med Clin North Am* 86(2):351–356, 2002
6. Schrier SL: Human erythrocyte G6PD deficiency: pathophysiology, prevalence, diagnosis, and management. *Compr Ther* 6:41–47, 1980
7. Paddock CD, Sumner JW, Comer JA, et al.: Rickettsia parkeri: A newly recognized cause of spotted fever rickettsiosis in the United States. *Clin Infect Dis* 38:805–811, 2004
8. Paddock CD, Childs JE: Ehrlichia chaffeensis: A prototypical emerging pathogen. *Clin Microbiol Rev* 16:37–64, 2003
9. Shore GM, Machado LJ, Huycke MM, et al.: Infections with Ehrlichia chaffeensis and Ehrlichia ewingii in persons coinfected with human immunodeficiency virus. *Clin Infect Dis* 33:1586–1594, 2001
10. Bekken JS, Dumler JS: Human granulocytic ehrlichiosis. *Clin Infect Dis* 31(2):554–560, 2000
11. Singh SK, Girschick HJ: Lyme borreliosis: From infection to autoimmunity. *Clin Microbiol Infect* 10:598–561, 2004
12. Stanek G, Strle F: Lyme borreliosis. *Lancet* 362:1639–1647, 2003
13. Steere AC: Lyme disease. *N Engl J Med* 345:115–125, 2001
14. Steere AC, Coburn J, Glickstein L: The emergence of Lyme disease. *J Clin Invest* 113:1093–1101, 2004
15. Belongia EA: Epidemiology and impact of coinfections acquired from Ixodes ticks. *Vector Borne Zoonotic Dis* 2:265–273, 2002
16. James AM, Liveris D, Wormser GP, Schwartz I, Montecalvo MA, Johnson BJ.: Borrelia lonestari infection after a bite by an Amblyomma americanum tick. *J Infect Dis* 183:1810–1814, 2001
17. Stromdahl EY, Williamson PC, Kollars TM Jr., Evan SR, Barry RK, Vince MA, Dobbs NA. Evidence of Borrelia lonestari DNA in Amblyomma americanum (Acari: Ixodidae) removed from humans. *J Clin Microbiol* 41:5557–5562, 2003
18. Dworkin MS, Schwan TG, Anderson DE Jr.: *Med Clin North Am* 86:417–433, 2002
19. Dworkin MS, Shoemaker PC, Fritz CL, Dowell ME, Anderson DE Jr.: The epidemiology of tick-borne relapsing fever in the United States. *Am J Trop Med Hyg* 66:753–758, 2002

20. Krause PJ: Babesiosis diagnosis and treatment. *Vector Borne Zoonotic Dis* 3:45–51, 2003

21. Zintl A, Mulcahy G, Skerrett HE, Taylor SM, Gray JS: Babesia divergens, a bovine blood parasite of veterinary and zoonotic importance. *Clin Microbiol Rev* 16:622–636, 2003

22. Evans ME, Gregory DW, Schaffner W, McGee ZA: Tularemia: A 30-year experience with 88 cases. *Medicine (Baltimore)* 64:251–269, 1985

23. Hayes EB, Dennis D, Feldman K: Tularemia—United States, 1990–2000. *Morb Mortal Wkly Rep* 51:182–184, 2002
    Goethert HK, Shani I, Telford 3rd: Genotypic Diversity of Francisella tularensis Infecting Dermacentor variabilis Ticks on Martha's Vineyard, Massachusetts. *J Clin Microbiol* 42(11):4968–4973, 2004

24. Buehler JW, Berkelman RL, Hartley DM, Peters CJ: Syndromic surveillance and bioterrorism-related epidemics. *Emerg Infect Dis* 9(10):1197–1204, 2003

25. Feldman KA, Stiles-Enos D, Julian K: Tularemia on Martha's Vineyard: Seroprevalence and occupational risk. *Emerg Infect Dis* 9:350–354, 2003

26. Lathrop SL, Matyas BT, McGuill M: An outbreak of primary pneumonic tularemia on Martha's Vineyard. *N Engl J Med* 345:1601–1606, 2001

27. Klasco R: Colorado tick fever. *Med Clin North Am* 86(2): 435–440, 2002

28. Change CC, Chomel BB, Kasten RW, Romano V, Tietze N: Molecular evidence of *Bartonella* spp. in questing adult Ixodes pacificus ticks in California. *J Clin Microbiol* 39: 1221–1226, 2001

29. Jacomo V, Kelly PJ, Raoult D: Natural history of Bartonella infections (an exception to Koch's postulate). *Clin Diagn Lab Immunol* 9:8–18, 2002

30. Spach DH, Koehler JE: Bartonella-associated infections. *Infect Dis Clin North Am* 12:137–155, 1998

31. Zaidi SA. Singer C: Gastrointestinal and hepatic manifestations of tickborne diseases in the United States. *Clin Infect Dis.* 34:1206–1212, 2002

32. Gritsun TS, Nuttall PA, Gould EA: Tick-borne flaviviruses. *Adv Virus Res* 61:317–371, 2003

33. Anonymous: Outbreak of Powassan encephalitis—Maine and Vermont, 1999–2001. *Morb Mortal Wkly Rep* 50:761–764, 2001

34. Greenstein P: Tick paralysis. *Med Clin North Am* 86:441–446, 2002

35. Donovan BJ, Weber DJ, Rublein JC, Raasch RH: Treatment of tick-borne diseases. *Ann Pharmacother* 36:1590–1597, 2002

36. Nadelman RB, Nowakowski J, Fish D, et al. (Tick Bite Study Group): Prophylaxis with single-dose doxycycline for the prevention of Lyme disease after an Ixodes scapularis tick bite. *N Engl J Med* 345:79–84, 2001

39

Fever in the Returning Traveler

Diane M. Birnbaumer

HIGH YIELD FACTS

1. For any patient presenting to the emergency department with fever, consider making it a habit to ask about travel.

2. In every febrile patient returning from travel to an area endemic for the diseases, consider malaria and/or dengue fever in the differential diagnosis of their illness.

3. Know the indications for admission in patients returning from travel who develop a fever.

CASE PRESENTATION

CC: Fever, malaise

HPI: A 42-year-old female presents complaining of 3 days of fever, malaise, and severe body aches. The patient states she has a headache during the fever, but it resolves when her fever resolves. She denies nausea, vomiting, diarrhea, abdominal pain, rash, cough, earache, sore throat, or cough, but states that she has severe body aches, particularly with the fever, that "wipe her out" and prevent her from even participating in her usual activities of daily living. She has not had any sick contacts, but volunteers the history that 5 days ago she returned from a trip to Turkey and India and stopped in the Caribbean on her way home. The trip ended 1 week prior to the onset of symptoms and she is concerned that her illness may be related to her recent travel.

PMH: Med, surg: None

Meds: Acetaminophen. States she did not take any medical prophylaxis on trip, nor did she get any immunizations prior to travel.

All: None

EXAM

VS: T = 103.5   RR = 20   HR = 130   BP = 120/70
O_2 Sat 99%

Gen: Nontoxic but very uncomfortable appearing 42-year-old female

Skin: Warm, dry, no lesions

HEENT: PERRL. EOMI. Anicteric, no conjunctival injection. TMs normal.

Oropharynx slightly dry, otherwise normal.

Neck: Supple, no meningeal signs.

Lungs: Clear

Cardiac: RRR, no murmurs, rubs, gallops

Abd: NABS, nontender.

Ext: No C/C/E

Neuro: A, Ox4. CN 3–12 intact. Motor 5/5 throughout, sensory intact throughout.

FNF normal. Gait normal.

EVALUATION

Labs: Normal CBC, chem-7, UA

CXR: Normal

What do you do now?

INTRODUCTION/EPIDEMIOLOGY

Emporiatrics: The science and health of travelers.

The quest to experience new cultures, climates, and environments compels 8 million Americans to explore developing countries annually. Ten million people, often immigrants, return to these countries to visit relatives. Associated with this travel is exposure to illnesses not usually found in North America. As many of these infectious diseases have an incubation period longer than the duration of travel, patients may not manifest symptoms of illness until after returning home. When seeking medical care their presenting complaints are often vague or nonspecific, and the history of travel may not be noted by either the patient or the medical care provider. An astute medical care provider will consider the possibility of travel-related infection in patients presenting with fever, diarrhea, or other nonspecific complaints. This is particularly important when treating patients who traveled to visit family members, as they may not think of their travel as a vacation or clue into the fact that they may be at risk for acquiring these travel-related diseases. These patients tend not to get adequate immunizations or take appropriate prophylactic medications for their travel (1).

There are literally dozens of infections that may be acquired by the traveler. This chapter will focus on two of the most important causes: malaria and dengue. Other infections seen in travelers, such as hepatitis, traveler's diarrhea and sexually transmitted diseases, are covered elsewhere in this book.

CLINICAL PRESENTATION

History

One of the most common presenting complaints in the patient with a travel-related disease is fever, which is sometimes recurrent. Other complaints in this patient population include respiratory problems (cough, shortness of breath), gastrointestinal illnesses (diarrhea, constipation, nausea, vomiting), rash, or symptoms typical to sexually transmitted diseases.

Unfortunately, patients presenting with travel-related diseases tend to seek medical care for these types of nonspecific complaints. Unless a history of recent travel is obtained, some important and potentially serious causes of the illness will not be considered. In addition, many patients will not volunteer a history of travel, as most develop their illness after returning home and may not connect their symptoms with their travel. Bearing this in mind, it is a useful habit to add a question about any recent travel when evaluating any patient with a nonspecific complaint and, in particular, those complaining of fever.

If the patient answers "yes" when asked about recent travel, an array of further questions need to be asked. These questions include:

1. Where did you travel? Did you have any stopovers during your travel?

2. How long were you there?

3. What type of travel did you do? Urban, rural, eco-travel?

4. What sort of activities did you do during your trip? Did you hike, camp, white-water raft, stay with indigenous people, etc?

5. Did you get any vaccinations before you left on your trip?

6. Did you take any prophylactic medications related to your trip? What were they? Exactly how did you take them, and for how long?

7. Did others in your travel group become ill?

8. Did you have any insect bites during your trip?

9. What did you eat/drink while you traveled?

10. Were you exposed to animals while you traveled?

11. What was your sexual activity during your travel? Did you have sexual contact with any of the local people?

12. When did your symptoms start in relation to your travel?

The answers to these questions help determine potential illnesses specific to the patient's travel and focus the treating physician on the most likely diseases the patient may have. Once the history of travel is obtained, the treating physician should determine diseases endemic to those areas. Accessing the Centers for Disease, Control and Pre-

vention (CDC-P) Web site (www.cdc.gov) or even calling the CDC-P (1-877-394-8747) is particularly useful for this information, as it changes frequently and is often not readily familiar to many practicing physicians.

In determining the cause of illness in the returned traveler, one of the most useful pieces of information is the timing of the symptoms in relation to the travel. Diseases can be divided into those that cause symptoms soon after infection versus those that cause symptoms as long as weeks to months after exposure (Table 39–1) (2).

Table 39–1. Travel-related Diseases Based on Incubation Period

Short incubation period (<28 days)	Arbovirus
	Bacterial dysentery
	Brucellosis
	Childhood viruses
	Dengue
	Epstein-Barr virus
	Hepatitis A
	Influenza
	Leptospirosis
	Malaria (no chemoprophylaxis)
	Plague
	Q fever
	Relapsing fever
	Rickettsial spotted fevers
	Rubella
	Rubeola
	Schistosomiasis
	Tularemia
	Typhoid fever
	Typhus
	Yellow fever
Long incubation period (>28 days)	African trypanosomiasis
	American trypanosomiasis
	Amoebiasis
	Brucellosis
	Filariasis
	Hepatitis B and C
	Leishmaniasis
	Malaria (partially immune or after chemoprophylaxis)
	Meliodosis
	Paragonimaisis
	Rabies
	Schistosomiasis
	Strongyloidiasis
	Tuberculosis

Examination

Examination of the returning traveler with a fever should be thorough, although often there is a paucity of helpful findings on exam. Particular attention should be paid to the vital signs, lymph node exam, skin exam, and examination for hepatomegaly and splenomegaly.

LABORATORY/DIAGNOSTIC TESTING

Which laboratory tests are ordered will largely depend on the disease suspected. Some laboratory tests may also lend diagnostic clues to certain diseases, particularly those that cause elevated eosinophil counts or positive parasitic blood smears.

In general, returning travelers with a fever should get a complete blood count with differential, a chemistry panel (electrolytes, blood urea nitrogen, and creatinine), serum glucose, a liver panel (AST, ALT, total bilirubin, and alkaline phosphatase), and a urinalysis. Particular attention should be paid to the absolute eosinophil count, which is considered elevated if over 500 eosinophils/mm^3. If the patient traveled to a malaria-endemic area, a thick and thin blood smear should also be sent; these smears may also be helpful in diagnosing borreliosis, babesiosis, and trypanosomiasis. A chest radiograph may be useful in patients with respiratory complaints. Other testing may also be sent as indicated, such as an erythrocyte sedimentation rate, stool studies (fecal occult blood, fecal leukocytes, stool for culture and sensitivity, and stool for ova and parasites), hepatitis serologies, coagulation studies, and specific serologic tests as indicated. Also, tests for sexually transmitted diseases (including HIV testing) may be indicated, and a PPD may also be placed.

DISPOSITION

Most returning travelers can be managed as outpatients as their workups progress. Admission is indicated in patients with suspected falciparum malaria, typhoid fever, and viral hemorrhagic fevers (Lassa, Ebola, Marburg, and Dengue Hemorrhagic Fevers), as well as in patients with the usual indications for admission.

SPECIFIC DISEASES: MALARIA

Introduction/Epidemiology

Malaria is endemic in over 100 countries, 92% of which are at risk for falciparum malaria, the most serious form of the parasite. Malaria tends to occur most commonly in countries along the equator (Fig. 39–1). Annually there are 300–500 million cases worldwide and 1.5–3.5 million deaths. Travelers to endemic areas are at moderate risk for acquiring infection (>1 case in 200 travelers but <1 in 10 travelers) (3, 4).

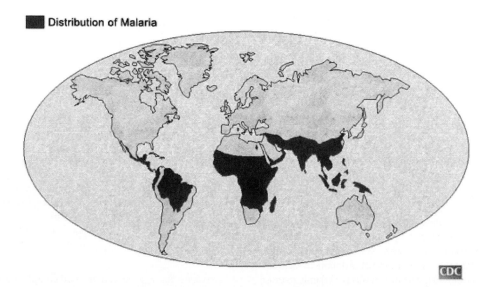

■ Distribution of Malaria

Fig. 39–1. Worldwide distribution of malaria (CDC).

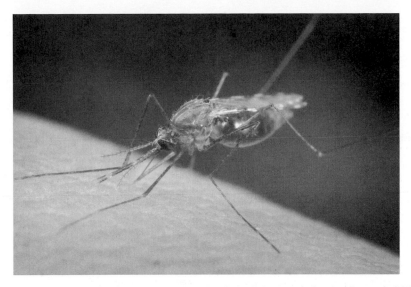

Fig. 39–2. Night-biting Anopheles mosquito responsible for malaria transmission (see "mosquito" TIFF).

Pathophysiology/Microbiology

Transmission of the parasite primarily occurs during the bite of the night-biting female Anopheles mosquito (Fig. 39–2), when sporozooities are injected into the bloodstream. The actual risk of infection varies significantly from season to season and whether the bite occurs in a rural or urban area. Once in the bloodstream, the sporozoites infect red blood cells, and the life cycle of the protozoan leads to red blood cell destruction. In addition to this erythrocytic stage, 2 species, *Plasmodium vivax* and *Plasmodium ovale*, also have an exoerythrocytic stage, where the parasites can rest quietly in the liver for years (Fig. 39–3).

Within the genus *Plasmodium* there are four species of malaria. *Plasmodium falciparum* is the most virulent form, primarily due to its ability to infect red blood cells of all ages. This species has a worldwide distribution in tropical regions as well as in sub-Saharan Africa. This form of malaria accounts for just over half of imported malaria (5, 6). *P. vivax* accounts for most of the remainder of imported malaria (just over 40%) (5, 6). It is prevalent in the tropics and is less virulent than *P. falciparum* because it only infected young red blood cells and reticulocytes. It has an exoerythrocytic stage where it becomes "dormant" as hypnozoities that rest in the liver. *P. ovale* is seen in western Africa and is relatively uncommon in North America, causing less than 5% of the imported malaria. Like *P. vivax*, it also has an exoerythrocytic stage. *P. malariae* is distributed worldwide, has no exoerythro-

cytic phase, and infects only mature red blood cells. It accounts for less than 5% of imported malaria.

Clinical Presentation

The incubation period of malaria is typically 8–30 days, so it tends to present as an acute febrile illness occurring less than a month after the traveler returns. However, this typically short incubation period can be longer in patients who acquire the infection despite taking chemoprophylaxis or in those who are already partially immune (7). *P. vivax* and *P. ovale*, due to their exoerythocytic hypnozoite stage, may present with symptoms as much as years after the primary infection, when the hypnozoites become active and reinfect the circulating red blood cells.

Clinically, the symptoms of malaria are notoriously nonspecific. The most common symptom is fever, occurring in 99% of patients (7). Early in the illness there is no specific pattern to the fever, but if the infection continues untreated for a prolonged period the fevers may develop a pattern suggestive of the species of malaria causing the infection. This cyclical pattern, when seen, develops in only one third of patients infected with malaria. Chills, rigors, and headaches occur in over three-quarters of patients (7). Malaise, myalgias, and backache occur in half, and nausea, vomiting, and/or diarrhea occur in about a third (7). Altered mental status occurs in one in ten, and suggests cerebral malaria, a dreaded complication of this infection found in patients infected with *P. falciparum* (5).

Malaria

(*Plasmodium* spp.)

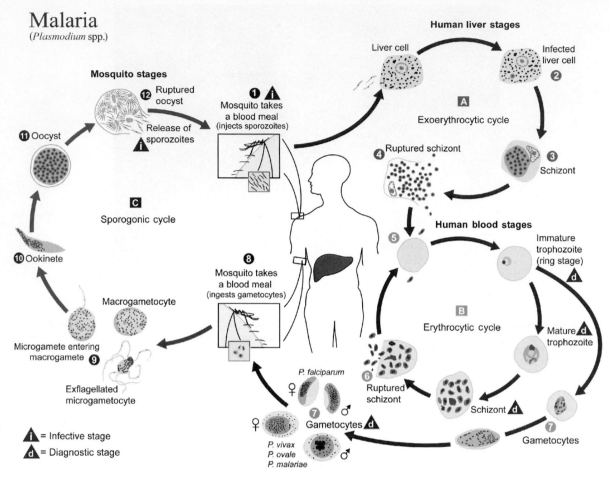

Fig. 39–3. Life cycle of the plasmodium species (see "life cycle" TIFF).

On examination, 80% of patients will have a fever, sometimes as high as 40°C. One in eight patients is jaundiced and may have abdominal tenderness (7). Hepatomegaly and splenomegaly are found in a third (7).

Laboratory/Diagnostic Testing

The most suggestive findings of malaria on routine blood testing are thrombocytopenia, seen in just under half of patients, and anemia, found in a third (7). The white blood cell count is normal in the majority of patients, although an elevated band count is seen in many. One-third of patients have an elevated bilirubin and three-quarters have an elevated lactate dehydrogenase level; both elevations are due to lysis of the infected red blood cells.

The definitive tests for malaria are thick and thin blood smears. These tests will be positive in over 90% of infected patients, but smears may need to be checked twice daily for 2–3 days during fever spikes to rule out the diagnosis (5). This fact is very important for physicians to understand so they do not rely on a single blood smear to rule out the diagnosis and order the multiple smears necessary to exclude the disease as the cause of the patient's symptoms.

Disposition

Although many patients with malaria can be treated as outpatients, those with suspected falciparum malaria need admission to the hospital. Findings suggestive of infection

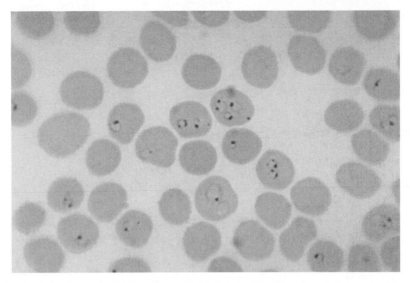

Fig. 39–4. Large intraerythrocytic parasite load seen in a patient infected with falciparum malaria(see multiple ring forms TIFF).

with this species include smears that show either a high parasite load (Fig. 39–4) or microgametocytes (Fig. 39–5), severe anemia, jaundice, altered mental status, and travel to endemic areas.

When malaria is suspected, it is prudent to consult an infectious disease specialist or to call the Centers for Disease Control and Prevention (CDC-P) for advice on how best to treat the infection. Treatment recommendations vary depending on the potential type of species involved and where the infection was acquired. Typically, nonfalciparum malaria (typically caused by *P. vivax*) is treated with chloroquine 10 mg/kg base (max 600 mg), then, once the patient tests negative for G-6-PD deficiency, is also treated with primaquine 0.25 mg/kg base daily for 14 days. This added treatment with primaquine treats the exoerythrocytic phase seen in infection with *P. vivax* or *P. ovale*, but patients must be evaluated for G-6-PD deficiency before this drug is given. If the patient has suspected

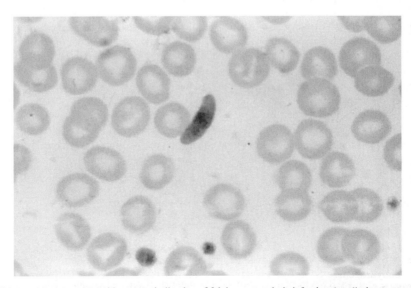

Fig. 39–5. Microgametocyte seen on thin smear, indicative of falciparum malaria infection (see "microgametocyte" TIFF).

Table 39–2. Imported Malaria

Imported Malaria—Summary Information				
Parasitology	*P. falciparum*	*P. vivax*	*P. ovale*	*P. malariae*
Incubation	12 days (8–25 days)	14 days (8–27 days)	15 days (9–17 days)	18 days (15–30 days)
Relapses?	No	Yes (exoerythocytic phase)	Yes (exoerythrocytic phase)	No
High parasite load	++	–	–	–
RBC preferences	All ages	Reticulocytes	Reticulocytes	Senescent
Clinical Presentation				
Mortality	++	+	–	–
Severe anemia	++	+	+	–
Cerebral malaria	++	–	–	–
Respiratory failure	++	–	–	–
Renal failure	+	–	–	+
Splenic rupture	–	+	–	–
Diagnosis				
Blood smear	RBC normal Multiple rings Banana gametocytes	Enlarged RBC Schuffner granules	Oval RBC Schuffner granules	RBC normal
Treatment Issues				
Chloroquine resistance?	Worldwide	Rare	None	None
Multidrug resistance?	++	None	None	None

nonfalciparum malaria acquired in an area of known chloroquine resistance, the patient may be treated with mefloquine or halofantrine.

Patients with suspected falciparum malaria need admission to the hospital. Treatment consists of IV quinidine 10 mg/kg base IV over 8 h (max 600 mg), then 15 mg/kg base IV over 24 h. These patients must be closely monitored for dysrhythmias and hypoglycemia.

Table 39–2 summarizes the most salient features of the four types of Plasmodium infection.

SPECIFIC DISEASES: DENGUE FEVER

Introduction/Epidemiology

The CDC-P considers dengue fever "the most important mosquito-borne viral disease infecting humans." The four serotypes of this single-stranded RNA flavivirus are found in the tropics worldwide. It is transmitted by the day-biting *Aedes aegypti* mosquito, which is found in both urban and rural areas. This mosquito frequently lives indoors in close proximity to humans; this indoor exposure has made environmental eradication programs difficult. There are 50–100 million cases of this disease annually, with 250,000–500,000 cases of dengue hemorrhagic fever and 24,000 deaths (8, 9). Over the past 30 years, incidence has increased dramatically, and air travel has imported cases of this infection to nonendemic countries such as the United States. For travelers, this is considered a moderate risk infection, occurring in less than 1 in 10 travelers but more than 1 in 200 (3).

Pathophysiology/Microbiology

There are four serotypes of flavivirus known to cause dengue fever. Although lifelong immunity develops after infection with one specific serotype, this immunity is specific to only that serotype, and there is minimal cross-immunity between serotypes. In fact, patients with a second infection of dengue fever are more likely to be seriously ill, a phenomenon suspected to be due to antibody-dependent enhancement, when antibodies from one serotype enhance infection with a second serotype.

Clinical Presentation

After infection with the dengue flavivirus, the vast majority of patients acquire the infection asymptomatically. When symptomatic, patients may present with one of four syndromes: undifferentiated febrile illness, dengue fever, dengue hemorrhagic fever, and dengue shock syndrome. Due to its short incubation period of 2–7 days, patients with symptomatic dengue infection present with an acute febrile illness occurring either during or soon after returning from travel.

Undifferentiated febrile illness

This syndrome is clinically indistinguishable from other viral infections and patients recover fully.

Dengue fever

Dengue fever can occur during either primary or secondary dengue infection. It is characterized by sudden onset of high fever, malaise, and a severe retroorbital headache. Patients also have conjunctival injection, arthralgias and myalgias, anorexia, and abdominal discomfort. Myalgias and arthralgias can be severe and give the disease its nickname, "breakbone fever" and this may be a clue to this disease. Some patients develop an erythematous, macular rash that starts on the trunk and spreads to the limbs and face. This facial flushing, often accompanied by conjunctival injection and puffiness of the eyelids, is known as "dengue facies." The fever in dengue fever tends to last for 2–7 days and often recurs for several days, resolves, and then returns. This biphasic pattern is known as "saddleback fever." Although some patients develop the more ominous syndromes of dengue hemorrhagic fever or dengue shock syndrome, most patients with dengue fever recover fully, but may have a prolonged recovery period.

Dengue hemorrhagic fever

Dengue hemorrhagic fever (DHF) is a relatively rare but potentially life-threatening syndrome that occurs most commonly in children under age 16 who live in areas endemic for the dengue flavivirus (10). Although DHF can be seen during primary infection with dengue, it is much more commonly seen during secondary infections, which is the reason that children in endemic areas are more at risk for this syndrome. The increased risk during secondary infection is thought to be due to antibody-dependent enhancement, where the antibody from one serotype enhances the infection with a second serotype.

DHF has several manifestations similar to dengue fever, but the addition of circulatory failure and hemorrhage make DHF more lethal. Like dengue fever, patients with DHF have intermittent high fever, severe headaches (often retroorbital), flushing, myalgias and arthralgias, vomiting, anorexia, and acute abdominal pain. The more serious bleeding manifestations that are associated with DHF include epistaxis, bleeding from the gums, petechiae and ecchymoses, hematemesis, melena, and vaginal bleeding in females.

Although hemorrhage is often part of the syndrome and lends it its name, the most concerning characteristic of DHF is plasma leakage, characterized by circulatory disturbances including hypotension, tachycardia, a narrow pulse pressure, and delayed capillary refill. Due to this plasma leakage pleural effusions and ascites may also be seen. Rarely, patients with DHF may develop complications of encephalopathy, encephalitis, liver failure, myocarditis, and disseminated intravascular coagulation (10–12).

Figure 39–6 shows the World Health Organization grades of severity of dengue hemorrhagic fever (13).

Grade I: No shock, only positive tourniquet test
Grade II: No shock, has spontaneous bleeding other than a positive
             tourniquet test
Grade III: Shock
Grade IV: Profound shock with unmeasurable blood pressure and/or pulse

Fig. 39–6. World Health Organization dengue hemorrhagic fever grading scale.

Table 39–3. Types of Dengue Infection

Undifferentiated febrile illness
Dengue fever
  Acute illness with two or more of the following:
    Headache, retro-orbital headache, myalgia, arthral-
    gia, rash, hemorrhagic manifestations, leukopenia
Dengue hemorrhagic fever
  Patients should have all of the following:
  Manifestations of hemorrhage (positive tourniquet
    test, petechiae, ecchymoses or purpura, or bleeding
    from gums, gastrointestinal tract, or other locations)
  Platelet count $<100,000/mm^3$
  Objective evidence of plasma leakage (pleural
    effusion, ascites, hemoconcentration of $>20\%$
    baseline)
Dengue shock syndrome
  Patients should have the following:
  Manifestations of dengue hemorrhagic fever,
    and either
  Pulse pressure <20 mm Hg, or
  Hypotension (SBP <80 mm Hg in children <5 years
    or <90 for those ≥ 5 years)

Dengue shock syndrome

Dengue shock syndrome is the most lethal form of dengue infection, with a mortality rate of 9–47% (14). These patients present in profound shock (systolic blood pressure less than 80 mm Hg and/or a pulse pressure <20 mm Hg) and require aggressive supportive management.

Table 39–3 summarizes the different forms of dengue infection.

Laboratory/Diagnostic Testing

Patients with suspected dengue infection should have blood sent for a complete blood count, electrolytes, blood urea nitrogen, creatinine, coagulation studies, liver function tests, and, if bleeding is apparent or the patient is felt to be at risk, for type and crossmatch.

In many patients with dengue infection laboratory results are normal (15, 16). In the more severe forms of the disease, leukopenia and thrombocytopenia (platelets $<100,000/mm^3$) may be seen, as may elevated liver function tests. Patients developing disseminated intravascular coagulation have abnormal coagulation studies.

Laboratory confirmation of dengue infection is done by various methods ranging from virus isolation to serologic testing to DNA amplification methods (17). These tests are not routinely available and are typically a "send out" study. As a result, this diagnosis is often made clinically.

Disposition

There is no specific pharmacologic treatment available to treat dengue infection, so management of this infection is supportive. If the patient does not have evidence of hepatitis, fever should be treated with acetaminophen. Aspirin and aspirin-containing agents should be avoided in children as their use in viral illnesses is associated with Reyes syndrome.

The most important issue in managing the more severe forms of dengue infection (DHF and dengue shock syndrome) is the early recognition and management of plasma leakage. Early signs include hemoconcentration, tachycardia, and a narrowing pulse pressure. The syndrome is obvious once the patient develops hypotension or overt bleeding. Patients should receive intravenous crystalloid with close monitoring of their vital signs, mental status, and urinary output. Patients may require liters of intravenous fluids, and physicians should not hesitate to use as much crystalloid as is necessary and can be used safely.

Bleeding complications from dengue such as gastrointestinal bleeding should be managed with transfusions of blood, fresh frozen plasma, and platelets as indicated. Controversy surrounds at which platelet level platelets should be transfused in patients with thrombocytopenia without evidence of bleeding, and there is no consensus on this issue. Patients with evidence of disseminated intravascular anticoagulation should be managed in the usual fashion.

Although patients with dengue fever can be managed as outpatients, a low threshold should be used when deciding if these patients need admission. Patients with DHF or dengue shock syndrome need admission, and children in whom dengue hemorrhagic fever is suspected should also be admitted. All admitted patients should be watched closely for development of either the significant bleeding complications or shock that may occur with the illness.

Recovery from dengue infection is prolonged, with fatigue often lasting for months after the illness. Patients with symptoms suggestive of dengue fever should be reported to the CDC.

Vaccine

Concerted effort is being made to develop an effective vaccine for dengue fever, but to date these efforts have not proven clinically fruitful. A major stumbling block is the necessity of developing a tetravalent vaccine that is equally effective against all four serotypes. This multivalent vaccine is necessary as secondary dengue infection is more commonly associated with the more severe forms of the disease due to antibody-dependent enhancement. Unless the vaccine induces an adequate antibody response to all four serotypes, the vaccine could actually increase the risk of more severe forms of dengue infection (16).

CASE OUTCOME

As the patient had traveled to areas where both dengue fever (the Caribbean) and malaria (Turkey and India) are endemic, the treating physician sent thick and thin blood smears to determine if the patient had malaria. The thin smear was read as "high degree of parasite load," causing the treating physician to be concerned about the possibility of falciparum malaria as the cause of the patient's illness. The physician admitted the patient to the hospital and consulted the infectious disease specialist on call, who worked with the primary care physician to determine the best way to treat the patient. The patient recovered without incident.

Web sites for information on travel-related disease are www.cdc.gov/travel (Centers for Disease Control and Prevention), www.who.int/inf-fs (World Health Organization), www.paho.org (Pan American Health Organization).

REFERENCES

1. Angell SY, Cetron MS: Health disparities among travelers visiting friends and relatives abroad. *Ann Intern Med* 142:67–73, 2005.
2. Re III LV, Gluckman SJ: Fever in the returned traveler. *AFP* 68:1343–1350, 2003.
3. *health Information for International Travel 2003–2004*. Atlanta, U.S. Department of Health and Human Services, Public Health Service, Centers for Disease Control and Prevention, National Center for Infectious Diseases, Division of Quarantine, 2003.
4. Bruni M, Steffen R: Impact of travel-related health impairments. *J Travel Med* 4(2):61–64, 1997.
5. Ryan ET, Wilson ME, Kain KC: Illness after international travel. *N Engl J Med* 347:505–516, 2002.
6. O'Brien D, et al: Fever in returned travelers: Review of hospital admissions for a 3-year period. *Clin Infect Dis* 33:603–609, 2001.
7. Dorsey G, et al: Difficulties in the prevention, diagnosis, and treatment of imported malaria. *Arch Intern Med* 160:2505–2510, 2000.
8. Jelinek T: Dengue fever in international travelers. *Clin Infect Dis* 31:144–147, 2000.
9. Gibbons RV, Vaughn DW: Dengue: An escalating problem. *BMJ* 324:1563–1566, 2002.
10. Rigau-Perez JG, et al: Dengue and dengue haemorrhagic fever. *Lancet* 352:971–977, 1998.
11. Guzman MG, Kouri G: Dengue: An update. *Lancet Infect Dis* 2:33–42, 2002.
12. Cam BV, et al: Prospective case-control study of encephalopathy in children with dengue hemorrhagic fever. *Am J Trop Med Hyg* 65:848–851, 2001.
13. World Health Organization: Prevention and control of dengue and dengue haemorrhagic fever: Comprehensive guidelines. WHO Regional Publication, SEARO, No. 29, 1999.
14. Malavige GN, et al: Dengue viral infections. *Postgrad Med J* 80:588–601, 2004.
15. Kalayanarooj S, et al: Early clinical and laboratory indicators of acute dengue illness. *J Infect Dis* 176:313–321, 1997.
16. Guzman MG, Kouri G: Dengue diagnosis, advances and challenges. *Int J Infect Dis* 8:69–80, 2004.
17. Shu PY, Huang JH: Current advances in dengue diagnosis. *Clin Diag Lab Immun* 11:642–650, 2004.

40

Immunizations

Michael E. Hagensee

HIGH YIELD FACTS

1. The Emergency Medicine physician must have a high suspicion for rabies as well as knowledge of what animals in his/her community are at risk for being rabid.

2. The Emergency Medicine physician should also know how to manage a dirty wound and the prophylaxis against tetanus.

3. Passive immunity, that is immune globulin, is indicated in the acute exposure setting for botulism, tetanus, hepatitis A and B, rabies, diphtheria, vaccinia, and varicella-zoster. For the rare cases of botulism and diphtheria, immune globulin products are made in horses and 10% of people who receive these products will develop serum sickness.

4. Vaccination against smallpox is much more common these days and the Emergency Medicine physician should be familiar with some of its complications and side effects.

5. The emergency department can administer pneumococcal and influenza virus vaccines to populations at risk including the elderly and those with chronic medical conditions.

Case

A 6-year-old boy who lives in a rural area presents to the emergency department in no acute distress. His parents are hysterical because a live bat was found in the boy's room earlier this morning. The boy's bedroom window was open and it is known that bats inhabit the area. Close physical examination reveals no clear bite marks on the boy and vital signs are normal. The parents are understandably anxious. What course of action is indicated?

COMMON VACCINES
Active and Passive

Immediate administration of both active and passive immunizations is critical in the care of the exposed patient.

The emergency medicine physician plays a vital role in identifying those potential exposures that require immediate administration of vaccines, some of which target rare but potentially morbid or fatal infectious diseases including those that require some time to procure. The goal of this chapter is to highlight several vaccines that are important for the Emergency Medicine physician's practice rather than an exhaustive review of all vaccines.

An active immunization is what is often referred to as a vaccine. Vaccines may be composed of inactivated pathogen(s) (inactivated polio vaccine, IPV; influenza virus, rabies virus), attenuated live pathogen(s) (oral polio vaccine, OPV; varicella-zoster virus vaccine, VZV), or subunit vaccines composed of purified protein (hepatitis B), toxoids (diphtheria, tetanus) or proteins conjugated to carriers to improve immunogenicity (pneumococcal; *Haemophilus influenzae* type B). These agents require the body to generate an immune response against the pathogen in order to confer protection. Passive immunizations are concentrated collections of immunoglobulins, some of which are pathogen specific. These immunizations are designed to provide immediate immunity and do not require the body to generate an immune response. A few of the passive immunological agents are actually produced in animals (e.g., botulism and diphtheria in horses) which can lead to an immune response against them, that is, serum sickness. There are very few of these products available and the diseases that they prevent are also relatively rare.

Tetanus (Td)

The dirty wound that is at risk for infection by *Clostridium tetani* is commonplace in the emergency department (ED) setting. In the United States, tetanus immunization in conjunction with diphtheria (the little "d" in the *Td* vaccine) is part of the universal childhood immunization schedule, therefore rendering the majority of the U.S. population at rather low risk for these disease entities. However, the adult tetanus booster recommended at 10-year intervals is less commonly administered, resulting in many potentially susceptible adults. Indeed, in a recent serological survey of women enrolled in the 3rd National Health and Nutrition Examination Survey (NHANES), only 41% of women over age 20 had adequate antitoxin levels for both tetanus and diphtheria (1). Overall, more than 95% of tetanus cases in the last decades have involved individuals over the age of 20 years. In addition, professional and recreational activities that potentially expose individuals to ground contact can increase risk for carpenters and

Table 40–1. Summary Guide to Tetanus Prophylaxis in Routine Wound Management

History of adsorbed tetanus toxoid (doses)	Clean, minor wounds	All other wounds*
Unknown or <3	Td+ only	Td+ TIG
≥3 doses &	No@ No	No** No

*Such as, but not limited to, wounds contaminated with dirt, feces, soil, and saliva; puncture wounds; avulsions; and wounds resulting from missiles, crushing, burns and frostbite.

+For children <7 years old; DTP (DT, if pertussis vaccine is contraindicated) is preferred to tetanus toxoid alone. For persons >= 7 years of age, Td is preferred to tetanus toxoid alone.

&If only three doses of fluid toxoid have been received, then a fourth dose of toxoid, preferably an adsorbed toxoid, should be given.

@Yes, if >10 years since last dose.

**Yes, if >5 years since last dose. (More frequent boosters are not needed and can accentuate side effects).

excavators, particularly those who reside in warm, rural areas. Typical at-risk injuries include abrasions, puncture wounds, and lacerations. Obtaining an immunization history is imperative as not all children have received the recommended newborn series of immunizations, especially with the influx of non-U.S.-born individuals and religious beliefs that preclude the use of vaccines.

In the ED, the patient may present with a dirty wound exposure and have an unclear vaccination history. Alternatively, in the setting of major trauma when preventative tetanus prophylaxis needs to be considered, the patient may be uncommunicative. When the clinical signs and symptoms of tetanus (i.e., increased muscle tone, dysphagia, and trismus) develop, it may be too late for any vaccine to work effectively and supportive measures are all that can be provided. Nonetheless, human tetanus immune globulin (TIG) should be administered even in advanced cases. The optimal dose is not known but routinely 250–500 units are given intramuscularly (IM). There are some theoretical reasons to administering the dose prior to manipulation of the wound and a part of the dose can be used to infiltrate the wound (2). TIG delivered intramuscularly may also be indicated in wounds that are not clean and minor as part of standard wound management (see below).

The routine active tetanus immunization (usually as part of combined diphtheria, tetanus, and acellular pertussis immunization) schedule for children is at 2 months, 4 months, and 6 months of age with booster doses at 15–18 months and 4–6 years of age. Tetanus toxoid with diphtheria toxoid (i.e., Td) is recommended at 11–12 years of age and every 10 years thereafter.

The routine passive tetanus immunization schedule for the nonimmunized adult includes three doses of Td

(tetanus toxoid and diphtheria toxoid). The first two doses should be 4 weeks apart and the third dose should be administered 6–12 months later. As with children, Td should then be administered every 10 years thereafter.

Wound management is summarized in Table 40–1 (3). Clean and minor wounds do not require TIG, but Td is indicated for those individuals

1. who have an unclear prior vaccination history
2. who are not yet fully immunized (less than three doses)
3. who have not had tetanus vaccination for over 10 years

Dirty wounds require intramuscular administration of TIG (250 units = prophylactic dose) only when no complete vaccination history is available. Td is also given for unclear vaccination history and to those whose most recent booster was more than 5 years ago. TIG is available from the CDC (see contact information above). The equine product tetanus antitoxin (TAT) is no longer recommended due to a side-effect profile which includes serum sickness and hypersensitivity reactions.

Botulism

Botulism is caused by toxins released from the gram-positive rod *Clostridium botulinum*. The toxins cleave important fusion proteins at the acetylcholine neuromuscular junction, resulting in flaccid paralysis. The major toxins that have effects on humans are A, B, E, and F. A typical family outbreak occurs after ingestion of poorly home-canned foods, particularly canned vegetables. Other potential food ingestions include homemade salsa, sautéed onions, and salted or fermented fish. Foodborne botulism usually develops within 3 days but can occur anywhere from 2 h until 8 days after ingestion. Inhalational botulism from a biowarfare weapon can occur within 3 days.

The Emergency Medicine physician must be aware of the presenting symptoms of botulism in order to act promptly and intervene with passive vaccination. The classic triad of acute, symmetrical, descending flaccid paralysis coupled with a clear sensorium and the absence of fever should significantly increase the suspicion for botulism. In addition, a common presentation includes a bulbar palsy that can manifest as diplopia, dysponia, and dysphagia. Gastrointestinal symptoms also include significant nausea, vomiting, and diarrhea and typically result from ingestion of food contaminated by infected stool. Wound botulism can occur when a wound is contaminated by *C. botulinum*.

Once botulism is suspected, prompt management is essential and consists of supportive care and administration of antitoxin. The antitoxin formulation is one of the few remaining horse-derived health care products and is a combination of antitoxins against toxins A, B, and E. It is available from the CDC 24-h hot line. The usual dose is 1 vial (10 cc consisting of 7500 IU of anti-A, 5500 IU of anti-B, and 8500 IU of anti-E), but in some centers where blood is measured for toxin activity, persistent activity precipitates administration of additional doses (4). Side effects of the antitoxin include serum sickness, fevers, and urticaria. Those sensitive to the antitoxin should receive the antitoxin slowly, usually over 3–4 h. A human antitoxin exists and is available only for infants and can be obtained through the California Department of Public Health. The military uses the *Fab* fragment of antibodies made against the seven strains of toxin from horses, and its efficacy has been excellent so far.

There is a preventative vaccine, the botulinum toxoid, which has been shown to generate a protective response in 97% of the soldiers who have received two doses. The regimen is administered at 0, 2, and 12 weeks and a booster dose is given at 1 year. This vaccine is used for immunizing high-risk laboratory and military personnel.

Diphtheria

Corynebacterium diphtheria is a gram-positive rod whose severe disease is associated with production of a toxin, tox+, which is carried on a bacteriophage. Universal administration of diphtheria toxin vaccination as one of the recommended childhood vaccines has greatly reduced the number of cases of diphtheria to a mere handful. However epidemics have occurred over the past 20 years and are usually associated with poor living conditions (i.e., Seattle in the 1980s and the Soviet Union in the 1990s). The

Table 40–2. Dosing of Diphtheria Antitoxin

Indication	Dose of Antitoxin
Laryngeal disease and less than 48 hour duration	20,000–40,000 units
Nasopharyngeal infections	40,000–60,000 units
Extensive disease >3 day duration	80,000–100,000 units
Presence of neck swelling (Bull neck)	

challenge for the Emergency Medicine physician is the identification of an acute presentation of the rare case of diphtheria and the need for quick diagnosis and use of diphtheria antitoxin. The onset of fever is gradual and the patient usually presents with a sore throat; dysphagia is appreciated in about 50% of cases. Patients can also present with toxic signs and symptoms such as tachycardia and vascular collapse. The presence of the pseudomembrane is the hallmark of pharyngeal diphtheria. It is usually gray-white in color, usually more extensive than group A streptococcal infection and classically bleeds when attempts are made to remove the pseudomembrane. Cutaneous diphtheria occurs mostly on extremities and tends to produce a grayish color over the skin. However, it does not respond to antitoxin therapy. Severe complications of diphtheria include myocarditis and polyneuritis with bulbar dysfunction. Diagnosis is initially dictated by clinical suspicion. The clinical microbiology lab needs to be alerted to the possibility of diphtheria so that the throat swab can be cultured on appropriate tellurite media.

Treatment must be initiated based on clinical suspicion alone (see Table 40–2). The diphtheria antitoxin is a horse-made product, so care must be taken to inquire about horse sensitivity and perform skin testing when indicated. The dose is based on the site of infection and the severity of symptoms (2).

Other Care Items

The diphtheria antitoxin is administered intravenously. Ten percent of patients will develop serum sickness. Careful observation for respiratory obstruction is necessary and, when present, early tracheotomy should be performed. Antibiotics have shown little benefit in the acute setting, but are recommended to prevent transmission.

Vaccination with the diphtheria toxoid is not recommended in acute cases and it is unclear when it should be administered to affected individuals. The DTP or DTaP is a part of the childhood vaccination series and >90% of the U.S. population has been vaccinated. The majority of the recent sporadic cases of diphtheria has been reported in elderly patients without a clear recent history of dT booster immunization. One should remember that the usual tetanus vaccination for adults also contains a reduced dose of diphtheria toxoid as well.

Invasive Pneumococcal Disease

Streptococcus pneumoniae is still the leading cause of bacterial pneumonia. In addition, *S. pneumoniae* is a common cause of bacterial meningitis, otitis media, and sinusitis. Patients with pneumococcal pneumonia usually present acutely ill with fever up to 103°F, an elevated pulse and respiratory rate, and shortness of breath with a productive cough. Signs of lung consolidation are common and lobar infiltrates are typically appreciated on chest x-ray. The Emergency Medicine physician certainly considers the diagnosis of pneumococcal pneumonia and bacteremia in many patients who present with pulmonary symptoms, fever, and an abnormal chest radiograph, and treatment protocols usually primarily target coverage of this organism. However, the emergency department can also be an important site for pneumococcal vaccination.

The current purified pneumococcal polysaccharide vaccine (Pneumovax-23) contains 23 of the most common serotypes associated with bacteremic pneumococcal pneumonia and it has been shown to be up to 81% effective in preventing invasive disease (but not pneumonia) in immuncomptetent adults. With the emergence of drug-resistant pneumococcus, vaccination efforts should be increased because many of the subtypes associated with antibiotic resistance are included in the vaccine. The following groups are felt to be at higher risk for pneumococcal disease: (1) children less than 2 years old, (2) those who lack a spleen or have hypersplenism, (3) those 65 years of age or older and those with HIV infection, chronic heart disease, chronic lung disease, renal failure, cirrhosis, or diabetes, (4) immunocompromised patients due to lymphoproliferative disorders, hematologic malignancies, or chronic steroid use, and (5) denizens of nursing homes and other long-term care facilities. A conjugate vaccine (to tetanus toxoid, Prevnar®) has recently been developed which contains seven serotypes. This is utilized in children (<2 years old) including those as young as 2 months of age.

Rabies

Rabies is a serious infection of the nervous system that requires prompt diagnosis and early initiation of treatment in order to prevent deadly consequences. Much of the exposure to rabies results from the bite of an infected animal; therefore, the role of the Emergency Medicine physician is usually to (1) immediately stabilize the victim of an animal bite, (2) ascertain the nature of the wound and the inflicting animal, (3) have knowledge of the epidemiology of rabies in the local environment including prevalence of disease and which animals are potential sources, (4) determine whether the inflicting animal can be captured and observed while quarantined for at least 10 days, (5) risk-stratify the patient, and (6) initiate the postexposure rabies vaccination if indicated.

Rabies is a relatively rare disease although many animals throughout the world can become infected and transmit this disease. The typical exposures come in two general forms. The urban form usually results from exposure to a diseased dog, cat, and other household pets. The sylvatic form results from exposure to wild animals such as raccoons, skunks, and bats. In general, the two types of exposure occur concomitantly, that is, areas where sylvatic sources of rabies increase lead to increased exposure in the domestic pets and an eventual increase in urban cases as well. Knowledge of the local potential rabid animals is critical along with worldwide variations in the sylvatic animals affected such as the wolf in Eastern Europe, mongoose in South Africa, and bat in North and South America. In the United States in 2002, rabies was found in raccoons (36.3%; 2891 cases), skunks (30.5%; 2433 cases), bats (17.2%; 1373 cases), foxes (6.4%; 508 cases), cats (3.8%; 299 cases), dogs (1.2%; 99 cases), and cattle (1.5%; 116 cases). In some regions, skunks are more commonly infected with rabies than raccoons (5).

A high index of suspicion is necessary since at least one young patient is reported to have acquired rabies without any clear exposure other than an outside bedroom window left open at a time when rabid bats were known to be in the community. Despite lack of any evidence of a bite, the child contracted rabies and died (6). In addition, up to one-third of bat-associated cases of rabies have no obvious exposure and only close examination delineates the bite site. Thus, at this point, such exposures require aggressive workup, and initiation of postexposure vaccination is recommended.

Clinically apparent rabies starts with mild symptoms including fatigue, anorexia, and fever. At this stage one should be looking for shaking or fasciculation at the bite site. More than half of people infected with rabies describe such symptoms. After this 3–4 day prodromal period, an encephalitic phase marked by a notable increase in motor activity occurs. This phase consists of agitation, excitement, increased alertness followed by confusion,

Table 40–3. Rabies Preexposure Prophylaxis Guide

Risk Category	Nature of Risk	Typical Populations	Preexposure Recommendations
Continuous	Virus present continuously often in high concentrations. Specific exposures likely to go unrecognized. Bite, nonbite, or aerosol exposure.	Rabies research laboratory workers;* rabies biologics production workers.	Primary course. Serologic testing every 6 months; booster vaccination if antibody titer is below acceptable level.+
Frequent	Exposure usually episodic, with source recognized, but exposure also might be unrecognized. Bite, nonbite, or aerosol exposure.	Rabies diagnostic lab workers,* spelunkers, veterinarians and staff, and animal-control and wildlife workers in rabies-enzootic areas.	Primary course. Serologic testing every 2 years; booster vaccination if antibody titer is below acceptable level.+
Infrequent (greater than population at large);	Exposure nearly always episodic with source recognized. Bite or nonbite exposure. Travelers visiting areas where rabies is enzootic and immediate access to appropriate medical care including biologics is limited.	Veterinarians and animal-control and wildlife workers in areas with low rabies rates. Veterinary students.	Primary course. No serologic testing or booster vaccination.
Rare (population at large)	Exposure always episodic with source recognized. Bite or nonbite exposure.	U.S. population at large, including persons in rabies-epizootic areas.	No vaccination necessary.

*Judgment of relative risk and extra monitoring of vaccination status of laboratory workers is the responsibility of the laboratory supervisor.
+Minimum acceptable antibody level is complete virus neutralization at a 1:5 serum dilution by the rapid fluorescent focus inhibition test. A booster dose should be administered if the titer falls below this level.

bizarre hallucinations, and disordered thought processes. Seizures, muscle spasms, and the classic opisthotonic posturing can be observed. Hypersensitivity to various stimuli including temperature, light, noise, and even gentle touch follows and increases in salivation, perspiration, and lacrimation are often noted.

Severe brainstem dysfunction ultimately develops with diplopia, facial palsies, and difficulty in swallowing. Laryngeal spasm creates a fear of drinking water (i.e., hydrophobia). The patient's behavior becomes increasingly unusual and erratic. Even with today's technological advances in critical care medicine, survival is rare. Diabetes insipidus, cardiac arrhythmias, vascular instability, and ARDS are often noted in the intensive care unit setting.

Initial management consists initially of local skin care and then ascertainment of the type of exposure. If the implicated animal is caught, then an early decision can be considered to quarantine the animal and watch for clinical signs of rabies (Table 40–3, 40–4) (7). Other management issues include the following:

1. Local skin care includes thorough cleaning of the wound and debridement as necessary. Generous use of soap and water is indicated and this can be followed by washing with 1–4% benzalkonium chloride. This approach has been shown to potentially increase survival by 50% (8).

2. Passive immunization with the human rabies immune globulin (HRIG) is available from the CDC and is now

Table 40–4. Rabies Postexposure Prophylaxis Guide – United States, 1999

Animal Type	Evaluation and Disposition of Animal	Postexposure Prophylaxis Recommendations
Dogs, cats, and ferrets	Healthy and available for 10 days observation Rabid or suspected rabid Unknown (e.g.,escaped)	Persons should not begin prophylaxis unless animal develops clinical signs of rabies.* Immediately vaccinate. Consult public health officials.
Skunks, raccoons, foxes and most other carnivores; bats	Regarded as rabid unless animal proven negative by laboratory tests+	Consider immediate vaccination.
Livestock, small rodents, lagomorphs (rabbits and hares), large (woodchucks and beavers), and other mammals	Consider individually.	Consult public health officials. Bites of rodents squirrels, hamsters, guinea pigs, gerbils, chipmunks, rats, mice, other small rodents, rabbits, and hares almost never require antirabies postexposure prophylaxis.

*During the 10-day observation period, begin postexposure prophylaxis at the first sign of rabies in a dog, cat, or ferret that has bitten someone. If the animal exhibits clinical signs of rabies, it should be euthanized immediately and tested.

+The animal should be euthanized and tested as soon as possible. Holding for observation is not recommended. Discontinue vaccine if immunofluorescence test results of the animal are negative.

indicated instead of antiquated horse serum. A total of 20 units per kg of the HRIG is given with at least 50% of the dose administered subdermally at the site of infection (Table 40–5) (7).

3. Active immunization with any of the three rabies vaccines (Tables 40–5 and 40–6, human diploid cell vaccine (HDCV), rabies vaccine absorbed (RVA), or purified chick embryo cell vaccine (PCEC) (7) is initiated on day 0 and given again on days 3, 7, 14, and 28 after exposure. The deltoid muscle is preferred because administration in the buttock results in decreased efficacy. One should not mix the vaccine and HRIG in the same syringe.

Preexposure Vaccination

Those who are at increased risk for exposure to either urban or sylvatic rabies (i.e., veterinarians, spelunkers, wildlife officers, rabies laboratorians, animal control officers, and travelers to areas where dog-associated rabies is endemic and health care is absent) should wear appropriate clothing and avoid interaction with potentially rabid animals (7). Preexposure vaccination is given on days 0,

7, and 21 or 28 and boosters are given annually thereafter (8). High-exposure individuals (i.e., rabies lab workers) need to have serum antibodies measured or receive booster doses every 6 months. Those at less but still significant exposure risk (i.e., forest rangers) should have antirabies antibody levels checked at 2-year intervals. Low levels should be boosted again with HVDC. Those vaccinated individuals who have received preexposure vaccination still need boosting doses of HDCV after exposure to rabies at days 0 and 3 although no HRIG is required (8).

Smallpox/Variola/Vaccinia Virus Vaccination

In 1980, the WHO declared that smallpox (variola major) had been eliminated worldwide due to an enormous immunization campaign. There are reportedly only two remaining sources of variola in two research laboratories: one in the United States and one in Russia. With the clear possibilities of biowarfare, there has been a growing concern that smallpox virus exists in a nonsecure location. If the expertise and equipment to grow stockpiles of this virus exist, the world population would be at great risk since routine vaccination has ceased for at least 20 years. This possibility has rekindled interest in the potential for

Table 40–5. Rabies Biologics – United States, 1999

Human Rabies Vaccine	Product Name	Manufacturer
Human diploid cell vaccine (HFCV)		Pasteur-Meriux Serum et Vaccins, Connaught Laboratories, Inc.
Intramuscular	Imovax Rabies	Phone: (800) VACCINE
Intradermal	Imovax Rabies I.D.	(822-2463)
Rabies vaccine adsorbed (RVA)	Rabies Vaccine	BioPort Corporation
Intramuscular	Adsorbed (RVA)	Phone: (517) 335-8120
Purified chick embryo cell vaccine (PCEC)	RabAvert	Chiron Corporation Phone: CHIRON8 (800) 244-7668
Intramuscular		
Rabies immune globulin (RIG)	Imogam Rabies-HT	Pasteur-Merieux Serum et Vaccins, Connaught Laboratories, Inc. Phone: (800) VACCINE (822-2463)
	BayRab	Bayer Corporation Pharmaceutical Div. Phone: (800) 288-8370

mass smallpox vaccination campaigns. Initially these efforts have focused on vaccination of hospital personnel who could then care for the potential victims of a variola bioweapon exposure.

The vaccinia virus is the agent used to vaccinate against variola. It is a virus that has been passed from cow to human and essentially represents a hybrid between them. Recent studies demonstrate about 90% sequence homology to variola. Thus the majority of antigens are shared, but there is enough difference to make vaccinia less toxic to humans. However, administration of vaccinia is not without risk and when given to an immunosuppressed individual, serious consequences can occur. The major side effects are as follows: (for a pictorial atlas of vaccinia side effects pictures see the CDC Web site www.cdc.gov/smallpox) (1) generalized vaccinia (1 in 5000 primary vaccinations) which is the appearance of a few pock-like lesions over the whole body which usually resolves spontaneously, (2) eczema vaccinatum that occurs in patients with previous or current eczema and

Table 40–6. Rabies Vaccination

Type of Vaccination	Route	Regimen
Primary	Intramuscular	HDCV, PCEC, or RVA; 1.0 mL (deltoid area), one each on days 0*, 7, and 21 or 28
	Intradermal	HDCV; 0.1 mL, one each on days 0*, 7, and 21 or 28
Booster	Intramuscular	HDCV, PCEC, or RVA; 1.0 mL (deltoid area), day 0* only
	Intradermal	HDCV, 0.1 mL, day 0* only

HDCV = human diploid cell vaccine; PCEC = purified chick embryo cell vaccine; RVA = rabies vaccine adsorbed.

*Day 0 is the day the first dose of vaccine is administered.

causes a severe skin reaction, (3) progressive vaccinia, which usually occurs in the immunosuppressed, is a progressive life-threatening tissue destruction at the vaccination site, and (4) postinfection encephalitis which affects 12 per million first-time vacinees and 2 per million revaccinated individuals. The latter causes fatal disease in 25% of individuals and 25% have long-term serious neurological sequelae. During the recent bioterrorist-motivated campaign for smallpox vaccinations, it became clear that vaccination either directly or indirectly caused myopericarditis (a total of 50 cases reports), that is, a rate of 0.01%. Young, Caucasian men were primarily affected within the first month after vaccination. Presentations included atypical chest pain and electrocardiographic evidence of diffuse ST segment elevation (9).

The vaccinia virus vaccination is administered in a unique fashion by skin scarification, that is, the vaccine is deposited on the skin and then a needle is used to inoculate the skin. In this manner, a pock-like lesion develops and when the scab falls off (about 2 weeks) the individual is considered to be immune to variola. Due to the above potential side effects and that vaccinated individuals shed live virus for 1–2 weeks, persons with known immunodeficiencies, history of eczema or related skin condition, or a family member with such history are instructed not to be immunized. For severe side effects other than the encephalitis, vaccinia immune globulin (VIG) can be administered (0.6 mL/kg), although this treatment has never been proven to be effective. VIG is derived from blood donors and processed according to good clinical practice guidelines for ensuring the quality of a reagent for human use. In adults, the dose is divided and given over 24–36 h, with repeat doses 3 days later (available from the CDC).

Recently, numerous investigators have noted the effectiveness of cidofovir for either side effects of vaccinia vaccination or treatment of variola (10–12). In addition, ether esters of cidofovir seem to remain extremely potent but are not orally bioavailable (13).

Hepatitis A

Hepatitis A is an RNA virus of the picornavirus family. Issues concerning hepatitis A infection are seen in the ED in two basic scenarios: (1) after acute high-risk exposure to patient with acute hepatitis A infection and (2) person who may be traveling to endemic areas that require hepatitis A vaccination. In the acute setting after exposure, the incubation period is 4 weeks and the infectious route is fecal-oral. Thus, hepatitis A infection occurs following consumption of infected food such as shellfish, milk products, as well as fecal-oral spread in institutional settings such as day care, nursing homes, and hospitals. Infected patients typically present with fever, anorexia, nausea, malaise, and jaundice.

Passive immunization with immune globulin is recommended for postexposure prophylaxis of close contacts of patients with acute hepatitis A infection (i.e., house, classroom) and for those who have consumed uncooked food handled by a patient with acute hepatitis A infection. All preparations of IG have adequate titers of anti-HAV to be effective. The dose is 0.02 mL/kg administered as soon as possible after exposure and may be effective up to 2 weeks after exposure. Larger doses are used for more extreme exposures. Of note, there have been no documented cases of HIV transmission as a result of immunoglobulin prophylaxis.

Active vaccination is recommended for those traveling to endemic HAV areas and staying for a prolonged period of time (>30 days). Other potential vacinees include military personnel, day care and nursing home workers, hepatitis A laboratory workers, children living in areas of the United States where hepatitis A rates are at least twice the national average, intravenous drug users, men who have sex with other men, individuals with chronic liver disease or recipient of a liver transplant, and people who require blood clotting concentrates (14). There are two vaccines approved (Havrix©, Vaqta©) for those over age 2 years and it takes effect about 1 month after inoculation (Table 40–7, (15)). The dose for adults is 1440 units that is, 1 mL given at time 0 and repeated 6–12 months later. The dose for children aged 2–18 years is 360 units. Vaccination provides protection for over 20 years. If travel to an endemic area is occurring sooner than 1 month, then immune globulin can be utilized at 0.02 mL/kg in conjunction with the first vaccine dose, albeit at a different anatomical site. Of note, a combined hepatitis A–B combination vaccine is now available (Twinrix©) (14) (Table 40–7) (15). Finally, a new aluminum-free hepatitis A vaccine, Epaval©, has been shown to effectively generate an antihepatitis immune response (16).

Hepatitis B

Similar to hepatitis A, hepatitis B cases present to the ED in two forms: (1) acute hepatitis associated with fever, right upper quadrant abdominal pain, jaundice and (2) acute exposure to someone with active hepatitis B infection. It is well recognized that hepatitis B is spread percutaneously, that is, through shared use of needles

Table 40–7. Hepatitis A and B Vaccination

Recommended Dosages and Schedules of Hepatitis A Vaccines

Vaccine	Age Group	Dose	Volume	# Doses	Schedule
Havrix (Glaxo-SmithKline)	2–18 years 19 years and older	720 El.U.* 1440 El.U.*	0.5 mL 1.0 mL	2 2	0, 6–12 mos. 0, 6–12 mos.
Vaqta (Merck & Co.)	2–18 years 19 years and older	25 U** 50 U**	0.5 mL 1.0 mL	2 2	0, 6–18 mos. 0, 6–18 mos.

*El.U. = Elisa Units.
**U = Units.

Recommended Dosages and Schedules of Hepatitis B Vaccines

Vaccine	Age Group	Dose	Volume	# Doses	Schedule*
Engerix-B (Glaxo-SmithKline)	0–19 years	10μg	0.5 ml	3	**Infants:** birth, 1–4, 6–18 mos. of age **Alternative for older children:** 0, 1–2, 4 mos.
	20 years & older	20μg	1.0 ml	3	0, 1, 6 mos.
Recombivax HB (Merck & Co.)	0–19 years	5μg	0.5 ml	3	**Infants:** birth, 1–4, 6–18 mos. of age **Alternative for older children:** 0, 1–2, 4 mos.
	11 thru 15 yrs.	10μg	1.0 ml	2	0, 4–6 mos.
	20 years & older	10μg	1.0 ml	3	0, 1, 6 mos.

*The schedule for hepatitis B vaccination is flexible and varies. Consult the ACIP statement on hepatitis B (11/91), AAP's *2003 Red Book*, or the package insert for details.

Note: For adult dialysis patients, the Engerix-B dose required is 40μg/2.0 ml (use the adult 20μg/ml formulation) on a schedule of 0, 1, 2, and 6 months. For Recombivax HB, a special formulation for dialysis patients is available. The dose is 40μg/1.0 ml and it is given on a schedule of 0, 1, and 6 months.

Combinations Using Hepatitis A and/or Hepatitis B Vaccines

Vaccine	Age Group	Antigens Used	Volume	# Doses	Schedule
Comvax* (Merck & Co.)	6 weeks thru 4 yrs.	Recombivax HB (5μg) combined with PedvaxHib	0.5 ml	3	2, 4, 12–15 mos. of age
Pediarix* (Glaxo-SmithKline)	6 weeks thru 6 yrs.	Engerix-B(10 g), Infanrix (DTaP), and IPV	0.5 ml	3	2, 4, 6 mos. of age
Twinrix* (Glaxo-SmithKline)	18 years & older	Havrix (720 El.U.) combined with Engerix-B (20μg)	1.0 ml	3	0, 1, 6 mos.

*Licensed combination vaccines may be used whenever any component of the combination is indicated and its other component(s) is/are not contraindicated. (CDC. Recommended Childhood Immunization Schedule—United States. *MMWR* 2004; Vol. 53, Q1–3 [16]).
The use of licensed combination vaccines is preferred over separate injection of their equivalent component vaccines. ("Combination Vaccines for Childhood Immunization," *MMWR,* 1999; Vol. 48, 1–15 [RR-5] 2).

particularly in the intravenous drug using population and (in the past) through blood transfusion. What is not as well appreciated is the number of hepatitis B infections acquired through sexual contact. Hepatitis B infection rate is high in health care workers, hemophiliacs, and others who require numerous blood transfusions, promiscuous gay men, and in neonates born in endemic areas of hepatitis B infection such as the Far East.

Active hepatitis B vaccination is recommended for universal use and is included in the childhood vaccination schedule. Despite this, only about 10–20% of high-risk individuals have received hepatitis B vaccination. There are two available hepatitis B vaccines, Recombivax-HB© and Engerix-B©, each containing hepatitis B surface antigen but in differing amounts (Table 40–7) (15). The vaccine is a three-shot series administered at 0, 1, and 6 months. The doses for the two FDA-approved products are provided below: it is possible to use these vaccinations interchangeably if necessary. In addition a new combined hepatitis A–B combination vaccine is available (Twinrix©) (14) (Table 40–7) (15).

For unvaccinated people who have experienced an exposure to hepatitis B, postexposure prophylaxis consists of hepatitis B immune globulin (HBIG) and immediate active hepatitis B vaccination. The dose of HBIG varies with the exposure: (1) to prevent vertical transmission, a 0.5 mL injection (IM) followed by the hepatitis B routine vaccine schedule is recommended; (2) to prevent infection after a percutaneous exposure (needle stick) or mucosal exposure (splashed in the face), the dose is 0.06 mL/kg (IM) administered immediately, followed by the hepatitis B routine vaccine schedule; and (3) to prevent an infection after a sexual exposure, the dose recommended is 0.06 mL/kg (IM) within 1 week, followed by the routine hepatitis B vaccine schedule. If both HBIG and the hepatitis B vaccine are to be given simultaneously, different injection sites are recommended. For use with the many other childhood vaccines, a new hexavalent vaccine is being developed and will potentially reduce the number of injections required in the growing infant.

VZV—Exposure

Varicella-zoster infection presents in classic ways. Primary varicella infection is manifest by vesicles distributed all over the body, typically in a dermatomal distribution. Varicella is a rather benign disease when contracted at an early age but becomes potentially more morbid in older individuals. Historically, the Emergency Medicine physician is usually involved in making the diagnosis of primary varicella infection in a child (i.e., chicken pox) and

herpes zoster (i.e., shingles) in an adult. Despite the advent of the live attenuated varicella vaccine, adults without a history of varicella infection may occasionally present to the ED after exposure to a person with primary varicella infection. These individuals may be candidates for passive immunization.

The exposures that may merit vaccination include household contacts, contact with playmates for >1 h, hospital contact, or contact with mother. Additional host factor indications include immunocompromised children, newborn infants with a mother with acute varicella infection 5 days predelivery and 2 days postdelivery, and premature babies. The formulations that can be administered are zoster immune globulin (ZIG) and Varicella-zoster IG (VZIG). VZIG is commonly used at a dose of 125 units/10 kg with a maximum dose of 625 units. A new form of VZIG is now available which can be given intravenously and appears to be very safe (17).

Influenza

Influenza is characterized by an acute respiratory illness with associated fever, headache, myalgia, and weakness. Superinfection with bacterial pathogens contributes significantly to the mortality of influenza. Types of influenza are classified according to its antigenic characteristics (A, B, or C), and the A viruses are characterized by changes in the hemagluttinin (H) or neuraminidase (N) proteins. Minor antigen changes are called drifts which lead to only a small increase in the cases of influenza. On the other hand, major changes in the H and N proteins, that is antigenic shifts, can lead to major pandemics leading to a great number of deaths. The last pandemic was in 1977 and there is concern for a new pandemic in the near future.

Vaccination is based on inactivated influenza viruses which are generally safe but may not always be immunogenic in the target populations, namely the young, the elderly, and those with chronic medical conditions that increase the risk for influenza-related mortality. Since the viruses are killed, these vaccines can be safely administered to the immunocompromised host including those with HIV infection. The composition of the trivalent vaccine usually includes two A strains and one B strain. The exact strains are chosen based on the prevalent strains in the population and the prediction of which strains will occur in the future. When accurately predicted, the vaccine is highly efficacious. The vaccine is best administered in the fall of the year of design. Even when effective, the at-risk populations are not always receiving vaccine. Therefore, the Emergency Medicine physician can greatly assist in increasing influenza virus vaccination rates. When at-risk patients come to the ED (e.g., the elderly) and are stabilized, they can be vaccinated if no contraindication exists.

The new cold-adapted live-attenuated influenza vaccine (FluMist$^{\copyright}$) is administered by nasal mist, and, unlike the inactivated vaccine, does not require a needle for administration. A single dose of 10^7 tissue culture infectious dose (TCID) with its yearly makeup of two influenza A strains and one influenza B strain is recommended for healthy individuals aged 9–49 years, and two doses are recommended for children 5–8 years old (18). Individuals who are outside these age groups, pregnant women, individuals with asthma or other reactive airway disease, those who use salicylates, those with history of Guillian-Barre syndrome, and those with hypersensitivity to eggs or other component of the vaccine should not receive this form of the influenza vaccine.

VACCINATION PRIMARILY FOR TRAVELERS

On occasion, the Emergency Medicine physician participates in immunization decisions for patients before international travel. There are various Web sites (e.g., CDC Web site http://www.cdc.gov, phone – 404-332-455, fax 404-332-4565) that can be accessed to assist with this task (see CDC site below), and physicians who practice travel medicine need to remain up to date on the most recent recommendations.

Several of the common travel-associated diseases and immunizations include the following:

Hepatitis A—see above

Yellow Fever. Travel to rural areas in South America and Africa. The yellow fever vaccine is composed of a live-attenuated 17D strain virus. Vaccination is effective for those older than 1 year, lasts about 10 years, and should be given 10 days prior to travel. This vaccine needs to be administered at least 3 weeks from the time of administration of typhoid vaccine.

Japanese encephalitis. Travel to rural China for >30 days.

This effective vaccine is formalin-inactivated and purified from mouse brain. Doses (1 mL) are given on days 0, 7, and 30. For children 1–3 years old, use 0.5 mL of vaccine.

Salmonella typhi. Travel to Latin-America, Asia, and Africa. The old heat-*killed* and phenol extract typhoid vaccines are no longer available because of limited effectiveness. The live oral, Ty21a vaccine is recommended and immunity is conferred for at least a few years. The

new purified Vi polysaccharide vaccine can be used in children and may provide longer duration of protection than the Ty21a vaccine.

REPORTING OF ADVERSE EFFECTS—VAERS (VACCINE ADVERSE EFFECTS REPORTING SYSTEM)

All vaccine-related adverse effects should be reported so that ongoing safety evaluations of all licensed vaccines can be done. The VAERS can be accessed in many ways:directly

http://www.vaers.com,FDA http://www.fda.gov/cber/vaers.htm, and CDC

http://www.cdc.gov/nip or the Vaccine Safety Datalink, rtc@cdc.gov.Also one can mail to Vaccine Adverse Event Reporting System, PO Box 1100, Rockville, MD 20849-1100.

CASE OUTCOME

The presence of a bat in the boy's room is a reason enough for suspicion to consider rabies postexposure prophylaxis with HRIG and rabies vaccine. Rabies is endemic in bats and unless the animal is caught, any possible wound should be cleansed and 50% of the HRIG dose administered to the bite site and 50% given IM (total dose is 20 units/kg). In addition, active rabies vaccination series should be administered in the deltoid muscle on days 0, 3, 7, 14, and 28.

REFERENCES

1. Kruszon-Moran DM, McQuillan GM, Chu SY: Tetanus and diphtheria immunity among females in the United States: Are recommendations being followed? *Am J Obstet Gynecol*190:1070–1076, 2004.
2. Keller MA, Stiehm ER: Passive immunity in prevention and treatment of infectious diseases. *Clin Microbiol Rev* 13:602–614, 2000.
3. Update on adult immunization. Recommendations of the Immunization Practices Advisory Committee (ACIP). *MMWR Recomm Rep* 40:1–94, 1991.
4. Robinson RF, Nahata MC: Management of botulism. *Ann Pharmacother* 37:127–131, 2003.
5. Krebs JW, Wheeling JT, Childs JE: Rabies surveillance in the United States during 2002. *J Am Vet Med Assoc* 223:1736–1748, 2003.

6. Messenger SL, Smith JS, Rupprecht CE: Emerging epidemiology of bat-associated cryptic cases of rabies in humans in the United States. *Clin Infect Dis*35:738–747, 2002

7. Human rabies prevention—United States, 1999. Recommendations of the Advisory Committee on Immunization Practices (ACIP). *MMWR Recomm Rep* 48:1–21, 1999.

8. Warrell MJ, Warrell DA: Rabies and other lyssavirus diseases. *Lancet* 363:959–969, 2004.

9. Cassimatis DC, Atwood JE, Engler RM, Linz PE, Grabenstein JD, Vernalis MN: Smallpox vaccination and myopericarditis: A clinical review. *J Am Coll Cardiol* 43:1503–1510, 2004.

10. Quenelle DC, Collins DJ, Kern ER: Cutaneous infections of mice with vaccinia or cowpox viruses and efficacy of cidofovir. *Antiviral Res* 63:33–40, 2004.

11. Bray M, Roy CJ: Antiviral prophylaxis of smallpox. *J Antimicrob Chemother* 54:1–5, 2004

12. Neyts J, Leyssen P, Verbeken E, De Clercq E: Efficacy of cidofovir in a murine model of disseminated progressive vaccinia. *Antimicrob Agents Chemother* 48:2267–2273, 2004.

13. Buller RM, Owens G, Schriewer J, Melman L, Beadle JR, Hostetler KY: Efficacy of oral active ether lipid analogs of cidofovir in a lethal mousepox model. *Virology* 318:474–481, 2004.

14. Craig AS, Schaffner W: Clinical practice. Prevention of hepatitis A with the hepatitis A vaccine. *N Engl J Med* 350:476–481, 2004.

15. Immunization Action Coalition 2005 http://www.immunize.org/.

16. Usonis V, Bakasenas V, Valentelis R, Katiliene G, Vidzeniene D, Herzog C: Antibody titres after primary and booster vaccination of infants and young children with a virosomal hepatitis A vaccine (Epaxal). *Vaccine*21:4588–4592, 2003.

17. Koren G, Money D, Boucher M, et al.: Serum concentrations, efficacy, and safety of a new, intravenously administered varicella zoster immune globulin in pregnant women. *J Clin Pharmacol* 42:267–274, 2002.

18. Belshe, RB, Mendelman PM: Safety and efficacy of live attenuated, cold-adapted, influenza vaccine-trivalent. *Immunol Allergy Clin North Am* 23:745–767, 2003.

41

HIV in the Emergency Department

Ronald D. Wilcox

HIGH YIELD FACTS:

1. Routine testing for HIV should be a part of medical care in areas of high prevalence in patients and targeted testing should be reserved for area of low prevalence; rapid testing in patients greater than 15 months of age should be confirmed with an ELISA and Western blot.

2. The acute retroviral syndrome presents similarly to infectious mononucleosis so emergency physicians must consider it in the differential diagnosis of a patient with fever.

3. Fever of unknown origin in HIV patients frequently is caused by mycobacterial infections; the required evaluation may be extensive but can be narrowed based on the patient's CD4 counts.

4. Opportunistic infections diagnosed in the emergency department may include bacterial pneumonias, *Pneumocystic jiroveci* pneumonia (formerly *P. carinii*), disseminated *Mycobacteria* avium/intracellulare, histoplasmosis, cytomegalovirus, retinitis, cryptococcal meningitis, brain masses, progressive multifocal leukoencephalopathy, and candidal esophagitis.

5. Many antiretroviral medications have significant toxicities that may require emergent evaluation or hospitalization.

CASE PRESENTATION

A 42-year-old man presents to the emergency department with a history of 20 pounds of weight loss over the past 2 months, generalized fatigue, and low-grade fever. His social history reveals the patient is an over-the-road truck driver who is married but has occasional casual sex partners outside his relationship. On physical examination he is noted to have bilateral cervical lymphadenopathy, whiteexudates on his buccal mucosa bilaterally, and hepatomegaly. The laboratory evaluationreveals a total protein of 10.2 with an albumin of 2.4, a white blood cell count of 3.4 with an absolute lymphocyte count of 840, and a hemoglobin level of 7.2. Additional laboratory ab-

normalities include an elevated LDH at 275 and an alkaline phosphatase of 874.

INTRODUCTION

Frequently the emergency department will be the initial place of medical care sought out by people infected with the human immunodeficiency virus (HIV) who are not aware of their serostatus. Up to 15% of all visits in some emergency departments are by the HIV-infected population whereas less than 1% of the population in the United States is infected. Despite the efforts for prevention of transmission, the annual "newly diagnosed" incidence continues to be approximately 40,000 cases per year in the United States, a figure that has not changed much in the past two decades. For these reasons, there are many important issues about which emergency physicians need to be aware. These include indications for HIV testing, the acute retroviral syndrome, the appropriate evaluation for fever of unknown origin in the HIV-infected patient, the standard presentations of common opportunistic infections, and the toxicities of the antiretroviral medications that may lead to an emergency department evaluation.

TESTING FOR HIV

The standard screening test for HIV used for patients older than 15 months of age is the enzyme-linked immunosorbent assay (ELISA). When the ELISA is positive, the Western Blot is then used to confirm the diagnosis, requiring the presence of three viral surface markers, p24, gp41, and gp 120/160, to be positive (2 of 3 in high-risk individuals).

Because the ELISA may yield false-positive results, the Western Blot must be performed before informing the patient. Late pregnancy, malignancies, connective tissue disorders, and recipients of experimental HIV vaccinations are a few known causes of false-positive results on ELISA. When a patient has a positive ELISA but only one band present on the Western Blot, the result is called "indeterminate." If a patient is tested during the first few months of infection (the "window period"), the result may be reported as indeterminate and the test should be repeated 6–12 weeks later if the patient is at risk (see next section for more information). Results usually take several days to weeks to return.

There are now available other forms of screening tests for HIV that utilize blood and saliva. The SUDS (single use diagnostic system) is another blood test that yields results within a few hours. The Oraquick test is a salivary test that screens for antibody against HIV. The Oraquick

Table 41–1. Indicators for HIV Testing

Constitutional	*Mycobacteria kansasii*
Unexplained fevers, bilateral lymphadenopathy, or	*Pneumocystis jiroveci* (formerly *P. carinii*) pneumonia
weight loss	Pseudomonal or rhodococcal pneumonia
Cutaneous	Two or more episodes of bacterial pneumonia in
Facial seborrheic dermatitis	past year
Molluscum contagiosum in an adolescent or older patient	Lymphocytic interstitial pneumonitis
Kaposi Sarcoma	Genitourinary
Varicella zoster (shingles) that crosses the midline or is	Any sexually transmitted disease, including gonorrhea,
multidermatomal	*Chlamydia*, pelvic inflammatory disease,
Eosinophilic folliculitis	nongonococcal urethritis, Trichomoniasis, genital
Cryptococcal skin lesions	human papilloma virus, syphilis, chancroid, LGV
Bacillary angiomatosis (looks similar to KS, caused by	Malignancies
Bartonella spp.)	Non-Hodgkin lymphoma
Gastrointestinal	Hodgkin disease
Oral candidiasis—three forms: pseudomembranous,	Cervical carcinoma
erythematous, and cheilosis	Anal carcinoma
Oral hairy leukoplakia	Kaposi sarcoma
Oral ulcerations	Laboratory abnormalities
Esophagitis—candidal, cytomegaloviral, herpetic,	Unexplained leukopenia (especially lymphopenia),
aphthous	anemia, or thrombocytopenia
Diarrhea lasting longer than 2 weeks	Unexplained proteinuria or hematuria
Diarrhea due to *Cryptosporidia, Isospora, Cyclospora*, or	Hypergammaglobulinemia
Microsporidiae	Reactive hyperplasia on lymph node biopsy
Hepatitis C	Pediatric indicators
Neurologic	Failure to thrive
Unexplained peripheral neuropathy	Developmental DELAYS
Dementia or encephalopathy	*All* children born to HIV+ mothers
Cytomegaloviral retinitis	Children born to mothers who were not tested for HIV
Ring-enhancing lesions on CT or MRI of brain	during pregnancy
Cardiac	Parotitis
Unexplained dilated cardiomyopathy	Hepatosplenomegaly
Pulmonary	Miscellaneous
Tuberculosis	Anyone who requests testing

and UniGold Recombigen are "rapid tests" that return with results within 20–30 minutes. The Oraquick is easy to use and interpret, similar to a pregnancy test, and has been used for global screening in some emergency departments with favorable results. A positive test with any of these tests requires confirmation with the standard ELISA/Western Blot (1).

Children less than 15 months of age will have received maternal antibodies across the placenta so the ELISA is not an appropriate screening test for this age group. In the United States the standard test for this age group is polymerase chain reaction (PCR) for HIV cDNA, the double-stranded DNA copy formed by reverse transcriptase from the viral RNA. For HIV-exposed infants, this test is obtained within the first 48 h after birth, between 3 and 6 weeks, between 6 and 12 weeks, and a fourth test between 12 and 24 weeks.

There are many clinical and laboratory indications for performing HIV testing (see Table 41–1). Additionally, every person with any sexually transmitted disease, and all pregnant women, should be offered HIV testing.

ACUTE RETROVIRAL SYNDROME

Pathophysiology

The acute retroviral syndrome (ARS), also called primary HIV infection, occurs during the first few weeks after the initial exposure and before seroconversion (formation of HIV antibodies as evidenced by a positive ELISA) has occurred. During this period there is very rapid viral replication, leading to high viral load (as measured by PCR of HIV RNA). The viral load frequently rises into the millions, and is accompanied with a rapid decline in

CD4+ cell counts. The body has not yet had the opportunity to form an immune response to the infection, allowing the virus to replicate quickly. As the body develops CD8+ lymphocytes of the cell-mediated immune system and antibodies to the virus of the humoral immune system, the viral load decreases and the symptoms frequently will diminish or subside (2–4). During this time period, the ELISA/Western Blot may be negative or classified as "indeterminate." The direct measurement of viral RNA (the viral load) may be performed at this time but it is not approved as a diagnostic test for HIV because of false positives.

Clinical Presentation

The symptoms of ARS have often been compared to those seen in acute infectious mononucleosis. In a study by Vanhems and co-workers, 378 people who presented with ARS from five different countries were studied. Ninety-four percent of the patients were male and 74% of the patients had a transmission risk factor of male-to-male sexual activity, 12% heterosexual activity, 9% intravenous drug use, and 5% unknown. The most common presenting feature was fever and was found in approximately 75% of patients. Other clinical features, in descending order of incidence, included fatigue, myalgia, macular erythematous skin rash, headache, pharyngitis, cervical adenopathy, night sweats, arthralgia, diarrhea, and inguinal adenopathy. The only difference in findings statistically significant when comparing genders was myalgias (male/female 50% versus 26%, $p = 0.03$). When comparing age groups, significant findings included lower incidence of pharyngitis in those over 37 years of age (46% versus 21%, $p = 0.001$) as well as the increased incidence of cervical lymphadenopathy in the age group younger than 28 years (51% versus 37%, $p = 0.03$). When comparing clinical manifestations with the route of infection, fever, mylagia, skin rash, pharyngitis, and diarrhea were less frequent in those infected by sharing needles as compared to those who acquired HIV sexually. The median duration of symptoms was approximately 13 days and was similar regardless of age, gender, or exposure category. The mean time between onset of symptoms and seroconversion was 50.2 days and also did not differ by age, gender, or exposure category (5). Other symptoms reported include thrush, oral or genital ulcerations, peripheral neuropathy, meningoencephalitis, thrombocytopenia, and rhabdomyolysis (6, 7).

Laboratory/Diagnostic Testing

Laboratory testing done during the time of acute infection will show a high HIV viral load (RNA PCR), a de-

creased CD4+ lymphocyte count, and an increased CD8+ lymphocyte count with a subsequent inversion of the CD4:CD8 ratio. Screening for ARS may initially be done by obtaining either a qualitative cDNA PCR or quantitative RNA PCR (viral load). Since neither test is approved for diagnosis, if either of these tests is positive a subsequent ELISA and Western Blot must still be performed within 6 weeks (6). A specific p24 antigen assay can also be obtained but this test is usually a send-out for most medical centers and can take several weeks to obtain the results.

Management

If ARS is suspected, it is important to have the patient placed on the highly active antiretroviral therapy (HAART) as soon as possible. Early therapy with antiretrovirals decreases the baseline viral load and improves the immune systems' response to the virus, thereby possibly slowing the progression to AIDS in the long term. A baseline resistance assay (genotype or phenotype) should also be obtained before starting HAART because some studies have shown that up to 25% of newly infected patients have a virus with resistance to at least one HIV medication (8). Because of the complexity of choosing an appropriate initial regimen, an infectious disease specialist or infection control personnel may be consulted to assist with the selection of the regimen.

Take home point: If you have a patient you think may have infectious mononucleosis and the rapid screening test for Epstein–Barr Virus is negative, consider going back to the patient to assess risk and perform the screening testing for HIV as appropriate.

FEVER OF UNKNOWN ORIGIN IN HIV
Pathophysiology/Clinical Presentation

In the HIV-infected patient there are different criteria for fever of unknown origin (FUO) than for the non-HIV-infected patient. The criteria that have been proposed include fever $\geq 38.3°C$ for more than 4 weeks duration for outpatients, fever $\geq 38.3°C$ more than 3 days duration for inpatients, fever $\geq 38.3°C$ without a diagnosis after 3 days of appropriate investigation, including negative cultures after at least 2 days of incubation (9).

Laboratory/Daignostic Testing

Before commencing on any expensive medical evaluation, one should (as always) perform a thorough history and physical examination with attention given to the medications the patient takes, including herbal supplements and over-the-counter medications, as well as a comprehensive social history. The most common cause worldwide (over 50% in one study) of FUO in HIV-infected patients is mycobacterial infection, including (in descending order of frequency) *M. tuberculosis* (MTB), *M. avium-intracellulare* complex (MAC), and other nontuberculous mycobacteria but the differential of FUO will vary geographically. Disseminated MAC is a more common cause of FUO than MTB in the HIV-infected population in the United States. Laboratory abnormalities may provide clues such as elevations in LDH may suggest *Pneumocystis jiroveci* (formerly *P. carinii*) pneumonia (*PcP*), non-Hodgkin lymphoma (NHL), extrapulmonary tuberculosis, or extracerebral toxoplasmosis. Increased alkaline phosphatase levels may be the only manifestation of disseminated MAC.

A skin rash or oral ulceration may suggest disseminated histoplasmosis. Connective tissue disorders are relatively uncommon as causes of FUO in this population. The initial evaluation in the emergency department will be similar to that done for the non-HIV-infected patient who has fever without an obvious source, including obtaining blood cultures, chest radiography, and urinalysis and culture.

A normal chest radiograph does not exclude either PcP or pulmonary TB since up to 5% of patients will have a relatively normal initial chest x-ray. HIV-positive patients who present with cough and/or fever should be placed in respiratory isolation until pulmonary TB has been excluded. Additional evaluation is guided by the patient's CD4 count and percentage because most opportunistic infections occur when the patient's CD4 counts fall below 200 cells/mL or the CD4% is less than 14%. (The CD4 count can often be estimated—if the patient has thrush it is likely the CD4 count is <200 cells/mL.) If skin lesions are present, biopsy may be performed with examination for bacteria, mycobacteria, fungi, syphilis, histology, and viral inclusions. If a patient has unilateral lymphadenopathy, fine needle aspiration is a rapid procedure and may be performed; care must be taken not to create a chronic sinus in the event of mycobacterial disease. The likely causes for FUO are based on the patients' CD4 count. For those with CD4 counts >300 cells/mL, pulmonary TB is the most common cause. When the CD4 count drops to 200–300 cells/mL, both Hodgkin and non-Hodgkin lymphomas enter the differential diagnosis, as do Kaposi Sarcoma (KS) and extrapulmonary tuberculosis. For those with CD4 counts between 100 and 200 cells/mL, one must also consider esophageal candidiasis, PcP, HIV encephalitis, and wasting syndrome. Patients with CD4 counts between 50 and 100 copies/mL are at increased risk of developing visceral leishmaniasis, toxoplasmic encephalitis, disseminated cryptococcosis or endemic mycoses (such as histoplasmosis or coccidioidomycosis), and progressive multifocal leukoencephalopathy (PML). For the most immunosuppressed (CD4 count ≤50 cells/mL), the likelihood of disseminated MAC, cytomegalovirus (CMV) retinitis, and primary central nervous system (CNS) lymphoma greatly increases (10).

The medical evaluation includes acid fast bacilli (AFB) blood cultures for disseminated MTB or MAC; a computed tomography (CT) or magnetic resonance imaging (MRI) of the brain with contrast to evaluate for primary CNS lymphoma, toxoplasmic encephalitis, or PML; abdominal CT to assess for disseminated mycobacterial infection, histoplasmosis, or malignancy such as NHL or KS; a serum and/or cerebral spinal fluid cryptococcal antigen assay; a dilated fundoscopic examination to assess for CMV retinitis; and a buffy coat or urine sample for histoplasma antigen. Radionuclide imaging, especially a gallium scan, may be helpful in evaluating for PcP or MTB or lymphoma. Paranasal sinus films may be useful as may echocardiography in patients who inject illicit drugs (10, 11).

Take home point: When an HIV-positive patient presents with fever, assessment of the possible cause is based on the CD4 count and accompanying symptoms or laboratory abnormalities. In the emergency department, the standard microbiological evaluation is helpful and emergency physicians may also wish to include AFB blood cultures, fungal assays, or radiologic imaging, such as CT of the brain or abdomen. Patients with cough or an abnormality on chest radiograph should be placed in respiratory isolation pending evaluation for pulmonary TB.

COMMON PRESENTATIONS OF OPPORTUNISTIC INFECTIONS

Lobar Infiltrate

When an HIV-infected patient presents with fever and cough, community-acquired pneumonia (CAP) is frequently the cause. Patients with CD4 counts <200 cells/mL have bacterial pneumonias at approximately 20 times the incidence as immunocompetent patients. The most causative organisms are the same as in the immunocompetent population, including *Streptococcus pneumoniae* and *Haemophilus influenzae*. If a patient is not responding as expected to standard antibiotic treatment directed at the above organisms, therapy should be expanded to cover *Pseudomonas aeruginosa*, an organism not commonly associated with CAP (12). *Rhodococcus equi*, a bacterium associated with causing bronchopneumonia in foal horses, is also a causative organism in this population, although rare. If a lobar infiltrate is not improving despite good bacterial coverage, other considerations would include Cryptococcosis, Aspergillosis, Blastomycosis, Coccidioidomycosis, Nocardia, *Mycobacteria tuberculosis*, and nontuberculous species (i.e., *M. kansasii*), non-Hodgkin lymphoma, and *Pneumocystis jiroveci* (formerly *P. carinii*). Empyema and accompanying bacteremia are also more common in patients with HIV and bacterial pneumonias.

Take home point: HIV-infected patients with abnormal chest radiography should be placed in respiratory isolation until the presence of pulmonary TB is excluded. Empiric antibiotic therapy directed toward the common pathogens of community-acquired pneumonia should be administered (see Chapter 10) with the consideration of providing adequate coverage against the Pseudomonas species.

Interstitial Infiltrate

The typical radiologic presentation of *Pneumocystis jiroveci* pneumonia is an interstitial or reticulo-nodular infiltration most concentrated in the perihilar regions extending outward, resulting in a "bat wing" appearance. PcP can also appear as a lobar infiltrate, a diffuse pattern similar to miliary TB, or even a completely normal chest radiograph. The patient usually will report a gradually increasing shortness of breath, especially with ambulation or exertion. There may also be present a nonproductive cough or a cough that is productive of clear to white sputum; purulent sputum is usually suggestive of a bacterial pneumonia or superinfection with the PcP. Fever is usually low grade. Physical examination may reveal no abnormalities or dry inspiratory crackles or inspiratory "squeaks." Laboratory evaluation will frequently show an elevation in LDH and possibly hypoxemia on an arterial blood gas. Pulse oximetry may show normal saturation at rest but will show quick desaturation with minimal ambulation or exertion. Diagnosis is done by obtaining an early morning induced sputum for stain but the yield on this test is dependent on the quality of the specimens obtained by the personnel at each institution. If the induced sputum is negative, bronchoscopy with broncho-alveolar lavage can be performed with approximately 95% sensitivity. A gallium scan can also be useful in the evaluation, with the lungs having significant uptake of the radionuclide in the setting of PcP or tuberculosis. If PcP is suspected, the ther-

apeutic agent of choice is trimethoprim/sulfamethoxazole (Bactrim, Septra), dosed at 20 mg/kg/day orally (divided every 6–8 h) for mild disease and 15 mg/kg/day IV (divided every 6–8 h) for a minimum of 21 days of therapy. If a patient is intolerant to sulfamethoxazole, IV pentamidine dosed at 4 mg/kg/day may also be used for moderate-to-severe disease (13).

Other alternative treatments for mild-to-moderate disease include atovaquone (Mepron), dapsone with trimethoprim, clindamycin with primaquine, or trimetrexate. If the patient's room air PaO_2 is less than 70, or the A-a O_2 gradient is greater than 30, adjunctive therapy with corticosteroids should be used; the dosage of prednisone is 40 mg orally twice daily for 5 days, then 40 mg daily for 5 days, then 20 mg daily for 11 days. The steroids must be added within the first 72 h of starting therapy to be effective.

There are many other causes of interstitial pulmonary infiltrates that must be considered, especially viral causes such as influenza or cytomegalovirus or varicella zoster or severe acute respiratory syndrome (SARS).

The atypical bacteria such as *Mycoplasma* or *Chlamydia* or *Legionella* can present similarly, as can infection with tuberculosis and some of the nontuberculous mycobacteriae. If a patient does not respond as expected to standard therapy for PcP, then the evaluation should be expanded to assess for other causes.

Take home point: If a patient presents with a nonproductive, or minimally productive, cough, desaturates easily with minimal exertion, and has an interstitial infiltrate on chest radiograph, treatment should be started for PcP empirically while further evaluation for diagnosis is performed.

Fever and Anemia

There are many causes of fever with anemia in HIV-infected patients but the two most common causes are disseminated *Mycobacteria avium-intracellulare* complex (MAC) and disseminated histoplasmosis. MAC is a ubiquitous organism with an unknown transmission mechanism. In the non-HIV-infected patients, the disease usually presents as either lymphadenitis (especially in children) or pulmonary disease (especially in the elderly). In the AIDS patients, especially those with CD4 counts <100 cells/mL, the common presentation is bone marrow suppression (as evidenced by anemia or neutropenia), fever, wasting or weight loss, fatigue, hepatosplenomegaly with transaminitis, and possibly lymphadenopathy, especially intraabdominal. Pulmonary MAC in unusual in the HIV-infected host. An elevated alkaline phosphatase is a frequent indication of the possible presence of MAC. MAC may also cause small bowel infection with subsequent diarrhea as well as an ascending cholangitis. Diagnosis is usually by blood cultures for acid fast bacilli but the organism may also be cultured from sputum, stool, bone marrow aspirate, or biopsy. Treatment consists of a macrolide, such as clarithromycin 500 mg twice daily or azithromycin 500–600 mg once daily, plus ethambutol 15 mg/kg daily. Rifabutin may be added but dosage will need to be altered based on the HAART therapy the patient is receiving (14).

Disseminated histoplasmosis presents in a similar manner to disseminated MAC but may also include oral ulcerations or a maculopapular rash. The most sensitive test for diagnosis is a urinary histoplasma antigen assay, but it may also be found in a buffy coat assay for antigen in the serum, on biopsy of a skin or oral lesion, and on bone marrow aspirate.

Treatment is usually with itraconazole or amphotericin B; the itraconazole suspension is better absorbed than the capsules and should be used whenever possible (15).

If the patient with anemia and fever also has renal insufficiency, mental status changes, or thrombocytopenia, thrombotic thrombocytopenic purpura (TTP) must be considered. TTP is increased in incidence in the HIV-positive population. There is also a possible association of TTP development in AIDS patients with CD4 counts <200 cells/mL who receive valacyclovir (Valtrex) although further investigation of this possible association is ongoing.

Take home point: HIV-infected patients who present with fever and anemia should have AFB blood cultures drawn and may be placed on empiric therapy targeting MAC. If a rash or oral lesion is also present, the possibility of histoplasmosis must also be considered. Patients with mental status changes, decreased platelets, or renal insufficiency must be evaluated for TTP.

"Floaters" or Visual Loss

Patients with low CD4 counts, especially counts <50 cells/mL, are at high risk for the development of cytomegaloviral (CMV) retinitis. The usual initial complaint for these patients is the presence of "floaters" or dark spots in their visual fields that slowly move. Patients may also note some loss of vision in particular fields or unilaterally due to retinal detachment. Fundoscopic examination may reveal "ketchup and mustard" lesions on the retina due to hemorrhagic events and exudates or possible "flare" lesions. A similar disease also seen in HIV-positive patients is progressive outer retinal necrosis, most commonly caused by the varicella zoster virus. The standard treatment for CMV retinitis at this time is valganciclovir (Valcyte) dosed at 900 mg p.o. BID for 21 days then 900 mg p.o. daily for suppressive therapy, which has been shown to have equal efficacy with IV ganciclovir (16). If a patient is unable to tolerate oral medications, IV ganciclovir, foscarnet, or cidofovir are other treatment options.

Take home point: Immunosuppressed patients with visual changes should have a dilated fundoscopic examination to evaluate for CMV retinitis.

Headache or Seizure

HIV-infected patients who present with headache or seizure should have radiologic evaluation of their head to evaluate for meningeal inflammation, masses or "ring-enhancing lesions" with either a contrast-enhanced CT or MRI. Evaluation for meningitis should be of primary concern; if the headache is new in onset and rapidly progressive, treatment for possible bacterial meningitis must be started as soon as the diagnosis is considered and then a lumbar puncture performed when possible after imaging. Antimicrobial therapy for bacterial meningitis must include coverage for *Listeria monocytogenes* in patients with lower CD4 lymphocyte counts. If the headache is more insidious with progression over several days to weeks, a chronic meningitis may be involved, such as cryptococcal or tuberculous meningitis. A cryptococcal antigen of both the serum and cerebral spinal fluid (CSF) should be obtained as well as an India ink stain of the CSF; the CSF should also be sent for fungal culture. It is very important to obtaining an opening pressure when performing the lumbar puncture since many patients with cryptococcal meningitis may have markedly elevated intracranial pressures >50 cm H_2O and may require serial lumbar punctures to relieve the pressure. Therapy can be either with 600–800 mg fluconazole daily for mild disease, or for moderate-to-severe disease, amphotericin B given at 0.7 mg/kg daily for a total of 500–1000 mg of treatment; if using a liposomal or lipid-complex form of amphotericin, the usual dosage is 5–7.5 mg/kg daily for a total for 2 weeks. Flucytosine may be added for synergy with amphotericin; levels must be monitored and the addition of this medication has been shown to sterilize cultures faster and decrease the incidence of relapse but not to change the overall morbidity or mortality of the disease (17). Tuberculous meningitis usually presents insidiously and commonly causes dysfunction of cranial nerves since the inflammation is commonly centered over the basal ganglia.

Table 41–2. Mnemonic for Ring-Enhancing Lesions of the Brain in HIV

MAGIC

M—metastases or malignancies

A—abscesses—most commonly toxoplasma but includes mycobacteriae, *Cryptococcus*, *Aspergillus*, bacterial, *Bartonella*, *Nocardia*

G—glioma

I—infections—including cytomegalovirus, herpes simplex, and progressive multifocal leukoencephalopathy (PML)

C—cysticercosis or cancer (primary CNS lymphoma)

HIV-infected patients who present with seizures frequently have lesions seen on radiographic imaging of the brain. The most common cause of a ring-enhancing lesion for an HIV-positive patient not on trimethoprim/sulfamethoxazole is toxoplasmic encephalitis. The next most common cause is a primary central nervous system lymphoma (PCNSL), usually caused by the Epstein-Barr virus. Other causes in this population include metastatic disease from another primary cancer, bacterial or mycobacterial abscess, nocardia abscess, aspergillus, or cryptococcal abscess, glioma, viral infections such as cytomegalovirus, J-C virus, or neurocysticercosis (see Table 41–2 for the MAGIC mnemonic). If not already assessed, the patient should have a toxoplasma IgG level drawn and started on empiric therapy for toxoplasmosis with either sulfadiazine and pyrimethamine (plus folinic acid) or clindamycin and pyrimethamine (plus folinic acid). If CT shows only a single lesion, an MRI with gadolinium should be obtained. If the toxoplasma antibody is negative or there is only a single lesion on MRI, neurosurgery should be consulted to consider a brain biopsy. If there are multiple lesions seen on scan, empiric toxoplasmosis therapy is given for 2 weeks and the brain is reimaged at that time; if there is no improvement, a biopsy is necessary (18).

Take home points: HIV-infected patients who present with either headache or seizures should have radiographic imaging performed, with contrast, of the brain. If the onset of symptoms is rapid, antimicrobial therapy, including coverage for Listeriosis, should be initiated quickly. If the onset is slow in progression, the patient should be evaluated for cryptococcal, or tuberculous, meningitis. If a brain lesion is evident, treatment should be given empirically for toxoplasmosis as further evaluation is accomplished.

Altered Mental Status

Patients may present to the emergency department with complaints of increasing memory loss or a family member may report a change in the personality of the patient. HIV-infected patients must be evaluated with radiographic imaging of the brain with contrast to assess for ring-enhancing lesions (see previous section), progressive multifocal leukoencephalothy, cerebral atrophy, encephalopathy, and meningeal enhancement.

Progressive multifocal leukoencephalopathy (PML) is caused by the J-C papovavirus. The clinical presentation of PML may include alterations in personality, short-term memory loss, hemianopsia, hemiplegia, or new onset seizures. Diagnosis is suggested by "white matter disease that crosses the midline" as seen on MRI with gadolinium. The diagnosis is confirmed by PCR of the CSF for the J-C virus. HIV dementia is usually a diagnosis of exclusion but may be suggested by cerebral atrophy and an elevated beta-2-microglobulin level and HIV viral load in the CSF. Treatment for PML is HAART that has good penetration into the CSF; therefore an HIV primary care provider or infectious disease specialist should be contacted to develop an appropriate treatment regimen (19, 20). Herpes encephalitis often presents differently in AIDS patients than in immunocompetent patients; instead of a rapid onset of delirium, patients with CD4 counts <200 cells/mL may present with an insidious onset of altered mental status over several weeks. MRI of the brain may demonstrate diffuse enhancement, and not just of the temporal lobe as is the classical radiographic finding. Diagnosis is done by PCR of the CSF.

Treatment for herpes encephalitis, regardless of HIV status, is with intravenousacyclovir 10–12 mg/kg/dose given every 8 h.

Take home point: Patients with HIV who present with altered mental status should have the standard evaluation, but should also have an MRI with gadolinium of their brain as well as examination of the CSF by PCR for JC and herpes simplex viruses.

Dysphagia or Odonophagia

Esophagitis is a common problem for patients with low CD4 lymphocyte counts. The most common cause is candidal esophagitis, which presents as either painful or difficult swallowing. This is usually a clinical diagnosis based on symptoms and perhaps the presence of oral candidiasis. Empiric treatment is with fluconazole (400 mg orally as a loading dose, then 200 mg orally daily for 13 days). Alternative therapies include ketoconazole, itraconazole, voriconazole, posiconazole, amphotericin B, and caspofungin. If there is no improvement within 3 days, the patient will need further evaluation such as endoscopy or a barium swallow study. Other causes of dysphgia/odonophagia in HIV-infected patients include cytomegalovirus, herpes simplex, and aphthous ulcerations.

TOXICITIES OF ANTIRETROVIRAL THERAPIES

Weakness/Myalgias

When a patient presents with generalized weakness or myalgias while on HIV therapy, lactic acidosis must be ruled out since it is has a high mortality rate. Asymptomatic hyperlactatemia is a common occurrence (9–16%) but only 1% of these have a level >5 mmol/L. Studies suggest that women are at increased risk for development of lactic acidosis. A review by Arenas-Pinto et al. presented 90 cases of antiretroviral induced lactic acidosis of which 53% were female. Lactic acidosis is frequently accompanied by hepatic steatosis, possibly with transaminitis, and occasional pancreatitis. In addition to the generalized weakness, patients often report nonspecific gastrointestinal complaints such as nausea, vomiting, and abdominal pain. Patients have also been noted to report dyspnea. The nucleoside reverse transcriptase inhibitors (nRTIs) have been associated with the production of lactic acidosis by the inhibition of mitochondrial DNA (mtDNA), leading to impairment of oxidative phosphorylation and dependence on anaerobic metabolism with conversion of pyruvate to lactate (21). In a review of 58 cases (50 from the literature) by Tripuraneni et al., there was a 52% mortality rate. The peak venous lactate was the best predictor for mortality ($p < 0.001$, OR 1.23) with the median peak lactate level of 9.8 mmol/L in survivors and 23 mmol/L in nonsurvivors. Although the use of stavudine (d4T, Zerit) has had the strongest correlation in multiple studies with the development of lactic acidosis, didanosine (ddI, Videx or Videx EC), or zidovudine (AZT, Retrovir) as causative agents for lactic acidosis were associated with a higher mortality (57% for ddI and 73% for AZT versus 14% for d4T). There is no standard accepted treatment for the nRTI-induced lactic acidosis except removal of the causative agent(s), possibly with substitution with tenofovir (TDF, Viread) or abacavir (ABC, Ziagen), although there are case reports of improvement with treatment with riboflavin, co-enzyme Q, and carnitine (22). Zidovudine (AZT) has also been associated with the develop-

ment of skeletal muscle myopathies due to mitochondrial toxicity; this can be assessed by measurement of a CK level.

Take home point: If a patient on nRTI therapy presents with abdominal complaints, dyspnea or weakness, obtain a serum bicarbonate level; if decreased, then measure the lactate level on free-flowing blood. If the level is >2.5 mmol/L, stop HIV therapy and consider supplementation with riboflavin or co-enzyme Q or carnitine.

Peripheral Neuropathy

Distal symmetric polyneuropathy (DSP) occurs in over 30% of patients with AIDS. The usual presentation is "burning feet" as well as numbness or paresthesias, usually starting in the distal lower extremities. The upper extremities are not usually involved until the neuropathy has ascended to the level of the knees. Patients have decreased ankle deep tendon reflexes as compared to the patellar reflexes. A patient may have a concurrent vacuolar myelopathy as evidenced by increased patellar reflexes with decreased Achilles reflexes. Vibratory thresholds are increased and temperature and pinprick sensations are usually decreased. This neuropathy may be caused by HIV itself, but can also be associated with the use of the nRTIs, in particular the "D drugs," which include stavudine (d4T), didanosine (ddI), and zalcitabine (ddC, Hivid). The mechanism is thought to be due to toxicity to the mitochondrial DNA. The occurrence is usually dose-dependent and, when used together, there is an additive effect. Other medications that may be involved include vincristine for the treatment of malignancies, isoniazid (INH) for the treatment of TB, and thalidomide for the treatment of oral aphthous ulcerations. The diagnosis is made clinically, although small or absent sural nerve action potentials may be found, and sural nerve biopsy may show segmental demyelination and axonal degeneration. Epidermal skin biopsy analysis may also aid in the diagnosis. Treatment initially consists of decreasing, or discontinuing, the dose of the offending medication. Nonsteroidal antiinflammatory agents or acetaminophen may be used. Anticonvulsants, most commonly gabapentin, and lamotrigine have also been shown to be effective in DSP due to neurotoxic medications. Lidocaine patches, or gels, have been used by some clinicians with encouraging effects. Occasionally, when none of the previously mentioned treatments have been able to control the pain to a level acceptable to the patient, a mixture of long-acting and short-acting narcotics may be needed (23).

Take home point: If an HIV-infected patient presents with complaints of peripheral neuropathic pain, first assess the use of potentially neurotoxic agents and contact the patient's primary health care provider to discuss any dosing alterations. Control of symptoms may be attempted initially with nonsteroidal antiinflammatories or acetaminophen.

Anemia/Neutropenia

Frequently HIV-infected patients suffer from anemia, due to medication toxicities, opportunistic infections, or HIV infection of the stem cells in the bone marrow. Zidovudine (AZT) is associated with the development of macrocytosis in all patients who take it but causes anemia in up to 23% of patients. Patients who have a deficiency of glucose-6-phosphodiesterase (G-6-PD) may develop hemolysis due to medications frequently used in treating HIV infection, such as trimethoprim/sulfamethoxazole or dapsone for PcP prophylaxis, or primaquine for PcP treatment. Assessment for G-6-PD deficiency cannot be done during hemolysis; levels will be reported as normal. Indinavir (IND) has also been reported to cause hemolytic anemia in a few patients. Neutropenia may also develop with zidovudine (AZT), lamivudine (3TC, Epivir), or trimethoprim/sulfamethoxazole due to suppression of production in the bone marrow.

The use of pyrimethamine in the treatment of toxoplasmosis will also lead to neutropenia if the patient is not co-administered folinic acid. Assessment must be done regarding the timing of the development of the anemia, or neutropenia, and the initiation of any HIV medications. Treatment consists of discontinuation of the causative agent. The patient's primary health care provider may assist in choosing an alternative antiretroviral regimen. If discontinuation is not desired, then stimulation of the bone marrow may be achieved with the use of erythropoetin or filgrastim injections (24).

Take home point: When an HIV-infected patient presents with anemia, or neutropenia, carefully assess their medications and identify those that may cause hemolysis. Substitution of the offending agent is the usual course of therapy.

Stomatitis

Oral ulcerations can be caused by herpes simplex, cytomegalovirus, histoplasmosis, non-Hodgkin lymphoma, aphthous ulcerations, or medications. Three to seven percent of patients who take zalcitabine (ddC, Hivid) develop oral ulcerations. The ulcerations are painful and appear either similar to those of herpetic stomatitis with an erythematous base or as aphthous ulcerations. Nevi-

rapine (NVP, Viramune) has also been associated with the development of oral ulcerations with an incidence of 4%. Additionally, abacavir (ABC, Ziagen) hypersensitivity reaction has been associated with oral ulcerations in severe cases (see section below) (24).

Pancreatitis

Patients may present to the emergency department with complaints of nausea, vomiting, and sharp abdominal pain. Patients with HIV infection frequently have elevations of serum amylase and it is usually from a salivary source; therefore a serum lipase level must be measured to evaluate for pancreatitis in this population. Didanosine (ddI) is the HIV medication that has the strongest association with pancreatitis and is thought to be due to mitochondrial toxicity. This occurs in elderly patients more commonly than younger patients. The co-administration of ribavirin, such as in the treatment of hepatitis C, increases the likelihood of pancreatitis. Stavudine (d4T), abacavir (ABC), and lamivudine (3TC) have also been reported to be associated with this condition, although rarely. Most of the protease inhibitors as well as stavudine (d4T) and efavirenz (EFV, Sustiva) have been associated with the development of hypertriglyceridemia, which may lead to pancreatitis. Pentamidine, when given systemically for the treatment of *Pneumocystis jiroveci*, may cause pancreatitis in 1–10% of patients (24). Treatment for pancreatitis includes discontinuation of the offending agent, rest for the gastrointestinal tract, and good hydration.

Take home point: When a patient with HIV has pancreatitis as measured by an elevation in the serum lipase, carefully review the patients' medications to assess for the use of agents associated with the development of pancreatitis, especially didanosine (ddI, Videx or Videx EC) and ribavirin.

Jaundice

There are two protease inhibitors associated with the development of jaundice: atazanavir (ATV, Reyataz) and indinavir (IND, Crixivan). These medications block the UGT enzyme that conjugates indirect bilirubin to direct bilirubin to allow excretion through the biliary system. Although over 40% of patients who take the standard dosage of atazanavir (ATV) develop hyperbilirubinemia, only approximately 5% develop clinical jaundice with scleral icterus and change in skin color. The patient can be advised that, in most cases, the jaundice will improve with time. Hyperbilirubinemia develops in 14% of patients taking indinavir (IND) but clinical jaundice occurs in only a small percentage (1–2%) (25, 26).

Take home point: If an HIV-infected patient presents with jaundice, assess the use of indinavir (IND, Crixivan), and atazanavir (ATV, Reyataz). If the patient is taking neither one, the standard laboratory evaluation should be performed, including evaluation of liver function and assessment for hemolytic anemia.

Renolithiasis

When an HIV-infected patient presents with hematuria and flank pain and is found to have a renolith, a careful medication history must be obtained to find if the patient is taking indinavir (IND, Crixivan). The renolith is made of the indinavir itself and will dissolve frequently without surgical intervention. The incidence is higher in pediatric patients taking the medication (29%) as compared to adults (12.4%). In the event of renolith formation, the indinavir should be held (along with the other antiretrovirals) for 1–3 days, and the patient should be instructed to increase their oral fluid intake. Patients on indinavir should be instructed to imbibe at least 48–64 ounces of water daily with an increase when spending time in an environment that may predispose them to dehydration (25).

Abacavir Hypersensitivity

Abacavir (ABC, Ziagen) use has been associated with development of a hypersensitivity reaction (HSR) in 5–8% of patients. The reaction is characterized by symptoms from *at least two* of the following groups: (1) fever, (2) rash, usually maculopapular or urticarial but erythema multiforme has been reported, (3) gastrointestinal, including nausea, vomiting, abdominal pain, or diarrhea, (4) respiratory, including dyspnea, pharyngitis, and cough, and (5) constitutional, including malaise, fatigue, or muscle aches. The most common presenting symptoms are fever (66%), rash (61%), and malaise (60%). Other findings have also included lymphadenopathy and mucous membrane lesions such as conjunctivitis and oral ulcerations. Patients may report an increase in severity of symptoms after taking a dose of abacavir (ABC). If the patient discontinues and then resumes taking the medication, severe symptoms, including hypotension and death, may develop within hours. Most cases occur within the first 2 weeks after initiation of therapy, with median time to onset of 9 days, and almost 90% occur within the first 6 weeks. Studies have suggested a genetic link to the development of abacavir HSR, linking HLA-B57 in Caucasians and

Hispanics but not in Black patients. If a patient is suspected of having abacavir HSR, the patient should *never* be placed on abacavir (Ziagen) or an abacavir-containing medication (Epzicom, Trizivir) again (27–29).

Take home point: When a patient presents with a flu-like or viral-like illness, assess if the patient is taking abacavir, or an abacavir-containing medication (Ziagen, Epzicom, Trizivir). If so, discontinue all antiretroviral medications. Symptoms should improve, or resolve, within 24 h.

CASE OUTCOME

Because the patient had thrush, anemia, leukopenia, and hypergammaglobulinemia, an OraQuick test was done in the emergency department with positive results. An ELISA and Western Blot were ordered for confirmation. The patient was treated for thrush; AFB blood cultures were drawn and the patient was discharged home. He was reevaluated 3 weeks later in the HIV outpatient clinic and found to have a CD4 count of 22 cells/ml and an HIV viral load of >750,000 copies/mL.

Mycobacterium avium-intracellulare complex was cultured from his blood. He was placed on treatment for MAC infection and a HAART regimen of a protease inhibitor plus two nRTIs. Six months later he reported an improvement in symptoms and he demonstrated an excellent response to HAART with an impressive elevation in his CD count of over 100.

REFERENCES

1. Beckwith CG, Simmons E, Lally MA, et al.: Testing for HIV infection: Should it be routine? *Res Staff Phys* 50(4):9–15, 2004.
2. Cooper DA, et al.: Acute AIDS retrovirus infection. Definition of a clinical illness associated with seroconversion. *Lancet* 537–540, 1985.
3. Cooper DA, et al.: Antibody response to human immunodeficiency virus after primary infection. *J Infect Dis* 155(6): 1113–1118, 1987.
4. Cooper DA, et al.: Characterization of T lymphocyte responses during primary infection with human immunodeficiency virus. *J Infect Dis* 157(5):889–896, 1988.
5. Vanhems P, Routy JP, Hirschel B, et al.: Clinical features of acute retroviral syndrome differ by route of infection but not by gender and age. *J Acquir Immune Defic Syndr* 31(3): 318–321, 2002.
6. Rosenberg E, Cotton D: Primary HIV infection and the acute retroviral syndrome. *AIDS Clin Care* 9(3):19, 23–25, 1997.

7. McDonagh CA, Holman RP: Primary human immunodeficiency virus type 1 infection in a patient with acute rhabdomyolysis. *South Med J* 96(10):1027–1030, 2003.

8. Eron JJ: The role of resistance testing in treatment-naïve HIV-infected individuals. *Resistance Testing in HIV: An In-Depth Series* presented by Clinical Care Options for HIV, 2004.

9. Durack DT, Street AC: Fever of unknown origin: Reexamined and redefined. *Curr Clin Top Infect Dis* 11:35–51, 1991.

10. Mayo J, Collazos J, Martinez E: Fever of unknown origin in the HIV-infected patient: New scenario for an old problem. *Scand J Infect Dis* 29:327–336, 1997.

11. Mayo J, Collazos J, Martinez E: Fever on unknown origin in the setting of HIV infection: Guidelines for a rational approach. *AIDS Patient Care STDs* 12(5):373–378, 1998.

12. Wolff AJ, O'Donnell AE: HIV-related pulmonary infections: A review of the recent literature. *Curr Opin Pulm Med* 9(3): 210–214, 2003.

13. Barry SM, Johnson MA: Pneumocystis carinii pneumonia: A review of current issues in diagnosis and management. *HIV Med* 2:123–132, 2001.

14. Benson CA: Mycobacterium avium complex and other atypical mycobacterial infections, in Dolin R, Masur H, Saag MS (eds.): *AIDS Therapy, 1st ed.* New York, Churchill Livingstone, 1999; pp 375–391.

15. Saidinejad M, Burns MM, Harper MB: Disseminated histoplasmosis in a nonendemic area. *Ped Inf Dis J* 23(8): 781–782, 2004.

16. Martin DF, Sierra-Madero J, Walmsley S, et al.: A controlled trial of valganciclovir as induction therapy for cytomegalovirus retinitis. *N Engl J Med* 2002 346(15):1119–1126, 2004.

17. Powderly WG: Current approach to the acute management of cryptococcal infections. *J Infect* 41:18–22, 2000.

18. Wilcox RD, Dalovisio JR, Figueroa JE: Seizures in a patient with HIV infection. *Infect Med* 17:398–406, 2000.

19. Berger JR, Pall L, Lanska D, Whiteman M: Progressive multifocal leukoencephalopathy in patients with HIV infection. *J Neurovirol* 4:59–68, 1998.

20. Antinori A, Ammassari A, De Luca A, et al.: Diagnosis of AIDS-related focal brain lesions: A decision making analysis based on clinical and neuroradiologic characteristics combined with polymerase chain reaction assays in CSF. *Neurology* 48:687–694, 1997.

21. Tripuraneni NS, Smith PR, Weedon J, et al.: Prognostic factors in lactic acidosis syndrome caused by nucleoside reverse transcriptase inhibitors: Report of eight cases and review of the literature. *AIDS Patient Care STDs* 18(7):379–384, 2004.

22. Arenas-Pinto A, Grant AD, Edwards S, Weller IVD: Lactic acidosis in HIV infected patients: A systematic review of published cases. *Sex Transm Infect* 79:340–344, 2003.

23. Simpson DM: Selected peripheral neuropathies associated with human immunodeficiency virus infection and antiretroviral therapy. *J Neurovir* 8(Suppl. 2): 33–41, 2002.

24. Lacy CF, Armstrong LL, Goldman MP, Lance LL: *Drug Information Handbook, 2002-2003.*

25. Package insert from Merck & Co. for indinavir (Crixivan), issued January 2002.

26. Package insert from Bristol-Myers-Squibb for atazanavir (Reyataz), issued June 2003.

27. Hetherington S, McGuirk S, Powell G, et al.: Hypersensitivity reactions during therapy with the nucleoside reverse transcriptase inhibitor abacavir. *Clin Ther* 23:1603–1614, 2001.

28. Package insert from GlaxoSmithKline for abacavir (Ziagen), issued July 2003.

29. Hughes A, Mosteller M, Bansal A, et al.: Association of genetic variations in HLA-B region with hypersensitivity in some, but not all, populations. *Pharmacogenetics* 5: 203–211, 2004.

INDEX

Page number followed by *f* indicates a figure; *t* indicates table